Understanding Complementary and Alternative Medicine

Understanding Complementary and Alternative Medicine

Edited by **Brendon Gould**

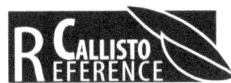

R CALLISTO REFERENCE

New York

Published by Callisto Reference,
106 Park Avenue, Suite 200,
New York, NY 10016, USA
www.callistoreference.com

Understanding Complementary and Alternative Medicine
Edited by Brendon Gould

International Standard Book Number: 978-1-63239-666-2 (Hardback)

The publisher's policy is to use permanent paper from mills that operate a sustainable forestry policy. Furthermore, the publisher ensures that the text paper and cover boards used have met acceptable environmental accreditation standards.

Trademark Notice: Registered trademark of products or corporate names are used only for explanation and identification without intent to infringe.

Printed in the United States of America.

Contents

Preface IX

Chapter 1 **Tualang Honey Protects against BPA-Induced Morphological Abnormalities and Disruption of ERα, ERβ, and C3 mRNA and Protein Expressions in the Uterus of Rats** 1
Siti Sarah Mohamad Zaid, Normadiah M. Kassim and Shatrah Othman

Chapter 2 **Influence of the Alcohol Present in a Phytotherapic Tincture on Male Rat Lipid Profiles and Renal Function** 19
Fernanda Coleraus Silva, Juliete Gomes de Lara de Souza, Alana Meira Reichert, Renata Prestes Antonangelo, Rodrigo Suzuki, Ana Maria Itinose and Carla Brugin Marek

Chapter 3 **Hypocholesterolemic and Antiatherosclerotic Potential of *Basella alba* Leaf Extract in Hypercholesterolemia-Induced Rabbits** 30
Gunasekaran Baskaran, Shamala Salvamani, Azrina Azlan, Siti Aqlima Ahmad, Swee Keong Yeap and Mohd Yunus Shukor

Chapter 4 **Anti-Inflammatory Activity of Triterpenes Isolated from *Protium paniculatum* Oil-Resins** 37
Patrícia D. O. de Almeida, Ana Paula de A. Boleti, André Luis Rüdiger, Geane A. Lourenço, Valdir Florêncio da Veiga Junior and Emerson S. Lima

Chapter 5 **In Vitro Pharmacological Activities and GC-MS Analysis of Different Solvent Extracts of *Lantana camara* Leaves Collected from Tropical Region of Malaysia** 47
Mallappa Kumara Swamy, Uma Rani Sinniah and Mohd. Sayeed Akhtar

Chapter 6 **Effects of *Cordyceps sinensis* on the Expressions of NF-κB and TGF-β1 in Myocardium of Diabetic Rats** 56
You-you Gu, Huan Wang, Su Wang, Hua Gao and Ming-cai Qiu

Chapter 7 **Phytochemical Profile and Biological Activity of *Nelumbo nucifera*** 62
Keshav Raj Paudel and Nisha Panth

Chapter 8 **Luoyutong Treatment Promotes Functional Recovery and Neuronal Plasticity after Cerebral Ischemia-Reperfusion Injury in Rats** 78
Ning-qun Wang, Li-ye Wang, Hai-ping Zhao, Ping Liu, Rong-liang Wang, Jue-xian Song, Li Gao, Xun-ming Ji and Yu-min Luo

Chapter 9 **The Consumption of Bicarbonate-Rich Mineral Water Improves Glycemic Control** 90
Shinnosuke Murakami, Yasuaki Goto, Kyo Ito, Shinya Hayasaka, Shigeo Kurihara, Tomoyoshi Soga, Masaru Tomita and Shinji Fukuda

Chapter 10   **Fuyuan Decoction Enhances SOX9 and COL2A1 Expression and Smad2/3 Phosphorylation in IL-1β-Activated Chondrocytes**   100
Yudi Zhang, Rongheng Li, Yu Zhong, Sihan Zhang, Lingyun Zhou and Shike Shang

Chapter 11   **Strong Manual Acupuncture Stimulation of "Huantiao" (GB 30) Reduces Pain-Induced Anxiety and p-ERK in the Anterior Cingulate Cortex in a Rat Model of Neuropathic Pain**   109
Xiao-mei Shao, Zui Shen, Jing Sun, Fang Fang, Jun-fan Fang, Yuan-yuan Wu and Jian-qiao Fang

Chapter 12   **Acupuncture for Lateral Epicondylitis: A Systematic Review**   120
Hongzhi Tang, Huaying Fan, Jiao Chen, Mingxiao Yang, Xuebing Yi, Guogang Dai, Junrong Chen, Liugang Tang, Haibo Rong, Junhua Wu and Fanrong Liang

Chapter 13   **Berberine in Combination with Insulin has Additive Effects on Titanium Implants Osseointegration in Diabetes Mellitus Rats**   133
Li Lu, Huang Zhijian, Li Lei, Chen Wenchuan and Zhu Zhimin

Chapter 14   **Diuretic Properties and Chemical Constituent Studies on *Stauntonia brachyanthera***   141
Xuan Li Liu, Dan Dan Wang, Zi Hao Wang and Da Li Meng

Chapter 15   **AHCC Activation and Selection of Human Lymphocytes via Genotypic and Phenotypic Changes to an Adherent Cell Type: A Possible Novel Mechanism of T Cell Activation**   149
Loretta Olamigoke, Elvedina Mansoor, Vivek Mann, Ivory Ellis, Elvis Okoro, Koji Wakame, Hajime Fuji, Anil Kulkarni, Marie Francoise Doursout and Alamelu Sundaresan

Chapter 16   **The Preventive Effect on Ethanol-Induced Gastric Lesions of the Medicinal Plant *Plumeria rubra*: Involvement of the Latex Proteins in the NO/cGMP/K$_{ATP}$ Signaling Pathway**   158
Nylane Maria Nunes de Alencar, Rachel Sindeaux Paiva Pinheiro, Ingrid Samantha Tavares de Figueiredo, Patrícia Bastos Luz, Lyara Barbosa Nogueira Freitas, Tamiris de Fátima Goebel de Souza, Luana David do Carmo, Larisse Mota Marques and Marcio Viana Ramos

Chapter 17   **Effects of "Danzhi Decoction" on Chronic Pelvic Pain, Hemodynamics, and Proinflammatory Factors in the Murine Model of Sequelae of Pelvic Inflammatory Disease**   168
Xiaoling Bu, Yanxia Liu, Qiudan Lu and Zhe Jin

Chapter 18   **Oleanolic Acid Attenuates Insulin Resistance via NF-κB to Regulate the IRS1-GLUT4 Pathway in HepG2 Cells**   180
Ming Li, Zongyu Han, Weijian Bei, Xianglu Rong, Jiao Guo and Xuguang Hu

Chapter 19   **Chemical Components and Cardiovascular Activities of *Valeriana* spp.**   189
Heng-Wen Chen, Ben-Jun Wei, Xuan-Hui He, Yan Liu and Jie Wang

Chapter 20   **Antibacterial and Cytotoxic Activity of Compounds Isolated from *Flourensia oolepis***   200
Mariana Belén Joray, Lucas Daniel Trucco, María Laura González, Georgina Natalia Díaz Napal, Sara María Palacios, José Luis Bocco and María Cecilia Carpinella

Chapter 21   **Identification of a Potential Target of Capsaicin by Computational Target Fishing**   **211**
Xuan-yi Ye, Qing-zhi Ling and Shao-jun Chen

Chapter 22   **Tiao He Yi Wei Granule, a Traditional Chinese Medicine, against Ethanol-Induced**
Gastric Ulcer in Mice   **217**
Jinfu Yao

Chapter 23   **Saw Palmetto Extract Inhibits Metastasis and Antiangiogenesis through STAT3**
Signal Pathway in Glioma Cell   **225**
Hong Ding, Jinglian Shen, Yang Yang and Yuqin Che

Chapter 24   **Additional Effects of Back-Shu Electroacupuncture and Moxibustion in**
Cardioprotection of Rat Ischemia-Reperfusion Injury   **234**
Seung Min Kathy Lee, Kang Hyun Yoon, Jimin Park, Hyun Soo Kim, Jong Shin Woo,
So Ra Lee, Kyung Hye Lee, Hyun-Hee Jang, Jin-Bae Kim, Woo Shik Kim, Sanghoon
Lee and Weon Kim

Permissions

List of Contributors

Preface

Complementary and alternative medicine is a parallel field to medical science for the diagnose and treatment of an array of diseases and disorders. Some common practices under the umbrella of complementary and alternative medicine are accupuncture, homeopathy, ayurvedic medicine, chiropractic, etc. The aim of this book is to present researches that have transformed this discipline and aided its progress. Although complementary and alternative medicines lack scientific bases, large populations of people have firm belief in these forms. This book unravels the recent studies in these fields. It provides significant information of this discipline to help develop a good understanding of the latest advances within these areas. The readers would gain knowledge that would broaden their perspective about complementary and alternative medicines.

Various studies have approached the subject by analyzing it with a single perspective, but the present book provides diverse methodologies and techniques to address this field. This book contains theories and applications needed for understanding the subject from different perspectives. The aim is to keep the readers informed about the progress in the field; therefore, the contributions were carefully examined to compile novel researches by specialists from across the globe.

Indeed, the job of the editor is the most crucial and challenging in compiling all chapters into a single book. In the end, I would extend my sincere thanks to the chapter authors for their profound work. I am also thankful for the support provided by my family and colleagues during the compilation of this book.

Editor

Tualang Honey Protects against BPA-Induced Morphological Abnormalities and Disruption of ERα, ERβ, and C3 mRNA and Protein Expressions in the Uterus of Rats

Siti Sarah Mohamad Zaid,[1,2] Normadiah M. Kassim,[1] and Shatrah Othman[3]

[1]Department of Anatomy, Faculty of Medicine, University of Malaya, 50603 Kuala Lumpur, Malaysia
[2]Department of Environmental Sciences, Faculty of Environmental Studies, Universiti Putra Malaysia,
 43400 Serdang, Selangor, Malaysia
[3]Department of Molecular Medicine, Faculty of Medicine, University of Malaya, 50603 Kuala Lumpur, Malaysia

Correspondence should be addressed to Shatrah Othman; shatraho@um.edu.my

Academic Editor: Omer Kucuk

Bisphenol A (BPA) is an endocrine disrupting chemical (EDC) that can disrupt the normal functions of the reproductive system. The objective of the study is to investigate the potential protective effects of Tualang honey against BPA-induced uterine toxicity in pubertal rats. The rats were administered with BPA by oral gavage over a period of six weeks. Uterine toxicity in BPA-exposed rats was determined by the degree of the morphological abnormalities, increased lipid peroxidation, and dysregulated expression and distribution of ERα, ERβ, and C3 as compared to the control rats. Concurrent treatment of rats with BPA and Tualang honey significantly improved the uterine morphological abnormalities, reduced lipid peroxidation, and normalized ERα, ERβ, and C3 expressions and distribution. There were no abnormal changes observed in rats treated with Tualang honey alone, comparable with the control rats. In conclusion, Tualang honey has potential roles in protecting the uterus from BPA-induced toxicity, possibly accounted for by its phytochemical properties.

1. Introduction

Bisphenol A (BPA) (2,2-bis(4-hydroxyphenyl)) is one of the most ubiquitous environmental endocrine disrupting chemicals (EDC) in the world. It is widely used in industries as plasticizer for the production of polycarbonate plastics epoxy resins and as nonpolymer additive to other plastics [1]. It has received significant worldwide attention due to its exposure to human through leaches from the inner lining of food and beverage containers, plastic bottles, dental sealants, water supply pipes, and adhesives [2].

Many studies have revealed the negative effects of BPA on the development of the reproductive system in humans and laboratory animals [3, 4]. BPA has been detected in the serum and follicular and amniotic fluids [5], fetal serum [6], milk of nursing mothers [7], and urine [8, 9]. These reports suggest that humans are routinely exposed to BPA. Thus, it

has fueled additional concern in human minds about BPA on their health.

Numerous studies have reported that BPA could induce morphological and functional alterations of the female genital system, particularly on the uterus [3, 10]. The main function of uterus is regulated by cyclic changes of sexual steroid hormones, and for this reason, it is widely used as a classical target organ to determine estrogenic effects of BPA [11]. BPA was shown to cause uterine disruptions by influencing the expression and distribution of estrogen receptor-α (ERα) and estrogen receptor-β (ERβ) [12]. BPA was also reported to reduce uterine immunity via dysregulation of complement C3 expression that caused ascending infections in the female reproductive tract [13]. Study by Xiao et al. (2011) has found that prenatal exposure to BPA could adversely affect transportation and preimplantation of the embryo from disturbance in the uterine receptivity that lead to infertility in female rats [14]. Furthermore, BPA has been reported to promote oxidative stress and inflammation in the female reproductive tract which might contribute to the morphological and functional abnormalities [15].

Natural compounds with antioxidant properties have been extensively studied as a means to counter disease-associated oxidative stress [16]. With these concerns in mind, we used a natural product with high antioxidant content, namely, Tualang honey (Agromas, Malaysia) as a possible potential therapeutic agent to counter the deleterious effects of BPA. Previous scientific studies have claimed that Tualang honey has the capability to ameliorate oxidative stress in renal and pancreas of streptozotocin-induced diabetic rats [17], reverse atrophic uterus and vagina [18], and to improve osteoporotic bone [19] in postmenopausal animal model. In addition, Tualang honey has the capability to protect against cigarette-induced damage on testis [20] and to counter the proliferation of oral squamous cell carcinomas (OSCC) [21], human osteosarcoma [21], and keloid fibroblasts [22].

Tualang honey, a dark brownish honey has been reported to contain more than 200 substances including sugars, amino acids, vitamins, minerals, enzymes, organic acids, and phytochemicals. The primary content of Tualang honey is inverted sugars that consist of fructose 29.6%, glucose 30%, sucrose 0.6%, and maltose 7.9% as well as a small amount of complex mixture of other saccharides (disaccharides, trisaccharides, and oligosaccharides) [23]. It also contains high total phenolic compounds (gallic, syringic, benzoic, trans-cinnamic, p-coumaric, and caffeic acids) and flavonoids (catechin, kaempferol, naringenin, luteolin, and apigenin) [24]. It has tremendous antioxidant properties with high radical scavenging and antioxidant activities [25]. The other compounds present in Tualang honey are stearic acids, furfural, acetic acid, 2-furylmethylketone, palmitic acid, ethyl linoleate, oleic acid, 2-hyroxy-2-cyclopenten-1-one, hyacinthine, and 5-methyl furfural [23].

The aims of our study were to investigate the effects of subchronic administration of BPA on the uterine morphology and function by determining the lipid peroxidation, protein distribution, and mRNA expressions of estrogen receptor-α, estrogen receptor-β, and complement C3. Consequently, investigation of the possible protective effects of Tualang honey against BPA-induced uterine toxicity is executed.

2. Material and Methods

2.1. Tualang Honey (Agromas, Malaysia). Tualang honey was purchased from the Federal Agricultural Marketing Authority (FAMA), under the Ministry of Agriculture and Agro-Based Industry, Malaysia. Tualang honey is wild multifloral honey collected from *Apis dorsata's* beehive that is built on a giant tree, *Koompassia excelsa* (locally known as Tualang tree), in the rain forest of Kedah, Malaysia. At Honey Processing Centre in Kuala Nerang, Kedah, the honey was processed through several stages (quality inspection, dehydration, packaging, and labeling). In brief, the honey was filtered to remove solid particles, concentrated in an oven at 40°C, and subjected to γ irradiation at 25 kGy at Sterilgamma (M) Sdn. Bhd.

(Selangor, Malaysia). The water concentration of the honey was standardized by FAMA at 18%.

2.2. Animal Model and Experimental Design. Female Sprague rats (P21) were obtained from the Animal Husbandry, Faculty of Medicine, University of Malaya. All the experimental design and procedures were conducted according to the National Institutes of Health guide for the care and use of Laboratory animals (NIH Publications number 8023, revised 1978) which has been approved by the Animal Care and Committee (ACUC) of the University of Malaya. Throughout the experimental period, the rats were maintained under the standard laboratory conditions (temperature 25 ± 2°C, 50 ± 15% relative humidity, and normal photoperiod of 12 h dark and 12 h light) and supplied *ad libitum* with water and commercial pellet diet (Gold Coin Feedmills Pte. Ltd., Malaysia). The rats were placed in stainless steel cages with wood bedding and water was supplied in glass bottles to minimize additional exposures endocrine disruptors. They were acclimatized to the laboratory environment for seven days prior to the commencement of the experiment. At 28 days of age, the rats were randomly divided into four groups ($n = 8$ in each group).

NC group (negative control) was administered with the vehicle (0.2 mL of corn oil). PC group (positive control) was administered with BPA (10 mg/kg body weight suspended in corn oil). THC group (Tualang honey control) was administered with Tualang honey (200 mg/kg body weight 30 min before administration of corn oil). TH group (Tualang honey + BPA) was administered with Tualang honey (200 mg/kg body weight 30 min before administration of BPA at 10 mg/kg body weight). The procedure was performed in the morning (between 09:00 and 10:00 AM) once daily by oral gavage (to mimic the most likely route of human exposure) for six consecutive weeks. Throughout the administration period, daily body weight was recorded. After the last treatment, the rats were sacrificed during their diestrous phase.

Once the rat was sacrificed, the wet weight of the whole uterus was recorded for uterotrophic response evaluation. The left horn of the uterus was immediately fixed in 10% buffered formalin for histopathological analysis. One half of the right horn of uterus was kept in phosphate buffer for malondialdehyde (MDA) determination while the other half was kept in RNAlater for mRNA extraction and subsequently stored in −80°C freezer until further analysis. The dose selection of BPA at 10 mg/g body weight was based on previous studies where BPA at this dose was reported to induce disruption on the morphological and biochemical parameters in the reproductive system [3, 26–28]. As for Tualang honey, it was freshly prepared daily to avoid oxidation of the antioxidants content. The dose of Tualang honey at 200 mg/kg body weight was based on previous study that showed positive biological effects on female reproductive organs and the dose was equal to one tablespoon which is routinely taken by an adult human [18].

2.3. Histopathological Evaluation. The uteri were fixed in 10% buffered formalin for 24 hours prior to further processing for histopathological examination. The uteri were trimmed accordingly, dehydrated through a graded series of increasing concentration of ethanol, cleared in xylene, and finally embedded in paraffin to form paraffin block. Subsequently, tissue sections of 5 μm thicknesses were obtained and mounted onto glass slides, deparaffinized in xylene, hydrated with water, and stained with hematoxylin and eosin (Sigma-Aldrich, USA). Once again, sections were dehydrated in a graded series of ethanol, cleared in xylene, and mounted with Canada Balsam (Sigma-Aldrich). All sections were analyzed for any morphological changes under a light microscope (Olympus CH-B145-2) attached to an image analyzer (NIS-Elements Advanced Research, Nikon, Japan). Representative micrographs were taken for future reference.

2.4. Histomorphometry. For histomorphometric analysis of the uterus, the tissue sections were reviewed and the clearest representative sections on each slide were photographed at ×20 and ×40 magnifications. The mean values of height of the luminal epithelial cells, thickness of the endometrium, and the myometrium layers were measured in six randomly chosen areas of the sections. All measurements (in μm) were manually determined by tracing the on-screen images using a computer-image analyzing program (NIS-Elements Advanced Research, Nikon, Japan).

2.5. Immunohistochemistry

2.5.1. Estrogen Receptor-α and Complement C3. The distribution of estrogen receptor-α and complement C3 in rat uteri was evaluated using ImmunoCruz Rabbit ABC staining system sc-2018 kit and ImmunoCruz Goat ABC staining system sc-2023 kit, respectively.

Briefly, tissue sections were deparaffinized, hydrated to water, boiled in 0.1 M sodium citrate buffer (pH 6.0) for 15 minutes, and incubated with 0.1%–1% of hydrogen peroxide for 10 minutes to quench the endogenous peroxidase activity. Nonspecific staining was blocked by incubating it in 1.5% blocking serum. Subsequently, the sections were incubated with primary antibody at 1 : 100 dilution of ERα (MC-20:sc-542, Santa Cruz Biotechnology, USA) or 1 : 100 dilution of C3 (V-20:sc-14612, Santa Cruz Biotechnology, USA) overnight at 4°C. On the following day, the sections were incubated with biotinylated secondary antibody for one hour and then incubated with AB enzyme reagent for another 30 minutes. Positive staining appeared (bluish in color) after incubation with peroxidase abstract for 10 minutes and, finally, the sections were counterstained with hematoxylin. The sections were then dehydrated through a graded series of ethanol, cleared in xylene and mounted with Canada Balsam (Sigma-Aldrich), and covered with glass coverslips before examination under light microscopy. The negative control tissue (not incubated with primary antibody) was included to ensure no false positive staining and for accurate interpretation of the staining results.

2.5.2. Estrogen Receptor-β. The distribution of estrogen receptor-β in uterus rats was evaluated using Rabbit Specific HRP/DAB (ABC) Detection IHC Abcam kit.

Briefly, the sections were deparaffinized, hydrated, boiled in 0.1 M sodium citrate buffer (pH 6.0) for 15 minutes, and incubated with hydrogen peroxide for 20 minutes to quench the endogenous peroxidase activity. Nonspecific staining was blocked by incubation in protein block. Subsequently, the sections were incubated with primary antibody at 1 : 200 dilution (ERβ antibody ab3576, Abcam, USA) overnight at 4°C. Next day, the sections were incubated with biotinylated secondary goat anti-polyvalent antibody for 30 minutes at room temperature. Positive staining developed after the incubation with DAB chromogen for 10 minutes, followed by counterstaining with haematoxylin. The sections were dehydrated in 2x 95% of ethanol, 2x 100%, and 3x xylenes for 10 seconds each. Finally, the sections were mounted with Canada Balsam (Sigma-Aldrich) and covered with glass coverslips for observation under light microscopy. The negative control tissue (not incubated with primary antibody) was included to ensure no false positive staining and accurate interpretation of the staining results.

2.5.3. Determination of Malondialdehyde (MDA) Levels. MDA levels of uterus were measured by the double heating method [29] using Thiobarbituric Acid Reactive Substances (TBARS) assay (OxiSelect TBARS assay kit, Cell Biolabs, USA). The uterus of each animal was homogenized in phosphate buffered saline (PBS) containing butylated hydroxytoluene (BHT). Subsequently, the uterine homogenate was centrifuged at 10,000 g for 5 minutes to collect the supernatant for the TBARS assay.

Briefly, 100 μL of samples and standards was mixed with 100 μL of SDS lysis solution in appropriate tubes and incubated for 5 minutes at room temperature. Then, 250 μL of TBA reagent was added to each tube followed by 60 minutes of incubation at 95°C. The tubes were cooled at room temperature in ice bath for five minutes. All the tubes were centrifuged at 3000 rpm for 15 minutes and 200 μL of the supernatant was transferred to a 96-well microplate for measurement of absorbance using a spectrophotometer at 532 nm wavelength. The concentration of MDA was calculated using the absorbance coefficient of the MDA-TBA complex and expressed as micromoles per microgram protein (μM/μg protein).

2.6. mRNA Expression of ERα, ERβ, and Complement C3

2.6.1. Purification of Total RNA. Purification of total RNA of uterus was performed using RNeasy Protect Mini Kit, Qiagen, USA. 30 mg of tissue samples of uteri was disrupted and homogenized in Buffer RLT. The lysate was centrifuged at maximum speed (12000 rpm). The supernatant were transferred into a new 1.5 mL tube and one volume of 70% of ethanol was added. This sample was transferred into an RNeasy spin column and centrifuged and the flow-through was discarded. Subsequently, buffer RPE was added to the RNeasy spin column and centrifuged for one minute at 10000 rpm and the flow-through was again discarded. This step was repeated but centrifugation was performed for a longer period of two minutes.

TABLE 1: Sequences of primers and references for TaqMan-PCR.

Gene	Forward primer	Reverse primer	References (accession number)
Estrogen receptor-α	5′-AAGCTGGCCTGACTCTGCAG-3′	5′-GCAGGTCATAGAGAGGCACGA-3′	Spreafico et al. [31] (X61098)
Estrogen receptor-β	5′-CTCTGTGTGAAGGCCATGAT-3′	5′-GGAGATACCACTCTTCGCAATC-3′	Kuiper et al. [32] (U57439)
Complement C3	5′-CTGTACGGCATAGGGATATCACG-3′	5′-ATGCTGGCCTGACCTTCAAGA-3′	Misumi et al. [33] (X52477)

Finally, the spin column was placed in a new 1.5 mL tube, added with 30 μL of RNase-free water, and centrifuged at 10000 rpm for one minute to elute the RNA. Finally, measurement of the concentration and purity of RNA was done by using a NanoDrop (BioTek, USA) at $OD_{260/280}$ while the quality assessment was performed via denaturing agarose gel electrophoresis. The RNA was kept at −20°C until further analysis.

2.6.2. Reverse Transcription of RNA to cDNA. Reverse transcription (RT) of RNA to single-stranded cDNA was done using the Applied Biosystems Kit, USA. Equal amounts of RNA (300 ng) from each sample were reverse-transcribed into cDNA. Each RT reaction mix consisted of 2x RT buffer (10 μL), 1 μL of reverse transcriptase, nuclease-free water, and RNA sample made up to a total volume of 20 μL. The reaction mixes were briefly centrifuged to spin down the contents and eliminate air bubbles. Finally, the tubes were placed in a programmed thermal cycler (Thermo Scientific) for 60 minutes at 37°C followed by five minutes at 95°C.

2.6.3. Quantitative Real-Time PCR of Selected Genes. Quantitative real-time PCR of selected genes was carried out using Applied Biosystems Kit, USA. The PCR reaction mix (reaction size of 20 μL) was prepared in triplicate. Each PCR reaction mix consists of 20x TaqMan Gene Expression Assay (1 μL), 2x TaqMan Gene Expression Master Mix (10 μL), cDNA template (4 μL), and RNase-free water (5 μL). The endogenous control gene used in this study was β-actin mRNA. In order to ensure specific amplification, three types of controls (water only, reaction without primers, and templates derived without reverse transcriptase) were included in the PCR reaction. The prepared PCR reaction mix was inverted to mix the reaction components, followed by brief centrifugation. Twenty μL of PCR reaction mix was transfer to each appropriate 96-well reaction plate and briefly centrifuged.

Finally, the plate was placed in the StepOne Plus Real-Time PCR system (Applied Biosystems, USA), followed by automated amplification of the genes of interest. The point at which exponential amplification of the PCR products begins (values for cycle threshold: CT) was determined using the Applied Biosystems software. Relative abundances of the target mRNA were calculated using the $2^{-\Delta\Delta CT}$ method [30]. The experiment was repeated three times to ensure the validity of the results. The relative mRNA expression levels for each selected gene were calculated in terms of the β-actin internal control. The sequences of primer used for the amplification of gene are shown in Table 1.

2.7. Statistical Analysis. All statistical evaluations were performed with Statistical Package for Social Sciences (SPSS Inc. Chicago, Illinois, USA, version 18.0 for Windows). Firstly, Shapiro-Wilk W test was performed to test whether all results followed a normal distribution (normally distributed if P value was greater than 0.05). Parametric variables were analyzed using One-way analysis of variance (ANOVA) followed by Bonferroni test for multiple comparisons to identify significant differences between groups. Values were reported as Mean ± SEM. $P < 0.05$ was considered significant.

3. Results

3.1. Body Weight and Uterine Weight. In toxicological studies, analysis of body weight and the weight of selected organs is a sensitive indicator for adverse effects of chemical exposure. In particular, analysis of normalization of absolute organ weight to body weight (relative organ weight) is a more accurate analytical endpoint for the identification of harmful effects of a toxic agent on the organ weights. The changes in body weight gain and uterine relative weight of animals in all experimental groups are shown in Table 2 and Figures 1(a) and 1(b), respectively.

To determine whether BPA exposure induces changes in body weight as a result of toxicity effects, the body weight of all rats was monitored throughout the experimental period. Although changes in the body weight gain were not statistically significant between BPA-exposed group and all the other groups, six weeks of subchronic exposure to BPA in the PC group had caused a slight increment (17.3%) in the body weight gain compared to the control animals (NC group). Similar increment (16.55%) in body weight gain was also noted in rats concurrently treated with BPA and Tualang honey (TH group). The changes in body weight gain for Tualang honey treated alone (THC group) rats were comparable to the control rats (NC group).

Similarly, the changes in uterine weight were recorded at the end of the administration period since this could be used as an indicator for any changes in the normal functions. After six weeks of BPA exposure (PC group), significant decline was observed in the uterine relative weight by 25% compared to the control rats (NC group). However, concurrent treatment

TABLE 2: Body weight gain, uterine relative weight, malondialdehyde (MDA) level, and uterine histomorphometry parameters in all experimental groups.

Group	Body weight gain (g)	Uterine relative weight (wet weight/body weight)	Malondialdehyde (MDA) level (μM/μ protein)	Height of luminal epithelial cells (μm)	Thickness of endometrium (μm)	Thickness of myometrium (μm)
NC	78.88 ± 14.61	1.89 ± 0.12[bbb]	0.0037 ± 0.00026[bbb]	30.51 ± 1.37[bbb,c]	571.87 ± 19.14[bb]	299.18 ± 16.86[bb]
PC	99.25 ± 9.90	1.41 ± 0.04[aaa,c,d]	0.0074 ± 0.00053[aaa,c,ddd]	18.88 ± 0.81[aaa,cc,ddd]	486.74 ± 10.15[aa,cc,ddd]	228.39 ± 8.91[aa,c,dd]
THC	89.5 ± 10.64	1.83 ± 0.07[bb]	0.0036 ± 0.00089[bbb]	28.23 ± 0.48[a,bbb]	574.25 ± 19.45[bbb]	299.26 ± 9.92[bb]
TH	92.5 ± 4.62	1.73 ± 0.04[b]	0.0049 ± 0.00064[b]	26.86 ± 0.68[bbb]	546.30 ± 3.78[b]	284.51 ± 16.63[bb]

Data are expressed as Mean ± SEM.
(1) [a] $P < 0.05$ and [aa] $P < 0.01$ versus NC (negative control).
(2) [b] $P < 0.05$, [bb] $P < 0.01$, and [bbb] $P < 0.001$ versus PC (BPA 10 mg/kg).
(3) [c] $P < 0.05$ and [cc] $P < 0.01$ versus TH (Tualang honey 200 mg/kg + BPA 10 mg/kg).
(4) [d] $P < 0.05$, [dd] $P < 0.01$, and [ddd] $P < 0.001$ versus THC (Tualang honey 200 mg/kg).

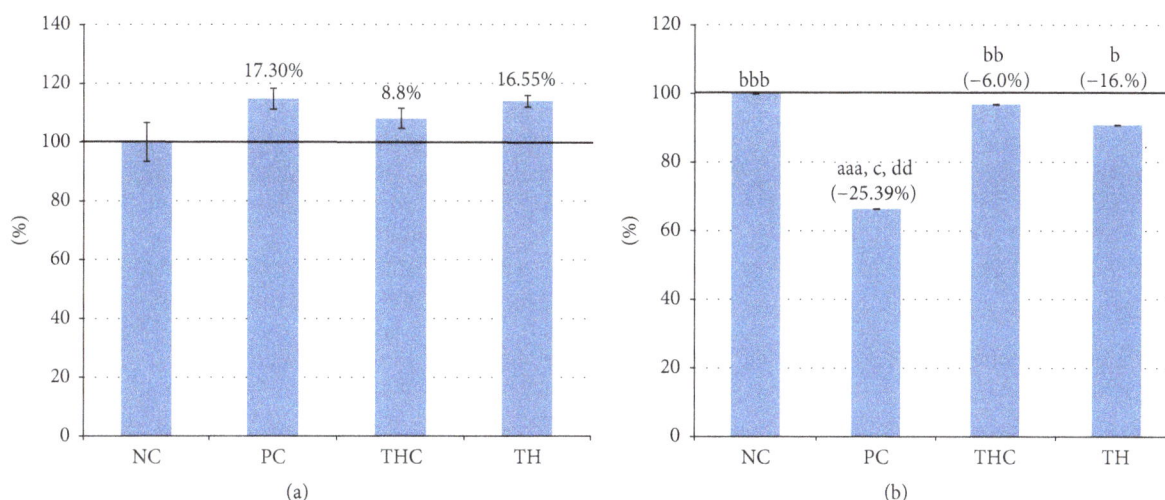

FIGURE 1: (a) Changes in body weight gain. Body weight gains were not statistically different among all experimental groups. (b) Uteri relative weights in all experimental groups. BPA exposure which caused a significant decline in body weight was observed (PC group), while concurrent treatment of BPA with Tualang honey (TH group) significantly prevented the reduction in the relative body weight. Data are expressed as Mean ± SEM. (1) [aaa] $P < 0.001$ versus NC (negative control). (2) [b] $P < 0.05$, [bb] $P < 0.01$, and [bbb] $P < 0.001$ versus PC (BPA 10 mg/kg). (3) [c] $P < 0.05$ versus TH (Tualang honey 200 mg/kg + BPA 10 mg/kg). (4) [dd] $P < 0.01$ versus THC (Tualang honey 200 mg/kg).

of rats with BPA and Tualang honey (TH group) had significantly prevented this effect. The uterine relative weight in rats treated with Tualang honey alone (THC group) was comparable to the control rat (NC group), reflecting that Tualang honey itself has no deleterious effect on the uterus weight.

3.2. Malondialdehyde (MDA) Level.
Lipid peroxides are unstable primary products of lipid peroxidation which decompose to the stable form malondialdehyde (MDA). Measurement of the MDA levels as the end product of lipid peroxidation is a widely accepted assay and is considered to be a crucial index of oxidative stress associated with organ pathophysiology in animals.

As shown in Table 2 and Figure 2, a significant increase in the MDA level by 49.7% was noted in rats exposed to BPA (PC group) as compared to the control rats (NC group). However, concurrent treatment of BPA with Tualang honey had led

to significant reduction in the MDA levels (TH group). The MDA level was not affected by Tualang honey treatment alone (THC group) and the value is comparable to the normal rats (NC group).

3.3. Uterine Histomorphometry Analysis.
As shown in Table 2 and Figures 3(a), 3(b), and 3(c), BPA exposure had caused a significant reduction in all histomorphometric parameters (including luminal epithelial cells and thickness of the endometrium and myometrium layers) (PC group) when compared to all the other groups (NC, TH, and THC groups).

In the BPA-exposed rats (PC group), the reductions were to 38.11%, 14.88%, and 23.66% in luminal epithelial cells height and endometrial and myometrial thickness, respectively. Interestingly, consistent with the reduction of the uterine relative weight, concurrent treatment of rats with BPA and Tualang honey (TH group) significantly prevented the

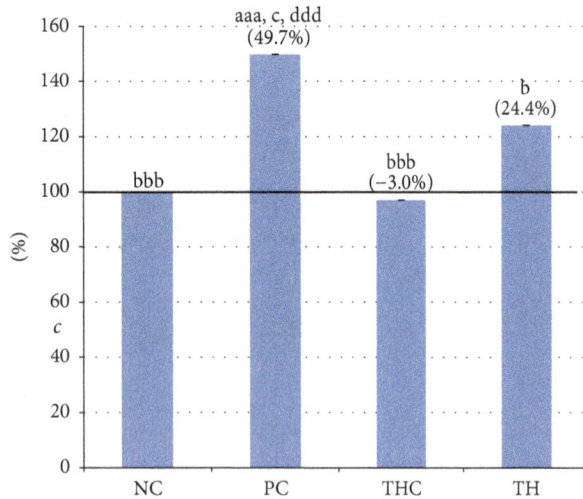

FIGURE 2: Levels of malondialdehyde (MDA) in all experimental groups. Malondialdehyde level was significantly increased in BPA-exposed rats (PC group), while concurrent treatment of BPA with Tualang honey (TH group) has significantly prevented the increment effect of BPA. Data are expressed as Mean ± SEM. (1) $^{aaa}P < 0.001$ versus NC (negative control). (2) $^{b}P < 0.05$, $^{bbb}P < 0.001$ versus PC (BPA 10 mg/kg). (3) $^{c}P < 0.05$ versus TH (Tualang honey 200 mg/kg + BPA 10 mg/kg). (4) $^{ddd}P < 0.001$ versus THC (Tualang honey 200 mg/kg).

reduction in these parameters. Meanwhile, the values of these parameters in the three groups were comparable to each other.

3.4. Morphology of the Uterus.

Morphological analysis of the representative uteri from sections of all groups is shown in Figure 4. The morphological changes were consistent with the histomorphometric analysis.

In the control rats (NC group), normal histological appearance was observed (Figures 4(A), 4(B), and 4(C)). The luminal epithelial cells were made up of tall pseudostratified columnar epithelium, cylindrical in shape with well-rounded nuclei, and rested on a prominent basement membrane. The lamina propria was intact with healthy endometrial glands and high cellular content in the stroma. A number of mitotic figures were visible in glandular epithelial cells. The myometrium appeared to be normal. The histological appearances of the endometria in rats treated with Tualang honey alone (THC group) were comparable to the control rats (NC group) (Figures 4(G), 4(H), and 4(I)).

The uterus of BPA-exposed rats (PC group) exhibited disruptive changes as shown in Figures 4(D), 4(E), and 4(F), when compared to the control rats (NC group). The luminal epithelial cells were shorter, the stroma had less cell population and appeared disorganized, and some cells were distorted and had irregular-shaped nuclei. Some of the nuclei had more condensed chromatin. There were very little interstitial intracellular spaces between the stroma cells. The endometrial glands appeared unhealthy by being smaller in size and lined by shrunken and distorted epithelial cells with irregularly shaped nuclei and some pyknotic nuclei, which are

less organized and reduced in number. The smooth muscle bundles of the myometrium which were also seen smaller and shrunken with the organizations of the inner circular and outer longitudinal smooth muscle fibers looked disintegrated.

In comparison with BPA-exposed rats (PC group), the uterine morphology of the Tualang honey (TH group) (Figures 4(J), 4(K), and 4(L)) showed slightly improved surface epithelium, but had healthy looking stromal cell population with larger stromal cells and relatively more interstitial spaces between cells compared to the PC group. The endometrial glands looked normal, lined by glandular epithelium, very much comparable to the NC group. Moreover, the myometrium also appeared normal.

3.5. ERα, ERβ, and C3 Protein Distribution.

The representative uterine tissue sections were stained using immunohistochemical technique to evaluate cell specific changes in the ERα, ERβ, and complement C3 proteins. These proteins are localized in the nuclei of epithelial and stromal cells of the uterus.

In general, the staining intensity of ERα protein receptor expression in all representative uterine sections was highest in the luminal and glandular epithelial cells but lower staining intensity was found in the cells of endometrial stroma (about 50 to 80%) (Figure 5). Among all groups, the most pronounced immunostaining intensity was observed in the control rats (NC groups) (Figures 5(C) and 5(D)) and the Tualang honey alone treated rats (THC group) (Figures 5(G) and 5(H)). As expected, lower immunostaining intensity was observed in BPA-exposed rats (PC group) (Figures 5(E) and 5(F)) and in rats with concurrent treatment with Tualang honey (TH group) (Figures 5(I) and 5(J)).

As shown in Figure 6, the immunostaining patterns and intensities of ERβ were different from the ERα. Comparable immunostaining intensities were observed in rats of NC group (Figures 6(C) and 6(D)), THC group (Figures 6(G) and 6 (H)), and TH group (Figures 6(I) and 6(J)), while there was less immunostaining intensity in all compartments (namely, luminal and glandular epithelial cells and stroma) in the BPA-exposed rats (PC group).

For complement C3 protein expression, the immunostaining intensity was highest in both the control rats (NC group) and Tualang honey alone treated rats (THC group) (Figures 7(C), 7(D) and 7(G), 7(H), resp.). There was less immunostaining intensity in the BPA-exposed rats (PC group) (Figures 7(E) and 7(F)) while there was slightly higher intensity of staining in the stroma of rats with concurrent treatment with Tualang honey (TH group) (Figures 7(I) and 7(J)).

3.6. ERα, ERβ, and C3 mRNA Expression.

The changes in mRNA expression of estrogen-related genes were measured to support the immunohistochemistry analysis. The ERα, ERβ, and complement C3 mRNA expression are shown in Figures 8(a), 8(b), and 8(c).

As shown in Figure 8(a), BPA exposure in PC group animals significantly downregulated the ERα mRNA expression by approximately 4-fold as compared to the control rats (NC

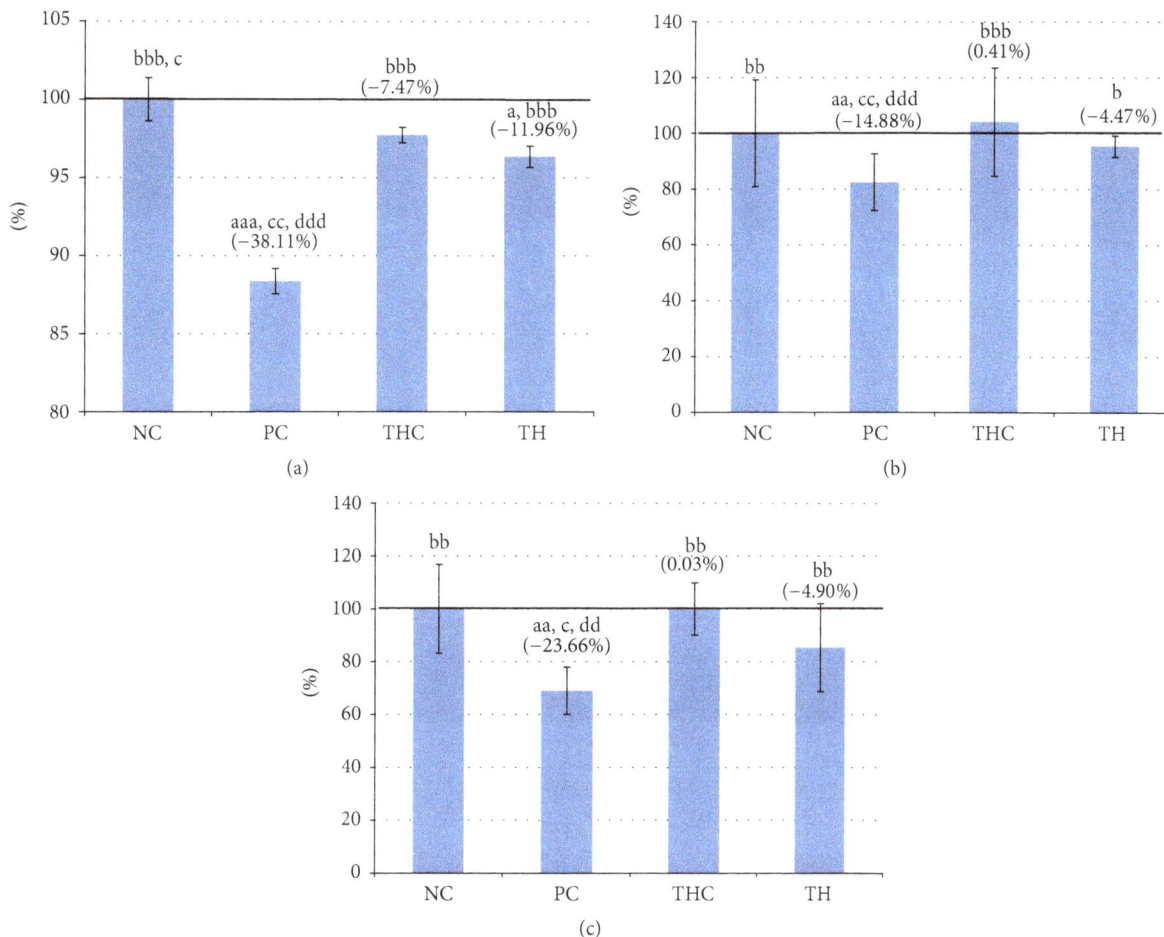

FIGURE 3: (a) Height of luminal epithelial cells of uterus in all experimental groups. BPA-induced reduction in luminal epithelial height (PC group) was significantly prevented by concurrent treatment with Tualang honey (TH group). Data are expressed as Mean ± SEM. (1) $^a P < 0.05$ and $^{aaa} P < 0.001$ versus NC (negative control). (2) $^{bbb} P < 0.001$ versus PC (BPA 10 mg/kg). (3) $^c P < 0.05$ and $^{cc} P < 0.01$ versus TH (Tualang honey 200 mg/kg + BPA 10 mg/kg). (4) $^{ddd} P < 0.001$ versus THC (Tualang honey 200 mg/kg). (b) Thickness of endometrium of uterus in all experimental groups. BPA-induced reduction in thickness of the endometrium layer (PC group) was significantly prevented by concurrent treatment with Tualang honey (TH group). Data are expressed as Mean ± SEM. (1) $^{aa} P < 0.01$ versus NC (negative control). (2) $^b P < 0.05$, $^{bb} P < 0.01$, and $^{bbb} P < 0.001$ versus PC (BPA 10 mg/kg). (3) $^c P < 0.05$ versus TH (Tualang honey 200 mg/kg + BPA 10 mg/kg). (4) $^{ddd} P < 0.001$ versus THC (Tualang honey 200 mg/kg). (c) Thickness of myometrium of uterus in all experimental groups. BPA-induced reduction in the thickness of the myometrium layer (PC group) was significantly prevented by concurrent treatment with Tualang honey (TH group). Data are expressed as Mean ± SEM. (1) $^{aa} P < 0.01$ versus NC (negative control). (2) $^{bb} P < 0.01$ versus PC (BPA 10 mg/kg). (3) $^c P < 0.05$ versus TH (Tualang honey 200 mg/kg + BPA 10 mg/kg). (4) $^{dd} P < 0.01$ versus THC (Tualang honey 200 mg/kg).

group). However, the magnitude was reduced to 3-fold by concurrent treatment with Tualang honey (TH group). In contrast, treatment with Tualang honey (THC group) showed 1.5-fold induction in the ERα mRNA expression compared to the control group.

Figure 8(b) shows a dissimilar pattern of ERβ mRNA expression compared to ERα mRNA expression. As compared to the control rats (NC group), the expression of ERβ was significantly upregulated by approximately 1.4-fold in BPA-exposed rats (PC group) and this was reduced to 1.1-fold by concurrent treatment of Tualang honey (TH group). This indicates that concurrent treatment with Tualang honey was able to reduce the ERβ mRNA expression in BPA-exposed

rats by 80%. Meanwhile, Tualang honey alone (THC group) had no effect on the ERβ mRNA expression with the value of expression comparable to the control rats (NC group).

As shown in Figure 8(c), BPA exposure (PC group) caused dramatic suppression of the complement C3 mRNA expression by almost 90% as compared to the control rats (NC group). Surprisingly, this effect was completely reversed with concurrent treatment with Tualang honey (TH group). In fact, the C3 mRNA expression in the Tualang honey group (TH group) was 1.8-fold higher than the control rats (NC group). Tualang honey alone had no effect on the C3 mRNA expression with the value of expression comparable to the control rats (NC group).

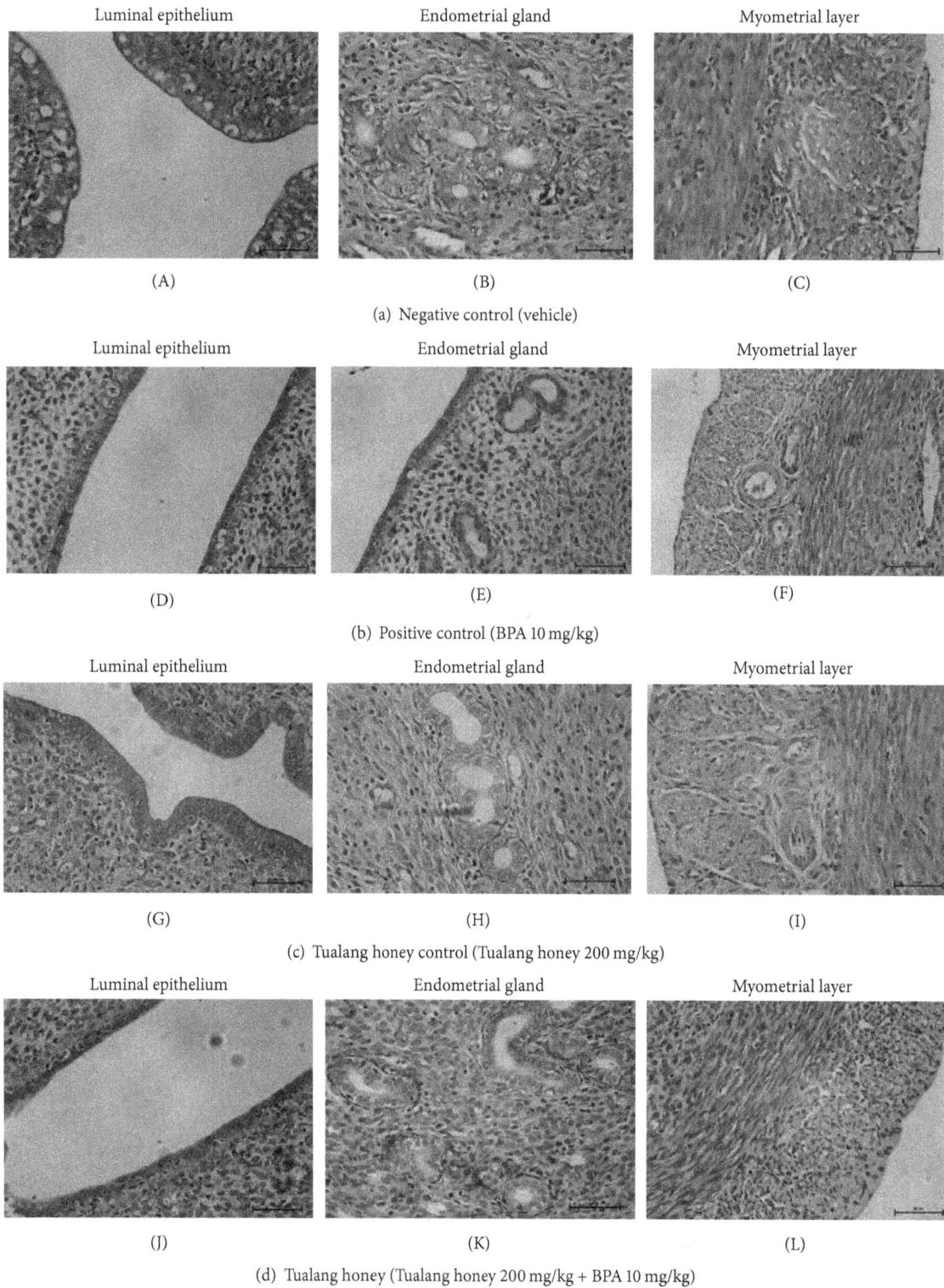

Luminal epithelium   Endometrial gland   Myometrial layer

(A)   (B)   (C)

(a) Negative control (vehicle)

Luminal epithelium   Endometrial gland   Myometrial layer

(D)   (E)   (F)

(b) Positive control (BPA 10 mg/kg)

Luminal epithelium   Endometrial gland   Myometrial layer

(G)   (H)   (I)

(c) Tualang honey control (Tualang honey 200 mg/kg)

Luminal epithelium   Endometrial gland   Myometrial layer

(J)   (K)   (L)

(d) Tualang honey (Tualang honey 200 mg/kg + BPA 10 mg/kg)

FIGURE 4: Representative sections of uteri from all experimental groups (H&E, ×40). Normal histological appearance was observed in control group (NC group) ((A), (B), and (C)). Significant disruptive morphological changes were observed in BPA-exposed rats (PC group) ((D), (E), and (F)). The uterus of rat treated with Tualang honey alone (THC group) ((G), (H), and (I)) was comparable to the control group, while concurrent treatment of rats with BPA and Tualang honey (TH group) ((J), (K), and (L)) showed partial prevention of tissues damage from the toxic effect of BPA.

(a) Negative control (vehicle) without primary antibody

(b) Negative control (vehicle)

(c) Positive control (BPA 10 mg/kg)

(d) Tualang honey control (Tualang honey 200 mg/kg)

(e) Tualang honey (Tualang honey 200 mg/kg + BPA 10 mg/kg)

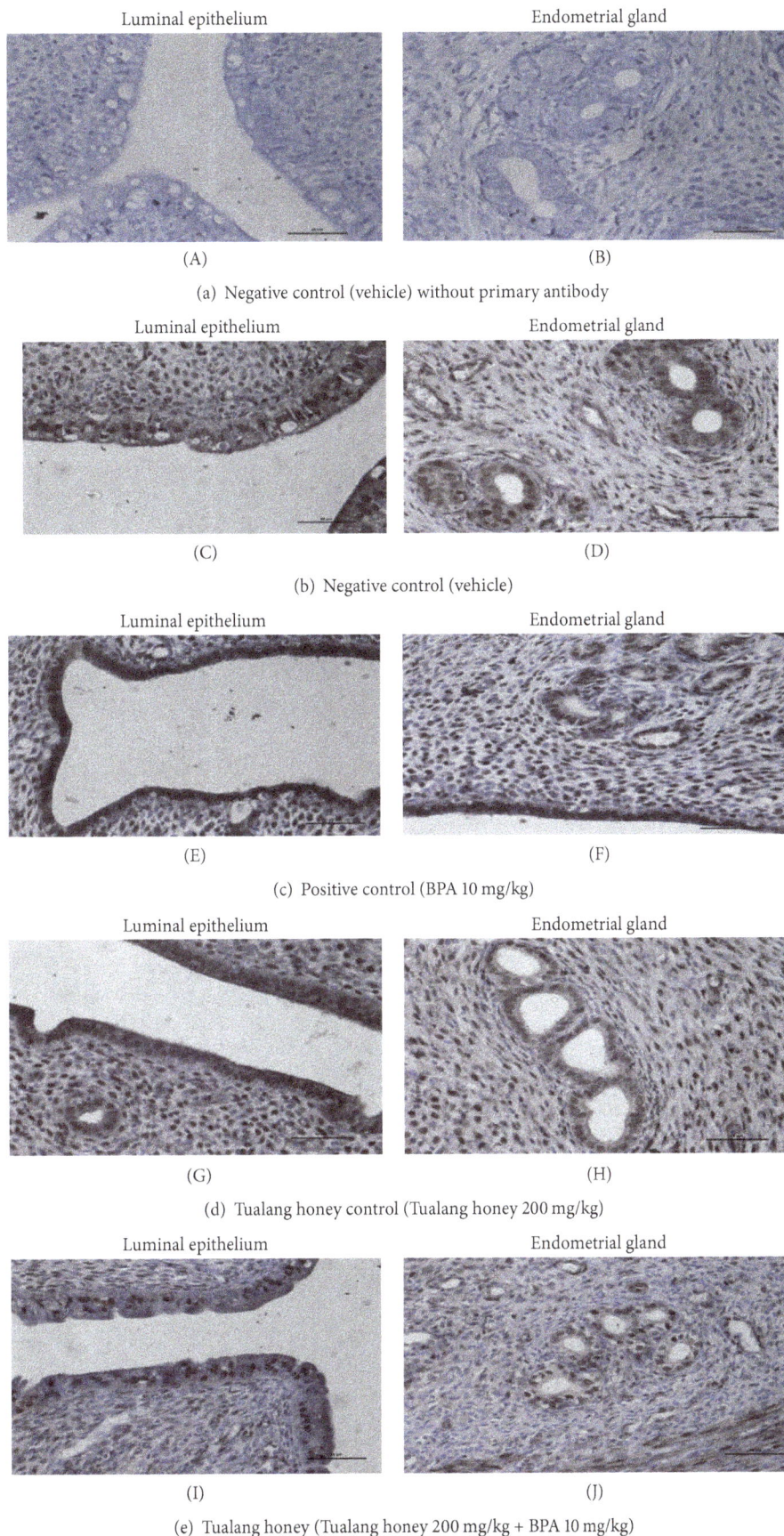

FIGURE 5: Representative sections of uteri showing the immunohistological localization of ERα in all experimental groups (×40). The most pronounced immunostaining intensity in both control ((C), (D)) (NC groups) and Tualang honey treated alone ((G), (H)) (THC groups) rats. Lower immunostaining intensity in BPA-exposed rats ((E), (F)) (PC group) was observed. Concurrent treatment with Tualang honey TH group ((I), (J)) also showed similar immunostaining intensity with these BPA-exposed rats.

Luminal epithelium

Endometrial gland

(A)

(B)

(a) Negative control (vehicle) without primary antibody

Luminal epithelium

Endometrial gland

(C)

(D)

(b) Negative control (vehicle)

Luminal epithelium

Endometrial gland

(E)

(F)

(c) Positive control (BPA 10 mg/kg)

Luminal epithelium

Endometrial gland

(G)

(H)

(d) Tualang honey control (Tualang honey 200 mg/kg)

Luminal epithelium

Endometrial gland

(I)

(J)

(e) Tualang honey (Tualang honey 200 mg/kg + BPA 10 mg/kg)

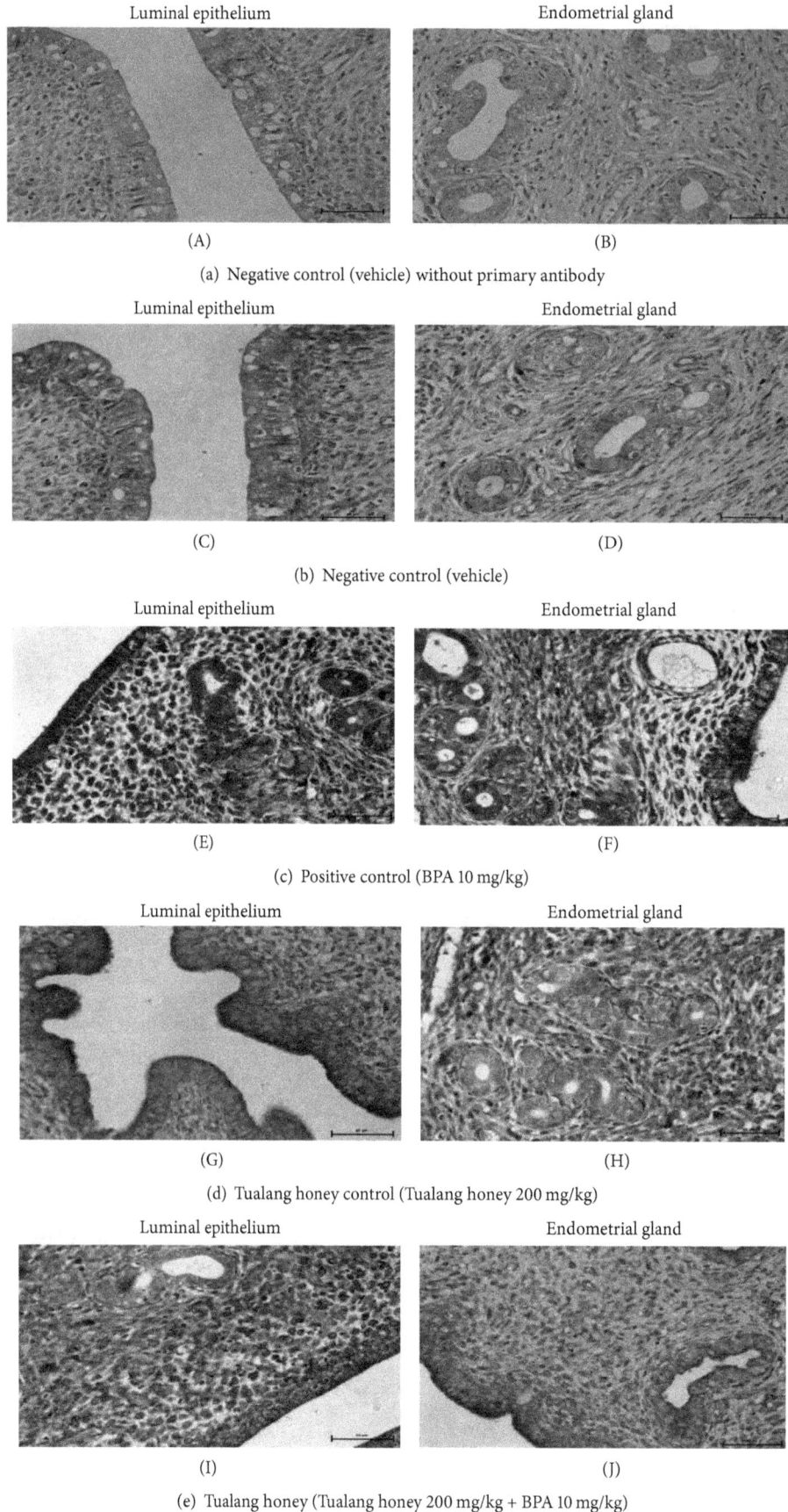

FIGURE 6: Representative sections of uteri showing the immunohistological localization of ERβ in all experimental groups (×40). The most pronounced immunostaining intensity was observed in BPA-exposed rats ((E), (F)) (PC group). Comparable immunostaining intensities were observed in NC ((C), (D)), THC ((G), (H)), and TH ((I), (J)) groups.

Luminal epithelium　　　　　　　　　　Endometrial gland

(A)　　　　　　　　　　　　　　　　(B)

(a) Negative control (vehicle) without primary antibody

Luminal epithelium　　　　　　　　　　Endometrial gland

(C)　　　　　　　　　　　　　　　　(D)

(b) Negative control (vehicle)

Luminal epithelium　　　　　　　　　　Endometrial gland

(E)　　　　　　　　　　　　　　　　(F)

(c) Positive control (BPA 10 mg/kg)

Luminal epithelium　　　　　　　　　　Endometrial gland

(G)　　　　　　　　　　　　　　　　(H)

(d) Tualang honey control (Tualang honey 200 mg/kg)

Luminal epithelium　　　　　　　　　　Endometrial gland

(I)　　　　　　　　　　　　　　　　(J)

(e) Tualang honey (Tualang honey 200 mg/kg + BPA 10 mg/kg)

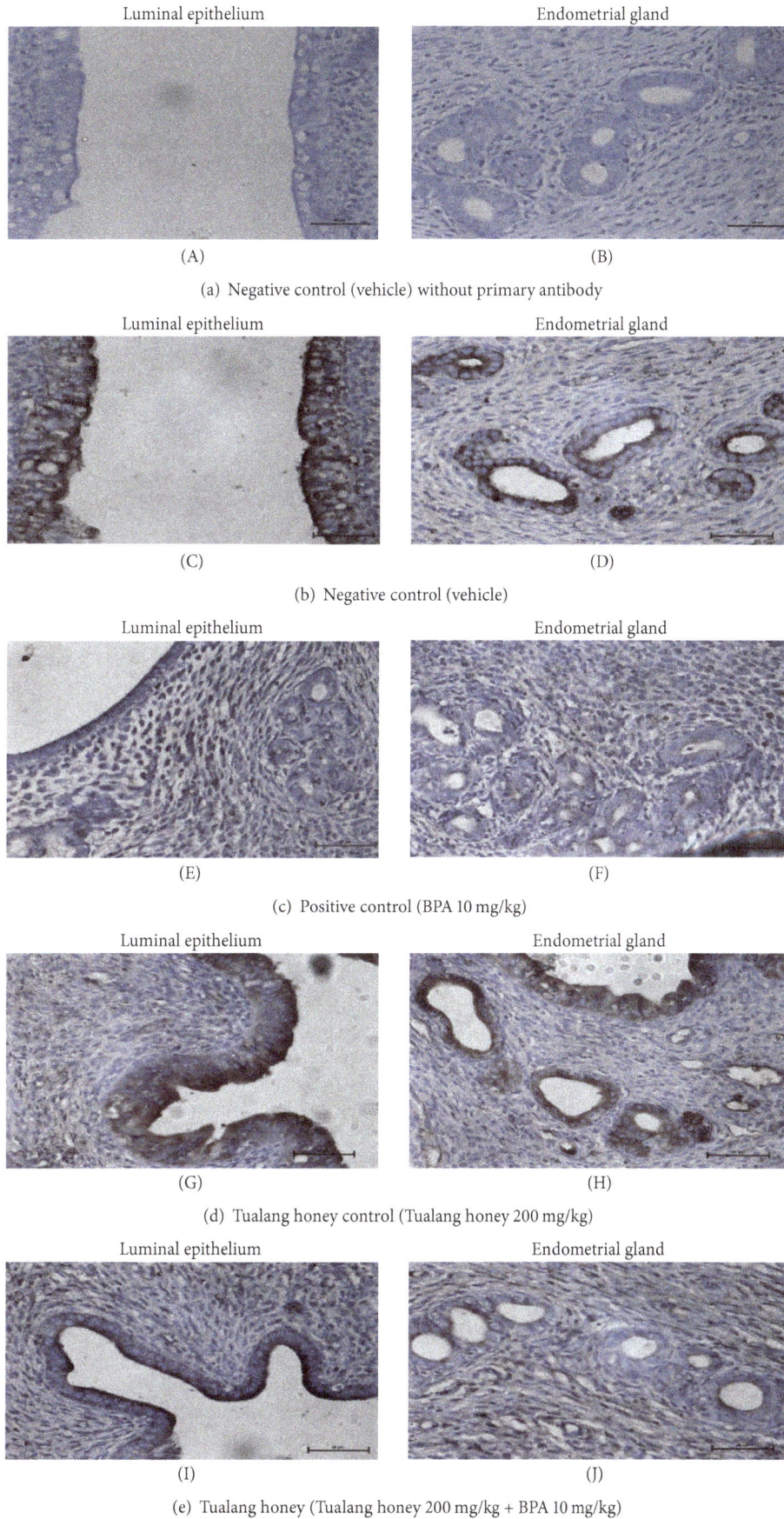

FIGURE 7: The lowest intensity of immunostaining was observed in BPA-exposed animals (PC group) ((E), (F)). However, higher intensity of color in stroma was noted with concurrent treatment with Tualang honey (TH group) ((I), (J)). Compared to the PC and TH groups, the highest and comparable immunostaining intensity were observed in NC group ((C), (D)) and THC group ((G), (H)).

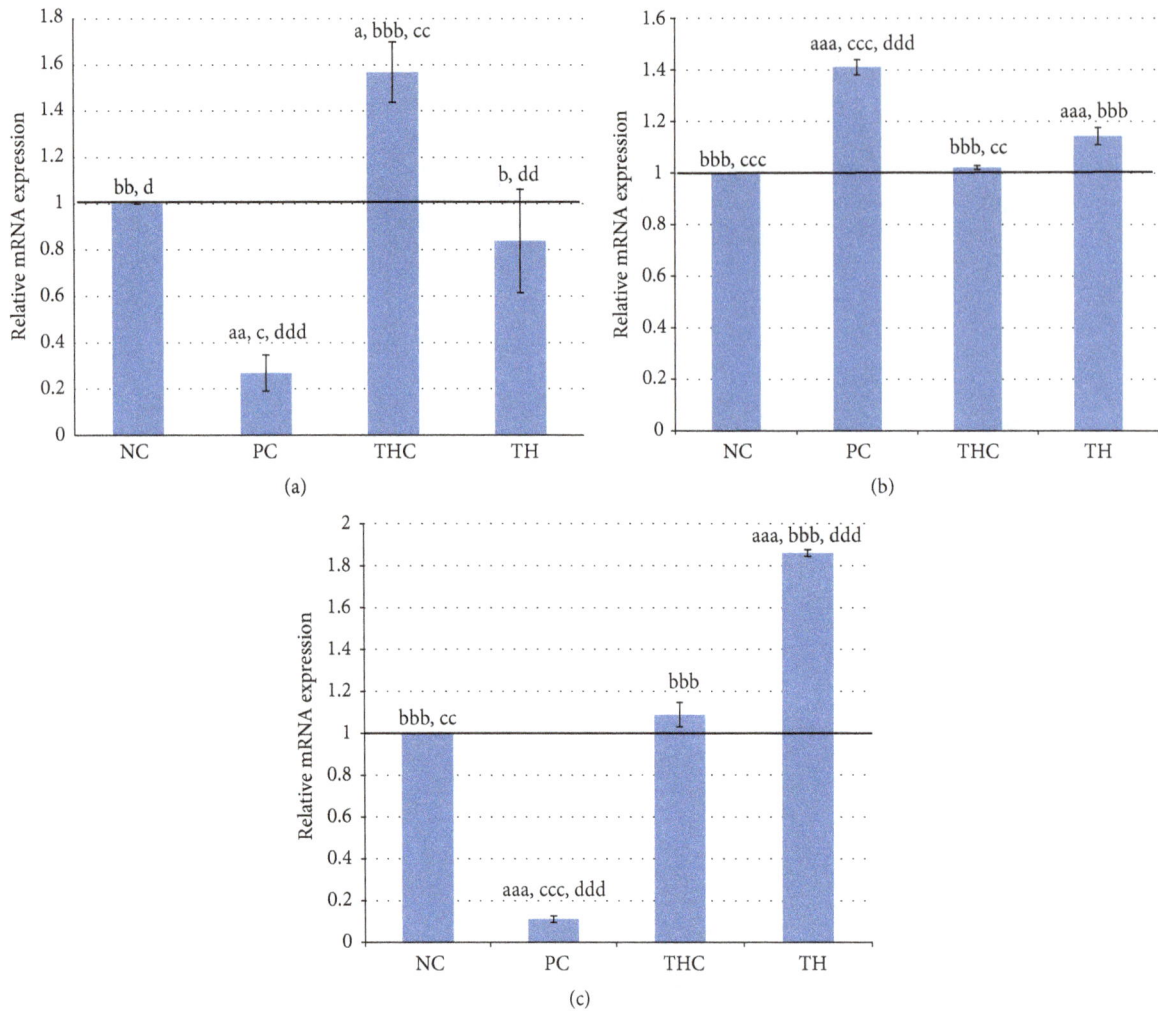

FIGURE 8: (a) Quantitative real-time PCR of ERα in all experimental groups. ERα mRNA expression was significantly downregulated in the rats exposed to BPA (PC group) (4-fold) as compared to the control animals (NC group). However, the decline was reversed (3-fold) by concurrent treatment with Tualang honey (TH group). Data are expressed as Mean ± SEM. (1) $^{a}P < 0.05$ and $^{aa}P < 0.01$ versus NC (negative control). (2) $^{b}P < 0.05$, $^{bb}P < 0.01$, and $^{bbb}P < 0.001$ versus PC (BPA 10 mg/kg). (3) $^{c}P < 0.05$ and $^{cc}P < 0.01$ versus TH (Tualang honey 200 mg/kg + BPA 10 mg/kg). (4) $^{d}P < 0.05$, $^{dd}P < 0.01$, and $^{ddd}P < 0.001$ versus THC (Tualang honey 200 mg/kg). (b) Quantitative real-time PCR of ERβ in all experimental groups. Compared to the control rats (NC group), the expression of ERβ was significantly upregulated (1.4-fold) in BPA-exposed rats (PC group) and this is reduced to 1.1-fold by concurrent treatment of Tualang honey (TH group). Data are expressed as Mean ± SEM. (1) $^{aaa}P < 0.001$ versus NC (negative control). (2) $^{bbb}P < 0.001$ versus PC (BPA 10 mg/kg). (3) $^{cc}P < 0.01$ and $^{ccc}P < 0.001$ versus TH (Tualang honey 200 mg/kg + BPA 10 mg/kg). (4) $^{ddd}P < 0.001$ versus THC (Tualang honey 200 mg/kg). (c) Quantitative real-time PCR of complement C3 in all experimental groups. BPA exposure (PC group) caused a significant downregulation of the amount of complement C3 mRNA (9-fold) as compared to the control rats (NC group). This effect was completely reversed by concurrent treatment with Tualang honey (TH group). Data are expressed as Mean ± SEM. (1) $^{aaa}P < 0.001$ versus NC (negative control). (2) $^{bbb}P < 0.001$ versus PC (BPA 10 mg/kg). (3) $^{cc}P < 0.01$ and $^{ccc}P < 0.001$ versus TH (Tualang honey 200 mg/kg + BPA 10 mg/kg). (4) $^{ddd}P < 0.001$ versus THC (Tualang honey 200 mg/kg).

4. Discussion

BPA, as an endocrine disrupting chemical (EDC), has the capability to mimic, enhance, or inhibit the activity of natural estrogen and to disrupt the functions of estrogen nuclear hormone receptors in a diverse set of target tissues [8, 13, 15, 34]. Thus, exclusively defining BPA as an environmental estrogen or selective estrogen receptor modulator (SERM) is indeed inaccurate [2].

In the last few decades, a considerable amount of evidence has been accumulated which demonstrates the fact that young women may be at high risk of reproductive infertility due to continuous exposure to numerous BPA products in their daily lives [35]. With this concern in mind, our present study had investigated the disruptive effects of BPA on the female reproductive physiology with special reference to the morphology, oxidative markers, and protein and molecular changes that occur in the rat uterus. In addition, the potential protective roles of Tualang honey as a natural product in reducing the disruptive effects of BPA on the above-mentioned selected parameters were evaluated. The mechanisms of the translational and transcription factors in estrogen receptors were also investigated. In addition to the classical *in vivo* tool (uterotrophic assay), more sensitive tools such as the analysis of gene transcription and protein expression were adopted to investigate the molecular responses due to BPA exposure.

In toxicology study, the differences in body and organ weights between untreated and treated animals can be a reliable indicator for the toxicity effects of the test compounds [36]. In the present study, the toxicology data showed that the effects of BPA appear to be very specific to the uterus as the reduction in weight seems to affect the uterus itself, without having significant effects on the whole body weight. These current results are in agreement with a previous report by Ashby et al. [37]. In contrast, others have shown that BPA exposure in rodent animals was reported to be associated with weight gain [38–40].

BPA is one of the suggested EDCs that induce reactive oxygen species (ROS) that play important roles in the pathology of female reproductive diseases such as uterine endometriosis [35]. Furthermore, lipid peroxidation (LPO) is a process of interaction between reactive oxygen species (ROS) and the cellular membrane that induces damage to cellular macromolecules and DNA [41]. Since malondialdehyde (MDA) is a secondary product of LPO, it is generally accepted as an oxidative stress marker [42]. The relationship between oxidative stress and infertility among women has been proven in several scientific studies [43, 44]. Epidemiological data showed that higher levels of reactive oxygen species (ROS) and lower antioxidant levels were detected in infertile women compared to fertile women [45, 46]. In the present study, the uterine MDA level in BPA-exposed animals was significantly higher compared to the normal control animals. The results could be due to lipid peroxidation process by BPA and this result correlated well with the histopathological, immunohistochemical, and gene expression analyses.

Treatment with Tualang honey in BPA-exposed rats significantly reduced the uterine MDA levels. This observation could be due to the antioxidant effects of Tualang honey which cause reduction in the number of free radicals. This explanation is based on several published data that reported Tualang honey as an effective antioxidant in reducing the MDA levels in human subjects and animal models [17, 47].

In addition to that, striking morphologic changes of the uterus (disruption of the normal structure of the luminal epithelium, endometrium, myometrium, and glandular epithelial cells) associated with oxidative stress were apparent in BPA-exposed rats compared to the controls. These morphological changes could be related to the potential direct actions of BPA on the DNA itself that results in alteration of gene expression. BPA-induced DNA damage has been evidently reported, in both *in vivo* and *in vitro* studies [48, 49]. This is because BPA can be oxidized to bisphenol-o-quinone that covalently binds to deoxyguanosine to form DNA adducts. Subsequently, DNA adducts cause improper

and incomplete replication that leads to the formation of atypical cells.

Interestingly, the disruptive effects of BPA on the uterine morphology were partially reduced following concurrent treatment with Tualang honey. The improvement could be, again, accounted for by the high natural antioxidant contents in Tualang honey in addition to the carbohydrates, amino acids, proteins, organic acids, vitamins, and various phytochemicals [24, 50]. In the natural state, cells of our body are capable of maintaining the normal equilibrium of antioxidant-oxidative stress balance by neutralizing or directly diminishing the oxidative damage by means of enzymatic and nonenzymatic antioxidants [51]. Evidently, Tualang honey contains nonenzymatic antioxidants such as vitamins E and C with their interactive effects as lipophilic and hydrophilic free-radical scavengers, respectively [52] hence possibly explaining the improvement observed in treated rats.

Vitamin E resides mainly in the cell membranes, thus playing an important role in the maintenance of cell membranes [53]. Meanwhile, the major function of vitamin C is as a scavenger of free radicals in the extracellular fluid, deceiving radicals in the aqueous phase, protecting biomembranes from peroxidase impairment, and regenerating tocopherol (vitamin E) from tocopheroxyl radicals in the membrane [54]. Several studies have found that both antioxidants can mitigate adverse pathological impacts by minimizing the genotoxicity and cytotoxicity effects in the cells [55–57]. Flavonols (quercetin and kaempferol) with weak estrogenic activities are attributed to the decrease in the intracellular reactive oxygen species (ROS) by a mechanism that involves estrogen receptors [58]. Thus, in our study, the antioxidant properties of Tualang honey could be contributing to the protective effects in cells by trapping and inactivating of free radicals as observed in the improvement of the heterogeneous cell types of the uterus (stromal, luminal epithelium, endometrial glands, and smooth muscle).

Nonetheless, the morphological recovery following treatment with Tualang honey in BPA-exposed uterus seems to be partial. This may be due to the presence of other reactive oxygen species that could also be in play to cause the disruptive effects. Moreover, even after removal of BPA, the inactive detoxifying proteins/enzymes may require a certain period of time to recover, as supported by Chevallet et al. [59].

Other findings in our study which are also in line with previous studies showed that BPA can disrupt the development, growth, and functions of the uterus by interrupting the regulation of mRNA expression and protein distribution of ERα, ERβ, and complement C3 [12, 13, 60]. Estrogen receptor (ER) is a member of steroid receptor superfamily, a ligand-activated enhancer protein that is activated by the hormone estrogen (17β-estradiol) and is able to regulate gene transcription via estrogen responsive elements [61]. Unfortunately, it can also be activated by other compounds including endocrine disrupting chemical such as BPA [62]. The ER is encoded by two subtype genes, namely, ERα and ERβ, that function as a signal transducer and a transcription factor in modulating the expression of target genes [63]. The endogenous estrogen (17β-estradiol) has a lower binding affinity to ERβ than ERα [34] but both receptors share similarity in terms of transactivation via estrogen responsive element (ERE) [64]. In contrast, they possess dissimilar functions with regard to their roles in transcription activation, which depend very much on the ligands and their responsive elements [65].

BPA is considered weak environmental estrogen since its binding affinity to ERα and ERβ is estimated to be 10,000-fold lower than the endogenous estrogen, with a relative binding affinity of 6-fold higher in ERβ compared to ERα [34, 62]. On the other hand, in some cell types, BPA exhibits estradiol-like agonist activity via ERβ and a mixed agonist/antagonist activity via ERα [15]. Both subtypes contain a ligand-dependent transactivation domain, named AF2 (Activation Function 2), for activation of transcription of target genes by the recruitment of transcriptional cofactors steroid receptor coactivator-1 (SRC-1) and transcriptional intermediary factor-2 (TIF-2) [66]. The disruptive role of BPA in this pathway significantly increases the recruitment of these cofactors [67]. This could be a possible explanation for our present data that showed significant upregulation in the expression of mRNA and higher protein distribution of ERβ in BPA-exposed animals (PC group) as compared to the control rats.

In our study, besides the role of lipid peroxidation, the upregulation of ERβ in BPA-exposed animals could be attributed to the disruptive effects in the uterus. A report in 2000 by Weihua et al. revealed that, in the uterus, ERβ acts as a modulator of ERα-mediated gene transcription [68]. The role of ERβ is as a transdominant repressor that inhibits the ERα transcriptional activity [69]. The inhibitory effects are due to the ability of ERβ to form heterodimers with ERα, which in turn regulate the functions of estrogen receptors [70]. Thus, unlike ERα, ERβ does not have classic uterotrophic effects but rather disruptive effects on ERα.

Other studies via crystallography structure analysis and computer modeling studies have found that BPA has higher binding affinity to ERRγ to ERα [71, 72]. ERRγ is an orphan nuclear receptor that belongs to the ERR family (estrogen receptor-related) [73]. Although both ERα and ERRγ receptors share similar sequence homology, 17β-estradiol does not associate to ERRγ [74]. The BPA-ERRγ interaction was suggested to trigger heterodimerization between ERα and ERRγ which results in suppression of the transcriptional activity of the ERα [71]. Similarly, Huppunen and Aarnisalo also reported that the modulation of BPA as an inhibitor on ERα signaling is also via ERRγ [75]. Such interaction could be an explanation for our present data that showed significant downregulation of mRNA expression and lower protein distribution of ERα in BPA-exposed animals (PC group) compared to the control normal animals. In addition, the ERα mRNA expression was also significantly higher in Tualang honey treated rats. However, the protein distribution did not differ much from the normal control rats. Hence, these results suggest that Tualang honey is likely to modulate the ERα mRNA expression at the transcriptional level but not at the translational level.

Complement C3 is involved in innate immunity. The crucial role of C3 is to regulate any activation of host cell damage by promoting phagocytosis, initiating local inflammatory responses against pathogens, and to instruct appropriate adaptive immune response towards antigens for a humoral response [76]. In 2004, Seidlová-Wuttke et al. have used quantitative RT-PCR analysis to investigate the effects of BPA on C3 mRNA transcription in rat uterus [13]. According to the authors, estradiol treatment significantly upregulated the C3 mRNA expression. Interestingly, the effect was not mimicked by BPA exposure where downregulation of C3 mRNA expression was observed. This effect was also observed in our present study. However, concurrent treatment with Tualang honey was able to significantly increase the C3 expression, indicating some improvement in the innate immune system. Interestingly, the mRNA expression in Tualang honey treated rats was also significantly higher compared to the control animals. This could be due to higher activation of transcriptional activity C3 induced by certain bioactive compounds that oppose the disturbance effects of BPA on the innate immune system. However, the protein distribution in Tualang honey treated rats did not differ much from the BPA-exposed rats. Hence, these results suggest that Tualang honey is likely to modulate the C3 mRNA expression at the transcriptional level but not at the translational level.

The improvements of protein and molecular levels of ERα, ERβ, and C3 in BPA-exposed animals treated by Tualang honey could be explained by the fact that Tualang honey contains high nutritional profile antioxidants including flavonoids, specifically flavonols [58]. The two main naturally occurring flavonols, namely, quercetin and kaempferol share structural similarities with 17β-estradiol and hence may potentially have weak estrogenic effects [58]. Evidence from our previous study have shown that besides the ability to scavenge oxidants and free radicals [19], biologically active estrogen-like compounds in Tualang honey also improved the atrophy state of uterus and vagina [18]. In addition, our previous findings also found that the potential competitive binding of these compounds also contributed to the improvement of the hypothalamic-pituitary axis function in BPA-exposed animals [77] as also supported by an earlier study [78].

The effects of lipid peroxidation of BPA on DNA damage have also been extensively tested in *in vivo* and *in vitro* studies [79–81]. The antigenotoxicity effects of Tualang honey were reported to occur via several mechanisms: the upregulation of double stranded DNA repair enzymes [82], reduction of cyclobutane pyrimidine dimers and 8-oxo-dG-positive cells (biomarkers of DNA damage) [83], and induction of apoptosis [84]. Similar protective mechanisms against DNA damage have been suggested in studies on Buckwheat honey and honey from arid regions that are also in line with the current Tualang honey findings [85, 86].

5. Conclusions

In conclusion, Tualang honey has potential roles in reducing BPA-induced uterine disruption, possibly accounted for by its phytochemical properties. In view of this, Tualang honey could be suggested as a promising natural product candidate in reducing the toxicity effects of BPA in the uterus. Thus, further investigation is warranted to establish precise and better understanding of the roles of phytochemical compounds in

Tualang honey that account for the reduction in BPA-induced uterine toxicity.

Abbreviations

BPA: Bisphenol A
OSCC: Oral squamous cell carcinomas
ERα: Estrogen receptor-alpha
ERβ: Estrogen receptor-beta
MDA: Malondialdehyde
TBARS: Thiobarbituric Acid Reactive Substances
PBS: Phosphate buffered saline
BHT: Butylated hydroxytoluene
RNA: Ribonucleic acid
cDNA: Complementary deoxyribonucleic acid
PCR: Polymerase chain reaction
NC: Negative control group
PC: Positive control group
TH: Tualang honey + BPA group
THC: Tualang honey control.

Conflict of Interests

The authors declare there is no conflict of interests.

Acknowledgments

The authors would like to acknowledge University of Malaya for providing a postgraduate research grant (no. PG087-2012B), Universiti Putra Malaysia, and Ministry of Higher Education, Malaysia, for their financial assistance to the first author Siti Sarah Mohamad Zaid. Sincere thanks are due to all the staff of the Department of Anatomy, Faculty of Medicine, University of Malaya.

References

[1] N. Von Goetz, M. Wormuth, M. Scheringer, and K. Hungerbühler, "Bisphenol a: How the most relevant exposure sources contribute to total consumer exposure," *Risk Analysis*, vol. 30, no. 3, pp. 473–487, 2010.

[2] Y. B. Wetherill, B. T. Akingbemi, J. Kanno et al., "In vitro molecular mechanisms of bisphenol A action," *Reproductive Toxicology*, vol. 24, no. 2, pp. 178–198, 2007.

[3] A. Suzuki, A. Sugihara, K. Uchida et al., "Developmental effects of perinatal exposure to bisphenol-A and diethylstilbestrol on reproductive organs in female mice," *Reproductive Toxicology*, vol. 16, no. 2, pp. 107–116, 2002.

[4] Y. J. Yang, Y.-C. Hong, S.-Y. Oh et al., "Bisphenol A exposure is associated with oxidative stress and inflammation in post-menopausal women," *Environmental Research*, vol. 109, no. 6, pp. 797–801, 2009.

[5] H.-W. Kuo and W.-H. Ding, "Trace determination of bisphenol A and phytoestrogens in infant formula powders by gas chromatography-mass spectrometry," *Journal of Chromatography A*, vol. 1027, no. 1-2, pp. 67–74, 2004.

[6] Y. Sun, M. Wada, O. Al-Dirbashi, N. Kuroda, H. Nakazawa, and K. Nakashima, "High-performance liquid chromatography with peroxyoxalate chemiluminescence detection of bisphenol A migrated from polycarbonate baby bottles using 4-(4,5-diphenyl-1H-imidazol-2-yl)benzoyl chloride as a label," *Journal of Chromatography B: Biomedical Sciences and Applications*, vol. 749, no. 1, pp. 49–56, 2000.

[7] C. Brede, P. Fjeldal, I. Skjevrak, and H. Herikstad, "Increased migration levels of bisphenol A from polycarbonate baby bottles after dishwashing, boiling and brushing," *Food Additives & Contaminants*, vol. 20, no. 7, pp. 684–689, 2003.

[8] J. C. Gould, L. S. Leonard, S. C. Maness et al., "Bisphenol A interacts with the estrogen receptor α in a distinct manner from estradiol," *Molecular and Cellular Endocrinology*, vol. 142, no. 1-2, pp. 203–214, 1998.

[9] M. V. Maffini, B. S. Rubin, C. Sonnenschein, and A. M. Soto, "Endocrine disruptors and reproductive health: the case of bisphenol-A," *Molecular and Cellular Endocrinology*, vol. 254-255, pp. 179–186, 2006.

[10] C. M. Markey, P. R. Wadia, B. S. Rubin, C. Sonnenschein, and A. M. Soto, "Long-term effects of fetal exposure to low doses of the xenoestrogen bisphenol-A in the female mouse genital tract," *Biology of Reproduction*, vol. 72, no. 6, pp. 1344–1351, 2005.

[11] P. Diel, T. Schulz, K. Smolnikar, E. Strunck, G. Vollmer, and H. Michna, "Ability of xeno- and phytoestrogens to modulate estrogen-sensitive genes in rat uterus: estrogenicity profiles and uterotrophic activity," *Journal of Steroid Biochemistry and Molecular Biology*, vol. 73, no. 1-2, pp. 1–10, 2000.

[12] G. Schönfelder, K. Friedrich, M. Paul, and I. Chahoud, "Developmental effects of prenatal exposure to bisphenol A on the uterus of rat offspring," *Neoplasia*, vol. 6, no. 5, pp. 584–594, 2004.

[13] D. Seidlová-Wuttke, H. Jarry, and W. Wuttke, "Pure estrogenic effect of benzophenone-2 (BP2) but not of bisphenol a (BPA) and dibutylphtalate (DBP) in uterus, vagina and bone," *Toxicology*, vol. 205, no. 1-2, pp. 103–112, 2004.

[14] S. Xiao, H. Diao, M. A. Smith, X. Song, and X. Ye, "Preimplantation exposure to bisphenol A (BPA) affects embryo transport, preimplantation embryo development, and uterine receptivity in mice," *Reproductive Toxicology*, vol. 32, no. 4, pp. 434–441, 2011.

[15] T. Kurosawa, H. Hiroi, O. Tsutsumi et al., "The activity of bisphenol A depends on both the estrogen receptor subtype and the cell type," *Endocrine Journal*, vol. 49, no. 4, pp. 465–471, 2002.

[16] H. Kabuto, S. Hasuike, N. Minagawa, and T. Shishibori, "Effects of bisphenol A on the metabolisms of active oxygen species in mouse tissues," *Environmental Research*, vol. 93, no. 1, pp. 31–35, 2003.

[17] O. O. Erejuwa, S. A. Sulaiman, M. S. Wahab, K. N. S. Sirajudeen, M. S. M. D. Salleh, and S. Gurtu, "Antioxidant protection of Malaysian tualang honey in pancreas of normal and streptozotocin-induced diabetic rats," *Annales d'Endocrinologie*, vol. 71, no. 4, pp. 291–296, 2010.

[18] S. S. M. Zaid, S. A. Sulaiman, K. N. M. Sirajudeen, and N. H. Othman, "The effects of Tualang honey on female reproductive organs, tibia bone and hormonal profile in ovariectomised rats—animal model for menopause," *BMC Complementary and Alternative Medicine*, vol. 10, article 82, 2010.

[19] S. S. Zaid, S. A. Sulaiman, N. H. Othman et al., "Protective effects of Tualang honey on bone structure in experimental postmenopausal rats," *Clinics*, vol. 67, no. 7, pp. 779–784, 2012.

[20] M. Mohamed, S. A. Sulaiman, H. Jaafar, and K. N. Salam, "Antioxidant protective effect of honey in cigarette smoke-induced testicular damage in rats," *International Journal of Molecular Sciences*, vol. 12, no. 9, pp. 5508–5521, 2011.

[21] A. A. Ghashm, N. H. Othman, M. N. Khattak, N. M. Ismail, and R. Saini, "Antiproliferative effect of Tualang honey on oral squamous cell carcinoma and osteosarcoma cell lines," *BMC Complementary and Alternative Medicine*, vol. 10, article 49, 2010.

[22] S. N. S. Mohamad, S. H. Ahmad, and H. G. Siew, "Antiproliferative effect of methanolic extraction of Tualang honey on human keloid fibroblasts," *BMC Complementary and Alternative Medicine*, vol. 11, no. 82, pp. 1–8, 2011.

[23] S. Ahmed and N. H. Othman, "Review of the medicinal effects of tualang honey and a comparison with Manuka honey," *Malaysian Journal of Medical Sciences*, vol. 20, no. 3, pp. 6–13, 2013.

[24] M. Mahaneem, K. N. S. Sirajudeen, M. Swamy, and S. Y. Nik, "Studies on antioxidant properties of Tualang honey," *African Journal of Traditional, Complementary and Alternative Medicines*, vol. 7, no. 1, pp. 59–63, 2010.

[25] M. I. Khalil, N. Alam, M. Moniruzzaman, S. A. Sulaiman, and S. H. Gan, "henolic acid composition and antioxidant properties of Malaysian honeys," *Journal of Food Science*, vol. 76, no. 6, pp. C921–C928, 2011.

[26] S. Anjum, S. Rahman, M. Kaur et al., "Melatonin ameliorates bisphenol A-induced biochemical toxicity in testicular mitochondria of mouse," *Food and Chemical Toxicology*, vol. 49, no. 11, pp. 2849–2854, 2011.

[27] K. Okuda, M. Takiguchi, and S. Yoshihara, "In vivo estrogenic potential of 4-methyl-2,4-bis(4-hydroxyphenyl)pent-1-ene, an active metabolite of bisphenol A, in uterus of ovariectomized rat," *Toxicology Letters*, vol. 197, no. 1, pp. 7–11, 2010.

[28] Y. Li, W. Zhang, J. Liu et al., "Prepubertal bisphenol A exposure interferes with ovarian follicle development and its relevant gene expression," *Reproductive Toxicology*, vol. 44, pp. 33–40, 2014.

[29] H. H. Draper and M. Hadley, "Malondialdehyde determination as index of lipid peroxidation," *Methods in Enzymology*, vol. 186, pp. 421–431, 1990.

[30] K. J. Livak and T. D. Schmittgen, "Analysis of relative gene expression data using real-time quantitative PCR and the $2^{-\Delta\Delta C_T}$ method," *Methods*, vol. 25, no. 4, pp. 402–408, 2001.

[31] E. Spreafico, E. Bettini, G. Pollio, and A. Maggi, "Nucleotide sequence of estrogen receptor cDNA from Sprague-Dawley rat," *European Journal of Pharmacology: Molecular Pharmacology*, vol. 227, no. 3, pp. 353–356, 1992.

[32] G. G. J. M. Kuiper, E. Enmark, M. Pelto-Huikko, S. Nilsson, and J.-Å. Gustafsson, "Cloning of a novel estrogen receptor expressed in rat prostate and ovary," *Proceedings of the National Academy of Sciences of the United States of America*, vol. 93, no. 12, pp. 5925–5930, 1996.

[33] Y. Misumi, M. Sohda, and Y. Ikehara, "Nucleotide and deduced amino acid sequence of rat complement C3," *Nucleic Acids Research*, vol. 18, no. 8, p. 2178, 1990.

[34] G. G. J. M. Kuiper, B. Carlsson, K. Grandien et al., "Comparison of the ligand binding specificity and transcript tissue distribution of estrogen receptors alpha and beta," *Endocrinology*, vol. 138, no. 3, pp. 863–870, 1997.

[35] B. Yi, H. Kasai, H.-S. Lee, Y. Kang, J. Y. Park, and M. Yang, "Inhibition by wheat sprout (*Triticum aestivum*) juice of bisphenol A-induced oxidative stress in young women," *Mutation Research/Genetic Toxicology and Environmental Mutagenesis*, vol. 724, no. 1-2, pp. 64–68, 2011.

[36] M. J. Wolfsegger, T. Jaki, B. Dietrich, J. A. Kunzler, and K. Barker, "A note on statistical analysis of organ weights in non-clinical toxicological studies," *Toxicology and Applied Pharmacology*, vol. 240, no. 1, pp. 117–122, 2009.

[37] J. Ashby, H. Tinwell, P. A. Lefevre, R. Joiner, and J. Haseman, "The effect on sperm production in adult Sprague-Dawley rats exposed by gavage to bisphenol A between postnatal days 91–97," *Toxicological Sciences*, vol. 74, no. 1, pp. 129–138, 2003.

[38] C. M. Markey, M. A. Coombs, C. Sonnenschein, and A. M. Soto, "Mammalian development in a changing environment: exposure to endocrine disruptors reveals the developmental plasticity of steroid-hormone target organs," *Evolution and Development*, vol. 5, no. 1, pp. 67–75, 2003.

[39] B. S. Rubin, M. K. Murray, D. A. Damassa, J. C. King, and A. M. Soto, "Perinatal exposure to low doses of bisphenol A affects body weight, patterns of estrous cyclicity, and plasma LH levels," *Environmental Health Perspectives*, vol. 109, no. 7, pp. 675–680, 2001.

[40] K. L. Howdeshell, A. K. Hotchkiss, K. A. Thayer, J. G. Vandenbergh, and F. S. Vom Saal, "Environmental toxins: exposure to bisphenol A advances puberty," *Nature*, vol. 401, no. 6755, pp. 763–764, 1999.

[41] M. Güney, B. Oral, H. Demirin et al., "Evaluation of caspase-dependent apoptosis during methyl parathion-induced endometrial damage in rats: ameliorating effect of vitamins E and C," *Environmental Toxicology and Pharmacology*, vol. 23, no. 2, pp. 221–227, 2007.

[42] R. Aslan, M. R. Sekeroglu, M. Tarakcioglu, and H. Koylu, "Investigation of malondialdehyde formation and antioxidant enzyme activity in stored blood," *Haematologia*, vol. 28, no. 4, pp. 233–237, 1997.

[43] T. Suzuki, N. Sugino, T. Fukaya et al., "Superoxide dismutase in normal cycling human ovaries: immunohistochemical localization and characterization," *Fertility and Sterility*, vol. 72, no. 4, pp. 720–726, 1999.

[44] M. Jozwik, S. Wolczynski, M. Jozwik, and M. Szamatowicz, "Oxidative stress markers in preovulatory follicular fluid in humans," *Molecular Human Reproduction*, vol. 5, no. 5, pp. 409–413, 1999.

[45] Y. Wang, J. Goldberg, R. K. Sharma, A. Agarwal, and T. Falcone, "Importance of reactive oxygen species in the peritoneal fluid of women with endometriosis or idiopathic infertility," *Fertility and Sterility*, vol. 68, no. 5, pp. 826–830, 1997.

[46] G. Polak, M. Koziol-Montewka, M. Gogacz, I. Blaszkowska, and J. Kotarski, "Total antioxidant status of peritoneal fluid in infertile women," *European Journal of Obstetrics Gynecology and Reproductive Biology*, vol. 94, no. 2, pp. 261–263, 2001.

[47] N. Shafin, Z. Othman, R. Zakaria, and N. H. Nik Hussain, "Tualang honey supplementation reduces blood oxidative stress levels/activities in postmenopausal women," *ISRN Oxidative Medicine*, vol. 2014, Article ID 364836, 4 pages, 2014.

[48] A. Atkinson and D. Roy, "In vivo DNA adduct formation by bisphenol A," *Environmental and Molecular Mutagenesis*, vol. 26, no. 1, pp. 60–66, 1995.

[49] J. S. Edmonds, M. Nomachi, M. Terasaki, M. Morita, B. W. Skelton, and A. H. White, "The reaction of bisphenol A 3,4-quinone with DNA," *Biochemical and Biophysical Research Communications*, vol. 319, no. 2, pp. 556–561, 2004.

[50] R. K. Kishore, A. S. Halim, M. S. N. Syazana, and K. N. S. Sirajudeen, "Tualang honey has higher phenolic content and

greater radical scavenging activity compared with other honey sources," *Nutrition Research*, vol. 31, no. 1, pp. 322–325, 2011.

[51] B. Oral, M. Guney, H. Demirin et al., "Endometrial damage and apoptosis in rats induced by dichlorvos and ameliorating effect of antioxidant vitamins E and C," *Reproductive Toxicology*, vol. 22, no. 4, pp. 783–790, 2006.

[52] S. S. M. Zaid, S. Othman, and N. M. Kassim, "Potential protective effect of Tualang honey on BPA-induced ovarian toxicity in prepubertal rat," *BMC Complementary and Alternative Medicine*, vol. 14, article 509, 12 pages, 2014.

[53] H. W. G. Baker, J. Brindle, D. S. Irvine, and R. J. Aitken, "Protective effect of antioxidants on the impairment of sperm motility by activated polymorphonuclear leukocytes," *Fertility and Sterility*, vol. 65, no. 2, pp. 411–419, 1996.

[54] V. Kumar, A. Rani, A. K. Dixit, D. Pratap, and D. Bhatnagar, "A comparative assessment of total phenolic content, ferric reducing-anti-oxidative power, free radical-scavenging activity, vitamin C and isoflavones content in soybean with varying seed coat colour," *Food Research International*, vol. 43, no. 1, pp. 323–328, 2010.

[55] A. S. A. Harabawy and Y. Y. I. Mosleh, "The role of vitamins A, C, E and selenium as antioxidants against genotoxicity and cytotoxicity of cadmium, copper, lead and zinc on erythrocytes of Nile tilapia, *Oreochromis niloticus*," *Ecotoxicology and Environmental Safety*, vol. 104, no. 1, pp. 28–35, 2014.

[56] A. S. Y. Hounkpatin, R. C. Johnson, P. Guedenon et al., "Protective effects of vitamin C on haematological parameters in intoxicated wistar rats with cadmium, mercury and combined cadmium and mercury," *International Research Journal of Biological Sciences*, vol. 1, no. 8, pp. 76–81, 2012.

[57] M. Shaban El-Neweshy and Y. Said El-Sayed, "Influence of vitamin C supplementation on lead-induced histopathological alterations in male rats," *Experimental and Toxicologic Pathology*, vol. 63, no. 3, pp. 221–227, 2011.

[58] A. Wattel, S. Kamel, R. Mentaverri et al., "Potent inhibitory effect of naturally occurring flavonoids quercetin and kaempferol on in vitro osteoclastic bone resorption," *Biochemical Pharmacology*, vol. 65, no. 1, pp. 35–42, 2003.

[59] M. Chevallet, E. Wagner, S. Luche, A. Van Dorsselaer, E. Leize-Wagner, and T. Rabilloud, "Regeneration of peroxiredoxins during recovery after oxidative stress: only some overoxidized peroxiredoxins can be reduced during recovery after oxidative stress," *Journal of Biological Chemistry*, vol. 278, no. 39, pp. 37146–37153, 2003.

[60] L. Vigezzi, V. L. Bosquiazzo, L. Kass, J. G. Ramos, M. Muñoz-de-Toro, and E. H. Luque, "Developmental exposure to bisphenol A alters the differentiation and functional response of the adult rat uterus to estrogen treatment," *Reproductive Toxicology*, vol. 52, no. 1, pp. 83–92, 2015.

[61] C. M. Klinge, "Estrogen receptor interaction with estrogen response elements," *Nucleic Acids Research*, vol. 29, no. 14, pp. 2905–2919, 2001.

[62] H. Hiroi, O. Tsutsumi, M. Momoeda, Y. Takai, Y. Osuga, and Y. Taketani, "Differential interactions of bisphenol A and 17beta-estradiol with estrogen receptor alpha (ERalpha) and ERbeta," *Endocrine Journal*, vol. 46, no. 6, pp. 773–778, 1999.

[63] J. F. Couse and K. S. Korach, "Estrogen receptor null mice: what have we learned and where will they lead us?" *Endocrine Reviews*, vol. 20, no. 3, pp. 358–417, 1999.

[64] P. Pace, J. Taylor, S. Suntharalingam, R. C. Coombes, and S. Ali, "Human estrogen receptor β binds DNA in a manner similar to and dimerizes with estrogen receptor α," *Journal of Biological Chemistry*, vol. 272, no. 41, pp. 25832–25838, 1997.

[65] K. Paech, P. Webb, G. G. J. M. Kuiper et al., "Differential ligand activation of estrogen receptors ERα and ERβ at AP1 sites," *Science*, vol. 277, no. 5331, pp. 1508–1510, 1997.

[66] J. J. Voegel, M. J. S. Heine, C. Zechel, P. Chambon, and H. Gronemeyer, "TIF2, a 160 kDa transcriptional mediator for the ligand-dependent activation function AF-2 of nuclear receptors," *The EMBO Journal*, vol. 15, no. 14, pp. 3667–3675, 1996.

[67] E. J. Routledge, R. White, M. G. Parker, and J. P. Sumpter, "Differential effects of xenoestrogens on coactivator recruitment by estrogen receptor (ER) α and ERβ," *Journal of Biological Chemistry*, vol. 275, no. 46, pp. 35986–35993, 2000.

[68] Z. Weihua, S. Saji, S. Mäkinen et al., "Estrogen receptor (ER) beta, a modulator of ERalpha in the uterus," *Proceedings of the National Academy of Sciences of the United States of America*, vol. 97, no. 11, pp. 5936–5941, 2000.

[69] J. M. Hall and D. P. McDonnel, "The estrogen receptor β-isoform (ERβ) of the human estrogen receptor modulates ERα transcriptional activity and is a key regulator of the cellular response to estrogens and antiestrogens," *Endocrinology*, vol. 140, no. 12, pp. 5566–5578, 1999.

[70] K. Pettersson, K. Grandien, G. G. J. M. Kuiper, and J.-Å. Gustafsson, "Mouse estrogen receptor β forms estrogen response element-binding heterodimers with estrogen receptor α," *Molecular Endocrinology*, vol. 11, no. 10, pp. 1486–1496, 1997.

[71] A. Matsushima, Y. Kakuta, T. Teramoto et al., "Structural evidence for endocrine disruptor bisphenol A binding to human nuclear receptor ERRγ," *Journal of Biochemistry*, vol. 142, no. 4, pp. 517–524, 2007.

[72] T. Nose and Y. Shimohigashi, "A docking modelling rationally predicts strong binding of bisphenol A to estrogen-related receptor γ," *Protein and Peptide Letters*, vol. 15, no. 3, pp. 290–296, 2008.

[73] V. Giguère, "To ERR in the estrogen pathway," *Trends in Endocrinology and Metabolism*, vol. 13, no. 5, pp. 220–225, 2002.

[74] S. Takayanagi, T. Tokunaga, X. Liu, H. Okada, A. Matsushima, and Y. Shimohigashi, "Endocrine disruptor bisphenol A strongly binds to human estrogen-related receptor gamma (ERRgamma) with high constitutive activity," *Toxicology Letters*, vol. 167, no. 2, pp. 95–105, 2006.

[75] J. Huppunen and P. Aarnisalo, "Dimerization modulates the activity of the orphan nuclear receptor ERRα," *Biochemical and Biophysical Research Communications*, vol. 314, no. 4, pp. 964–970, 2004.

[76] A. Sahu and J. D. Lambris, "Structure and biology of complement protein C3, a connecting link between innate and acquired immunity," *Immunological Reviews*, vol. 180, no. 1, pp. 35–48, 2001.

[77] S. S. Zaid, S. Othman, and N. M. Kassim, "Potential protective effect of Tualang honey on BPA-induced ovarian toxicity in prepubertal rat," *BMC Complementary and Alternative Medicine*, vol. 14, article 509, 2014.

[78] M. G. L. Hertog, P. C. H. Hollman, M. B. Katan, and D. Kromhout, "Intake of potentially anticarcinogenic flavonoids and their determinants in adults in The Netherlands," *Nutrition and Cancer*, vol. 20, no. 1, pp. 21–29, 1993.

[79] D. Tiwari, J. Kamble, S. Chilgunde et al., "Clastogenic and mutagenic effects of bisphenol A: an endocrine disruptor," *Mutation Research: Genetic Toxicology and Environmental Mutagenesis*, vol. 743, no. 1-2, pp. 83–90, 2012.

[80] T. Iso, T. Watanabe, T. Iwamoto, A. Shimamoto, and Y. Furuichi, "DNA damage caused by bisphenol A and estradiol through estrogenic activity," *Biological and Pharmaceutical Bulletin*, vol. 29, no. 2, pp. 206–210, 2006.

[81] H.-J. Wu, C. Liu, W.-X. Duan et al., "Melatonin ameliorates bisphenol A-induced DNA damage in the germ cells of adult male rats," *Mutation Research*, vol. 752, no. 1-2, pp. 57–67, 2013.

[82] N. S. Yaacob and N. F. Ismail, "Comparison of cytotoxicity and genotoxicity of 4-hydroxytamoxifen in combination with *Tualang* honey in MCF-7 and MCF-10A cells," *BMC Complementary and Alternative Medicine*, vol. 14, article 106, 2014.

[83] I. Ahmad, H. Jimenez, N. S. Yaacob, and N. Yusuf, "Tualang honey protects keratinocytes from ultraviolet radiation-induced inflammation and DNA damage," *Photochemistry and Photobiology*, vol. 88, no. 5, pp. 1198–1204, 2012.

[84] N. S. Yaacob, A. Nengsih, and M. N. Norazmi, "Tualang honey promotes apoptotic cell death induced by tamoxifen in breast cancer cell lines," *Evidence-Based Complementary and Alternative Medicine*, vol. 2013, Article ID 989841, 9 pages, 2013.

[85] J. Zhou, P. Li, N. Cheng et al., "Protective effects of buckwheat honey on DNA damage induced by hydroxyl radicals," *Food and Chemical Toxicology*, vol. 50, no. 8, pp. 2766–2773, 2012.

[86] H. M. Habib, F. T. Al Meqbali, H. Kamal, U. D. Souka, and W. H. Ibrahim, "Bioactive components, antioxidant and DNA damage inhibitory activities of honeys from arid regions," *Food Chemistry*, vol. 153, pp. 28–34, 2014.

Influence of the Alcohol Present in a Phytotherapic Tincture on Male Rat Lipid Profiles and Renal Function

Fernanda Coleraus Silva,[1] Juliete Gomes de Lara de Souza,[1]
Alana Meira Reichert,[1] Renata Prestes Antonangelo,[2] Rodrigo Suzuki,[1]
Ana Maria Itinose,[3] and Carla Brugin Marek[1]

[1]Laboratory of Cellular Toxicology, State University of Western Paraná, Rua Universitária 1619, 85819110 Cascavel, PR, Brazil
[2]Department of Veterinary Medicine, Dynamic Union of the Faculty Falls, 85852010 Foz do Iguaçu, PR, Brazil
[3]Assistance Center in Toxicology (CEATOX), Hospital University of Western Paraná, Avenida Tancredo Neves 3224,
 85806470 Cascavel, PR, Brazil

Correspondence should be addressed to Carla Brugin Marek; carla.marek@unioeste.br

Academic Editor: Yuewen Gong

This study evaluated the influence of the alcohol present in a formulation of the antiophidic phytotherapic tincture, Específico-Pessôa, on rat blood biochemical and hematological parameters, and on organ histology. Three groups of rats were treated orally for 10, 15, or 30 days; one group received the tincture, the other received alcohol alone, and the third was a control group. The results of this study indicated that cholesterol levels were significantly increased after 10 days in the alcohol and tincture groups, although these decreased after 30 days in the tincture group. Triglyceride levels were significantly reduced after 15 days in the tincture group and after 30 days in the alcohol and tincture groups. A higher creatinine level was observed in the alcohol and tincture groups after 15 and 30 days. The uric acid levels in these groups were reduced at 10 and 30 days, although this metabolite was elevated at 15 days in the alcohol group. Hydropic multifocal degeneration with lymphohistiocytic infiltration and some polymorphonuclear cells was observed in the livers of rats treated with either the tincture or alcohol. These data demonstrate the importance of considering the potential actions of the alcohol present in pharmaceutical formulations.

1. Introduction

It is well known that the therapeutic effects of medicines can be influenced by other substances, particularly by alcohol [1]. Although some studies have shown beneficial effects of moderate alcohol consumption on the risk for cardiac disease [2], other studies had shown increased risks for liver cirrhosis, neuromuscular disorders, and cancers [3, 4]. The recreational use of alcohol usually involves the ingestion of alcoholic beverages such as beers, wines, and spirits. However, non-recreational exposure can also occur in certain populations due to the ingestion of herbal medications containing alcohol in the formulation.

The use of alcohol is sometimes necessary to extract bioactive substances from plants [5] and it is common for traditional and folk medicines to have a high alcohol content; this may be >10%. It is possible that alcohol may interfere with the metabolism and mechanisms of action of the bioactive compounds present in herbal medicines. Some studies have investigated the pharmacokinetic and pharmacodynamic mechanisms involved in the interactions between alcohol and various drug classes [5, 6]; however few studies have investigated the influence of alcohol on the actions of compounds present in phytotherapic tinctures. This is an important issue in toxicology.

The phytotherapic tincture, Específico-Pessôa, has been used for more than 30 years as a supportive therapy for snake bites, particularly in the north and northeast of Brazil [7, 8]. This is a hydroalcoholic extract of the root of a plant commonly known as "cabeça-de-negro." Four Brazilian plant species are designated as "cabeça-de-negro": *Cayaponia tayuya* (Kell.) Cogn., *Cayaponia espelina* Cogn., *Annona*

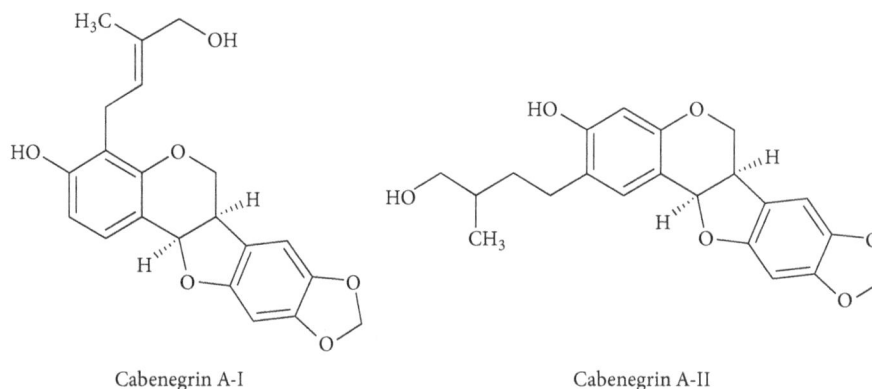

Cabenegrin A-I   Cabenegrin A-II

FIGURE 1: Structure of two pterocarpans isolated and identified in Específico-Pessôa phytotherapic tincture by Nakagawa et al. (1982) [7].

coriacea (Mart.), and *Wilbrandia* sp. [9]. There are reports of Específico-Pessôa tincture use as a supportive therapy and as the only form of treatment in certain regions [8]. There are few studies of the constituents of this tincture and most of these have focused on pterocarpans. The antiophidic effects of Específico-Pessôa have been suggested to arise from the actions of two pterocarpans, cabenegrin A-I and cabenegrin A-II (Figure 1), which were first isolated and identified by Nakagawa et al. (1982) [7]. Our previous research found that Específico-Pessôa altered body weight and the lipid profile in rats; some of these changes may be due to the alcohol present in the formulation [10]. Despite the widespread use of herbal medicines, there is little information in the literature about the possible pharmacodynamic effects of the alcohol present in these extracts. Therefore, the purpose of this study was to investigate the effects of the recommended dose of Específico-Pessôa on biochemical and hematological parameters at different time-points (10, 15, and 30 days) and to determine the contribution of alcohol to these effects. These times were chosen to reflect common tincture treatment periods.

2. Materials and Methods

2.1. Extract and Formulation. The phytotherapic tincture employed in the present work was purchased from a local drugstore (Cascavel, Brazil). This Específico-Pessôa was a hydroalcoholic extract manufactured in Ceará, Brazil (Register number 262, Department of Public Health of Rio de Janeiro). The usual adult dosage is 1.0 mL diluted in 14.0 mL of water, one to three times daily.

2.2. Animals. Adult male Wistar rats weighing 220–280 g were provided by the Central Animal Facility of the University and were fed *ad libitum* with a standard laboratory diet (Nuvilab). They were housed in propylene cages at $22 \pm 2°C$ in a room with a 12 h light/dark cycle. The experimental protocols and procedures used in the present study were approved by the Ethics Committee of the Western Paraná State University (Cascavel, Brazil) for the care and use of laboratory animals (Approval number 17/2014-CE).

2.3. Alcohol Assay. The alcohol content of the phytotherapic Específico-Pessôa tincture was measured using the method described by Widmark (1964) [11]. Essentially, alcohol was oxidized using dichromate and the excess dichromate was determined iodometrically. The result was expressed as $mg\ alcohol \cdot mL^{-1}$ tincture.

2.4. Experimental Procedure. All animals were treated once daily by oral gavage at a dosing volume of $0.25\ mL \cdot kg^{-1}$ body weight for 10, 15, or 30 days. One milliliter of the phytotherapic tincture (containing $165\ mg\ alcohol \cdot mL^{-1}$) was diluted with 14 mL water to produce the concentration recommended by the guide provided with the tincture. The alcohol (ethyl alcohol, 99.9% pure) was supplied by Merck and was diluted in water to match the concentration present in the tincture. The animals were randomly allocated to nine experimental groups with five animals in each:

> [Con10], [Con15], and [Con30] groups received normal water for 10, 15, and 30 days, respectively.
>
> [EP10] received $0.25\ mL \cdot kg^{-1}$ body weight of phytotherapic tincture for 10 days.
>
> [EP15] received $0.25\ mL \cdot kg^{-1}$ body weight of phytotherapic tincture for 15 days.
>
> [EP30] received $0.25\ mL \cdot kg^{-1}$ body weight of phytotherapic tincture for 30 days.
>
> [Alc10] received $2.77\ mg \cdot kg^{-1}$ body weight of alcohol for 10 days.
>
> [Alc15] received $2.77\ mg \cdot kg^{-1}$ body weight of alcohol for 15 days.
>
> [Alc30] received $2.77\ mg \cdot kg^{-1}$ body weight of alcohol for 30 days.

The $2.77\ mg \cdot kg^{-1}$ corresponds to the amount of alcohol that is present in the phytotherapic tincture. Water and food were freely available to the animals. Their general behavior was observed at 5 min, 30 min, 1 h, 2 h, 4 h, and 6 h following gavage. The behavioral observations included changes in respiration (slow or rapid shallow breathing), locomotion, tremor (rhythmic or repetitive limb movements), convulsion, hyperexcitability, reduced activity, ataxia (difficulty in walking and jumping), piloerection, drowsiness (closing the eyelids followed by eye immobility and sometimes bowing of the head), ptosis (eyelids partly closed), drooling, diarrhea, and abdominal constrictions. The body weight of the animals was monitored daily. At the end of the study, all rats were deprived of food for 12 h, anesthetized for blood collection, and subsequently sacrificed by an overdose of ketamine + xylazine anesthesia. Their organs were carefully dissected and removed for weighing, macroscopic examination, and histopathological analysis.

2.5. Collection of Blood and Biochemical Determinations. Blood samples were obtained by intracardiac puncture under ketamine + xylazine. Blood samples for biochemical analyses were centrifuged at 2,500 ×g for 10 min, and the levels of uric acid (UA), albumin, cholesterol, creatinine, glucose, high-density lipoprotein- (HDL-) cholesterol, low-density lipoprotein- (LDL-) cholesterol, lactate dehydrogenase (LDH), triglycerides, and urea were measured using commercial kits from Bioliquid (Brazil). Alanine aminotransferase (ALT), aspartate aminotransferase (AST), and gamma glutamyltransferase (GGT) levels were assayed using diagnostic reagent kits supplied by Ortho-Clinical Diagnostics VITROS 5.1 FS. All assays were performed in accordance with the manufacturers' instructions and protocols.

2.6. Hematological Analysis. All blood samples were analyzed as described by Lewis et al. (2012) [12] to determine the fraction of whole blood composed of red blood cells (hematocrit), the number of white blood cells, and the percentage of each type of white blood cell. The total level of hemoglobin and number of blood platelets were also determined using the Abbott hematology analyzer CELL-DYN Ruby. May-Grunwald-Giemsa staining was conducted using a commercial kit from Bioliquid (Brazil).

2.7. Organ Weights and Histopathological Analyses. The brain, heart, liver, lungs, and kidneys of all of the animals were examined macroscopically. The organs were weighed and preserved in 10% formalin. Tissue slides were prepared and stained with hematoxylin and eosin prior to microscopic examination.

2.8. Statistical Analysis. Data are expressed as the mean ± the standard error of the mean (SEM). The significance of differences between treated groups and the respective controls was evaluated using one-way analysis of variance (ANOVA) followed by Dunnett's test. Statistical significance was accepted at $P < 0.05$. GraphPad Prism 3 software was used for statistical analysis.

3. Results

The administration of alcohol or phytotherapic tincture led to drowsiness in all rats on each treatment day; this effect was reversible and lasted for up to 4 h.

3.1. Treatment for 10 Days. The [Alc10] and [EP10] groups gained less body weight than the [Con10] group, which increased from 233 ± 2.03 g to 270 ± 4.58 g. The [EP10] animals increased from 236 ± 8.03 g to 257 ± 4.16, corresponding to 56.4% of the control group weight gain; this was less than the [Alc10] group (224 ± 0.58 g to 253 ± 5.93 g, 79.8% of control), $P < 0.05$, Figure 2(a). No changes were observed in the macroscopic and histopathological analyses in these groups. Table 1 shows that the organ weight ratios did not differ between the groups. Rats treated with alcohol or phytotherapic tincture showed an elevated cholesterol level; Figure 3(a) shows that this increased by 25% in the [Alc10] group and by 26% in the [EP10] group ($P < 0.05$ for both groups, as compared with [Con10]). The levels of triglyceride, LDL-cholesterol, and HDL-cholesterol remained unchanged in the [Alc10] and [EP10] groups, as compared with the [Con10] group ($P > 0.05$) (Figure 3(c), Table 2). Both [Alc10] and [EP10] groups showed a significantly lower UA level ($P < 0.05$; Figure 4(b)) than the [Con10] group and there was no significant difference between the [Alc10] and [EP10] groups in this respect ($P > 0.05$). The other biochemical and hematological parameters showed no significant differences between the study groups (Tables 2 and 3, resp.).

3.2. Treatment for 15 Days. The body weight gain of rats in the [EP15] group was approximately 37% lower than that observed in the [Con15] group ($P < 0.001$; Figure 2(b)). There was no difference in the body weight gain in the [EP15] (32 ± 3.69 g) and [Alc15] (33 ± 2.59 g) groups. No macroscopic alterations and/or differences in organ weight ratios were observed in the [EP15] or [Alc15] groups, as compared with [Con15] (Table 1). However, microscopic examination of the liver of rats in the [EP15] or [Alc15] groups showed hydropic multifocal degeneration with lymphohistiocytic infiltrate and some polymorphonuclear cells (Figure 5). Blood analysis (Figure 3(c)) showed a significant 36% decrease in the triglyceride level in the [EP15] group, as compared with [Con15] ($P < 0.05$), but no effect on cholesterol, LDL-cholesterol, or HDL-cholesterol levels ($P > 0.05$) (Figure 3(a), Table 2). The lipid profile was not significantly altered in the [Alc15] group. Creatinine was significantly increased in both the [EP15] and [Alc15] groups ($P < 0.01$; Figure 4(a)). There was a significant increase in the UA level of the [Alc15] group ($P < 0.05$; Figure 4(b)). The remaining biochemical parameters were not affected and the hematological parameters remained unchanged (Tables 2 and 3).

3.3. Treatment for 30 Days. The final body weight gain and organ weight ratios did not differ significantly between the [EP30] and [Con30] groups (Figure 2(c), Table 1). The [Alc30] group showed a significantly lower increase in body weight ($P < 0.05$). No macroscopic differences between the organs of each study group were observed. Microscopic examination of the [EP30] and [Alc30] livers showed hydropic multifocal degeneration with lymphohistiocytic infiltrate and some polymorphonuclear cells (Figure 5). The [EP30] group had significantly lower levels of cholesterol and triglyceride; these were decreased by 8% ($P < 0.05$) and

TABLE 1: Effects of the indicated treatments on organ weight ratios in male rats.

Treatment	Group	Brain	Heart	Liver	Lung	Kidney
10 days	Control	0.667 ± 0.016	0.402 ± 0.012	3.41 ± 0.039	0.516 ± 0.020	0.845 ± 0.031
	EP	0.622 ± 0.015	0.371 ± 0.014	3.28 ± 0.163	0.545 ± 0.035	0.730 ± 0.019
	Alcohol	0.652 ± 0.012	0.398 ± 0.023	3.37 ± 0.015	0.523 ± 0.03	0.746 ± 0.018
15 days	Control	0.581 ± 0.035	0.433 ± 0.051	3.11 ± 0.118	0.565 ± 0.026	0.821 ± 0.027
	EP	0.634 ± 0.027	0.392 ± 0.018	3.45 ± 0.119	0.546 ± 0.021	0.908 ± 0.026
	Alcohol	0.672 ± 0.024	0.421 ± 0.021	3.61 ± 0.054	0.579 ± 0.026	0.916 ± 0.036
30 days	Control	0.552 ± 0.006	0.370 ± 0.007	3.03 ± 0.143	0.576 ± 0.017	0.726 ± 0.031
	EP	0.554 ± 0.014	0.372 ± 0.024	2.99 ± 0.074	0.580 ± 0.019	0.772 ± 0.012
	Alcohol	0.736 ± 0.015	0.378 ± 0.012	3.06 ± 0.062	0.579 ± 0.033	0.730 ± 0.015

EP, Específico-Pessôa phytotherapic tincture. Values represent the mean ± SEM of 5 animals.

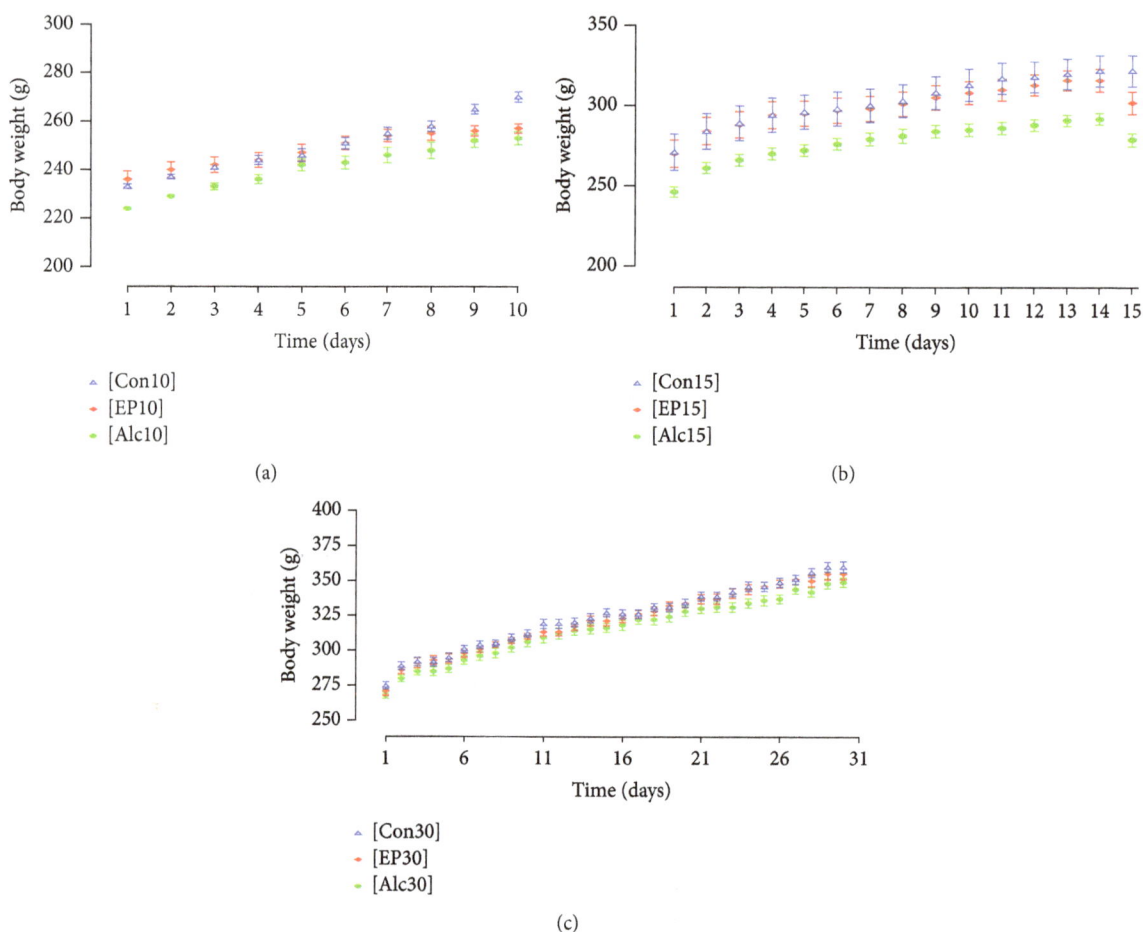

FIGURE 2: Body weights of male rats administered the indicated treatments for (a) 10 days, (b) 15 days, or (c) 30 days. Each point represents the mean ± SEM of 5 rats.

30% ($P < 0.01$), respectively, as compared with [Con30]. The [Alc30] group had a reduced triglyceride level only ($P < 0.01$; Figures 3(a) and 3(c)). The [EP30] and [Alc30] groups showed elevated creatinine ($P < 0.01$) and reduced UA ($P < 0.01$) levels (Figure 4). The other biochemical and hematological parameters remained unchanged (Tables 2 and 3).

4. Discussion

Although there are controversies in this area, alcohol is known to cause both acute and chronic physiological effects. Several factors may contribute to the nature and intensity of these effects, including the alcohol dose, rate of intake, and

(a)

(b)

(c)

(d)

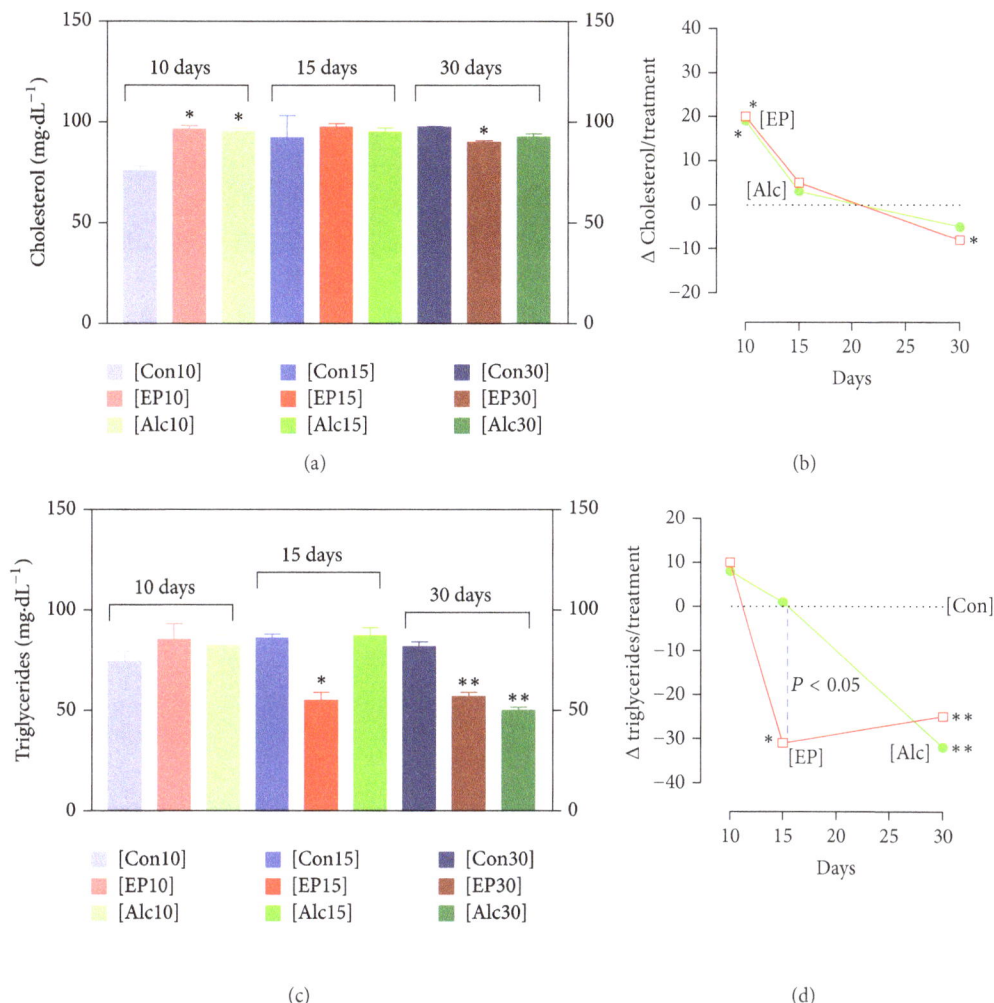

FIGURE 3: Plasma lipid profiles of male rats administered the indicated treatments for the indicated times. (a) Cholesterol levels, (b) the difference between the cholesterol level in the indicated group and that of the control group. (c) Triglyceride levels, (d) the difference between the triglyceride level in the indicated group and that of the control group. Each point represents the mean ± SEM of 5 rats. $^{*}P < 0.05$; $^{**}P < 0.01$, as compared to the respective control group. The P values refer to Dunnett's test. - - - represents a significant difference between the [EP15] and [Alc15] groups ($P < 0.05$).

type of drink [13, 14]. While many studies have investigated different types of alcoholic beverages, the alcohol present in pharmaceutical formulations has been largely ignored. The present study showed that although pterocarpans may have beneficial effects, regular exposure to the alcohol present in this type of phytotherapic tincture may lead to serious biochemical alterations.

Drowsiness was the first effect observed and this was due to alcohol. The depressant effect of alcohol on the central nervous system is well characterized [15, 16]. Some reductions in body weight gain were observed in rats treated with alcohol and to a lesser extent in those treated with phytotherapic tincture. Interestingly, previous studies using this phytotherapic tincture in rats at a dose of 0.75 mL·kg^{-1} for 10 days led to an increase in body weight gain [10]. Alcohol-mediated effects on body weight gain have been observed by other authors and both decreases and increases have been reported, according to the amount of alcohol

exposure [17, 18]. The effects of alcohol on the processes of absorption, digestion, utilization, storage, and excretion of proteins, vitamins, and minerals may partially explain these findings [19]. Furthermore, pterocarpans also affect body weight gain. A study with male C57BL/6J mice showed that pterocarpan-enriched soy leaf extract suppressed body weight gain [20]. A separate study of C57BL/6J mice treated with soy leaf extracts found a decrease in body weight gain and fat accumulation in white adipose tissue *via* several mechanisms related to adipogenesis and fat oxidation in this tissue [21]. In the present study, it is unclear why the [EP30] group showed a weight gain that was similar to that of the [Con30] group. Further studies will be required to investigate the interactions between alcohol and pterocarpans and the effects of these on weight gain.

The lipid profiles were affected differently in rats exposed to [EP] or [Alc] for different lengths of time. These findings were consistent with previous studies indicating that both

(a)

(b)

(c)

(d)

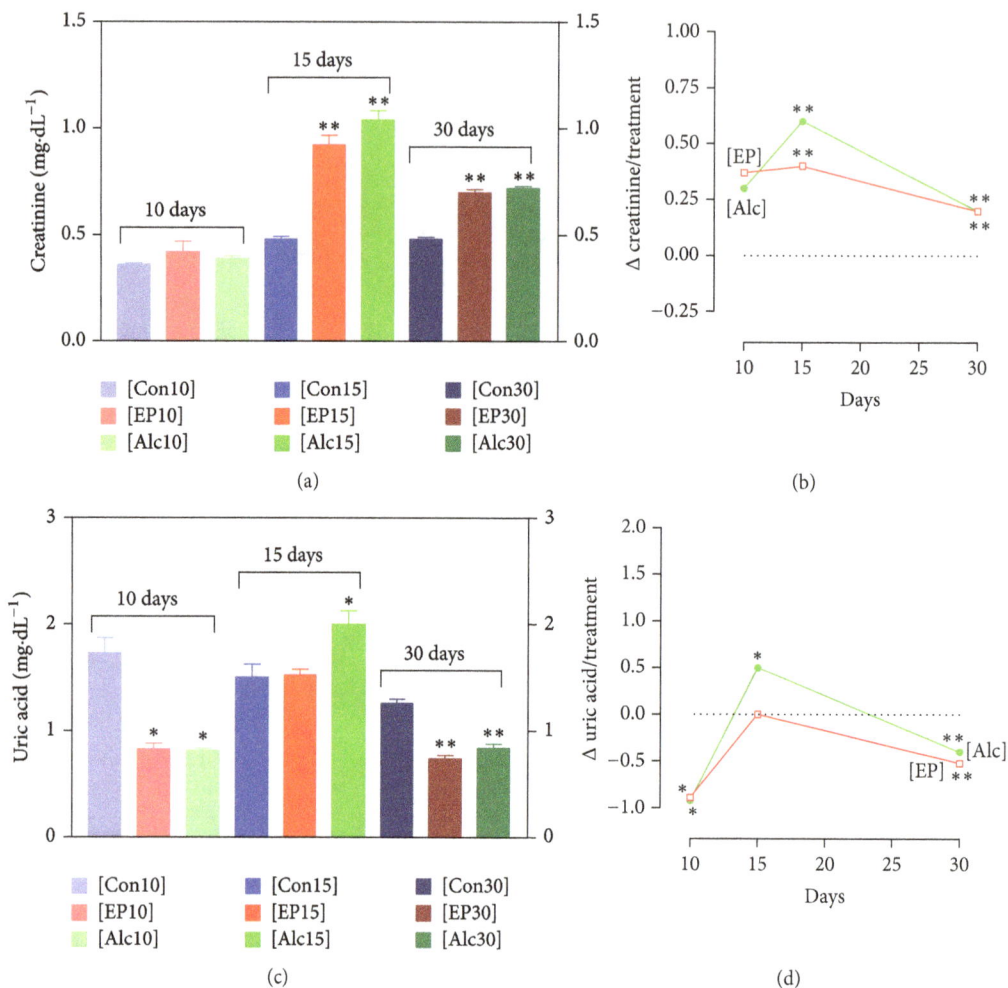

FIGURE 4: Plasma renal function measures in male rats administered the indicated treatments for the indicated times. (a) Plasma creatinine level, (b) the difference between the creatinine level in the indicated group and that of the control group. (c) Plasma uric acid level, (d) the difference between the uric acid level in the indicated group and that of the control group. Each point represents the mean $\pm$ SEM of 5 rats. $^{*}P < 0.05$; $^{**}P < 0.01$, as compared to the respective control group. The P values refer to Dunnett's test.

alcohol [22, 23] and pterocarpans [24] affected hepatic metabolism. The effects on cholesterol levels were similar in the [EP] and [Alc] groups, while these treatments produced different effects on triglyceride levels at 15 days. The increase of cholesterol levels by approximately $20\,mg\cdot dL^{-1}$ in the [EP10] and [Alc10] groups may reflect increased absorption of dietary cholesterol or altered protein metabolism. Some authors have reported a relationship between alcohol and both increased cholesterol levels and protein metabolism; this reflects channeling of peripheral amino acids to hepatic protein synthesis [25] and induction of cholesterol uptake [26] by alcohol. The mechanisms involved in the reduction of cholesterol levels by pterocarpans include acyl-CoA cholesterol acyltransferase (ACAT) inhibition. The hepatic cholesteryl ester level also has a direct effect on the concentration of liver triglycerides, limiting both the mobilization and secretion of triglycerides [27]. Studies of ACAT inhibitors have shown that they influence, perhaps indirectly, triglyceride levels [27, 28]. We observed significant decreases in the triglyceride

levels in the [EP15] and [EP30] groups. This reduction in the triglyceride level may have been indirectly affected by pterocarpans-mediated ACAT inhibition. However, this hypothesis requires further study since we did not measure ACAT activity or the levels of hepatic cholesteryl esters and triglycerides.

Although markers of liver function were not changed, microscopic tissue examination revealed hydropic multifocal degeneration with slight lymphohistiocytic infiltration and some polymorphonuclear cells in [EP15], [EP30], [Alc15], and [Alc30] groups. These findings suggest that although pterocarpans have been reported to have hepatoprotective effects [24, 29], alcohol toxicity may override these. Regular exposure to alcohol is associated with a variety of secondary effects, some of which relate to hepatocyte homeostasis and lipid metabolism. The observed hydropic degeneration suggested that alcohol altered cellular Na^{+} and fluid homeostasis, leading to increased intracellular water [30]. The excess reducing equivalents generated during the biotransformation

TABLE 2: Effect of the indicated treatments on biochemical parameters in male rats.

Parameter	Control	EP	Alcohol
10-day treatment			
Albumin (g·dL^{-1})	2.80 ± 0.01	2.68 ± 0.09	2.70 ± 0.07
ALT (U·L^{-1})	45.6 ± 4.08	47.0 ± 6.01	48.9 ± 5.18
AST (U·L^{-1})	79.8 ± 12.30	81.5 ± 9.25	80.0 ± 13.07
Cholesterol (mg·dL^{-1})	75.8 ± 5.32	96.3 ± 3.18*	95.3 ± 2.56*
Creatinine (mg·dL^{-1})	0.36 ± 0.01	0.42 ± 0.09	0.39 ± 0.03
GGT (U·L^{-1})	<10	<10	<10
Glucose (mg·dL^{-1})	72 ± 13.50	80 ± 12.80	83 ± 11.90
HDL (mg·dL^{-1})	43.8 ± 3.09	54.7 ± 3.84	47.3 ± 3.17
LDL (mg·dL^{-1})	24.6 ± 2.58	30.8 ± 4.50	21.7 ± 0.88
LDH (mg·dL^{-1})	348 ± 52.30	319 ± 48.70	352 ± 31.30
Triglycerides (mg·dL^{-1})	74.5 ± 9.87	85.3 ± 13.60	82.5 ± 10.50
Urea (mg·dL^{-1})	36.3 ± 0.99	32.3 ± 5.17	36.8 ± 1.80
Uric acid (mg·dL^{-1})	1.73 ± 0.32	0.83 ± 0.08*	0.82 ± 0.04*
15-day treatment			
Albumin (g·dL^{-1})	2.80 ± 0.16	2.52 ± 0.07	2.62 ± 0.08
ALT (U·L^{-1})	48.0 ± 7.60	48.8 ± 3.41	51.2 ± 4.27
AST (U·L^{-1})	80.2 ± 14.00	83.7 ± 12.04	81.1 ± 11.20
Cholesterol (mg·dL^{-1})	92.3 ± 18.90	97.4 ± 3.94	95.0 ± 4.48
Creatinine (mg·dL^{-1})	0.48 ± 0.03	0.92 ± 0.10**	1.04 ± 0.10**
GGT (U·L^{-1})	<10	<10	<10
Glucose (mg·dL^{-1})	89 ± 12.40	93 ± 6.67	122 ± 9.40
HDL (mg·dL^{-1})	54.4 ± 6.00	55.5 ± 2.53	55.4 ± 1.66
LDL (mg·dL^{-1})	28.5 ± 1.70	28.8 ± 1.65	22.8 ± 1.31
LDH (mg·dL^{-1})	357 ± 59.60	208 ± 43.20	349 ± 59.70
Triglycerides (mg·dL^{-1})	86.0 ± 3.51	55.0 ± 7.91*	87.3 ± 6.94‡
Urea (mg·dL^{-1})	36.3 ± 1.49	30.4 ± 2.48	32.4 ± 1.12
Uric acid (mg·dL^{-1})	1.50 ± 0.25	1.52 ± 0.12	2.00 ± 0.28*
30-day treatment			
Albumin (g·dL^{-1})	2.82 ± 0.02	2.66 ± 0.10	2.74 ± 0.07
ALT (U·L^{-1})	49.32 ± 10.04	47.1 ± 8.17	51.0 ± 9.13
AST (U·L^{-1})	83.0 ± 7.38	84.1 ± 9.90	85.3 ± 10.02
Cholesterol (mg·dL^{-1})	97.5 ± 0.65	90.0 ± 1.96*	92.5 ± 3.43
Creatinine (mg·dL^{-1})	0.48 ± 0.02	0.70 ± 0.03**	0.72 ± 0.02**
GGT (U·L^{-1})	<10	<10	<10
Glucose (mg·dL^{-1})	74 ± 10.50	88 ± 10.80	90 ± 13.90
HDL (mg·dL^{-1})	56.2 ± 1.11	57.0 ± 3.70	57.0 ± 3.39
LDL (mg·dL^{-1})	26.3 ± 2.33	23.3 ± 2.73	28.8 ± 1.20
LDH (mg·dL^{-1})	322 ± 40.00	331 ± 90.70	371 ± 27.80
Triglycerides (mg·dL^{-1})	81.8 ± 5.02	56.8 ± 4.80**	50.0 ± 3.91**
Urea (mg·dL^{-1})	36.0 ± 1.38	34.6 ± 1.33	38.4 ± 1.29
Uric acid (mg·dL^{-1})	1.26 ± 0.87	0.74 ± 0.07**	0.84 ± 0.09**

ALT, alanine aminotransferase; AST, aspartate aminotransferase; EP, Específico-Pessôa phytotherapic tincture; GGT, gamma glutamyltransferase; HDL, high-density lipoprotein cholesterol; LDL, low-density lipoprotein cholesterol, LDH, lactate dehydrogenase. ALT, AST, and GGT values represent the mean ± SEM of 3 animals. The other parameters represent the mean ± SEM of 5 animals. ‡$P < 0.05$ for the comparison between the EP and alcohol groups. *$P < 0.05$, **$P < 0.01$ for the comparison with the relevant control group. The P values represent Dunnett's test.

of alcohol by alcohol dehydrogenase and aldehyde dehydrogenase in the liver increases the NADH/NAD$^+$ ratio, affecting citrate cycle activity, and consequently reducing fatty acid oxidation. Furthermore, the increased NADH level favors fatty acid synthesis [31]. These effects promote hepatic fat accumulation. Moreover, repeat alcohol administration can also promote inflammation, as indicated by the presence of infiltrate. Interactions between alcohol and the proteins and

TABLE 3: Effect of the indicated treatments on hematological parameters in male rats.

Parameter	Control	EP	Alcohol
10-day treatment			
Hemoglobin (g/dL)	14.7 ± 0.70	15.4 ± 1.20	16.1 ± 0.21
Total red blood cells ($10^6/\mu$L)	8.2 ± 0.41	9.4 ± 0.80	9.1 ± 0.34
Total white blood cells ($10^3/\mu$L)	5.2 ± 0.36	5.4 ± 0.88	5.1 ± 0.70
Neutrophils (%)	25.6 ± 1.65	25.2 ± 2.18	25.3 ± 1.21
Lymphocytes (%)	71.0 ± 1.13	70.2 ± 2.34	72.0 ± 1.78
Eosinophils (%)	0.40 ± 0.28	0.60 ± 0.90	0.40 ± 0.88
Monocytes (%)	3.0 ± 0.43	3.8 ± 1.12	2.30 ± 0.31
Basophils (%)	0.0 ± 0.0	0.20 ± 0.20	0.0 ± 0.0
Packed cell volume (%)	47.2 ± 0.47	49.6 ± 2.10	48.6 ± 0.54
Mean corpuscular volume (fL)	58.0 ± 3.63	54.1 ± 4.90	53.9 ± 1.91
Mean corpuscular Hb (pg)	18.1 ± 1.49	17.0 ± 2.20	18.0 ± 0.57
Mean corpuscular Hb (%)	31.1 ± 1.52	31.4 ± 2.80	33.4 ± 0.12
15-day treatment			
Hemoglobin (g/dL)	16.1 ± 0.23	16.0 ± 0.20	16.5 ± 0.13
Total red blood cells ($10^6/\mu$L)	8.9 ± 0.04	7.6 ± 0.24	8.1 ± 0.98
Total white blood cells ($10^3/\mu$L)	4.8 ± 0.03	4.2 ± 0.41	5.5 ± 1.09
Neutrophils (%)	22.5 ± 3.51	23.2 ± 2.53	16.4 ± 6.48
Lymphocytes (%)	74.5 ± 3.51	72.8 ± 6.52	78.3 ± 2.31
Eosinophils (%)	0.0 ± 0.0	0.0 ± 0.0	0.0 ± 0.0
Monocytes (%)	3.0 ± 1.00	4.0 ± 0.72	5.30 ± 2.41
Basophils (%)	0.0 ± 0.0	0.0 ± 0.0	0.0 ± 0.0
Packed cell volume (%)	47.2 ± 0.62	46.4 ± 0.21	47.2 ± 1.00
Mean corpuscular volume (fL)	54.2 ± 0.04	59.9 ± 5.40	63.0 ± 1.31
Mean corpuscular Hb (pg)	18.6 ± 0.33	20.7 ± 1.87	21.6 ± 0.62
Mean corpuscular Hb (%)	34.3 ± 0.50	34.6 ± 0.23	34.3 ± 0.40
30-day treatment			
Hemoglobin (g/dL)	15.8 ± 0.11	16.1 ± 0.32	16.4 ± 0.09
Total red blood cells ($10^6/\mu$L)	7.4 ± 0.58	7.4 ± 0.31	7.5 ± 1.34
Total white blood cells ($10^3/\mu$L)	6.8 ± 0.38	5.7 ± 0.59	7.0 ± 0.71
Neutrophils (%)	33.2 ± 4.91	27.6 ± 3.52	22.6 ± 2.55
Lymphocytes (%)	64.0 ± 4.53	69.2 ± 4.56	75.8 ± 2.70
Eosinophils (%)	0.60 ± 0.60	0.20 ± 0.20	0.0 ± 0.0
Monocytes (%)	1.8 ± 1.03	2.8 ± 1.21	1.6 ± 0.48
Basophils (%)	0.4 ± 0.20	0.20 ± 0.20	0.0 ± 0.0
Packed cell volume (%)	45.4 ± 0.17	46.6 ± 0.68	48.0 ± 1.03
Mean corpuscular volume (fL)	64.0 ± 6.63	63.5 ± 2.45	63.8 ± 1.71
Mean corpuscular Hb (pg)	22.3 ± 2.34	21.9 ± 0.90	21.9 ± 0.27
Mean corpuscular Hb (%)	34.8 ± 0.32	34.5 ± 0.21	34.4 ± 0.62

EP, Específico-Pessôa phytotherapic tincture; Hb, hemoglobin. Values represent the mean ± SEM of 5 animals.

enzymes of the hepatic interstitial tissue affect the antioxidant defense mechanism and increase generation of reactive oxygen species, which may produce an inflammatory response [32]. The accumulation of fat and cholesterol deposits [33] also reduces liver function. Some authors consider that this deterioration is progressive, starting with some lipid profile changes, followed by a potentially compensatory phase, and finally resulting in liver failure. Moreover, this progressive liver deterioration may be responsible for the disappearance of hyperlipidemia found in some cases of chronic alcohol intake [34, 35]. This could explain our blood and hepatic tissue findings in animals treated for 30 days.

In addition to its effects on the liver, alcohol alters the structure, function, regulation, and metabolism of the kidneys [36, 37]. Chronic exposure to alcohol affects renal filtration [38] and increases blood urea nitrogen and creatinine levels; some authors have recently argued that it exerts an indirect nephrotoxic effect by activating leukocytes [39]. Although this was not observed microscopically in the present study, creatinine levels were elevated in the [EP15]

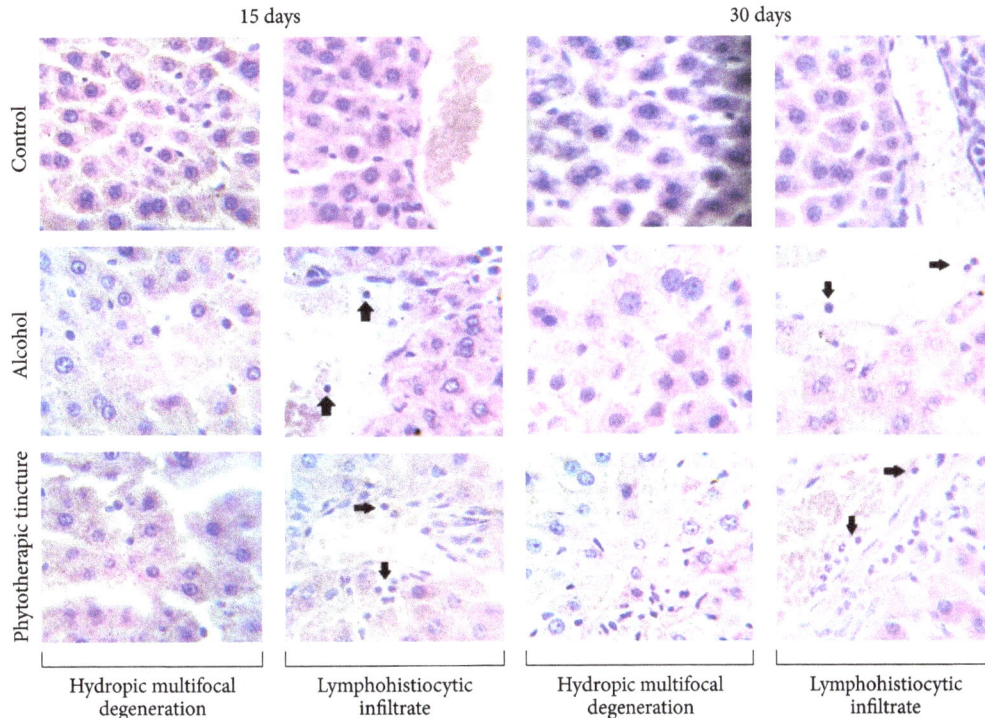

FIGURE 5: Histopathological analysis of liver tissue from rats in the indicated treatment groups. No pathological changes were observed in control rats.

and [EP30] groups, suggesting possible early kidney damage, although there was no change in circulating urea levels. This renal damage may be due to the alcohol present in the phytotherapic tincture, since the [Alc] groups showed the same pattern. Another important finding that requires further study is the reduced UA levels observed in the [Alc] and [EP] groups treated for 10 and 30 days. Alcohol has previously been shown to induce hyperuricemia [40]; this effect was noted in the [Alc15] group, but not in the [EP15] group, indicating that pterocarpans attenuated the hyperuricemic effect of alcohol in rats at this time-point by an unknown mechanism. The UA level is controlled by the rate of endogenous and exogenous purine breakdown into UA and the rate of UA excretion [41]; any factor that alters liver or kidney function may influence blood UA levels [42]. Further studies could explore the mechanisms underlying the observed changes in UA levels.

5. Conclusion

The data presented here demonstrate that the alcohol present in a phytotherapic tincture can alter the lipid profile and renal function in rats and cause liver damage. These data have important repercussions because toxicity studies generally focus on the safety of the active ingredients; this study demonstrates the importance of considering the potential actions of the alcohol present in pharmaceutical formulations. It is noteworthy that even at the relatively low dose of 2.77 mg alcohol·kg^{-1} body weight continuous exposure to this amount of alcohol could cause significant changes

in some biochemical parameters. This is important because phytotherapic tinctures are usually considered nontoxic and are used without medical supervision.

Conflict of Interests

The authors have declared no conflict of interests.

Acknowledgments

The authors thank the Araucária Foundation for financial support. They would like to thank Editage (http://www.editage.com.br/) for English language editing.

References

[1] W. L. Adams, "Interactions between alcohol and other drugs," International Journal of the Addictions, vol. 30, no. 13-14, pp. 1903–1923, 1995.

[2] M. Krenz and R. J. Korthuis, "Moderate ethanol ingestion and cardiovascular protection: from epidemiologic associations to cellular mechanisms," Journal of Molecular and Cellular Cardiology, vol. 52, no. 1, pp. 93–104, 2012.

[3] G. Pöschl and H. K. Seitz, "Alcohol and cancer," Alcohol & Alcoholism, vol. 39, no. 3, pp. 155–165, 2004.

[4] M. J. Barnes, T. Mündel, and S. R. Stannard, "The effects of acute alcohol consumption and eccentric muscle damage on neuromuscular function," Applied Physiology, Nutrition and Metabolism, vol. 37, no. 1, pp. 63–71, 2012.

[5] R. Weathermon and D. W. Crabb, "Alcohol and medication interactions," *Alcohol Research and Health*, vol. 23, no. 1, pp. 40–54, 1999.

[6] S. E. Ferreira, M. T. de Mello, M. Vinicius Rossi, and M. L. O. Souza-Formigoni, "Does an energy drink modify the effects of alcohol in a maximal effort test?" *Alcoholism: Clinical and Experimental Research*, vol. 28, no. 9, pp. 1408–1412, 2004.

[7] M. Nakagawa, K. Nakanishi, L. L. Darko, and J. A. Vick, "Structures of cabenegrins A-I and A-II, potent anti-snake venoms," *Tetrahedron Letters*, vol. 23, no. 38, pp. 3855–3858, 1982.

[8] S. V. Pierini, D. A. Warrell, A. de Paulo, and R. D. G. Theakston, "High incidence of bites and stings by snakes and other animals among rubber tappers and Amazonian Indians of the Jurua valley, Acre State, Brazil," *Toxicon*, vol. 34, no. 2, pp. 225–236, 1996.

[9] G. C. G. Militão, S. M. Pinheiro, I. N. F. Dantas et al., "Bioassay-guided fractionation of pterocarpans from roots of *Harpalyce brasiliana* Benth," *Bioorganic & Medicinal Chemistry*, vol. 15, no. 21, pp. 6687–6691, 2007.

[10] A. M. Reichert, C. B. Marek, A. M. Itinose et al., "Biochemical alterations induced by phytotherapic tincture with antiophidic activity in male Wistar rats," *African Journal of Pharmacy and Pharmacology*, vol. 8, no. 28, pp. 737–746, 2014.

[11] E. M. P. Widmark, "Blood alcohol," in *Chemical Methods of Medical Investigation*, A. G. Merck, Ed., p. 7275, E. Merck KG, Darmstadt, Germany, 10th edition, 1964.

[12] S. M. Lewis, B. J. Bain, B. L. Bates, and M. A. Laffan, *Dacie and Lewis Practical Haematology*, Churchill Livingstone, London, UK, 11th edition, 2012.

[13] G. Corrao, V. Bagnardi, A. Zambon, and S. Arico, "Exploring the dose-response relationship between alcohol consumption and the risk of several alcohol-related conditions: a meta-analysis," *Addiction*, vol. 94, no. 10, pp. 1551–1573, 1999.

[14] M. J. Dry, N. R. Burns, T. Nettelbeck, A. L. Farquharson, and J. M. White, "Dose-related effects of alcohol on cognitive functioning," *PLoS ONE*, vol. 7, no. 11, Article ID e50977, 2012.

[15] S. Darbra, G. Prat, M. Pallares, and N. Ferre, "Tolerance and sensitization to the hypnotic effects of alcohol induced by chronic voluntary alcohol intake in rats," *Journal of Psychopharmacology*, vol. 16, no. 1, pp. 79–83, 2002.

[16] I. Imam, "Alcohol and the central nervous system," *British Journal of Hospital Medicine*, vol. 71, no. 11, pp. 635–639, 2010.

[17] C. Larue-Achagiotis, A. M. Poussard, and J. Louis-Sylvestre, "Alcohol drinking, food and fluid intakes and body weight gain in rats," *Physiology & Behavior*, vol. 47, no. 3, pp. 545–548, 1990.

[18] K. Lauing, R. Himes, M. Rachwalski, P. Strotman, and J. J. Callaci, "Binge alcohol treatment of adolescent rats followed by alcohol abstinence is associated with site-specific differences in bone loss and incomplete recovery of bone mass and strength," *Alcohol*, vol. 42, no. 8, pp. 649–656, 2008.

[19] I. O. MacDonald, O. J. Olusola, and U. A. Osaigbovo, "Effects of chronic ethanol administration on body weight, reduced glutathione (GSH), malondialdehyde (MDA) levels and glutathione-s-transferase activity (GST) in rats," *New York Science Journal*, vol. 3, no. 4, p. 3947, 2010.

[20] U.-H. Kim, J.-H. Yoon, H. Li et al., "Pterocarpan-enriched soy leaf extract ameliorates insulin sensitivity and pancreatic β-cell proliferation in type 2 diabetic mice," *Molecules*, vol. 19, no. 11, pp. 18493–18510, 2014.

[21] H. Li, J.-H. Kang, J.-M. Han et al., "Anti-obesity effects of soy leaf via regulation of adipogenic transcription factors and fat oxidation in diet-induced obese mice and 3T3-L1 adipocytes," *Journal of Medicinal Food*, vol. 18, no. 8, pp. 899–908, 2015.

[22] S. K. Das, L. Dhanya, S. Varadhan, S. Mukherjee, and D. M. Vasudevan, "Effects of chronic ethanol consumption in blood: a time dependent study on rat," *Indian Journal of Clinical Biochemistry*, vol. 24, no. 3, pp. 301–306, 2009.

[23] M. C. F. Toffolo, A. S. de Aguiar-Nemer, and V. A. da Silva-Fonseca, "Alcohol: effects on nutritional status, lipid profile and blood pressure," *Journal of Endocrinology and Metabolism*, vol. 2, no. 6, pp. 205–211, 2012.

[24] H. Matsuda, T. Morikawa, F. Xu, K. Ninomiya, and M. Yoshikawa, "New isoflavones and pterocarpane with hepato-protective activity from the stems of *Erycibe expansa*," *Planta Medica*, vol. 70, no. 12, pp. 1201–1209, 2004.

[25] A. C. K. Goldberg, F. G. Eliaschewitz, and E. C. R. Quintao, "Origin of hypercholesterolemia in chronic experimental nephrotic syndrome," *Kidney International*, vol. 12, no. 1, pp. 23–27, 1977.

[26] M. A. Latour, B. W. Patterson, R. T. Kitchens, R. E. Ostlund Jr., D. Hopkins, and G. Schonfeld, "Effects of alcohol and cholesterol feeding on lipoprotein metabolism and cholesterol absorption in rabbits," *Arteriosclerosis, Thrombosis, and Vascular Biology*, vol. 19, no. 3, pp. 598–604, 1999.

[27] H. M. Alger, J. Mark Brown, J. K. Sawyer et al., "Inhibition of acyl-coenzyme A: cholesterol acyltransferase 2 (ACAT2) prevents dietary cholesterol-associated steatosis by enhancing hepatic triglyceride mobilization," *The Journal of Biological Chemistry*, vol. 285, no. 19, pp. 14267–14274, 2010.

[28] S. M. Post, J. Paul Zoeteweij, M. H. A. Bos et al., "Acyl-coenzyme A:cholesterol acyltransferase inhibitor, avasimibe, stimulates bile acid synthesis and cholesterol 7α-hydroxylase in cultured rat hepatocytes and *in vivo* in the rat," *Hepatology*, vol. 30, no. 2, pp. 491–500, 1999.

[29] M. S. Abdel-Kader, "Preliminary pharmacological study of the pterocarpans macckian and trifolirhizin isolated from the roots of *Ononis vaginalis*," *Pakistan Journal of Pharmaceutical Sciences*, vol. 23, no. 2, pp. 182–187, 2010.

[30] U. del Monte, "Swelling of hepatocytes injured by oxidative stress suggests pathological changes related to macromolecular crowding," *Medical Hypotheses*, vol. 64, no. 4, pp. 818–825, 2005.

[31] C. Henrique Lopez, J. Constantin, D. Gimenes, F. Suzuki-Kemmelmeier, and A. Bracht, "Heterogenic response of the liver parenchyma to ethanol studied in the bivascularly perfused rat liver," *Molecular and Cellular Biochemistry*, vol. 258, no. 1-2, pp. 155–162, 2004.

[32] M. A. K. Abdelhalim and B. M. Jarrar, "Histological alterations in the liver of rats induced by different gold nanoparticle sizes, doses and exposure duration," *Journal of Nanobiotechnology*, vol. 10, article 5, 2012.

[33] B. Thoolen, R. R. Maronpot, T. Harada et al., "Proliferative and nonproliferative lesions of the rat and mouse hepatobiliary system," *Toxicologic Pathology*, vol. 38, no. 7, pp. 5S–81S, 2010.

[34] E. Baraona and C. S. Lieber, "Effects of ethanol on lipid metabolism," *Journal of Lipid Research*, vol. 20, no. 3, pp. 289–315, 1979.

[35] M. Sozio and D. W. Crabb, "Alcohol and lipid metabolism," *American Journal of Physiology—Endocrinology and Metabolism*, vol. 295, no. 1, pp. E10–E16, 2008.

[36] L. Tussey and M. R. Felder, "Tissue-specific genetic variation in the level of mouse alcohol dehydrogenase is controlled

transcriptionally in kidney and posttranscriptionally in liver," *Proceedings of the National Academy of Sciences of the United States of America*, vol. 86, no. 15, pp. 5903–5907, 1989.

[37] M. Epstein, "Alcohol's impact on kidney function," *Alcohol Health & Research World*, vol. 21, no. 1, pp. 84–91, 1997.

[38] S. L. White, K. R. Polkinghorne, A. Cass, J. E. Shaw, R. C. Atkins, and S. J. Chadban, "Alcohol consumption and 5-year onset of chronic kidney disease: the AusDiab study," *Nephrology Dialysis Transplantation*, vol. 24, no. 8, pp. 2464–2472, 2009.

[39] C. Latchoumycandane, L. E. Nagy, and T. M. McIntyre, "Chronic ethanol ingestion induces oxidative kidney injury through taurine-inhibitable inflammation," *Free Radical Biology and Medicine*, vol. 69, pp. 403–416, 2014.

[40] D.-H. Kang, T. Nakagawa, L. Feng et al., "A role for uric acid in the progression of renal disease," *Journal of the American Society of Nephrology*, vol. 13, no. 12, pp. 2888–2897, 2002.

[41] H. K. Choi and G. Curhan, "Beer, liquor, and wine consumption and serum uric acid level: the Third National Health and Nutrition Examination survey," *Arthritis Care & Research*, vol. 51, no. 6, pp. 1023–1029, 2004.

[42] G. Bugdayci, Y. Balaban, and O. Sahin, "Causes of hypouricemia among outpatients," *Laboratory Medicine*, vol. 39, no. 9, pp. 550–552, 2008.

Hypocholesterolemic and Antiatherosclerotic Potential of *Basella alba* Leaf Extract in Hypercholesterolemia-Induced Rabbits

Gunasekaran Baskaran,[1] Shamala Salvamani,[1] Azrina Azlan,[2]
Siti Aqlima Ahmad,[1] Swee Keong Yeap,[3] and Mohd Yunus Shukor[1]

[1]Department of Biochemistry, Faculty of Biotechnology and Biomolecular Sciences, Universiti Putra Malaysia (UPM),
43400 Serdang, Selangor, Malaysia
[2]Department of Nutrition and Dietetics, Faculty of Medicine and Health Sciences, Universiti Putra Malaysia (UPM),
43400 Serdang, Selangor, Malaysia
[3]Institute of Bioscience, Universiti Putra Malaysia (UPM), 43400 Serdang, Selangor, Malaysia

Correspondence should be addressed to Mohd Yunus Shukor; mohdyunus@upm.edu.my

Academic Editor: Dolores García Giménez

Hypercholesterolemia is the major risk factor that leads to atherosclerosis. Nowadays, alternative treatment using medicinal plants gained much attention since the usage of statins leads to adverse health effects, especially liver and muscle toxicity. This study was designed to investigate the hypocholesterolemic and antiatherosclerotic effects of *Basella alba* (*B. alba*) using hypercholesterolemia-induced rabbits. Twenty New Zealand white rabbits were divided into 5 groups and fed with varying diets: normal diet, 2% high cholesterol diet (HCD), 2% HCD + 10 mg/kg simvastatin, 2% HCD + 100 mg/kg *B. alba* extract, and 2% HCD + 200 mg/kg *B. alba* extract, respectively. The treatment with *B. alba* extract significantly lowered the levels of total cholesterol, LDL, and triglycerides and increased HDL and antioxidant enzymes (SOD and GPx) levels. The elevated levels of liver enzymes (AST and ALT) and creatine kinase were noted in hypercholesterolemic and statin treated groups indicating liver and muscle injuries. Treatment with *B. alba* extract also significantly suppressed the aortic plaque formation and reduced the intima: media ratio as observed in simvastatin-treated group. This is the first *in vivo* study on *B. alba* that suggests its potential as an alternative therapeutic agent for hypercholesterolemia and atherosclerosis.

1. Introduction

Hypercholesterolemia is closely associated with atherosclerosis, which is the principal cause of mortality in world population. Hypercholesterolemia is characterized by increased serum concentrations of low-density lipoprotein (LDL) and triglycerides (TG) [1]. Accumulation of oxidized LDL leads to atherosclerotic plaque formation which contributes to stroke, myocardial infarction, and cardiovascular diseases (CVDs) [2]. It is well known that the hypocholesterolemic drugs are effective in lowering LDL but the long term consumption causes adverse effects such as liver and muscle injuries, rhabdomyolysis, myopathy, and acute renal failure. Thus, the investigation and usage of natural products from plant origin

in treating various diseases including CVDs have gained much attention [3, 4].

The potential of medicinal plants that exhibit hypocholesterolemic and antiatherosclerotic effects is still largely unexplored and could be an effective and safe alternative strategy for the treatment of hypercholesterolemia. In previous study, we have screened the HMG CoA reductase inhibitory activity of 25 medicinal plants extracts. *Basella alba* (*B. alba*) extract showed the highest enzyme inhibition, about 74% [5].

B. alba is known as Indian spinach and Remayung locally and belongs to the family of Basellaceae. *B. alba* is a wildly cultivated vegetable that has been used from ancient time due to its various pharmacological activities such as antifungal, antiulcer, anticonvulsant, antihypertensive, and many more activities [6]. In Asian countries, the stem and leaf of *B. alba* have been employed as traditional medicine to treat dysentery, skin diseases, hemorrhages, anemia, constipation, gonorrhea, and cancer [7–9].

There are no *in vivo* reports on the effects of *B. alba* on hypercholesterolemia up to date. Therefore, the present study was aimed at investigating the hypocholesterolemic and antiatherosclerotic properties of *B. alba* in hypercholesterolemic rabbits and also at determining the antioxidant capacity of this extract.

2. Materials and Methods

2.1. Preparation of B. alba Methanol Extract. *B. alba* leaf was purchased from a local market in Seri Kembangan, Selangor, Malaysia. A voucher specimen was deposited in the Institute of Bioscience, Universiti Putra Malaysia (voucher number SK 2087/12). *B. alba* leaf was washed thoroughly and air-dried at room temperature for overnight. The leaf was grounded using a blender (MX 8967, Panasonic) and subjected to methanol 50% (v/v) distillation for 48 hours. After filtration, the leaf extract was isolated using a separatory funnel. The crude methanolic extract of *B. alba* was concentrated using rotary evaporator (Heidolph) under reduced pressure at $40°C$ and freeze-dried at $-40°C$ for further analysis.

2.2. Animals and Experimental Design. Twenty male New Zealand white rabbits weighing 1.5–1.8 kg were purchased from local supplier. The animal studies were performed according to guidelines approved by the Institutional Animal Care and Use Committee (IACUC) of Universiti Putra Malaysia (UPM/IACUC/AUP-R011/2013). The rabbits were placed individually in stainless steel cages and were fed standard rabbit pellets for 1 week for acclimatization. Throughout the study, all the rabbits were kept in a 12 h light-dark cycle room with almost constant temperature at $23–25°C$.

The *in vivo* study was carried out for 12 weeks. The rabbits were randomly divided into 5 groups ($n = 4$): Group 1: control rabbits fed with standard diet for 12 weeks; Group 2: rabbits fed with 2% high cholesterol diet (HCD) for 12 weeks; Group 3: rabbits fed with 2% HCD for 8 weeks and treatment with simvastatin (10 mg/kg) for 4 weeks; Group 4: rabbits fed with 2% HCD for 8 weeks and treatment with *B. alba* extract (100 mg/kg) for 4 weeks; and Group 5: rabbits fed with 2% HCD for 8 weeks and treatment with *B. alba* extract (200 mg/kg) for 4 weeks.

The high cholesterol diet was prepared by dissolving 2% cholesterol (USP grade, anhydrous; Sigma Chemical Co., Missouri, USA) in 99% chloroform and sprayed on standard pellets. Butylated hydroxyanisole (0.02% of diet) was dissolved in chloroform to reduce oxidation of cholesterol. The chloroform was evaporated by exposing the diets in well-ventilated fume hoods at room temperature for overnight. The diets were vacuum-packed and stored in $-20°C$ freezer. All the rabbits received about 150 g pellets per day, with or without cholesterol supplementation, and water was provided *ad libitum*. Food and water consumption were recorded daily, while the body weight was measured every 2 weeks.

Blood samples were collected at 0, 4, 8, and 12th week via ear marginal vein using 23-gauge butterfly needle and 3 mL syringes into EDTA and heparinised tubes. At the end of the study, the rabbits were euthanized with overdose of sodium pentobarbital through intravenous injection.

2.3. Measurement of Serum Lipids. Serum total cholesterol (TC), LDL, HDL, and triglycerides (TG) levels were determined using Roche kit (Penzberg, Germany) and measured spectrophotometrically using Hitachi chemistry analyzer (Tokyo, Japan).

2.4. Liver and Muscle Test. The serum levels of ALT, AST, and creatine kinase (CK) were evaluated by enzymatic kit (Randox Laboratories, Crumlin, UK) using Hitachi chemistry analyzer (Tokyo, Japan).

2.5. Antioxidant Activities. Superoxide Dismutase (SOD) activity was measured by RANSOD kit (Randox Laboratories, Crumlin, UK) using Vitalab Selectra Analyzer (Merck, Darmstadt, Germany). The collected erythrocytes were washed four times with NaCl solution (0.9%, 3 mL) by centrifugation at 1000 ×g for 10 min. Cold distilled water was added up to 2 mL to the packed erythrocytes, vortexed for 10 s, and incubated at $4°C$ for 15 min. The lysate was then diluted with phosphate buffer (pH 7, 0.01 mol/L) and mixed thoroughly. The absorbance of the mixture was determined at 505 nm. The Glutathione Peroxidase (GPx) activity was measured by diluting 0.05 mL serum with 2 mL of RANSEL kit diluting agent (Randox Laboratories, Crumlin, UK) and the mixture was read at 340 nm using Vitalab Selectra Analyzer (Merck, Darmstadt, Germany).

2.6. Histological Analysis. The aortic arch of the rabbits was removed, cleaned, dried, and fixed in 10% neutral buffer formalin. The tissues were embedded in paraffin, cut in $5 \mu m$ sections, and stained with hematoxylin and eosin. The atherosclerotic lesion was analyzed for the thickness of intima, media, and intima: media ratio of 4 rabbits per group under a light microscope equipped with image analyzer system (Olympus, Germany).

2.7. Statistical Analysis. The data obtained are expressed as mean ± SD. All groups were analyzed using SPSS program version 19.0. One-way analysis of variance (ANOVA) followed by Dunnett's post hoc test for multiple comparisons among the groups was performed. The difference between groups was considered to be statistically significant when $p < 0.05$.

3. Results

3.1. Effect of B. alba Extract on Body Weight. In Table 1, rabbits fed with 2% cholesterol diet for 12 weeks showed significant increase ($p < 0.05$) in body weight compared to the normal control. Treatment with simvastatin and *B. alba* (100 and 200 mg/kg) for 4 weeks managed to reduce the body weight compared to the untreated hypercholesterolemic rabbits.

TABLE 1: Changes on body weight of rabbits between different groups.

Group	Body weight (kg)		
	Initial	Final	Change
G1	1.61 ± 0.16	2.22 ± 0.09	0.61 ± 0.13
G2	1.65 ± 0.17	2.55 ± 0.13	0.90 ± 0.06*
G3	1.63 ± 0.10	2.31 ± 0.14	0.68 ± 0.08
G4	1.75 ± 0.15	2.48 ± 0.13	0.73 ± 0.10
G5	1.84 ± 0.06	2.54 ± 0.16	0.70 ± 0.19

G1: normal control, G2: hypercholesterolemic control, G3: simvastatin-treated (10 mg/kg), G4: *B. alba* extract-treated (100 mg/kg), and G5: *B. alba* extract-treated (200 mg/kg). All data are presented as the mean ± SD ($n = 4$ for each group). *Significantly different from others ($p < 0.05$).

3.2. Effect of B. alba Extract on Serum Lipid Profile. As shown in Table 2, serum levels of TC, LDL, and TG were significantly higher ($p < 0.05$) in rabbits fed with HCD compared to the normal diet group after 8 weeks. There were significant decreases ($p < 0.05$) in the level of TC, LDL, and TG at week 12, after 4 weeks of treatment with simvastatin and *B. alba* extract. Administration with 10 mg/kg of simvastatin, used as a positive control, significantly decreased 58.9, 51.1, and 40.9% in TC, LDL, and TG levels, respectively. Administration of *B. alba* at 100 and 200 mg/kg decreased TC level by 49 and 54.2%, respectively, LDL level by 45 and 50.1%, respectively, and TG level by 34.9 and 39.7%, respectively. The TC, LDL, and TG lowering effects of *B. alba* (200 mg/kg) were not significantly different with simvastatin. *B. alba* at dose of 200 mg/kg has significantly higher hypocholesterolemic effect than that of 100 mg/kg. Meanwhile, the HDL level of hypercholesterolemic control rabbits was significantly lower ($p < 0.05$) compared to the normal control and treatment groups at week 12. Treatment with simvastatin and *B. alba* (100 and 200 mg/kg) showed significant increase ($p < 0.05$) in HDL levels, 31.7, 39.6, and 53.4%, respectively. *B. alba* (200 mg/kg) increases the HDL level more effectively than simvastatin.

3.3. Evaluation of Liver and Muscle Injuries. The hypercholesterolemia-induced rabbits showed significant increase ($p < 0.05$) in ALT, AST, and CK levels as presented in Table 3. The results revealed that the treatment with *B. alba* extract (100 and 200 mg/kg) significantly decreased ($p < 0.05$) ALT (40.5 and 44.9%, resp.), AST (37.3 and 43.7%, resp.), and CK (24.2 and 22.8%, resp.) levels while the treatment with simvastatin (10 mg/kg) showed significant elevation ($p < 0.05$) in the levels of ALT (61.4%), AST (64.1%), and CK (34%).

3.4. Evaluation of Serum Antioxidant Levels. As shown in Table 4, the hypercholesterolemic control showed significant reduction ($p < 0.05$) in the levels of SOD and GPx throughout the study. *B. alba*-treated rabbits (100 and 200 mg/kg) caused significant increase ($p < 0.05$) in SOD by 5 and 5.4%, respectively, and GPx by 15 and 21%, respectively. Meanwhile, simvastatin-treated groups showed significant reduction ($p < 0.05$) in SOD and GPx, 4 and 19%, respectively.

3.5. Effect of B. alba Extract on Atherosclerotic Lesion. The atherosclerotic changes in aortic intimal surface of 5 groups are shown in Figure 1. Normal control group (G1) showed healthy aorta with uniform thickness and intact endothelial lining. On the other hand, hypercholesterolemic control group (G2) caused alteration in the aortic wall with the appearance of a large atheromatous plaque and demonstrated a remarkable intimal thickening of aorta. In contrast, treatment with simvastatin (G3) and *B. alba* (G4 and G5) revealed significant decrease in the thickening of intima and no plaques were detected in the aortic walls. Table 5 summarizes the thickness of intima, media, and intima/media ratio of the 5 groups at week 12. The hypercholesterolemic control group showed significant difference ($p < 0.05$) with the highest value of intima and media thickness and intima/media ratio compared to other groups. On the other hand, significant reductions ($p < 0.05$) were noted in the thickness of intima and media as well as intima/media ratio of simvastatin and *B. alba* (100 and 200 mg/kg) treated groups compared to the hypercholesterolemic control group. There was no significant difference ($p < 0.05$) in the intima/media ratio between simvastatin and *B. alba* (200 mg/kg) treated groups.

4. Discussion

This is the first report that demonstrates the oral administration of *B. alba* extract in hypercholesterolemia-induced rabbits. Rabbit is a good model to study hypercholesterolemia and atherosclerosis since its lipoprotein profile and metabolism are more similar to humans than that of rat or mouse [10]. In the present study, simvastatin, a potent hypocholesterolemic drug, was used as a positive control because it has known mechanism of action in inhibiting HMG-CoA reductase [11].

HCD feeding showed significant elevation of TC, LDL, and TG, which increase lipid peroxidation and influence the development of atherosclerosis, in agreement with several studies [12]. In contrast, a significant decrease noted in serum HDL in hypercholesterolemic rabbits was also reported by Ismail et al. [4]. The rabbits administered simvastatin or *B. alba* extract had reduction in body weight and serum levels of TC, LDL, and TG and significant increase noted in HDL levels.

LDL cholesterol is a primary target of atherosclerosis risk-reduction therapy. Excess LDL is mostly deposited in arterial wall and becomes a main component of atherosclerotic plaque formation, while HCD feeding has been reported to reduce fatty acid oxidation, resulting in the increase of serum TG which is considered as another risk factor for CVDs [13]. In our study, *B. alba* extract (100 and 200 mg/kg) elicited beneficial effects by attenuating the level of cholesterol including LDL and TG of the treated rabbits. *B. alba* extract (200 mg/kg) reduces TC, LDL, and TG levels as effectively as simvastatin.

HDL plays an essential role in protecting the membranes against oxidative damage. HDL is involved in the uptake and transport of cholesterol to the liver through reverse cholesterol transport process [14]. Epidemiological and clinical

TABLE 2: Levels of total cholesterol, LDL, triglycerides, and HDL in serum of rabbits from various groups.

	G1	G2	G3	G4	G5
Total cholesterol (mg/dL)					
Baseline	39.45 ± 2.95^a	39.33 ± 3.38^a	44.37 ± 3.87^a	41.41 ± 4.58^a	42.30 ± 4.33^a
Week 4	42.66 ± 2.67^a	472.65 ± 4.54^b	480.83 ± 5.18^b	506.92 ± 9.57^b	467.08 ± 8.35^b
Week 8	46.14 ± 4.06^a	1104.98 ± 33.32^c	1112.70 ± 28.33^c	1002.53 ± 11.51^b	1038.85 ± 12.35^b
Week 12	53.57 ± 2.70^a	1326.91 ± 19.47^d	456.56 ± 5.23^b	510.99 ± 8.14^c	475.12 ± 10.94^b
LDL level (mg/dL)					
Baseline	26.48 ± 0.72^a	31.19 ± 0.97^a	25.39 ± 0.43^a	29.02 ± 1.13^a	27.03 ± 0.82^a
Week 4	33.92 ± 0.55^a	426.15 ± 4.52^b	440.66 ± 3.39^b	421.68 ± 3.95^b	435.94 ± 2.57^b
Week 8	38.79 ± 0.77^a	1157.09 ± 13.85^d	1056.66 ± 15.38^c	1001.23 ± 12.40^b	1081.04 ± 4.06^c
Week 12	45.96 ± 1.01^a	1259.60 ± 15.43^d	515.83 ± 14.03^b	547.39 ± 12.81^c	539.27 ± 13.05^b
Triglyceride level (mg/dL)					
Baseline	110.13 ± 4.55^a	116.46 ± 3.68^b	106.88 ± 6.28^a	114.39 ± 5.36^b	107.56 ± 7.58^a
Week 4	132.83 ± 7.84^a	340.63 ± 8.74^c	331.84 ± 4.97^b	349.42 ± 3.41^b	329.74 ± 6.95^b
Week 8	156.38 ± 8.80^a	654.58 ± 15.16^b	650.96 ± 18.35^b	639.52 ± 16.04^b	661.12 ± 18.81^b
Week 12	166.03 ± 5.81^c	869.57 ± 15.38^d	384.30 ± 14.63^a	416.14 ± 16.73^b	398.53 ± 10.66^a
HDL level (mg/dL)					
Baseline	45.65 ± 0.758^b	$41.53 \pm 5.27^{a,b}$	38.27 ± 0.71^a	46.02 ± 1.15^b	39.83 ± 5.30^a
Week 4	$46.94 \pm 1.09^{b,c}$	$38.13 \pm 5.28^{a,b}$	37.30 ± 0.78^a	44.31 ± 1.10^c	37.09 ± 5.27^a
Week 8	47.45 ± 1.15^c	34.33 ± 5.18^a	$36.37 \pm 2.66^{a,b}$	38.51 ± 3.35^b	35.88 ± 3.92^a
Week 12	47.25 ± 0.45^c	28.27 ± 7.21^a	47.93 ± 2.51^c	53.78 ± 3.45^b	55.05 ± 1.26^b

G1: normal control, G2: hypercholesterolemic control, G3: simvastatin-treated (10 mg/kg), G4: *B. alba* extract-treated (100 mg/kg), and G5: *B. alba* extract-treated (200 mg/kg). All data are presented as the mean $\pm$ SD (n = 4 for each group). One-way ANOVA was performed followed by Dunnett's *post hoc* test for multiple comparisons. Within a week, values sharing the same superscript letters are not significantly different from each other ($p < 0.05$).

TABLE 3: Levels of ALT, AST, and CK in serum of rabbits from various groups.

	G1	G2	G3	G4	G5
ALT (U/L)					
Baseline	21.22 ± 1.27^a	20.30 ± 1.47^b	23.20 ± 1.37^b	21.43 ± 1.53^b	22.45 ± 0.75^b
Week 4	21.05 ± 2.79^a	43.10 ± 4.67^b	47.75 ± 1.79^c	$44.85 \pm 1.44^{b,c}$	46.18 ± 0.51^c
Week 8	24.62 ± 1.65^a	63.75 ± 3.48^b	64.98 ± 6.99^b	67.85 ± 1.36^b	69.75 ± 1.48^b
Week 12	29.15 ± 1.07^a	91.80 ± 4.45^c	104.85 ± 4.53^d	40.35 ± 2.24^b	38.43 ± 2.28^b
AST (U/L)					
Baseline	29.65 ± 1.23^b	29.65 ± 4.06^b	28.18 ± 3.86^b	25.93 ± 3.15^a	$27.13 \pm 4.16^{a,b}$
Week 4	32.97 ± 3.78^a	49.75 ± 8.63^b	$51.78 \pm 6.57^{b,c}$	47.68 ± 5.57^b	46.33 ± 1.33^b
Week 8	36.97 ± 1.09^a	67.48 ± 8.76^b	69.30 ± 8.17^b	67.65 ± 5.64^b	71.65 ± 2.84^b
Week 12	39.87 ± 2.37^a	95.77 ± 8.54^c	113.75 ± 4.46^d	42.38 ± 3.46^b	40.32 ± 4.00^b
CK (U/L)					
Baseline	540.30 ± 22.85^a	578.80 ± 20.72^a	556.23 ± 51.60^a	544.08 ± 35.39^a	569.30 ± 36.96^a
Week 4	555.50 ± 25.17^a	900.48 ± 75.95^b	886.55 ± 113.73^b	865.90 ± 88.06^b	881.45 ± 6.00^b
Week 8	579.02 ± 22.00^a	1466.00 ± 233.42^b	1562.13 ± 196.69^b	1325.28 ± 97.91^b	1362.88 ± 104.08^b
Week 12	597.80 ± 13.49^a	1931.48 ± 223.55^c	2093.95 ± 272.50^c	1004.30 ± 100.27^b	1051.03 ± 99.88^b

G1: normal control, G2: hypercholesterolemic control, G3: simvastatin-treated (10 mg/kg), G4: *B. alba* extract-treated (100 mg/kg), and G5: *B. alba* extract-treated (200 mg/kg). All data are presented as the mean $\pm$ SD (n = 4 for each group). One-way ANOVA was performed followed by Dunnett's *post hoc* test for multiple comparisons. Within a week, values sharing the same superscript letters are not significantly different from each other ($p < 0.05$).

studies have shown that low level of HDL plays a crucial role in the atherogenic process [15]; thus, therapeutic approach to increase the HDL level is widely encouraged [16]. Significant increase in HDL as shown in *B. alba*-treated rabbits is a desirable criterion for an ideal hypercholesterolemic agent since it reduces the atherosclerotic risk.

The liver is the primary organ that is responsible for maintaining the cholesterol homeostasis. The marker enzymes, ALT and AST, were evaluated to detect the liver damage while CK was used to diagnose the muscle injury. These enzymes were reported to leak into the blood circulation when their cell membranes were injured [17]. The levels of the enzymes

TABLE 4: Levels of antioxidant enzymes in serum of rabbits from various groups.

	G1	G2	G3	G4	G5
SOD (U/mL)					
Baseline	$5.88 \pm 0.17^{a,b}$	5.63 ± 0.25^{a}	5.93 ± 0.11^{b}	$5.72 \pm 0.15^{a,b}$	$5.84 \pm 0.12^{a,b}$
Week 4	5.98 ± 0.21^{c}	5.49 ± 0.34^{b}	5.61 ± 0.18^{b}	5.39 ± 0.30^{a}	5.33 ± 0.21^{a}
Week 8	6.05 ± 0.22^{c}	5.35 ± 0.29^{b}	5.25 ± 0.25^{b}	4.96 ± 0.17^{a}	5.10 ± 0.31^{a}
Week 12	6.20 ± 0.18^{c}	4.91 ± 0.20^{a}	5.04 ± 0.28^{a}	5.21 ± 0.73^{b}	5.38 ± 0.35^{b}
GPx (U/L)					
Baseline	1243.73 ± 91.21^{a}	1211.65 ± 101.19^{a}	1443.10 ± 55.78^{b}	1313.95 ± 232.95^{b}	1401.20 ± 171.33^{b}
Week 4	1330.85 ± 77.53^{c}	1198.58 ± 90.38^{a}	1351.83 ± 128.17^{c}	1277.18 ± 184.68^{b}	1274.78 ± 124.44^{b}
Week 8	1459.45 ± 175.80^{b}	1055.30 ± 62.23^{a}	1205.00 ± 82.15^{a}	1079.55 ± 213.70^{a}	1169.20 ± 82.50^{a}
Week 12	1595.35 ± 219.20^{c}	885.23 ± 43.84^{a}	975.53 ± 62.41^{a}	1241.63 ± 181.98^{b}	$1418.5 \pm 82.55^{b,c}$

G1: normal control, G2: hypercholesterolemic control, G3: simvastatin-treated (10 mg/kg), G4: *B. alba* extract-treated (100 mg/kg), and G5: *B. alba* extract-treated (200 mg/kg). All data are presented as the mean ± SD ($n = 4$ for each group). One-way ANOVA was performed followed by Dunnett's *post hoc* test for multiple comparisons. Within a week, values sharing the same superscript letters are not significantly different from each other ($p < 0.05$).

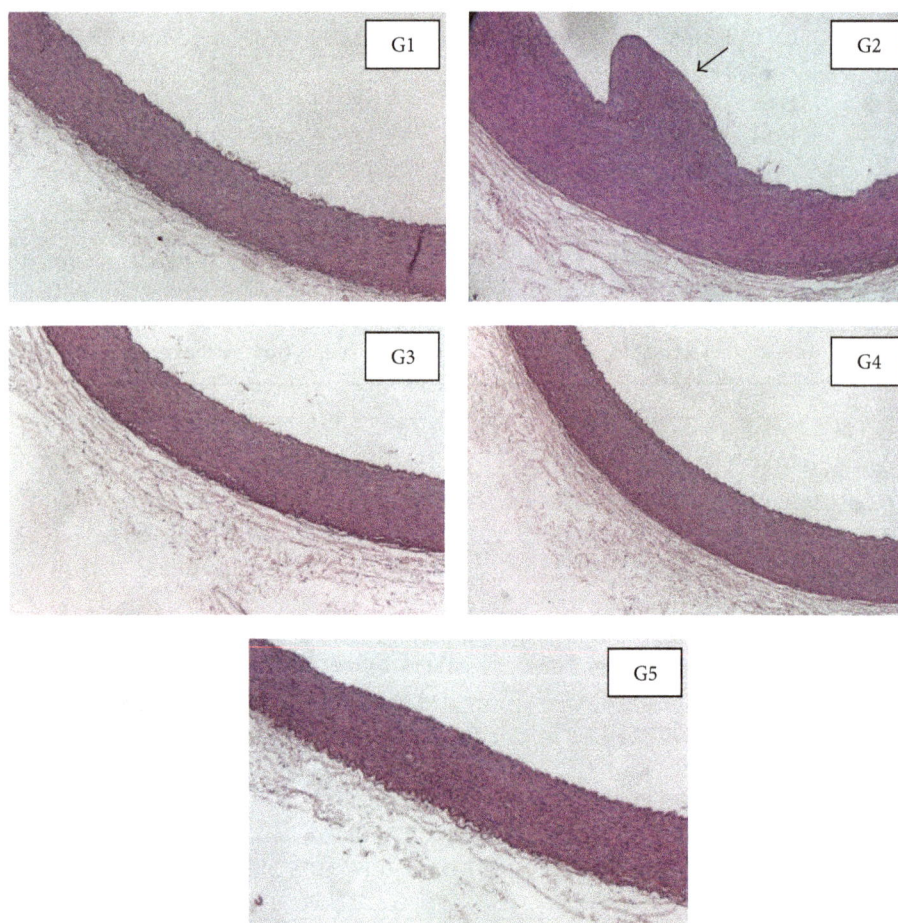

FIGURE 1: Representative photographs of rabbits' aortic arch from 5 groups stained with H&E. The aorta of a control hypercholesterolemic rabbit (G2) showing a large intimal plaque (arrow). G1: normal control, G2: hypercholesterolemic control, G3: simvastatin (10 mg/kg) treated, G4: *B. alba* extract (100 mg/kg) treated, and G5: *B. alba* extract (200 mg/kg) treated (Magnification 50x).

were found elevated in hypercholesterolemic control and simvastatin-treated rabbits compared to the normal group. This suggests high concentration of cholesterol and the usage of simvastatin caused liver and muscle damage [18, 19], whereas administration of *B. alba* extract for 4 weeks reduced the elevations of ALT, AST, and CK indicating its hepatic and muscle-protective effects.

Antioxidant enzymes (SOD and GPx) play essential roles in maintaining the physiological concentrations of oxygen and hydrogen peroxide by improving the dismutation of

Table 5: Thickness of intima, media, and intima/media ratio of experimental rabbits at week 12.

Groups	Intima thickness (μm)	Media thickness (μm)	Intima/media
G1	1045.439 ± 80.26[a]	3350.768 ± 213.40[a]	0.312 ± 0.039[a]
G2	4203.296 ± 160.96[d]	6004.708 ± 102.28[d]	0.700 ± 0.023[d]
G3	1585.270 ± 111.40[b]	3809.198 ± 160.44[b]	0.416 ± 0.035[b]
G4	1786.301 ± 104.59[c]	3978.398 ± 85.94[b,c]	0.449 ± 0.019[c]
G5	1720.678 ± 152.25[b]	4058.203 ± 181.25[c]	0.424 ± 0.033[b]

G1: normal control, G2: hypercholesterolemic control, G3: simvastatin-treated (10 mg/kg), G4: B. alba extract-treated (100 mg/kg), and G5: B. alba extract-treated (200 mg/kg). All data are presented as the mean ± SD ($n = 4$ for each group). One-way ANOVA was performed followed by Dunnett's post hoc test for multiple comparisons. Within a column, values sharing the same superscript letters are not significantly different from each other ($p < 0.05$).

oxygen radicals [20]. A decrease in the level of SOD and GPx was observed in simvastatin-treated and hypercholesterolemic control groups. A significant decrease in GPx activity in simvastatin-treated group was also noted by Trocha et al. [21]; this could be due to the reduced antioxidant capacity in the serum of the animal model.

High cholesterol diet alters the in vivo antioxidant status in blood by increasing the oxygen free radicals that cause lipid peroxidation [22]. In our present study, feeding hypercholesterolemic diet for 8 weeks leads to the reduction in the activities of SOD and GPx. Many reports have also proved that hypercholesterolemia diminishes the activity of SOD [23, 24] and GPx [25]. The reduced level of SOD and GPx activities is associated with increased risk of CVD [26, 27]. The data obtained in this study suggested that B. alba extract is capable of enhancing the activity of SOD and GPx in hypercholesterolemia-induced rabbits; the effect could be due to the presence of phenolic compounds. Indeed, plant polyphenols have been reported to regulate antioxidative status by ameliorating the activity of antioxidant enzymes [20]. Therefore, this suggests that B. alba extract is capable of improving the antioxidant status and could be beneficial in managing oxidative damage and preventing lipid peroxidation.

Oxidized LDL molecules are commonly found in subendothelial layers. The accumulation of oxidized LDL in macrophages can stimulate proliferation of monocytes, smooth muscle cells, and endothelial cells. When the scavenging receptor for oxidized LDL on macrophages is upregulated, it leads to foam cells formation which are the major component of fatty streaks. This contributes to atheromatous plaque formation and thickening of intimal layer [28, 29]. The histopathological examination of aorta correlates with the serum biochemical data. The level of hypercholesterolemia was directly proportional with the severity of atherosclerotic plaque as observed in the aorta of hypercholesterolemic control group. Simvastatin and B. alba-treated rabbits revealed a significant reduction in aortic plaque and intimal thickening. In general, B. alba treatment (200 mg/kg) showed no significant difference in intima/media ratio compared to simvastatin-treated group. This suggests that B. alba

extract (200 mg/kg) is as effective as simvastatin in treating atherosclerosis.

The mechanism by which B. alba inhibits the atherosclerotic plaque is not known but may be due to its antioxidant, hypocholesterolemic, and antiatherosclerotic effects such as decreasing oxidative stress, lowering the LDL level, reducing inflammation, and inhibiting macrophage accumulation. From the results obtained, it can be concluded that B. alba possesses therapeutic effects in treating hypercholesterolemia and atherosclerosis.

5. Conclusion

B. alba leaf extract could be an effective alternative treatment for hypercholesterolemia and atherosclerosis. The results from the present study showed that B. alba extract (200 mg/kg) effectively reduces the levels of TC, LDL, and TG and raised the level of HDL and antioxidants enzymes. B. alba leaf extract did not cause liver and muscle damage indicating that it is safe for consumption. B. alba successfully inhibited the atherosclerotic plaque formation in hypercholesterolemia-induced model. The finding from in vivo study is in good agreement with that of in vitro study with HMG CoA reductase, confirming the cholesterol lowering effect of B. alba. Further investigations are needed on the mechanisms of B. alba in inhibiting the atherosclerotic plaque formation. Isolation and identification of bioactive compounds of B. alba that are responsible for the observed effects are needed, which can be developed as a prophylactic agent against hypercholesterolemia and atherosclerosis.

Conflict of Interests

The authors declare that there is no conflict of interests regarding the publication of this paper.

Acknowledgments

This research is supported by University Putra Malaysia, Grant no. 9399800. Baskaran Gunasekaran is supported by Ministry of Education (MOE) of Malaysia.

References

[1] T. Yokozawa, E. J. Cho, S. Sasaki, A. Satoh, T. Okamoto, and Y. Sei, "The protective role of Chinese prescription Kangen-karyu extract on diet-induced hypercholesterolemia in rats," Biological and Pharmaceutical Bulletin, vol. 29, no. 4, pp. 760–765, 2006.

[2] S. K. Yeap, B. K. Beh, W. Y. Ho et al., "In vivo antioxidant and hypolipidemic effects of fermented mung bean on hypercholesterolemic mice," Evidence-Based Complementary and Alternative Medicine, vol. 2015, Article ID 508029, 6 pages, 2015.

[3] S. Salvamani, B. Gunasekaran, N. A. Shaharuddin, S. A. Ahmad, and M. Y. Shukor, "Antiartherosclerotic effects of plant flavonoids," BioMed Research International, vol. 2014, Article ID 480258, 11 pages, 2014.

[4] M. F. Ismail, M. Z. Gad, and M. A. Hamdy, "Study of the hypolipidemic properties of pectin, garlic and ginseng in

hypercholesterolemic rabbits," *Pharmacological Research*, vol. 39, no. 2, pp. 157–166, 1999.

[5] G. Baskaran, S. Salvamani, S. A. Ahmad, N. A. Shaharuddin, P. D. Pattiram, and M. Y. Shukor, "HMG-CoA reductase inhibitory activity and phytocomponent investigation of *Basella alba* leaf extract as a treatment for hypercholesterolemia," *Drug Design, Development and Therapy*, vol. 9, pp. 509–517, 2015.

[6] R. Adhikari, K. H. Naveen, and S. Shruthi, "A review on medicinal importance of *Basella alba* L.," *International Journal of Pharmaceutical Sciences and Drug Research*, vol. 4, no. 2, pp. 110–114, 2012.

[7] P. Kumar, "Indian spinach, *Basella alba* (PUI) succulent, branched, smooth, twining herbaceous vine," in *Best Nutrition*, PR Log-Global Press Release Distribution, 2010.

[8] H. Yasmin, M. A. Kaisar, M. M. R. Sarker, M. S. Rahman, and M. A. Rashid, "Preliminary anti-bacterial activity of some indigenous plants of Bangladesh," *Dhaka University Journal of Pharmaceutical Sciences*, vol. 8, no. 1, pp. 61–65, 2009.

[9] P. Balachandran and R. Govindarajan, "Cancer—an ayurvedic perspective," *Pharmacological Research*, vol. 51, no. 1, pp. 19–30, 2005.

[10] A. B. Waqar, T. Koike, Y. Yu et al., "High-fat diet without excess calories induces metabolic disorders and enhances atherosclerosis in rabbits," *Atherosclerosis*, vol. 213, no. 1, pp. 148–155, 2010.

[11] Y. Kureishi, Z. Luo, I. Shiojima et al., "The HMG-CoA reductase inhibitor simvastatin activates the protein kinase Akt and promotes angiogenesis in normocholesterolemic animals," *Nature Medicine*, vol. 6, no. 9, pp. 1004–1010, 2000.

[12] Y. Zhang, L. Li, J. You, J. Cao, X. Fu, and Y. Zhang, "Effect of 7-difluoromethyl-5, 4′-dimethoxygenistein on aorta atherosclerosis in hyperlipidemia ApoE$^{-/-}$ mice induced by a cholesterol-rich diet," *Development Theraphy*, vol. 7, pp. 233–242, 2013.

[13] O. A. Adaramoye, V. O. Nwaneri, K. C. Anyanwo, E. O. Farombi, and G. O. Emerole, "Possible anti-atherogenic effect of kolaviron (a *Garcinia kola* seed extract) in hypercholesterolaemic rats," *Clinical and Experimental Pharmacology and Physiology*, vol. 32, no. 1-2, pp. 40–46, 2005.

[14] J.-R. Nofer, B. Kehrel, M. Fobker, B. Levkau, G. Assmann, and A. V. Eckardstein, "HDL and arteriosclerosis: beyond reverse cholesterol transport," *Atherosclerosis*, vol. 161, no. 1, pp. 1–16, 2002.

[15] G. Assmann and A. M. Gotto Jr., "HDL cholesterol and protective factors in atherosclerosis," *Circulation*, vol. 109, no. 23, supplement 1, pp. 111–118, 2004.

[16] O. A. Adaramoye, O. Akintayo, J. Achem, and M. A. Fafunso, "Lipid-lowering effects of methanolic extract of *Vernonia amygdalina* leaves in rats fed on high cholesterol diet," *Vascular Health & Risk Management*, vol. 4, no. 1, pp. 235–241, 2008.

[17] F. Martinello, S. M. Soares, J. J. Franco et al., "Hypolipemic and antioxidant activities from *Tamarindus indica* L. pulp fruit extract in hypercholesterolemic hamsters," *Food and Chemical Toxicology*, vol. 44, no. 6, pp. 810–818, 2006.

[18] S. Bolkent, R. Yanardag, S. Bolkent, and M. M. Döger, "Beneficial effects of combined treatment with niacin and chromium on the liver of hyperlipemic rats," *Biological Trace Element Research*, vol. 101, no. 3, pp. 219–229, 2004.

[19] R. S. Scott, C. J. Lintott, and M. J. Wilson, "Simvastatin and side effects," *New Zealand Medical Journal*, vol. 104, no. 924, pp. 493–495, 1991.

[20] M. I. Kazeem, M. A. Akanji, M. T. Yakubu, and A. O. T. Ashafa, "Protective effect of free and bound polyphenol extracts from ginger (*Zingiber officinale* Roscoe) on the hepatic antioxidant and some carbohydrate metabolizing enzymes of streptozotocin-induced diabetic rats," *Evidence-Based Complementary and Alternative Medicine*, vol. 2013, Article ID 935486, 7 pages, 2013.

[21] M. Trocha, A. Merwid-Lad, E. Chlebda, M. Pieśniewska, T. Sozański, and A. Szelag, "Effect of simvastatin treatment on rat livers subjected to ischemia/reperfusion," *Pharmacological Reports*, vol. 62, no. 4, pp. 757–762, 2010.

[22] K. Prasad and J. Kalra, "Oxygen free radicals and hypercholesterolemic atherosclerosis: effect of vitamin E," *American Heart Journal*, vol. 125, no. 4, pp. 958–973, 1993.

[23] M. A. Mikail, I. A. Ahmed, M. Ibrahim et al., "*Baccaurea angulata* fruit inhibits lipid peroxidation and induces the increase in antioxidant enzyme activities," *European Journal of Nutrition*, pp. 1–10, 2015.

[24] I. Fki, M. Bouaziz, Z. Sahnoun, and S. Sayadi, "Hypocholesterolemic effects of phenolic-rich extracts of *Chemlali* olive cultivar in rats fed a cholesterol-rich diet," *Bioorganic and Medicinal Chemistry*, vol. 13, no. 18, pp. 5362–5370, 2005.

[25] J. Balkan, S. Doğru-Abbasoğlu, G. Aykaç-Toker, and M. Uysal, "The effect of a high cholesterol diet on lipids and oxidative stress in plasma, liver and aorta of rabbits and rats," *Nutrition Research*, vol. 24, no. 3, pp. 229–234, 2004.

[26] A. Crawford, R. G. Fassett, D. P. Geraghty et al., "Relationships between single nucleotide polymorphisms of antioxidant enzymes and disease," *Gene*, vol. 501, no. 2, pp. 89–103, 2012.

[27] B. Buijsse, D.-H. Lee, L. Steffen et al., "Low serum glutathione peroxidase activity is associated with increased cardiovascular mortality in individuals with low HDLc's," *PLoS ONE*, vol. 7, no. 6, Article ID e38901, 2012.

[28] L. Yao, J. E. Heubi, D. D. Buckley et al., "Separation of micelles and vesicles within lumenal aspirates from healthy humans: solubilization of cholesterol after a meal," *Journal of Lipid Research*, vol. 43, no. 4, pp. 654–660, 2002.

[29] V. M. Homer, A. D. Marais, F. Charlton et al., "Identification and characterization of two non-secreted PCSK9 mutants associated with familial hypercholesterolemia in cohorts from New Zealand and South Africa," *Atherosclerosis*, vol. 196, no. 2, pp. 659–666, 2008.

4

Anti-Inflammatory Activity of Triterpenes Isolated from *Protium paniculatum* Oil-Resins

Patrícia D. O. de Almeida,[1] **Ana Paula de A. Boleti,**[1] **André Luis Rüdiger,**[2] **Geane A. Lourenço,**[3] **Valdir Florêncio da Veiga Junior,**[2] **and Emerson S. Lima**[1]

[1]*Laboratório de Atividade Biológica, Faculdade de Ciências Farmacêuticas, Universidade Federal do Amazonas (UFAM), Avenida Gen. Rodrigo Otavio, No. 6200, 69077-000 Manaus, AM, Brazil*
[2]*Instituto de Ciências Exatas, Departamento de Química, Universidade Federal do Amazonas, Avenida Gen. Rodrigo Otavio, No. 6200, 69077-000 Manaus, AM, Brazil*
[3]*Laboratório de Farmacologia, Departamento de Ciências Fisiológicas, Instituto de Ciências Biológicas, Universidade Federal do Amazonas, Avenida Gen. Rodrigo Otavio, No. 6200, 69077-000 Manaus, AM, Brazil*

Correspondence should be addressed to Emerson S. Lima; eslima@ufam.edu.br

Academic Editor: Ken Yasukawa

Protium is the main genus of the Burseraceae family and one of the most common genera in South America, with an important species called "breu." Gum and oil-resins of this species are used as tonic and stimulant and for the treatment of ulcers and inflammation. The present study aims to isolate and investigate the anti-inflammatory activity of triterpene compounds isolated from oil-resin of *Protium paniculatum*. The pentacyclic triterpenes α,β-amyrin, acetylated α,β-amyrin, α,β-amyrone, and brein/maniladiol did not alter the viability of murine J774 macrophages ($IC_{50} > 20\,\mu g/mL$), with the exception of mixture of brein/maniladiol which showed moderate cytotoxic activity. Also it was observed that compounds at $10\,\mu g/mL$ inhibited more than 80% of production of NO$^\bullet$, although only α,β-amyrin was able to inhibit the production of TNF-α ($52.03 \pm 2.4\%$). The compounds inhibited the production of IL-6 and induced the production of IL-10 in murine J774 macrophages stimulated by LPS. α,β-Amyrone inhibited the expression of COX-2 and also inhibited the formation of paw or ear edema in rats and mice, having a quick and immediate effect. This study may provide the basis for future investigations on the therapeutic role of α,β-amyrone in treating inflammation.

1. Introduction

Inflammation is a defense reaction of the body, and a local response of living tissues to injury in mammalians aimed at eliminating or limiting the spread of an injurious agent [1]. The use of medicinal plants or their active components is becoming an increasingly attractive approach for treating various inflammatory disorders [2]. The origin of the anti-inflammatory properties of various phytomedicines can be explained by the presence of substances such as flavonoids, alkaloids, tannins, saponins, anthraquinones, triterpenoids, and other constituents which act as inhibitors of molecular targets and proinflammatory mediators in inflammatory responses [3].

Triterpenoids are constituents that have aroused great interest in recent years due to their pharmacological potential, with numerous therapeutic activities, such as anticancer, anti-inflammatory, antiviral, antibacterial, antifungal, antidiuretic, giardicidal, and acetylcholinesterase inhibitors [4–6]. α,β-Amyrin is a pentacyclic triterpene and constitutes the main component of the resin *Protium* sp. Furthermore, other compounds have been isolated from the resin *Protium* sp., and little is known about its anti-inflammatory properties [7].

In the last 10 years, studies have shown systemic anti-inflammatory action of α,β-amyrin associated with inhibition of the transcription factor NF-κB, inhibition of COX-2, and the production of proinflammatory cytokines [7, 8]. It was recently shown that δ-amyrone, a constituent which is

α-Amyrin

β-Amyrin

α-Amyrone

β-Amyrone

Brein

Maniladiol

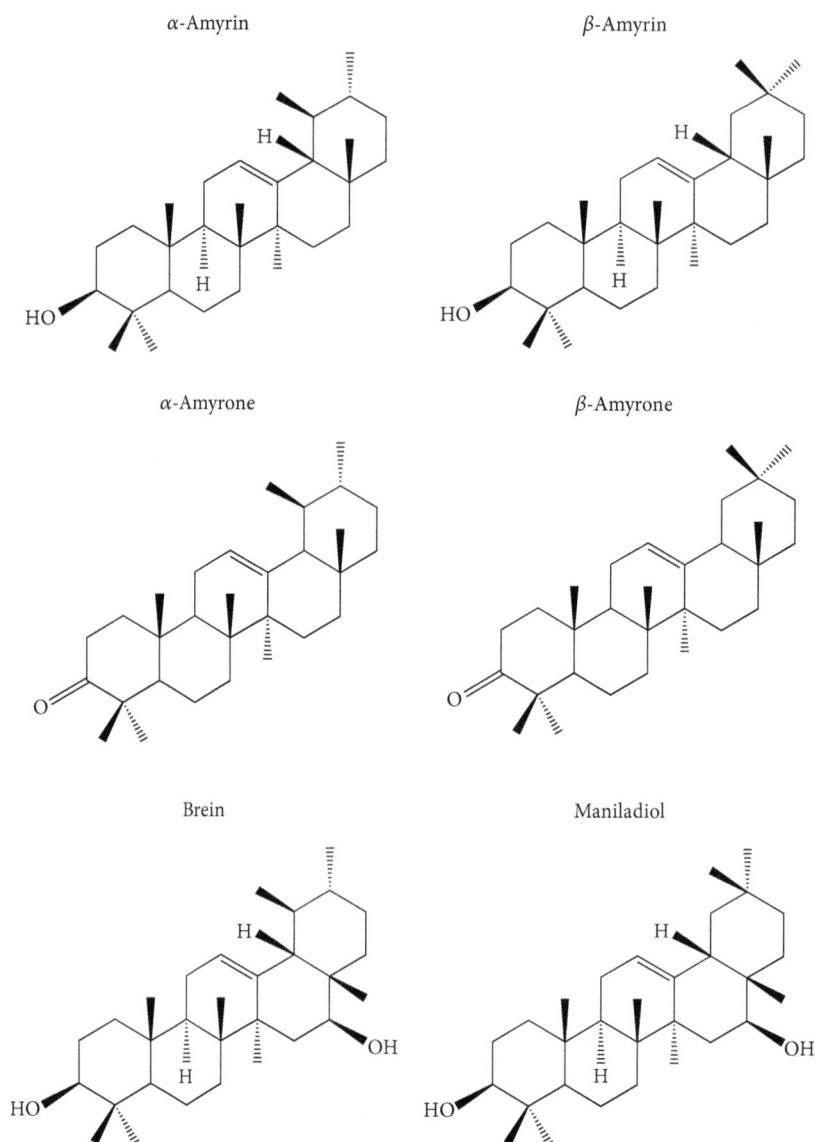

FIGURE 1: Chemical structure of the compounds isolated from *Protium* spp. resin.

extracted and separated from of *Sedum lineare* Thunb., inhibited the ear edema in xylene-induced mouse ear edema and also decreased the level of nitric oxide (NO), prostaglandin E2 (PGE2), interleukin-6 (IL-6), and leukocyte numbers in acetic acid-induced peritonitis *in vivo* [9].

Based on evidence that *Protium* species accumulate, mainly tetracyclic and pentacyclic triterpenoids were isolated from *Protium paniculatum* mixtures of triterpenoids brein/maniladiol and α,β-amyrin [10]. Synthetic derivatives, acetylated amyrin and α,β-amyrone, were obtained from α,β-amyrin. This study aims to evaluate the anti-inflammatory activity of triterpenoids cited, considering that there are few studies in the literature showing possible biological activity.

2. Methods

2.1. Plant Material. Oleoresin of *Protium paniculatum* var. *modestum* (PPM) was collected in Ducke Forest Reserve, 26,

Highway AM-010, Km 26, Manaus, AM, Brazil. The species was catalogued by the Flora Project of Ducke Reserve of the National Institute of Amazonian Research (Instituto Nacional de Pesquisas da Amazônia, INPA) and it was identified by Burseraceae taxonomists: Ph.D. Douglas C. Daly and Ph.D. José Eduardo L. S. Ribeiro. Voucher was deposited in the New York Botanical Garden (1413737) and the INPA herbarium (191303).

2.2. Extraction and Isolation. Mono- and dihydroxylated triterpenes were isolated from the insoluble material which resulted from PPM oleoresin hexanic extraction (Figure 1). Samples were solubilized with ethyl acetate (1008.9 mg); this material was submitted to gravity chromatography over silica gel (mesh: 70–230, $\varnothing_{column}$: 2.5 cm, and $m_{(SiO2)}$: 40 g) using dichloromethane (DCM) and ethyl acetate with gradient polarity. Ketones and acetyl derivatives were obtained from the amyrin mixture by chemical reactions. The data relating to isolations, identification, and reactions are described in Supplementary Material available online at http://dx.doi.org/10.1155/2015/293768.

2.3. Cell Culture.

The murine macrophage cell line J774 was kindly provided by Dr. Leda Quercia Vieira (Laboratory of Gnotobiology and Immunology, UFMG, MG, Brazil) and was cultured at 37°C in a humidified incubator with 5% CO_2 in RPMI-1640 medium containing 10% fetal bovine serum (FBS), 50 U/mL penicillin, and 50 μg/mL streptomycin (Invitrogen). Lipopolysaccharide (LPS) was prepared as a 1 mg/mL stock solution in sterile water and stored at −20°C. The triterpene compounds were added along with treatment with LPS.

2.4. Animals.

Female Wistar rats (200 g each) and Swiss mice (25–35 g) were previously housed in standard polypropylene cages under controlled conditions of temperature (22 ± 2°C) and 12 h light/dark cycle, with free access to diet and water. Mice were allowed to adapt to laboratory for at least 1 h before testing. All experimental procedures using animals were performed following international guidelines and approved by the Institutional Animal Ethics Committee (number 002/2013 CEEA/UFAM).

2.5. Cell Viability Assay.

The cytotoxicity of triterpenes compounds to the murine macrophage cell line J774 was determined by the Alamar Blue method as described by Nakayama and coworkers [11]. Briefly, adherent cells (5×10^3 cells/well) were grown in 96-well tissue culture plates and exposed to the triterpenes: α,β-amyrin, acetylated α,β-amyrin, α,β-amyrone, and brein/maniladiol (2.5; 5; and 10 μg/mL) for 24, 48, and 72 h. After incubation, the Alamar Blue solution (10 μL of 0.4% Alamar Blue (resazurin) in PBS) was added and the cells were incubated for 3 h at 37°C. Fluorescence was measured (excitation at 545 nm and emission at 595 nm) and expressed as a percentage of the cells in the control after background fluorescence was subtracted. Doxorubicin (5 μg/mL) was used as a positive control of cell death. The assays were performed in triplicate.

2.6. NO• Production Assay.

Nitric oxide (NO•) production by J774 cells was assayed by measuring the accumulation of nitrite in the culture medium using Griess reaction [12]. Briefly, after incubation of the cells (1×10^6 cells/mL) with triterpenes compounds in different concentrations of 2.5; 5; and 10 μg/mL, cells were incubated for 24 h with LPS (1 μg/mL), at 37°C in a 5% CO_2 incubator. Nitric oxide was measured as NO_2^- in culture supernatant by reaction with Griess reagent. Absorbance of the reaction product was determined at 560 nm using a microplate reader (DTX 800, Beckman). Sodium nitrite was used as a standard to calculate nitrite.

2.7. Measurement of Cytokines.

Macrophage cells (1×10^6 cells/mL) were incubated with the triterpenes compounds in a concentration of 10 μg/mL and then stimulated with 1 μg/mL of LPS. The culture supernatants were collected after 24 h of LPS stimulation. The levels of cytokines in the culture media were measured by flow cytometry (BD Cytometric Bead Array, CBA, Mouse Inflammation kit) according to the manufacturer's instructions.

2.8. Western Blot Analysis.

J774 cells were cultured in 96-well plates (1×10^6 cells per well) and incubated with α,β-amyrone in concentrations of 2.5; 5; and 10 μg/mL. Cells were stimulated with LPS (1 μg/mL) and incubated for 24 hours. After incubation, cells were washed with phosphate buffered saline and lysed with lysis buffer (Tris-HCl [50 mM, pH 7.5]), 150 mM NaCl, 0.5% nonidet P-40, 1 mM EGTA, 1 mM MgCl$_2$, 10% glycerol, and proteases inhibitors (cocktail of protease inhibitors EDTA-free, Roche; 1 mM PMSF). After 1 hour at 4°C, cell lysates were obtained by centrifugation at 10,000 g for 10 minutes. The total protein concentration in the lysates was measured by Bradford method [13], protein assay using bovine serum albumin as the standard.

Samples containing equal amounts of protein concentration were separated by 12% of sodium dodecyl sulfate-polyacrylamide gel electrophoresis and transferred to nitrocellulose membranes. Nonspecific binding was blocked with Tris-buffered saline with Tween 20 (1 M Tris-HCl [pH 7.5], 2.5 M NaCl, and 0.5% Tween 20) containing 5% nonfat milk for 2 hours at room temperature. The membranes were incubated overnight with the primary antibody [COX-2 and β-actin (abcam, ab52237, and ab8227, resp.)] diluted in Tris-buffered saline with Tween 20 (1 : 1.000 and 1 : 2.000, resp.) and then washed with Tris-buffered saline with Tween 20 and incubated with horseradish peroxidase-conjugated anti-immunoglobulin G antibody (goat anti-rabbit immunoglobulin G) as secondary antibody for 1 hour at room temperature. The immunoblots were visualized with a chemiluminescence detection kit, used according to the manufacturer's recommendations (SuperSignal West Pico Chemiluminescent Substrate, Prod # 34080, Thermo Scientific).

2.9. Carrageenan Induced Paw Edema Assay.

Paw edema was induced by intraplantar injection of 100 μL of 1% carrageenan into the right hind paw of rats as previously described [14]. Animal groups were treated with α,β-amyrone (10 and 5 mg/kg, v.o.) and indomethacin (10 mg/kg, v.o.) and the control animals received identical treatments with the vehicle, which was 3% Tween 80 (10 mg/kg) in saline in this study. After sixty minutes, the animals received an intraplantar injection of carrageenan. The paw volume was measured thereafter at "0 hours" and then at 1, 2, 3, 4, and 5 hours after carrageenan injection using a hydroplethysmometer (Panlab, SLU). The results are expressed as the increase in paw volume (mL) calculated by subtracting basal volume.

2.10. Ear Phenol-Induced Edema.

Inflammation was induced in Balb C mice (n = 5/group) by local administration of 20 μL of a solution of phenol diluted in acetone (10%) (group 1), administered after 20 μL α,β-amyrone solution at concentrations of 0.6 mg, 0.3 mg, and 0.1 mg or dexamethasone of 0.1 mg dissolved in acetone. Sixty minutes after application, mice were euthanized and both ears were removed. Circular

TABLE 1: Cell viability of J774 cells treated with 5, 10, and 20 μg/mL of isolated triterpenes for 24, 48, and 72 hours.

Concentration (μg/mL)	24 hours			48 hours			72 hours		
	20	10	5	20	10	5	20	10	5
	Mean ± SE	Mean ± SE	Mean ± SE	Mean ± SE	Mean ± SE	Mean ± SE	Mean ± SE	Mean ± SE	Mean ± SE
α,β-Amyrin	57.3 ± 1.9	86.4 ± 0.8	105.8 ± 2.3	36.4 ± 3.1	88,5 ± 2.8	110.0 ± 2.5	37.1 ± 3.5	88.7 ± 1.2	97.2 ± 1.8
Acetylated α,β-amyrin	87.1 ± 0.5	152.9 ± 0.7	124.4 ± 1.9	32.1 ± 2.4	99.5 ± 3.6	125.0 ± 1.7	47.7 ± 1.9	98.0 ± 2.9	103.5 ± 2.7
α,β-Amyrone	119.4 ± 0.5	153.8 ± 1.8	144.0 ± 0.78	81.9 ± 2.9	126.7 ± 0.7	133.5 ± 1.5	65.3 ± 1.7	102.0 ± 0.7	105.2 ± 3.5
Brein/maniladiol	40.6 ± 1.1	82.4 ± 1.9	97.2 ± 3.5	13.3 ± 2.0	47.6 ± 2.9	90.0 ± 1.2	5.4 ± 0.6	23.8 ± 3.1	80.2 ± 1.6
Indomethacin	100.1 ± 3.2	123.6 ± 2.9	117.5 ± 3.7	50.5 ± 2.8	100.8 ± 1.3	105.9 ± 0.8	57.9 ± 1.1	102.3 ± 1.7	103.8 ± 2.9
Doxorubicin	26.0 ± 0.4	27.3 ± 1.2	25.7 ± 2.6	9.3 ± 1.4	10.0 ± 0.1	10.1 ± 0.2	3.8 ± 0.7	3.9 ± 0.07	3.9 ± 0.1
DMSO	70.8 ± 0.7	108.6 ± 0.6	113.3 ± 0.6	38.9 ± 0.2	98.9 ± 2.7	109.5 ± 2.9	33.4 ± 2.3	98.6 ± 1.1	99.0 ± 1.3
Medium	106.1 ± 4.0	100.0 ± 9.7	101.30 ± 1.5	106.7 ± 1.8	101.9 ± 11.0	103.4 ± 2.1	99.9 ± 4.8	98.9 ± 3.4	95.4 ± 4.2

Notes. Data are presented as % mean ± standard error ($n = 3$). SE: standard error; DMSO: dimethyl sulfoxide.

sections were removed, using a biopsy punch with a diameter of 5 mm, and weight of the inflamed ears was compared with weight of the ear against-lateral not treated with the phlogistic agent. The increase in weight caused by the irritant was measured by subtracting the weight of the untreated left ear section from that of the treated right ear sections [15].

2.11. Statistical Analysis. Results are expressed as the means and standard deviations of triplicate measurements. Each experiment was performed at least three times. Differences between groups were assessed by one-way analysis of variance (ANOVA) followed by the Tukey *post hoc* test. A value of $P < 0.05$ indicated significance. Western blots are representative of 3 independent experiments.

Data obtained from animal experiments were expressed as the mean ± standard error of the mean (±SEM). Statistical differences between the treated and the control groups were analyzed statistically by analysis of variance (ANOVA) followed by Dunnett's test, in the tutorial Prisma 3.0. Results with [*]$P < 0.05$ and [**]$P < 0.01$ were considered significant.

3. Results

Before evaluating the anti-inflammatory effects of triterpenes isolated from *Protium paniculatum* on LPS-stimulated J774 macrophages, first the cytotoxic effects were investigated. Triterpenes did not exhibit a significant reduction in viability of macrophages compared with the positive control, showing $IC_{50} > 20\,\mu$g/mL, except that triterpene brein/maniladiol showed $IC_{50} = 16.02\,\mu$g/mL after 24 hours of treatment (Table 1).

Because NO$^\bullet$ is known to be a proinflammatory mediator in inflammatory disorders [16], we investigated whether triterpenes inhibit NO$^\bullet$ production in LPS-induced J774 cells. We measured the accumulation of nitrite in the culture media and found that triterpenes concentration-dependently inhibited nitrite levels in the conditioned media of LPS-induced cells. Figure 2 shows the inhibitory effect of triterpenes, α,β-amyrin, acetylated α,β-amyrin, α,β-amyrone, and brein/maniladiol, on NO$^\bullet$ production at concentration of 1.25–10 μg/mL. The triterpenes inhibited the production of NO$^\bullet$ at 98.34 ± 0.9%; 96.05 ± 0.8%; 99.86 ± 1.1%; and 75.43 ±

2.8%, at 10 μg/mL, respectively, and showed IC_{50} at 4.96 ± 0.2; 5.04 ± 0.12; 4.61 ± 0.08; and 6.49 ± 0.02 μg/mL at 10 μg/mL, respectively (Figures 2(a), 2(b), 2(c), and 2(d)). Indomethacin was used with the positive control of anti-inflammatory effect showing an inhibition of 86.31 ± 1.2% in NO$^\bullet$ production at 10 μg/mL (Figure 2(e)).

LPS induce production of proinflammatory cytokines such as the tumor necrosis factor-α (TNF-α) and IL-1 and IL-6 in cells. As shown in Figure 3, among the triterpenes evaluated, only the α,β-amyrin led to a significant decrease in TNF-α levels (52.03 ± 2.4%) at a concentration of 10 μg/mL (Figure 3(a)). However, the other triterpenes, with exception of acetylated α,β-amyrin, inhibited the production of IL-6. Figure 3(b) shows that α,β-amyrin, α,β-amyrone, brein/maniladiol, and indomethacin at a concentration of 10 μg/mL inhibited the IL-6 levels at 67.81±2.8%; 61.43±3.2%; 61.27±5.1%; and 64.24±2.8%, respectively. Furthermore only α,β-amyrone showed an inhibition in IL-10 level; an anti-inflammatory cytokine is secreted under different conditions of immune activation by a variety of cell types, including T cells, B cells, and monocytes/macrophages (Figure 3(c)).

Due to acetylation, α,β-amyrin did increase inhibition of NO$^\bullet$ and TNF-α, and despite the fact that brein/maniladiol showed potential anti-inflammatory activity, it exhibited moderate cytotoxicity activity in J774 murine macrophage cells. Moreover, it is a mixture that needs to be further isolated and characterized. For these reasons we evaluated only triterpene α,β-amyrone. Thus, the protein expression levels of the COX-2 in LPS-challenged cells with and without the treatment of α,β-amyrone were evaluated by western blotting (Figures 4(a) and 4(b)). Treatment with α,β-amyrone showed inhibited COX-2 expression in a concentration-dependent manner, reduced by approximately 90%, at concentrations of 5 or 10 μg/mL.

Figure 5 shows that oral administration of α,β-amyrone (5 and 10 mg/kg, $n = 5$) induced dose-dependent rat paw edema compared with animals receiving only saline. The edema was of rapid onset and relatively short duration (36.3 ± 1.6% and 54.5 ± 1.1%, resp.), after 1 hour of treatment compared to the edema after 3 hours (72.2 ± 1.3% and 79.1 ± 0.4%, resp.). In phenol-induced ear edema in a murine model, it was found that the triterpene α,β-amyrone exhibited significant

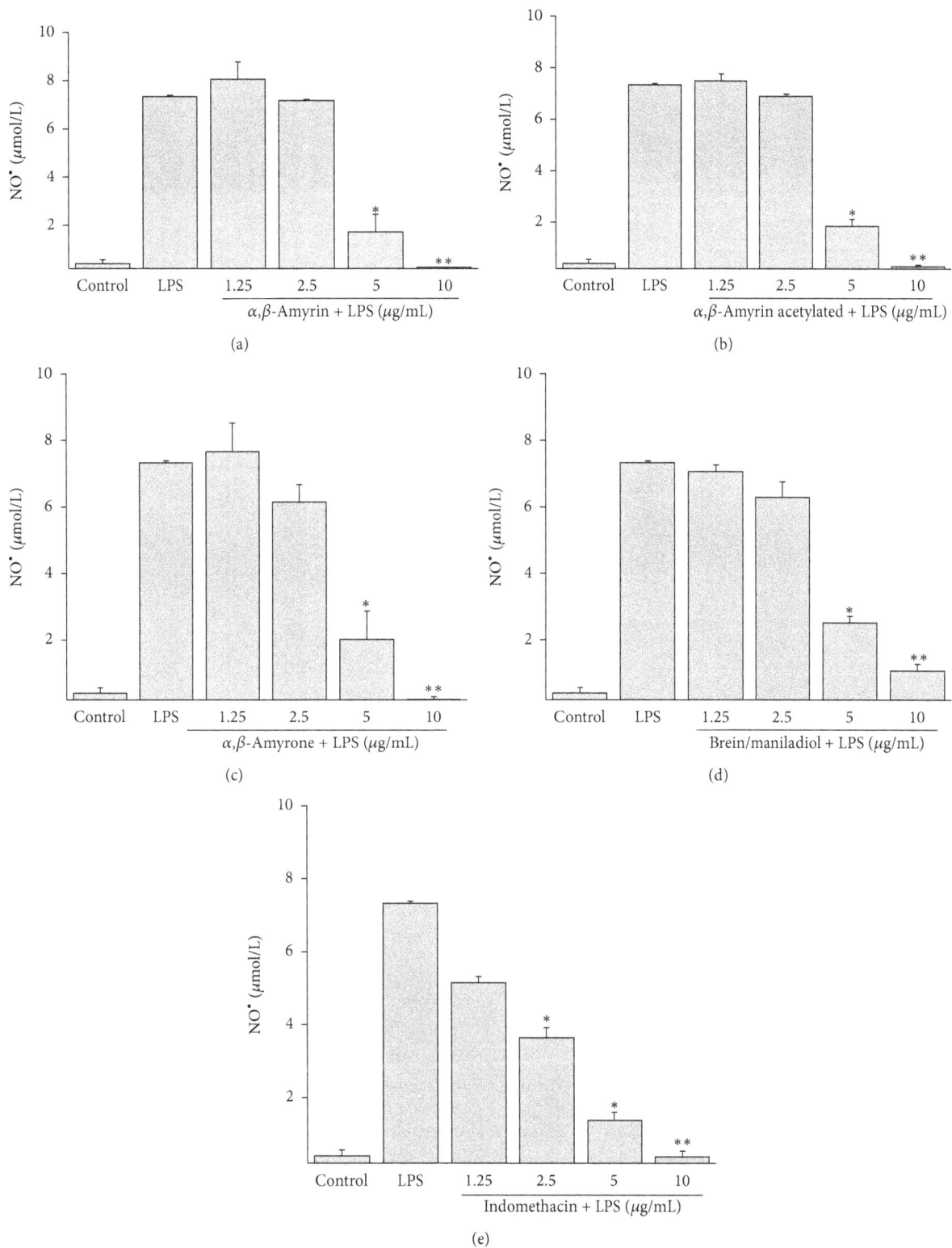

FIGURE 2: Effect of the isolated triterpenes on NO$^\bullet$ production in LPS-stimulated J774 cells. (a) α,β-amyrin (b) acetylated α,β-amyrin (c) α,β-amyrone (d) brein/maniladiol, and (e) indomethacin. Production of NO$^\bullet$ was assayed in culture supernatants of macrophages stimulated with LPS (1 μg/mL) for 24 h in the presence of the four compounds (1.25–10 μg/mL). The nitrite values are the mean $\pm$ SD from three independent experiments. Significance was determined using Student's-t-test ($^*P < 0.05$; $^{**}P < 0.01$ compared to LPS).

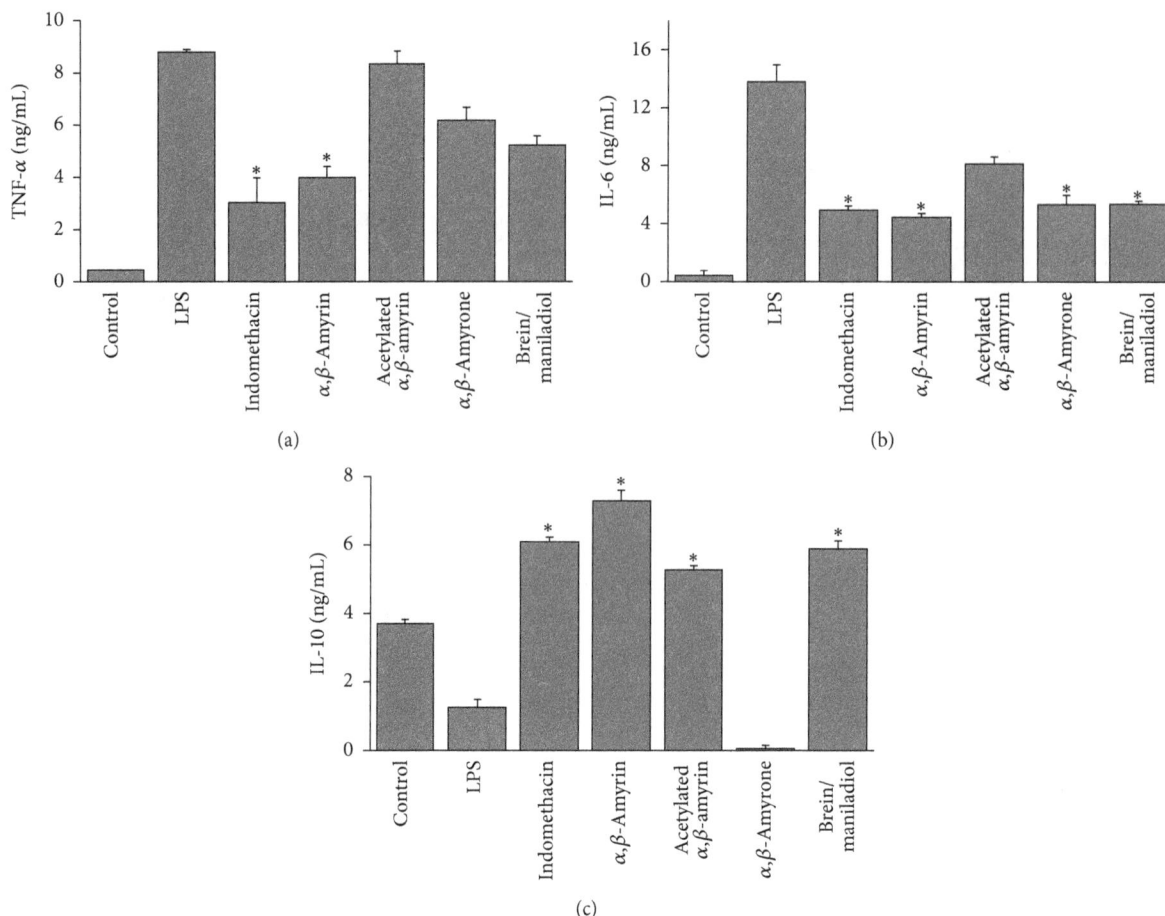

(a)

(b)

(c)

FIGURE 3: Effect of the isolated triterpenes on cytokine production in LPS-stimulated J774 cells. (a) TNF-α, (b) IL-6, and (c) IL-10. Indomethacin (10 μg/mL) was used as a standard. The production of cytokines was assayed in the culture supernatants of macrophages stimulated with LPS (1 μg/mL) for 24 h in the presence of the four compounds (10 μg/mL). Each value was the mean ± SD from three independent experiments. The significance was determined using Student's-t-test ($^*P < 0.05$ compared to LPS).

inhibition in ear edema formation in a dose-related manner. It caused 47% inhibition at the dose of 0.6 mg/kg body weight, respectively, compared with the standard drug dexamethasone where the inhibition was 36% at the dose of 0.1 mg/kg body weight Figure 5(b).

4. Discussion

The use of natural products, especially those derived from medicinal plants, is a traditional form of providing relief from illness. Over the years, natural products have contributed enormously to the development of important therapeutic drugs used currently in modern medicine [17, 18]. Recent studies have shown that the resin of *Protium* sp. displays marked anti-inflammatory activity, in different models of inflammation, with hepatoprotective potential, topical anti-inflammatory action, pancreatic injury, and colitis [5, 6, 18, 19].

Our study demonstrated for the first time the cytotoxic and anti-inflammatory effects of natural triterpenes α,β-amyrin, brein/maniladiol, and synthetic triterpenes acetylated α,β-amyrin and α,β-amyrone on LPS-stimulated J774

macrophages. The triterpenes did not exhibit a significant reduction in macrophage viability compared with the positive control, showing IC$_{50}$ > 20 μg/mL, except triterpene brein/maniladiol which showed IC$_{50}$ = 16.02 μg/mL in 24 hours of treatment. Similar results were observed by Siani et al. [20] who verified that essential oil obtained by steam distillation (leaves and resin) from *Protium* species at 100 μg/mL inhibited the proliferation of different cell lines, with 76–89% inhibition of J774 cells after 72 h of treatment. As noted, brein/maniladiol showed cytotoxic effects on J774 macrophages. Likewise, Ukiya et al. [7] showed that maniladiol isolated from the nonsaponifiable lipid fraction of the edible flower extract of *Chrysanthemum morifolium* exhibited moderate cytotoxicity in kidney cancer cell lines and accentuated activity in breast cancer.

NO$^{\bullet}$ plays an important role in various inflammatory conditions where it is produced by the inducible form of nitric oxide synthase (iNOS) from the amino acid L-arginine [21, 22]. NO$^{\bullet}$ in tissue is susceptible to manipulation by proinflammatory cytokines [23]. NO$^{\bullet}$ has important immune, cardiovascular, and neurological second messenger functions implicated in sepsis, cancer, and inflammation. A variety of

(a)

(b)

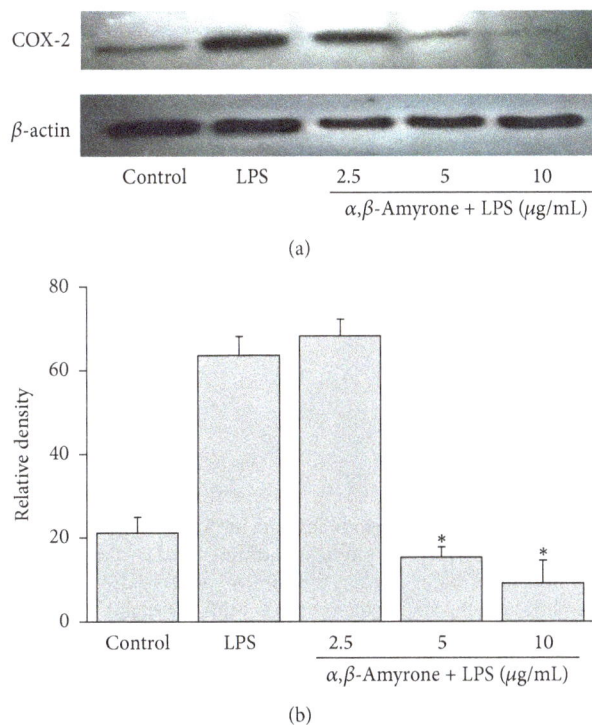

FIGURE 4: Effect of the triterpene α,β-amyrone isolated from *Protium* ssp. on COX-2 expression in LPS-stimulated J774 cells. (a) J774 cells were pretreated with concentrations of 2.5, 5, and 10 μg/mL of α,β-amyrone and LPS (1 μg/mL) for 24 h. The cells were lysed, and the lysates were analyzed by immunoblotting with an anti-COX-2 antibody. The blot was stripped and reprobed with an anti-actin antibody to confirm equal loading. (b) Relative density of COX-2 protein was performed using the ImageJ Software. The significance was determined using ANOVA ($^*P < 0.05$ compared to LPS).

stimuli, such as with LPS, TNF-α, and IFN-γ, can result in the production of a massive amount of NO$^\bullet$ by the activated macrophages which can participate in the pathological processes in several acute and chronic inflammatory disorders [24]. Our results suggest that triterpenes from *P. paniculatum* have dose-dependent anti-inflammatory activities related to their inhibition of NO$^\bullet$ in macrophages without affecting the viability of these cells.

Our results were better than those obtained by Siani et al. [20] who demonstrated that essential oil obtained from leaves and resin from *Protium* species at 100 μg/well, changed the NO$^\bullet$ production from stimulated mouse macrophage after 24 hours of pleurisy induction, in which the resin of *P. heptaphyllum* inhibited 74% and *P. strumosum* inhibited 46% of the NO$^\bullet$ production. In contrast, the triterpenes isolated from *Protium paniculatum*, α,β-amyrin, acetylated α,β-amyrin, α,β-amyrone, and brein/maniladiol, at a concentration of 10 μg/mL inhibited the production of NO$^\bullet$ at 98.34 $\pm$ 0.9%; 96.05 $\pm$ 0.8%; 99.86 $\pm$ 1.1%; and 75.43 $\pm$ 2.8%, respectively.

Furthermore, the media of IC$_{50}$ of triterpenes were similar with the media observed by Niu et al. [25] who evaluated their potential to inhibit the NO$^\bullet$ production induced by LPS

stimulation in RAW 264.7 macrophages of one new olean-13(18)-ene-3,12,19-trione, and two known oleanene triterpenes δ-amyrone and δ-amyrin acetate isolated from a petroleum ether fraction from an alcohol extract of the whole plant of *Sedum linear* Thunb., which exhibited values of IC$_{50}$ at 9.91 μM, 12.24 μM, and 43.34 μM, respectively.

Monocytes and macrophages are key players in inflammatory responses and are also major sources of proinflammatory cytokines and enzymes including tumor necrosis factor-α (TNF-α), interleukins (ILs), cyclooxygenase (COX), and nitric oxide synthase (NOS) [24, 26]. These genes of proinflammatory mediators are strongly induced during inflammation and are responsible for its initiation and persistence. TNF-α are cytokines that act as signaling molecules for immune cells and coordinate the inflammatory response [24]. In this study, among the triterpenes tested, only α,β-amyrin inhibited TNF-α production. This result corroborates with several studies of inhibitory effects of α,β-amyrin on TNF-α production in different models of inflammation [5, 8, 18, 27].

Interleukin-6 (IL-6) is one of the earliest and most important proinflammatory cytokines produced in response to inflammatory stimuli [28]. The presence of IL-6 in tissues is not an unusual occurrence, but its production can lead to uncontrolled exposure and subsequent chronic inflammation, and they are strongly associated with many types of cancer [29]. As our continuing research on anti-inflammatory agents, a number of plant extracts and natural products have been discovered to suppress the secretion of IL-6 in LPS-stimulated macrophages *in vitro* [28, 30]. Interestingly, all the triterpenes tested exerted inhibitory effects on IL-6 production at 10 μg/mL, except acetylated α,β-amyrin. Similar results were demonstrated by Lee et al. [31] who isolated seven flavonoids from the methanol extracts of *Psoralea corylifolia* (bakuchiol, bavachinin, neobavaisoflavone, corylifol A, corylin, isobavachalcone, and bavachin) and found that these compounds were able of inhibit IL-6 production by action of STAT3 promoter activity in Hep3B cells. These compounds also inhibited STAT3 phosphorylation induced by IL-6 in Hep3B cells.

Interleukin-10 (IL-10) is produced by activated macrophages and T cells and plays an important role in anti-inflammatory responses, including the inhibition of cytokine production (tumor necrosis factor-α, IL-6, and IL-12) in macrophages induced by lipopolysaccharide [31]. This study verified that triterpenes, except α,β-amyrone, showed induced IL-10 production. So, the decline of TNF-α accumulation in our study was consistent with findings in several studies demonstrating that IL-10 can suppress TNF-α production in human monocytes and macrophages or even cause diminished levels of TNF-α and IL-6 [32, 33].

Similar results were observed by Zdzisiñska et al. [34] who evaluated the immunomodulatory properties of triterpene betulin and its oxidized form, betulinic acid, as agents inducing cytokines examining human whole blood stimulated by mitogens (PHA). It was observed that triterpene betulin induced TNF-α production in a dose-dependent manner but did not induce the production of IL-10 and IFN-γ; these results suggest that secretion of IFN-γ, IL-10, and TNF-α can be regulated by different mechanisms or various

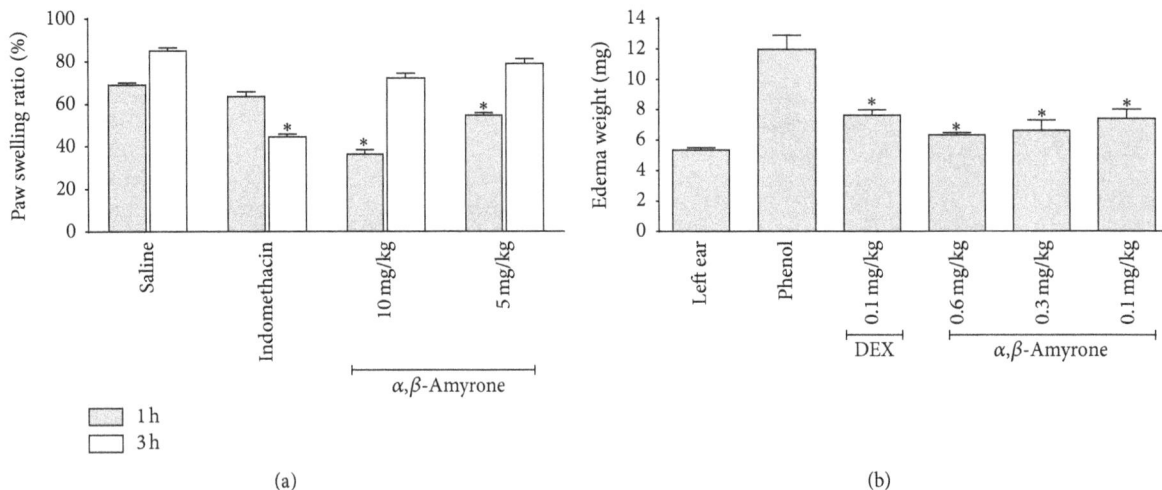

Figure 5: Effect of triterpene α,β-amyrone on rats paw edema induced by 1% of solution of carrageenan into the intraplantar surface of right hind paw and the effects of α,β-amyrone on mice ear edema induced by a phenol model. (a) α,β-amyrone was administered at concentrations of 5 and 10 mg/kg and the edema was measured at the indicated times. The effect of saline injected in the control group is also shown. (b) α,β-amyrone was administered at concentrations of 0.6, 0.3, and 0.1 mg/kg and dexamethasone of 0.1 mg/kg on mice ear edema induced by a phenol model. Data are expressed as mean ± standard error of five animals per group. The significance was determined using ANOVA and Dunnett's test ($^{*}P < 0.05$ compared with control group).

types of leukocytes in whole blood differ in their sensitivity to betulin, unlike, betulinic acid, which did not influence the TNF-α production but inhibited the production of IFN-γ and increased production of IL-10.

Cyclooxygenases are inducible enzymes that catalyze the production of prostaglandins, which contribute to the inflammatory process and tissue damage. It has been reported that COX-2 can also be activated by high concentrations of nitric oxide, contributing towards more intense inflammatory responses as seen in many chronic inflammatory disorders [22]. In the current study, we verified only Cox-2 expression of triterpene α,β-amyrone that was able to inhibit COX-2 in a concentration-dependent manner. Several natural products of plant origin have been shown to transmit their anti-inflammatory activities through suppression of COX-2; however, suppression of nitric oxide production is critical for this [22, 35]. In previous studies the ability of triterpene α,β-amyrin to inhibit COX-2 expression using a different model of inflammation is shown, as in the case of topic inflammation in rats and a colitis model [2, 18]. In accordance with the prepreliminary results α,β-amyrone was able to inhibit the production of NO$^{•}$, IL-6, and COX-2 expression, suggesting that the mechanism by which α,β-amyrone exerts its anti-inflammatory activity is the same mechanism by which α,β-amyrin acts, that is, by inhibiting the nuclear factor-kappa B (NF-κB).

The model of paw edema induced by carrageenan is an appropriate test and widely used for evaluating anti-inflammatory activity of different compounds [1]. Carrageenan induced hind paw edema is the standard experimental model of acute inflammation. Carrageenan is the phlogistic agent of choice for testing anti-inflammatory drugs as it is not known to be antigenic and is devoid of apparent systemic effects [36]. The present study of anti-inflammatory activity of α,β-amyrone against carrageenan induced paw edema shows that triterpenes have a significant effect on inflammation and markedly reduced the swelling at 10 μg/mL after 3 hours of treatment.

α,β-Amyrone showed the activity at concentrations of 10 and 5 mg/kg and showed a different effect of indomethacin, whereas α,β-amyrone showed a maximum effect in the first hour after administration of carrageenan with a decrease with respect to time, and indomethacin at a dose of 10 mg/kg showed increased activity after three hours of induction of inflammation, when the carrageenan starts to show its greatest inflammatory effect, decreasing effect in five hours, which indicates an effect faster than α,β-amyrone.

In the present study, the significant anti-inflammatory effect of topical application of triterpene α,β-amyrone in phenol-induced mouse ear edema was shown for the first time. Phenol is an irritant agent for stimulating contact dermatitis in mice [37, 38]. Skin keratinocyte membranes are ruptured upon direct contact with phenol, resulting in protein kinase C mediating release of inflammatory mediators such as IL-1α, TNF-α, and IL-8 [38–40]. The topical anti-inflammatory activity of α,β-amyrone was demonstrated by results showing that α,β-amyrone dose-dependently attenuated the phenol-induced ear edema with an effect as potent as dexamethasone and showing the property of this substance to penetrate the skin and exert its activity in deeper layers which could be indicator of its potential use in pharmaceutical formulations with anti-inflammatory properties. In addition, the anti-inflammatory activity of α,β-amyrone needs the additional studies which will provide clinical evidences in context of specific inflammatory inductions and/or microbial infection activity.

5. Conclusion

The triterpenes α,β-amyrin, acetylated α,β-amyrin, α,β-amyrone, and brein/maniladiol are capable of modulating an immune response. In particular, the triterpene α,β-amyrone showed no cytotoxic potential in J774 macrophages and exerted immunomodulatory activity at low concentrations, characterized by its inhibitory effects on the production of proinflammatory mediators such as NO$^\bullet$, IL-6, and COX-2 expression and inducing the production of anti-inflammatory cytokine IL-10, and reduced paw edema induced by carrageenan in rats, as well as reducing ear edema in mice.

Abbreviations

COX$_2$: Cyclooxygenase 2
Dexa: Dexamethasone
DMSO: Dimethyl sulfoxide
EDTA: Ethylenediaminetetraacetic acid
EGTA: Ethylene glycol tetraacetic acid
IL6: Interleukin-6
IL10: Interleukin-10
LPS: Lipopolysaccharide
MgCl$_2$: Magnesium chloride
NaCl: Sodium chloride
NF-κB: Nuclear factor kappa B
NO: Nitric oxide
PBS: Phosphate buffered saline
PMSF: Phenylmethanesulfonyl fluoride
TNFα: Tumor necrosis factor-α.

Disclosure

This study is part of the project of Regional Scientific Development/FAPEAM (DCR) of Professor Dr. Ana Paula de A. Boleti, developed in the laboratory of biological activities, Faculty of Pharmaceutical Sciences, Federal University of Amazonas, under the supervision of Professor Dr. Emerson S. Lima.

Conflict of Interests

Authors declare no conflict of interests.

Acknowledgments

The authors are grateful to Conselho Nacional de Desenvolvimento Científico e Tecnológico (CNPq) and Fundação de Amparo à Pesquisa do Estado do Amazonas (FAPEAM) for funding this research. Emerson S. Lima is a member of the INCT de Processos Redox em Biomedicina-Redoxoma (MCT/CNPq). Ana Paula de A. Boleti received a grant from DCR/CNPq/FAPEAM. Jim Hesson of AcademicEnglishSolutions.com revised the English.

References

[1] B. Patgiri, B. L. Umretia, P. U. Vaishnav, P. K. Prajapati, V. J. Shukla, and B. Ravishankar, "Anti-inflammatory activity of Guduchi Ghana (aqueous extract of Tinospora cordifolia Miers.)," AYU, vol. 35, no. 1, pp. 108–110, 2014.

[2] C. E. Vitor, C. P. Figueiredo, D. B. Hara, A. F. Bento, T. L. Mazzuco, and J. B. Calixto, "Therapeutic action and underlying mechanisms of a combination of two pentacyclic triterpenes, α and β-amyrin, in a mouse model of colitis," British Journal of Pharmacology, vol. 157, no. 6, pp. 1034–1044, 2009.

[3] K.-J. Soumaya, M. Dhekra, C. Fadwa et al., "Pharmacological, antioxidant, genotoxic studies and modulation of rat splenocyte functions by Cyperus rotundus extracts," BMC Complementary and Alternative Medicine, vol. 13, article 28, 2013.

[4] P. N. Bandeira, O. D. L. Pessoa, M. T. S. Trevisan, and T. L. G. Lemos, "Metabólitos secundários de Protium heptaphyllum March," Química Nova, vol. 25, no. 6, pp. 1078–1080, 2002.

[5] C. M. Melo, K. M. M. B. Carvalho, J. C. de Sousa Neves et al., "α,β-amyrin, a natural triterpenoid ameliorates L-arginine-induced acute pancreatitis in rats," World Journal of Gastroenterology, vol. 16, no. 34, pp. 4272–4280, 2010.

[6] I. Matos, A. F. Bento, R. Marcon, R. F. Claudino, and J. B. Calixto, "Preventive and therapeutic oral administration of the pentacyclic triterpene α,β-amyrin ameliorates dextran sulfate sodium-induced colitis in mice: the relevance of cannabinoid system," Molecular Immunology, vol. 54, no. 3-4, pp. 482–492, 2013.

[7] M. Ukiya, T. Akihisa, H. Tokuda et al., "Constituents of compositae plants. III. Anti-tumor promoting effects and cytotoxic activity against human cancer cell lines of triterpene diols and triols from edible chrysanthemum flowers," Cancer Letters, vol. 177, no. 1, pp. 7–12, 2002.

[8] K. A. B. S. da Silva, A. F. Paszcuk, G. F. Passos et al., "Activation of cannabinoid receptors by the pentacyclic triterpene α,β-amyrin inhibits inflammatory and neuropathic persistent pain in mice," Pain, vol. 152, no. 8, pp. 1872–1887, 2011.

[9] X. Niu, H. Yao, W. Li et al., "δ-Amyrone, a specific inhibitor of cyclooxygenase-2, exhibits anti-inflammatory effects in vitro and in vivo of mice," International Immunopharmacology, vol. 21, no. 1, pp. 112–118, 2014.

[10] A. L. Rüdiger and V. F. Veiga-Junior, "Chemodiversity of ursane- and oleanane-type triterpenes in amazonian burseraceae oleoresins," Chemistry & Biodiversity, vol. 10, no. 6, pp. 1142–1153, 2013.

[11] G. R. Nakayama, M. C. Caton, M. P. Nova, and Z. Parandoosh, "Assessment of the Alamar Blue assay for cellular growth and viability in vitro," Journal of Immunological Methods, vol. 204, no. 2, pp. 205–208, 1997.

[12] L. C. Green, D. A. Wagner, J. Glogowski, P. L. Skipper, J. S. Wishnok, and S. R. Tannenbaum, "Analysis of nitrate, nitrite, and [^{15}N]nitrate in biological fluids," Analytical Biochemistry, vol. 126, no. 1, pp. 131–138, 1982.

[13] M. M. Bradford, "A rapid and sensitive method for the quantitation of microgram quantities of protein utilizing the principle of protein-dye binding," Analytical Biochemistry, vol. 72, no. 1-2, pp. 248–254, 1976.

[14] C. A. Winter, E. A. Risley, and G. M. Nuss, "Carrageenin-induced edema in hind paw of the rat as an assay for anti-iflammatory drugs," Proceedings of the Society for Experimental Biology and Medicine, vol. 111, pp. 544–547, 1962.

[15] S. Kondo, S. H. Fujisawa, G. M. Shivji et al., "Interleukin-1 receptor antagonist suppresses contact hypersensitivity," Journal of Investigative Dermatology, vol. 105, no. 3, pp. 334–338, 1995.

[16] C. Nathan, "Nitric oxide as a secretory product of mammalian cells," The FASEB Journal, vol. 6, no. 12, pp. 3051–3064, 1992.

[17] Y.-J. Surh, J. K. Kundu, H.-K. Na, and J.-S. Lee, "Redox-sensitive transcription factors as prime targets for chemoprevention with anti-inflammatory and antioxidative phytochemicals," *Journal of Nutrition*, vol. 135, no. 12, pp. 2993–3001, 2005.

[18] R. Medeiros, M. F. Otuki, M. C. W. Avellar, and J. B. Calixto, "Mechanisms underlying the inhibitory actions of the pentacyclic triterpene α-amyrin in the mouse skin inflammation induced by phorbol ester 12-O-tetradecanoylphorbol-13-acetate," *European Journal of Pharmacology*, vol. 559, no. 2-3, pp. 227–235, 2007.

[19] F. A. Oliveira, M. H. Chaves, F. R. C. Almeida et al., "Protective effect of α- and β-amyrin, a triterpene mixture from *Protium heptaphyllum* (Aubl.) March. trunk wood resin, against acetaminophen-induced liver injury in mice," *Journal of Ethnopharmacology*, vol. 98, no. 1-2, pp. 103–108, 2005.

[20] A. C. Siani, M. F. S. Ramos, O. Menezes-De-Lima Jr. et al., "Evaluation of anti-inflammatory-related activity of essential oils from the leaves and resin of species of *Protium*," *Journal of Ethnopharmacology*, vol. 66, no. 1, pp. 57–69, 1999.

[21] G. Kojda and D. Harrison, "Interactions between NO and reactive oxygen species: pathophysiological importance in atherosclerosis, hypertension, diabetes and heart failure," *Cardiovascular Research*, vol. 43, no. 3, pp. 562–571, 1999.

[22] S. I. Abdelwahab, W. S. Koko, M. M. E. Taha et al., "In vitro and in vivo anti-inflammatory activities of columbin through the inhibition of cycloxygenase-2 and nitric oxide but not the suppression of NF-κB translocation," *European Journal of Pharmacology*, vol. 678, no. 1–3, pp. 61–70, 2012.

[23] S. J. Wimalawansa, "Nitric oxide: new evidence for novel therapeutic indications," *Expert Opinion on Pharmacotherapy*, vol. 9, no. 11, pp. 1935–1954, 2008.

[24] N. Verma, S. K. Tripathi, D. Sahu, H. R. Das, and R. H. Das, "Evaluation of inhibitory activities of plant extracts on production of LPS-stimulated pro-inflammatory mediators in J774 murine macrophages," *Molecular and Cellular Biochemistry*, vol. 336, no. 1-2, pp. 127–135, 2010.

[25] X.-F. Niu, X. Liu, L. Pan, and L. Qi, "Oleanene triterpenes from *Sedum lineare* Thunb," *Fitoterapia*, vol. 82, no. 7, pp. 960–963, 2011.

[26] G. Bonizzi and M. Karin, "The two NF-κB activation pathways and their role in innate and adaptive immunity," *Trends in Immunology*, vol. 25, no. 6, pp. 280–288, 2004.

[27] S. A. H. Pinto, L. M. S. Pinto, G. M. A. Cunha, M. H. Chaves, F. A. Santos, and V. S. Rao, "Anti-inflammatory effect of α, β-Amyrin, a pentacyclic triterpene from *Protium heptaphyllum* in rat model of acute periodontitis," *Inflammopharmacology*, vol. 16, no. 1, pp. 48–52, 2008.

[28] H. N. Ko, T.-H. Oh, J. S. Baik, C.-G. Hyun, S. S. Kim, and N. H. Lee, "Anti-inflammatory activities for the extracts and carpinontriols from branches of *Carpinus turczaninowii*," *International Journal of Pharmacology*, vol. 9, no. 2, pp. 157–163, 2013.

[29] D. R. Hodge, E. M. Hurt, and W. L. Farrar, "The role of IL-6 and STAT3 in inflammation and cancer," *European Journal of Cancer*, vol. 41, no. 16, pp. 2502–2512, 2005.

[30] S.-K. Yang, Y.-C. Wang, C.-C. Chao, Y.-J. Chuang, C.-Y. Lan, and B.-S. Chen, "Dynamic cross-talk analysis among TNF-R, TLR-4 and IL-1R signalings in TNFα-induced inflammatory responses," *BMC Medical Genomics*, vol. 3, article 19, 2010.

[31] S. W. Lee, B. R. Yun, M. H. Kim et al., "Phenolic compounds isolated from *Psoralea corylifolia* inhibit IL-6-induced STAT3 activation," *Planta Medica*, vol. 78, no. 9, pp. 903–906, 2012.

[32] H. Kuwata, Y. Watanabe, H. Miyoshi et al., "IL-10-inducible Bcl-3 negatively regulates LPS-induced TNF-α production in macrophages," *Blood*, vol. 102, no. 12, pp. 4123–4129, 2003.

[33] W. Chanput, J. Mes, R. A. M. Vreeburg, H. F. J. Savelkoul, and H. J. Wichers, "Transcription profiles of LPS-stimulated THP-1 monocytes and macrophages: a tool to study inflammation modulating effects of food-derived compounds," *Food & Function*, vol. 1, no. 3, pp. 254–261, 2010.

[34] B. Zdzisińska, W. Rzeski, R. Paduch et al., "Differential effect of betulin and betulinic acid on cytokine production in human whole blood cell cultures," *Polish Journal of Pharmacology*, vol. 55, no. 2, pp. 235–238, 2003.

[35] J. Tian, S. F. Kim, L. Hester, and S. H. Snyder, "S-nitrosylation/activation of COX-2 mediates NMDA neurotoxicity," *Proceedings of the National Academy of Sciences of the United States of America*, vol. 105, no. 30, pp. 10537–10540, 2008.

[36] A. Ganguly, Z. A. Mahmud, M. M. N. Uddin, and S. M. A. Rahman, "In-vivo anti-inflammatory and anti-pyretic activities of *Manilkara zapota* leaves in albino Wistar rats," *Asian Pacific Journal of Tropical Disease*, vol. 3, no. 4, pp. 301–307, 2013.

[37] H. Lim, H. Park, and H. P. Kim, "Inhibition of contact dermatitis in animal models and suppression of proinflammatory gene expression by topically applied flavonoid, wogonin," *Archives of Pharmacal Research*, vol. 27, no. 4, pp. 442–448, 2004.

[38] J. Mo, P. Panichayupakaranant, N. Kaewnopparat, S. Songkro, and W. Reanmongkol, "Topical anti-inflammatory potential of standardized pomegranate rind extract and ellagic acid in contact dermatitis," *Phytotherapy Research*, vol. 28, no. 4, pp. 629–632, 2014.

[39] J. L. Wilmer, F. G. Burleson, F. Kayama, J. Kanno, and M. I. Luster, "Cytokine induction in human epidermal keratinocytes exposed to contact irritants and its relation to chemical-induced inflammation in mouse skin," *Journal of Investigative Dermatology*, vol. 102, no. 6, pp. 915–922, 1994.

[40] R. A. Saraiva, M. K. A. Araruna, R. C. Oliveira et al., "Topical anti-inflammatory effect of *Caryocar coriaceum* Wittm. (Caryocaraceae) fruit pulp fixed oil on mice ear edema induced by different irritant agents," *Journal of Ethnopharmacology*, vol. 136, no. 3, pp. 504–510, 2011.

In Vitro Pharmacological Activities and GC-MS Analysis of Different Solvent Extracts of *Lantana camara* Leaves Collected from Tropical Region of Malaysia

Mallappa Kumara Swamy,[1] **Uma Rani Sinniah,**[1] **and Mohd. Sayeed Akhtar**[2]

[1]*Department of Crop Science, Faculty of Agriculture, Universiti Putra Malaysia (UPM), 43400 Serdang, Selangor, Malaysia*
[2]*Institute of Tropical Agriculture, Universiti Putra Malaysia (UPM), 43400 Serdang, Selangor, Malaysia*

Correspondence should be addressed to Mallappa Kumara Swamy; swamy.bio@gmail.com
and Uma Rani Sinniah; umarani@upm.edu.my

Academic Editor: Rahmatullah Qureshi

We investigated the effect of different solvents (ethyl acetate, methanol, acetone, and chloroform) on the extraction of phytoconstituents from *Lantana camara* leaves and their antioxidant and antibacterial activities. Further, GC-MS analysis was carried out to identify the bioactive chemical constituents occurring in the active extract. The results revealed the presence of various phytocompounds in the extracts. The methanol solvent recovered higher extractable compounds (14.4% of yield) and contained the highest phenolic (92.8 mg GAE/g) and flavonoid (26.5 mg RE/g) content. DPPH radical scavenging assay showed the IC_{50} value of 165, 200, 245, and 440 μg/mL for methanol, ethyl acetate, acetone, and chloroform extracts, respectively. The hydroxyl scavenging activity test showed the IC_{50} value of 110, 240, 300, and 510 μg/mL for methanol, ethyl acetate, acetone, and chloroform extracts, respectively. Gram negative bacterial pathogens (*E. coli* and *K. pneumoniae*) were more susceptible to all extracts compared to Gram positive bacteria (*M. luteus*, *B. subtilis*, and *S. aureus*). Methanol extract had the highest inhibition activity against all the tested microbes. Moreover, methanolic extract of *L. camara* contained 32 bioactive components as revealed by GC-MS study. The identified major compounds included hexadecanoic acid (5.197%), phytol (4.528%), caryophyllene oxide (4.605%), and 9,12,15-octadecatrienoic acid, methyl ester, (Z,Z,Z)- (3.751%).

1. Introduction

Nature has existed as a source of almost all drugs for many years and natural products were the only source of medicine for mankind ever since the ancient period. Herb based products play an important role in primary human health care as the majority (80%) of the global population rely on traditional medical practices [1, 2]. Most of the modern drugs are derived either from plant sources or from their derivatives for various medicaments and are extensively used in the pharma industry [2]. In addition to the prevailing health problems, emerging infectious diseases and disorders have seriously caused the world population to suffer with a high mortality rate. It is reported that about 50% of all fatality occurring in tropic countries is mainly due to the current infectious diseases [3]. Also, increase of antimicrobial resistance among the pathogens is a rising problem which is challenging the scientific advancement of the medical world [4]. This situation has prompted researchers to develop efficient new antimicrobial agents. Therefore, exploration of natural products as leads to discover new drug molecules is continuously made to understand their therapeutic potential with special reference to biological activities, efficiency, and safety aspects. Exploration of medicinal plants for curative purposes is mainly based on the available traditional information from the experts and local population [5, 6].

Lantana camara L. is a medicinal aromatic plant that belongs to the family Verbenaceae and occurs in most parts of the world as an evergreen notorious weed species. It is also considered as an ornamental garden plant. It is widely used in different traditional medical practices for treating various health problems. Different parts of the plant are used in treating various human ailments such as measles, chicken pox, tetanus, malaria, cancers, asthma, ulcers, fevers, eczema, skin rashes, cardiac disorders, and rheumatism [7, 8]. Also leaf extracts and essential oil of *L. camara* leaves possess larvicidal activities, antioxidant, anti-inflammatory, analgesic, antidiabetic, hypolipidemic, anthelmintic, wound healing, and antipyretic properties [9, 10]. The therapeutic potential of the plant is due to the occurrence of many bioactive phytocompounds such as terpenoids, alkaloids, flavonoids, phenolics, glycosides, and steroids as major phytoconstituents [11]. Some of the important bioactive compounds include quercetin, isorhamnetin, oleanolic acid, lantadene A, β-sitosterol pomonic acid, camaric acid, verbacosides, lantanoside, linaroside, octadecanoic acid, palmitic acid, and docosanoic acid. The essential oil from the leaves is rich in monoterpenes and sesquiterpenes [11–13]. Various factors including genetic, geographical location, plant parts, and environmental factors have been shown to influence the accumulation of phytochemical contents in different parts of *L. camara* and its essential oil composition [14–16]. Also, occurrence of varietal differences in phytoconstituents of *L. camara* has been documented by Sharma et al. [17]. More recently, in vitro study indicated the existence of chemical differences in methanol leaf extract of four varieties of *L. camara* collected from India and their antioxidant property was found to differ [8]. Certainly, more research efforts should be carried out to explore the potential benefits of *L. camara* for treating various health problems. Therefore, the present investigation was aimed at determining the phytochemical constituents and antioxidant and antimicrobial activities of different solvent extracts of *L. camara* leaves collected from the tropical region of Malaysia. Moreover, the bioactive components of the extracts were also identified using GC-MS analysis.

2. Materials and Methods

2.1. Plant Collection. *L. camara* plant material was collected from the forest area near Universiti Putra Malaysia, Serdang, Selangor, Malaysia, during the month of May 2015. Plant material was authenticated by N. A. P. Abdullah, Department of Crop Science, Universiti Putra Malaysia, Malaysia, and the voucher specimen (LC-102015) was deposited at the department. The leaves were detached from the collected materials, washed with water and dried under shade for 1 week, and finely powdered using electric blender. The powdered material was kept at room temperature for future use.

2.2. Preparation of Extracts. Five grams of powdered leaves was kept in a beaker to which 100 mL of various organic solvents (ethyl acetate, methanol, acetone, and chloroform) was added and thoroughly shaken. Later the mixture was placed at room temperature for 48 hrs and stirred 2-3 times a day. After filtering the mixture, the filtrate was evaporated to dryness using Rotavapor. The final extracts were weighed to determine the yield (%) and the dried extracts were stored at 4°C in a refrigerator for further studies.

2.3. Phytochemical Screening. The presence of various phytochemical constituents such as alkaloids, saponins, flavonoids, phenolics, anthraquinones, tannins, cardiac glycosides, steroids, and terpenoids was screened qualitatively by using standard procedures [18–20].

2.4. Determination of Total Phenolic and Flavonoid Contents. Total phenolic contents present in different solvent extracts were determined by using FC (Folin-Ciocalteu) colorimetric method as detailed by Salar and Seasotiya [21]. About 0.1 g of dried extract was suspended in 1 mL of the respective solvents and 0.1 mL of this solution was mixed thoroughly with 1 mL of sodium carbonate (20%) solution and 0.5 mL of 50% FC reagent. Thereafter, the solution was allowed to remain at room temperature for about 20 min to observe the color change. The absorbance was taken against the blank (water) at 730 nm. Using different concentrations of gallic acid, a standard calibration curve was generated. Total phenolic content was represented as mg of gallic acid equivalents (GAE) per gram of dried extract.

Total flavonoids content present in different solvent extracts was verified by the modified procedure of Zhishen et al. [22] using colorimeter. Briefly, 2 mL of distilled water was mixed well with 0.5 mL of solvent extract. Thereafter, 150 μL of $NaNO_2$ solution (5%) was added and kept for 5 min at room temperature. It was followed by adding 600 μL of $AlCl_3$ (10%) and 2 mL of NaOH (4%). After mixing thoroughly, the solution was made up to 5 mL with distilled water and set aside for 15 min at room temperature. By using water as blank, absorbance was measured at 510 nm. A standard calibration curve was generated using different concentrations of rutin. Total flavonoid content was articulated as mg of rutin equivalent (RE) per gram of dried extract.

2.5. Antioxidant Activity

2.5.1. Free Radical Scavenging Activity. The antioxidant activity of each extract was assessed using DPPH (1,1-diphenyl-2-picrylhydrazyl) free radical scavenging assay as explained by Mohanty et al. [23] with little modifications. In short, 0.3 mL of different extract at varied concentrations (100–1000 μg/mL) was mixed with 2 mL of 0.1 mM DPPH solution and incubated for 30 min under dark conditions at room temperature. Afterwards, using UV-visible spectrophotometer, the absorbance was taken at 517 nm against methanol (blank) while ascorbic acid served as a standard sample. The reaction mixture showing lower absorbance is an indication of higher activity of radical scavenging. The inhibition percentage of free radical scavenging was calculated based on the following formula:

$$\text{DPPH scavenging activity (\%)} = \frac{A\text{control} - A\text{sample}}{A\text{control}} \times 100. \tag{1}$$

For each extract, IC_{50} values (the minimum quantity of extract necessary for scavenging free radicals up to 50%) were calculated from the standard plot.

TABLE 1: Qualitative screening of phytochemicals present in different solvent extracts of *L. camara* leaves.

Phytochemicals	Ethyl acetate	Methanol	Chloroform	Acetone
Alkaloids	−	+	−	+
Flavonoids	+	+	+	+
Saponins	+	+	−	+
Phenolics	+	+	+	+
Tannins	−	−	+	−
Anthraquinones	+	−	−	+
Cardiac glycosides	+	+	+	+
Terpenoids	−	+	+	−
Steroids	−	+	−	−

Note: + = present, − = absent.

2.5.2. Hydrogen Peroxide (H_2O_2) Scavenging Activity. The potential capacity of different solvent extracts to scavenge H_2O_2 was carried out by the method outlined by Mohanty et al. [23]. In brief, various quantities of plant extract (100–1000 μg/mL) were prepared as detailed in previous experiment. By using phosphate buffer (pH 7.4), H_2O_2 solution (4 mM/L) was prepared. Varied amounts of plant extracts were mixed with 0.6 mL of H_2O_2 solution and kept for 30 min incubation at room temperature. The activity of H_2O_2 was analyzed by taking absorbance at 230 nm using phosphate buffer without H_2O_2 as blank solution. H_2O_2 scavenging activity (%) was calculated by using the following equation:

$$H_2O_2 \text{ scavenging activity } (\%)$$
$$= \frac{A\text{control} - A\text{sample}}{A\text{control}} \times 100. \quad (2)$$

For each extract, IC_{50} value (the minimum quantity of extract necessary for scavenging free radicals up to 50%) was calculated from the standard plot.

2.5.3. Determination of Antibacterial Activity. The antibacterial activities for the extracts were evaluated by using disc diffusion method. The experiment included both Gram positive (*Micrococcus luteus, Bacillus subtilis,* and *Staphylococcus aureus*) and Gram negative (*Escherichia coli* and *Klebsiella pneumoniae*) pathogenic strains of bacteria. One mg of each extract was dissolved in 1 mL of DMSO (dimethyl sulfoxide) and about 2.5, 5.0, and 10 μL of this solution were impregnated on sterilized filter paper discs (6 mm size). The discs were kept on the nutrient agar medium preinoculated uniformly with the known bacterial culture. The discs soaked with chloramphenicol (50 μL of 50 μg/mL) served as positive control while discs soaked with 50 μL DMSO served as negative control. All culture plates were kept in an incubator at 37°C for 24 h and the bacterial inhibition zone was recorded and expressed in mm. For each bacterial strain, the test was repeated 3 times.

2.6. GC-MS Analysis. GC-MS analysis of the active methanol extract of *L. camara* was carried out by using the GC-MS instrument (Model GCMS-QP2010 Ultra, Shimadzu Co., Japan) equipped with a capillary column DB-1 (0.25 μm film

× 0.25 mm i.d. × 30 m length). The instrument was operated in electron impact mode at ionization voltage (70 eV), injector temperature (230°C), and detector temperature (280°C). The carrier gas used was helium (99.9% purity) at a flow rate of 1 mL/min and about 1 μL of the sample was injected. The oven temperature was initially programmed at 80°C (isothermal for 5 min.) and then increased to 200°C at 5°C/min and finally to 280°C at 5°C/min (isothermal for 16 min). The identification of compounds from the spectral data was based on the available mass spectral records (NIST and WILEY libraries).

2.7. Statistical Analysis. All the data measured in each experiment included 3 replications ($n = 3$) and the results were represented as mean ± SD. The one-way analysis of variance (ANOVA) was performed to compare the data and Tukey's test was used to find out the statistically significant differences at $p < 0.05$ using statistical software, GraphPad Prism version 5.0.

3. Results and Discussion

The results of preliminary investigation on the phytochemicals present in different solvent extracts of *L. camara* are presented in Table 1. Different phytocompounds such as alkaloids, saponins, flavonoids, phenolics, anthraquinones, tannins, cardiac glycosides, steroids, and terpenoids were detected in the crude extracts. Flavonoids, phenolics, and cardiac glycosides were noticed in all solvent extracts used. Methanol extracts with 7 phytoconstituents were the best among the organic solvents evaluated in our study. Acetone extract showed the presence of 6 phytoconstituents while ethyl acetate and chloroform extracts contained 5 phytocompounds. All these identified phytochemicals are known to have a wide range of biological activities including antibacterial, antifungal, antiviral, antioxidant, and cytotoxic properties [19]. Understanding the occurrence of phytochemicals in medicinal plants is advantageous and presently, the discovery of new drug compounds or lead molecules from plants is mainly based on the systematic examination of different plant extracts or plant based products. Also, this preliminary knowledge can decipher a new source for economically valued chemical compounds [1, 23].

TABLE 2: Dry weight and total yield of different solvent extracts of *L. camara* leaves.

Solvent extracts	Weight of the extract (μg ± SD)	Yield (%)
Ethyl acetate	501.3 ± 3.5[b]	10.0
Methanol	721.3 ± 1.5[a]	14.4
Acetone	260.6 ± 4.0[c]	5.2
Chloroform	141.6 ± 2.5[d]	2.8

Note: each value is expressed as mean ± standard deviation (SD) (n = 3). Values in the column followed by a different letter superscript are significantly different ($p < 0.05$).

TABLE 3: Total phenolics and flavonoids content of different solvent extracts of *L. camara* leaves.

Solvent extracts	Total phenolic content (mg GAE/g) ± SD	Flavonoid content (mg RE/g) ± SD
Ethyl acetate	75.6 ± 0.9[b]	16.7 ± 0.6[c]
Methanol	92.8 ± 1.7[a]	26.5 ± 0.5[a]
Acetone	62.9 ± 1.7[c]	20.6 ± 0.3[b]
Chloroform	33.7 ± 0.5[d]	21.2 ± 0.8[b]

Note: each value is expressed as mean ± standard deviation (SD) (n = 3). Values in the column followed by a different letter superscript are significantly different ($p < 0.05$) and values having the same letters are not statistically significant ($p < 0.05$). GAE: gallic acid equivalent, RE: rutin equivalent.

The weight of the leaf extracts and their yield obtained from different solvent extracts of *L. camara* are presented in Table 2. Different solvents showed a significant influence on the total dry weight and yield of the extracts. Relatively, the extract from methanol resulted in superior extraction yield (14.4%) with 721.3 ± 1.5 μg of dry weight. The recovery of extractable constituents from different extracts remained in the following order of methanol > ethyl acetate > acetone > chloroform. Our results are in conformity with previous studies supporting the use of methanol as the best solvent to recover higher extractable compounds from various medicinal plants [23, 24]. Similarly, Anwar et al. [16] have stated that methanol as the best solvent for extraction from *L. camara*. Also, methanol was commonly employed by other researchers in *L. camara* for various biological studies [8, 25–27]. However, literature study shows that there are no available reports on the comparative yield analysis obtained from different solvent extracts till date. The existence of significant differences of dry weight of the extracts and yields between various organic solvents can be because of different polar nature of the solvents tested [24].

Polyphenols and flavonoids are the plant secondary metabolites occurring in several medicinal plants known to possess antimicrobial, antioxidant, antispasmodic, antidepressant, antitumor, antimutagenic, anti-inflammatory, and many other biological activities [27, 28]. In plants, these phenolic compounds provide defense against various pathogens, regulate cell division and growth, and help in pigmentation and many other metabolic pathways [29]. Therefore, we investigated the occurrence of total phenolic and flavonoid content in different organic solvent extracts (Table 3). The results clearly indicated the existence of statistically significant differences ($p < 0.05$) among the different extracts. The highest phenolic content (92.8±1.7 mg GAE/g) and flavonoid content (26.5 ± 0.5 mg RE/g) were observed in the methanol leaf extract of *L. camara*. On the other hand, ethyl acetate, acetone, and chloroform extract contained phenolic content of 75.6 ± 0.9, 62.9 ± 1.7, and 33.7 ± 0.5 mg GAE/g, respectively. Total flavonoid content in ethyl acetate, acetone, and chloroform extract was found to be 16.7 ± 0.6, 20.6 ± 0.3, and 21.2 ± 0.8 mg RE/g, respectively. Similarly, previous studies have shown the occurrence of rosmarinic and caffeic acid as the major phenolic compounds and few flavonoids such as 3,7-dimethoxy-, 3-methoxy-, and 3,7,4′-trimethoxy-quercetin, hispidulin, 3, pectolinarigenin 7-O-β-D-glucoside, and camaraside glycoside were evident in the plant extract

of *L. camara* [7, 11, 26]. Due to high polarity, methanol was found to exhibit better efficiency in extracting various polar phytocompounds (phenolics and flavonoids) from the leaves of *L. camara*. Both total phenolic and flavonoid contents obtained in our study were relatively much higher than the quantity obtained by earlier researchers in the same species but collected from geographically distant places [8, 16, 26]. However, total phenolic content was much lesser than the quantity (245.5 ± 3.5 mg gallic acid/g) as reported by Mahdi-Pour et al. [15] from methanol leaf extract of *L. camara* located in Kedah, Malaysia, and this difference can be attributed the influence of environmental factors and geographical location.

The formation of increased free radicals in human body may cause cell damage and induces various disorders such as cancer, myocardial infarction, atherosclerosis, and neurodegenerative disorders. However, antioxidant compounds derived from natural source or plants can repair these free radicals formed in cells and thereby, antioxidants are very useful in preventing various disorders [2, 15, 23]. The antioxidant capacities of either natural products or crude plant extracts are usually evaluated by making use of DPPH radical scavenging test [23]. In principal, the test depends on the capacity of DPPH free radicals reacting with plant metabolites such as phenolic and flavonoid compounds (H^+ donors) occurring in the sample. After the reaction, DPPH solution turns from purple to yellow color due to acquiring of a proton from the donor species. The intensity of color change directly relates to the scavenging ability of the biological sample [27]. Figure 1 shows the DPPH scavenging activity of *L. camara* leaf extracts in comparison to positive control (ascorbic acid). In all the solvent extracts, radical scavenging activity was found to be concentration dependent. The highest percentage of scavenging activity (86.4 ± 0.2 μg/mL) was observed in methanolic leaf extracts at 500 μg/mL concentration. The next best solvent extract was found to be acetone (80.5 ± 0.3 μg/mL) followed by ethyl acetate (72.4 ± 0.3 μg/mL) and chloroform (526.1 ± 0.3 μg/mL). However, the activities of all extracts were inferior to that of the ascorbic acid standard. The IC_{50} values of DPPH free radical scavenging activity were found to be in the following order: ascorbic acid (80 μg/mL) > methanol extract (165 μg/mL) > ethyl acetate (200 μg/mL) > acetone (245 μg/mL) > chloroform (440 μg/mL). These results are on a par with or even superior to that of reports by other researchers on several other crude extracts of the plant

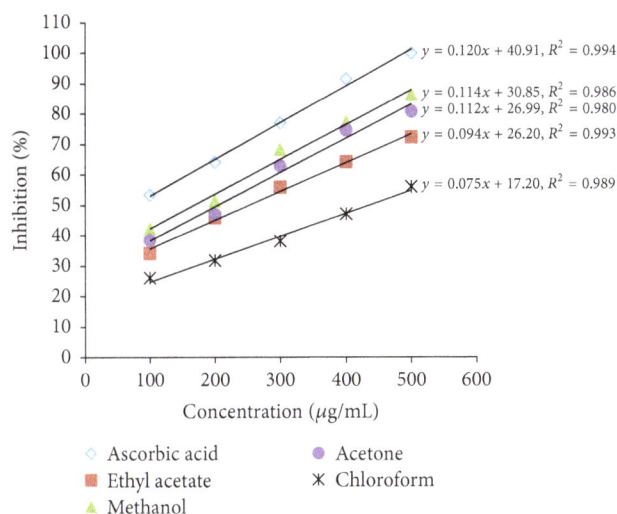

FIGURE 1: DPPH scavenging activities of various solvent extracts of *L. camara*.

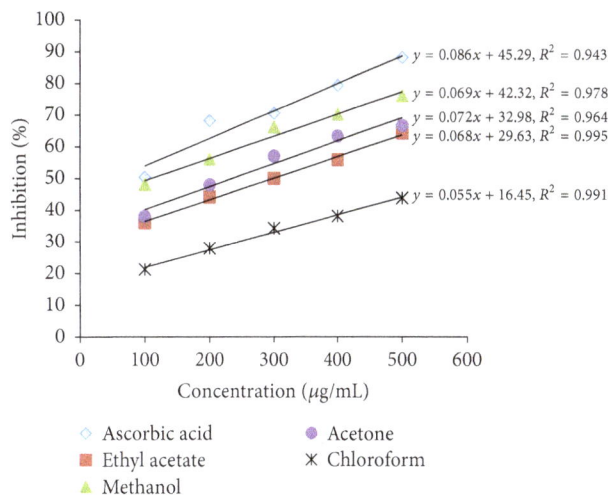

FIGURE 2: H$_2$O$_2$ scavenging activities of various solvent extracts of *L. camara*.

evaluated under the same conditions using DPPH assay [27]. The higher antioxidant potential of plant extracts is correlated to the occurrence of many antioxidant compounds especially polyphenols [23]. Although the antioxidant activity of *L. camara* leaf extracts by using DPPH assay was reported by earlier researchers [15, 16, 26], none of them compared the effects of different solvents on antioxidant potential. In our study, due to higher solubility of antioxidant compounds, the methanol extract exhibited increased radical scavenging activity compared to other solvent extracts. Similarly, other researchers have stated that free radical scavenging potential of plant extracts depends mainly on the occurrence of bioactive compounds, particularly polyphenols [8, 30].

In biological system, a large quantity of hydroxyl radicals is formed due to activation of immune cells which are known to be highly toxic radicals and causes extreme damage to all molecules occurring in live cells. These radicals can trigger cell toxicity and mutagenesis by damaging DNA nucleotides [8, 31]. Therefore, measuring hydroxyl radical scavenging activity can provide good information on the antioxidant potential of *L. camara* leaf extracts obtained by different solvents. The results of hydroxyl radicals inhibition obtained from our study are depicted in Figure 2. It is evident that, irrespective of the organic solvents used for extraction, the percent inhibition of hydroxyl radicals increased with the concentration of the extracts. At higher concentration of 500 μg/mL, the percentage of hydroxyl scavenging activity for ascorbic acid, ethyl acetate, methanol, acetone, and chloroform extracts was found to be 88.1 ± 0.4, 64.2 ± 1.0, 76 ± 0.3, 66.6 ± 0.5, and 43.7 ± 0.2%, respectively. The IC$_{50}$ value was found to be in the following order of ascorbic acid (60 μg/mL) > methanol (110 μg/mL) > ethyl acetate (240 μg/mL) > acetone (300 μg/mL) > chloroform (510 μg/mL). The lower the IC$_{50}$ value, the higher the scavenging activity and hence, methanol extract was found to possess superior antioxidant potential compared to other extracts tested. However, their effect was considerably lesser than the standard, ascorbic

acid. These results completely corroborate the earlier reports that have proved the existence of correlation between the antioxidant property and the concentration and composition of different plant metabolites occurring in the extracts [23, 32]. In our study, methanol extracts contained significantly higher quantity of phenolics (92.8 ± 1.7 mg GAE/g) and flavonoids (26.5 ± 0.5 mg RE/g) and hence possessed superior antioxidant potential compared to other solvent extracts.

At present, the increased prevalence of deadly diseases and microbes adapting to antibiotic resistance is a great concern in the medical world [33]. Hence, more research interest is shown by medical community towards the development or discovery of novel antimicrobial agents. Due to the severe side effects of several synthetic antibiotics, research preference is mainly focused on discovering plant based natural drugs [5, 34]. Since *L. camara* possessed numerous secondary metabolites, we evaluated the effects of their different solvent extracts against some common human pathogenic bacterial strains. The results of our study revealed that all solvent extracts of *L. camara* were effective against both Gram positive and Gram negative bacterial strains tested, but their efficacy varied (Table 4). With the increase in the concentration, there was an enhanced antibacterial activity irrespective of the solvent used for extraction. Gram negative bacteria were more susceptible to all extracts compared to Gram positive bacteria. In general, Gram negative bacteria are known to exhibit high resistance towards wide range of chemical agents and antibiotics compared to Gram positive bacteria. Besides, Gram negative bacteria are reported to be the most prevailing pathogens causing a large number of deaths [34, 35]. Thus, *L. camara* leaf extracts can be more beneficial in treating most of these Gram negative disease causing pathogens. Methanol extract had the highest inhibition activity against all the tested microbes when compared to any other solvent extracts. The methanol leaf extract exhibited the highest activity against *E. coli* (24.1 ± 0.4 mm) followed by *K. pneumoniae* (18.1 ± 0.4 mm) at higher concentration (10 μL/disc). *S. aureus* was also more vulnerable to methanol extract with 18.0 ± 0.4 mm

TABLE 4: Antibacterial activity of different solvent extracts of *L. camara* at different concentrations.

Solvent extracts (μL/disc)	Zone of inhibition (mm)				
	Escherichia coli	*Klebsiella pneumoniae*	*Micrococcus luteus*	*Bacillus subtilis*	*Staphylococcus aureus*
Ethyl acetate					
2.5	08.2 ± 0.8	06.9 ± 0.5	06.1 ± 0.7	10.0 ± 0.5	—
5.0	13.0 ± 0.9	08.3 ± 0.5	07.1 ± 0.3	13.8 ± 0.5	06.1 ± 0.1
10.0	12.0 ± 0.5	10.5 ± 0.8	07.0 ± 0.5	13.9 ± 0.4	10.6 ± 0.4
Methanol					
2.5	14.6 ± 0.5	08.2 ± 0.3	08.1 ± 0.7	10.0 ± 0.3	14.1 ± 0.2
5.0	18.2 ± 0.2	14.5 ± 0.5	12.2 ± 0.3	14.0 ± 0.6	16.1 ± 0.6
10.0	24.1 ± 0.4	18.1 ± 0.4	18.0 ± 0.5	16.1 ± 0.2	18.0 ± 0.4
Acetone					
2.5	16.1 ± 0.4	06.1 ± 0.6	07.9 ± 0.2	14.2 ± 0.3	05.8 ± 0.6
5.0	24.0 ± 0.4	10.1 ± 0.6	12.3 ± 0.2	15.9 ± 0.4	10.2 ± 0.2
10.0	28.2 ± 0.6	16.2 ± 0.2	12.2 ± 0.2	16.3 ± 0.4	12.2 ± 0.4
Chloroform					
2.5	10.6 ± 0.6	—	—	10.5 ± 0.9	—
5.0	12.9 ± 0.6	09.2 ± 0.2	06.8 ± 0.7	12.1 ± 0.7	07.2 ± 0.2
10.0	14.8 ± 0.3	11.4 ± 0.8	08.2 ± 0.2	12.4 ± 0.4	07.9 ± 0.2

Note: the negative control discs were soaked with 50 μL DMSO and the positive control discs with 50 μL (50 μg/mL) *chloramphenicol*. Each value represents the mean ± standard deviation (SD) of 3 replicates per treatment in 3 repeated experiments. "—" represents no activity.

of inhibition zone at 10 μL/disc concentration. Among the tested bacterial strains, *E. coli* and *B. subtilis* showed increased zone of inhibition to all the solvent extracts and were the most susceptible strains. Ethyl extract was also most effective against *B. subtilis* while other bacterial strains were moderately inhibited. Likewise, acetone and chloroform extracts were also effective in inhibiting *E. coli* and *B. subtilis*. However, at lower concentrations, ethyl acetate extract showed no inhibition against *S. aureus*. In contrast, chloroform extract was less effective to all bacteria and at lower concentration, it failed to show antibacterial activity. *L. camara* finds its application in many parts of the world to cure various human ailments [7]. Previously, researchers have reported the varied antimicrobial potential of this plant and thus our reports support these findings [13, 14]. These results substantiate the findings of Naz and Bano [26] where methanol extract of *L. camara* leaves showed the highest antimicrobial activity. However, this is the first ever attempt which emphasizes the influence of different solvent extracts on human pathogenic bacterial strains. Our study clearly indicated the existence of considerable differences in the antibacterial activity among the various solvent extracts evaluated. This could be due to varied phytochemical constituents present in different solvent extracts.

Further, we used GC-MS analysis to identify the bioactive compounds occurring in the most competent solvent extract of *L. camara*. GC-MS profiling was performed only for methanolic leaf extract due to the fact that it contained many phytochemicals and exhibited superior biological activities. The distinctive chromatogram of the methanolic leaf extract of *L. camara* is shown in Figure 3. The analysis separated and identified a total of 32 known compounds belonging to different chemical classes (Table 5). The major compounds

included hexadecanoic acid (5.197%), phytol (4.528%), caryophyllene oxide (4.605%), 9,12,15-octadecatrienoic acid, methyl ester, (Z,Z,Z)- (3.751%), 2,3-dihydro-2,5-dihydroxy-6-methyl-4H-pyran-4-one (2.954%), α-D-galactopyranoside, methyl (2.790%), coumaran (2.288%), germacrene-D (2.185%), bicyclo[5.2.0]nonane, 2-methylene-4,8,8-trimethyl (2.065%), spathulenol (1.888%), 1,2,3-propanetriol, 1-acetate (1.689%), propane-1,2,3-triol (1.1615), and 2,4(1H,3H)-pyrimidinedione, 5-methyl- (1.180%). Few other compounds identified in the extract are α-elemol, myristic acid, neophytadiene, furfuryl alcohol, propargyl alcohol, and acetic acid, fluoro-, ethyl ester. Many of these identified constituents are known to possess several pharmacological activities. Hexadecanoic acid, a major phytoconstituent of *L. camara* methanolic leaf extract, is known to possess strong antimicrobial activity [36]. The diterpene, phytol, is an important compound reported with antioxidant, cytotoxic, and antimicrobial properties [37]. Similarly a conjugated saponin, 2,3-dihydro-2,5-dihydroxy-6-methyl-4H-pyran-4-one, is reported to possess strong antioxidant, anticancer, and anti-inflammatory properties [38, 39]. Caryophyllene oxide, spathulenol, and germacrene-D are known to possess anticarcinogenic, anti-inflammatory, and antibacterial properties [2, 40]. As a biofumigant, coumaran is reported to act against insect pests found in stored food grains [41]. The compound 2,3-dihydro-2,5-dihydroxy-6-methyl-4H-pyran-4-one has been reported in plant extracts exhibiting antioxidant, antiproliferative, and anti-inflammatory properties [40]. More recently, anti-inflammatory and cytotoxicity activities of hexadecanoic acid, methyl ester have been reported by Othman et al. [42]. However, pharmacological activities of other compounds of *L. camara* methanolic leaf extract are yet to be determined. Therefore, we assume that the strong bioactivities exhibited

Total ion current (TIC) chromatogram

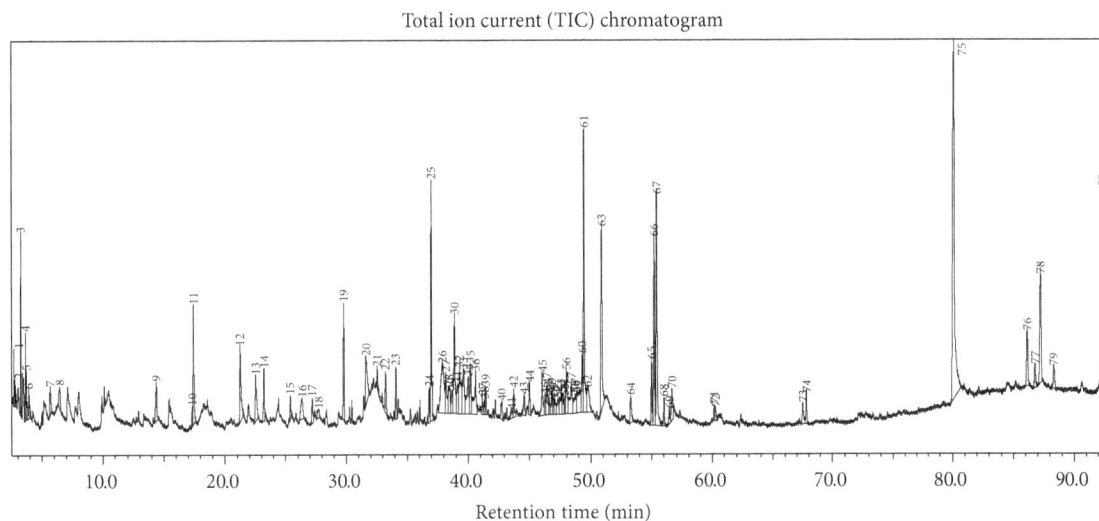

FIGURE 3: GC-MS chromatograph of methanolic leaf extract of *L. camara*.

TABLE 5: The major phytocompounds detected in the methanolic leaf extract of *L. camara* by GC-MS analysis.

S. number	Name of the compound	Peak number[*]	Retention time (min)	Area (%)
1	2-Propanone, 1-hydroxy-	1	2.703	0.481
2	Propane-1,2,3-triol	3	3.275	1.161
3	Propargyl alcohol	4	3.653	0.877
4	Acetic acid, fluoro-, ethyl ester	5	3.719	0.737
5	Furfuryl alcohol	7	5.672	0.750
6	2,4(1H,3H)-Pyrimidinedione, 5-methyl-	9	14.366	1.180
7	2,3-Dihydro-2,5-dihydroxy-6-methyl-4H-pyran-4-one	11	17.443	2.954
8	Coumaran	12	21.251	2.288
9	1,2,3-Propanetriol, 1-acetate	13	22.529	1.689
10	Cyclohexasiloxane, dodecamethyl-	14	23.200	0.978
11	4-Vinylguaiacol	15	25.393	0.809
12	Bicyclo[5.2.0]nonane, 2-methylene-4,8,8-trimethyl	19	29.798	2.065
13	Germacrene-D	21	32.547	2.185
14	Longifolene	22	33.22	0.889
15	4-Epi-cubedol	23	34.084	0.817
16	Caryophyllene oxide	25	36.995	4.605
17	α-D-Galactopyranoside, methyl	26	37.909	2.790
18	Humulene epoxide II	27	38.173	0.696
19	Spathulenol	30	38.886	1.888
20	α-Elemol	34	39.997	0.507
21	Myristic acid	42	43.751	0.652
22	Neophytadiene	45	46.059	0.820
23	3-Eicosyne	53	47.594	0.211
24	9-Octadecenoic acid (Z)-, methyl ester	60	49.296	0.093
25	Hexadecanoic acid, methyl ester	61	49.438	0.696
26	Hexadecanoic acid	63	50.888	5.197
27	9,12-Octadecadienoic acid (Z,Z)-, methyl ester	65	55.007	1.037
28	9,12,15-Octadecatrienoic acid, methyl ester, (Z,Z,Z)-	66	55.225	3.751
29	Phytol	67	55.426	4.528
30	Octadecanoic acid, methyl ester	68	56.428	0.330
31	9,12,15-Octadecatrienoic acid, (Z,Z,Z)-	70	56.640	1.019
32	Phthalic acid, di(2-propylpentyl) ester	74	67.804	0.688

[*]Peak number is represented in Figure 3.

by *L. camara* in this study are correlated to the occurrence of these bioactive compounds in the methanol solvent extract. However, further studies on the isolation, characterization, and biological evaluation of these identified compounds are necessary to confirm their potential benefits.

4. Conclusion

In conclusion, the present investigation clearly revealed that phytochemical composition of *L. camara* leaf extract varied with respect to different solvents. Total phenolic and flavonoid content significantly varied among the different solvent extracts. Methanol solvent extract of *L. camara* leaves contained more extractable metabolites compared to any other solvents. Moreover, all solvent extracts of *L. camara* showed considerable antioxidant and antimicrobial activity with varying differences due to differences in their phytochemical composition. Thus, our study suggests that methanol leaf extract of *L. camara* containing many bioactive compounds may possibly be utilized as a therapeutic source for developing beneficial drugs to manage various human diseases and disorders.

Disclosure

Mohd. Sayeed Akhtar is a coauthor.

Conflict of Interests

The authors declare that there is no conflict of interests.

Acknowledgments

The authors are highly grateful to the Department of Crop Science, Universiti Putra Malaysia, Malaysia, for providing research facilities and the Department of Biosciences, Universiti Putra Malaysia, Malaysia, for GC-MS analysis.

References

[1] Z. Gezahegn, M. S. Akhtar, D. Woyessa, and Y. Tariku, "Antibacterial potential of *Thevetia peruviana* leaf extracts against food associated bacterial pathogens," *Journal of Coastal Life Medicine*, vol. 3, no. 2, pp. 150–157, 2015.

[2] M. K. Swamy and U. R. Sinniah, "A Comprehensive review on the phytochemical constituents and pharmacological activities of Pogostemon cablin Benth.: an Aromatic Medicinal Plant of Industrial Importance," *Molecules*, vol. 20, no. 5, pp. 8521–8547, 2015.

[3] D. A. Lobo, R. Velayudhan, P. Chatterjee, H. Kohli, and P. J. Hotez, "The neglected tropical diseases of India and South Asia: review of their prevalence, distribution, and control or elimination," *PLoS Neglected Tropical Diseases*, vol. 5, no. 10, Article ID e1222, 2011.

[4] R. C. Moellering Jr., J. R. Graybill, J. E. McGowan Jr., and L. Corey, "Antimicrobial resistance prevention initiative-an update: proceedings of an expert panel on resistance," *American Journal of Infection Control*, vol. 35, no. 9, p. -S23, 2007.

[5] I. M. Ayoub, M. El-Shazly, M.-C. Lu, and A. N. B. Singab, "Antimicrobial and cytotoxic activities of the crude extracts of Dietes bicolor leaves, flowers and rhizomes," *South African Journal of Botany*, vol. 95, pp. 97–101, 2014.

[6] S. K. Mohanty, K. Malappa, A. Godavarthi, B. Subbanarasiman, and A. Maniyam, "Evaluation of antioxidant, in vitro cytotoxicity of micropropagated and naturally grown plants of Leptadenia reticulata (Retz.) Wight & Arn.-an endangered medicinal plant," *Asian Pacific Journal of Tropical Medicine*, vol. 7, no. 1, pp. S267–S271, 2014.

[7] E. L. Ghisalberti, "*Lantana camara* L. (Verbenaceae)," *Fitoterapia*, vol. 71, no. 5, pp. 467–486, 2000.

[8] S. Kumar, R. Sandhir, and S. Ojha, "Evaluation of antioxidant activity and total phenol in different varieties of *Lantana camara* leaves," *BMC Research Notes*, vol. 7, no. 1, p. 560, 2014.

[9] S. Patel, "A weed with multiple utility: lantana camara," *Reviews in Environmental Science and Biotechnology*, vol. 10, no. 4, pp. 341–351, 2011.

[10] T. Venkatachalam, V. K. Kumar, P. K. Selvi, A. O. Maske, and N. S. Kumar, "Physicochemical and preliminary phytochemical studies on the *Lantana camara* (L.) fruits," *International Journal of Pharmacy and Pharmaceutical Sciences*, vol. 3, no. 1, pp. 52–54, 2011.

[11] J. A. Parrotta, *Healing Plants of Peninsular India*, CABI International, New York, NY, USA, 2001.

[12] S. B. Yadav and V. Tripathi, "A new triterpenoid from Lantana camara," *Fitoterapia*, vol. 74, no. 3, pp. 320–321, 2003.

[13] A. Saraf, S. Quereshi, K. Sharma, and N. A. Khan, "Antimicrobial activity of *Lantana camara* L.," *Journal of Experimental Sciences*, vol. 2, no. 10, pp. 50–54, 2011.

[14] D. Ganjewala, S. Sam, and K. Hayat Khan, "Biochemical compositions and antibacterial activities of *Lantana camara* plants with yellow, lavender, red and white flowers," *EurAsian Journal of Biosciences*, vol. 3, no. 10, pp. 69–77, 2009.

[15] B. Mahdi-Pour, S. L. Jothy, L. Y. Latha, Y. Chen, and S. Sasidharan, "Antioxidant activity of methanol extracts of different parts of Lantana camara," *Asian Pacific Journal of Tropical Biomedicine*, vol. 2, no. 12, pp. 960–965, 2012.

[16] F. Anwar, N. Shaheen, G. Shabir, M. Ashraf, K. M. Alkharfy, and A.-H. Gilani, "Variation in antioxidant activity and phenolic and flavonoid contents in the flowers and leaves of Ghaneri (*Lantana camara* L.) as affected by different extraction solven," *International Journal of Pharmacology*, vol. 9, no. 7, pp. 442–453, 2013.

[17] O. P. Sharma, J. Vaid, and P. D. Sharma, "Comparison of lantadenes content and toxicity of different taxa of the lantana plant," *Journal of Chemical Ecology*, vol. 17, no. 11, pp. 2283–2291, 1991.

[18] J. B. Harborne, *Phytochemical Methods*, Chapman & Hall, London, UK, 1998.

[19] N. Pokharen, S. Dahal, and M. Anuradha, "Phytochemical and antimicrobial studies of leaf extract of *Euphorbia neriifolia*," *Journal of Medicinal Plants Research*, vol. 5, no. 24, pp. 5785–5788, 2011.

[20] M. Kumara Swamy, K. M. Sudipta, P. Lokesh et al., "Phytochemical screening and in vitro antimicrobial activity of *Bougainvillea spectabilis* flower extracts," *International Journal of Phytomedicine*, vol. 4, no. 3, pp. 375–379, 2012.

[21] R. K. Salar and L. Seasotiya, "Free radical scavenging activity, phenolic contents and phytochemical evaluation of different extracts of stem bark of *Butea monosperma* (Lam.) kuntze," *Frontiers in Life Science*, vol. 5, no. 3-4, pp. 107–116, 2011.

[22] J. Zhishen, T. Mengcheng, and W. Jianming, "The determination of flavonoid contents in mulberry and their scavenging effects on superoxide radicals," *Food Chemistry*, vol. 64, no. 4, pp. 555–559, 1999.

[23] S. K. Mohanty, K. Malappa, A. Godavarthi, B. Subbanarasiman, and A. Maniyam, "Evaluation of antioxidant, in vitro cytotoxicity of micropropagated and naturally grown plants of *Leptadenia reticulata* (Retz.) Wight & Arn.-an endangered medicinal plant," *Asian Pacific Journal of Tropical Medicine*, vol. 7, supplement 1, pp. S267–S271, 2014.

[24] B. Sultana, F. Anwar, and M. Ashraf, "Effect of extraction solvent/technique on the antioxidant activity of selected medicinal plant extracts," *Molecules*, vol. 14, no. 6, pp. 2167–2180, 2009.

[25] D. Bhakta and D. Ganjewala, "Effect of leaf positions on total phenolics, flavonoids and proanthocyanidins content and antioxidant activities in *Lantana camara* (L)," *Journal of Scientific Research*, vol. 1, no. 2, pp. 363–369, 2009.

[26] R. Naz and A. Bano, "Phytochemical screening, antioxidants and antimicrobial potential of *Lantana camara* in different solvents," *Asian Pacific Journal of Tropical Disease*, vol. 3, no. 6, pp. 480–486, 2013.

[27] C. L. Apetrei, C. Tuchilus, A. C. Aprotosoaie, A. Oprea, K. E. Malterud, and A. Miron, "Chemical, antioxidant and antimicrobial investigations of *Pinus cembra* L. bark and needles," *Molecules*, vol. 16, no. 9, pp. 7773–7788, 2011.

[28] A. Ghasemzadeh and N. Ghasemzadeh, "Flavonoids and phenolic acids: role and biochemical activity in plants and human," *Journal of Medicinal Plant Research*, vol. 5, no. 31, pp. 6697–6703, 2011.

[29] V. Lattanzio, V. M. Lattanzio, and A. Cardinali, "Role of phenolics in the resistance mechanisms of plants against fungal pathogens and insects," *Phytochemistry: Advances in Research*, vol. 661, pp. 23–67, 2006.

[30] J. Dai and R. J. Mumper, "Plant phenolics: extraction, analysis and their antioxidant and anticancer properties," *Molecules*, vol. 15, no. 10, pp. 7313–7352, 2010.

[31] R. Manian, N. Anusuya, P. Siddhuraju, and S. Manian, "The antioxidant activity and free radical scavenging potential of two different solvent extracts of *Camellia sinensis* (L.) O. Kuntz, *Ficus bengalensis* L. and *Ficus racemosa* L.," *Food Chemistry*, vol. 107, no. 3, pp. 1000–1007, 2008.

[32] P. Kuppusamy, M. M. Yusoff, N. R. Parine, and N. Govindan, "Evaluation of in-vitro antioxidant and antibacterial properties of *Commelina nudiflora* L. extracts prepared by different polar solvents," *Saudi Journal of Biological Sciences*, vol. 22, no. 3, pp. 293–301, 2015.

[33] E. M. Tekwu, A. C. Pieme, and V. P. Beng, "Investigations of antimicrobial activity of some Cameroonian medicinal plant extracts against bacteria and yeast with gastrointestinal relevance," *Journal of Ethnopharmacology*, vol. 142, no. 1, pp. 265–273, 2012.

[34] K. Canli, E. M. Altuner, and I. Akata, "Antimicrobial screening of *Mnium stellare*," *Bangladesh Journal of Pharmacology*, vol. 10, no. 2, pp. 321–325, 2015.

[35] M. V. Villegas and J. P. Quinn, "An update on antibiotic-resistant gram-negative bacteria," *Infections in Medicine*, vol. 21, no. 12, pp. 595–599, 2004.

[36] R. Preethi, V. V. Devanathan, and M. Loganathan, "Antimicrobial and antioxidant efficacy of some medicinal plants against food borne pathogens," *Advances in Biological Research*, vol. 4, no. 2, pp. 122–125, 2010.

[37] L. S. Wei, W. Wee, J. Y. F. Siong, and D. F. Syamsumir, "Characterization of anticancer, antimicrobial, antioxidant properties and chemical compositions of *Peperomia pellucida* leaf extract," *Acta Medica Iranica*, vol. 49, no. 10, pp. 670–674, 2011.

[38] J. O. Ban, I. G. Hwang, T. M. Kim et al., "Anti-proliferate and pro-apoptotic effects of 2,3-Dihydro-3,5- dihydroxy-6-methyl-4Hpyranone through inactivation of NF-κB in human colon cancer cells," *Archives of Pharmacal Research*, vol. 30, pp. 1455–1463, 2007.

[39] N. Sharma, K. W. Samarakoon, R. Gyawali et al., "Evaluation of the antioxidant, anti-inflammatory, and anticancer activities of Euphorbia hirta ethanolic extract," *Molecules*, vol. 19, no. 9, pp. 14567–14581, 2014.

[40] A. I. Hussain, F. Anwar, S. T. H. Sherazi, and R. Przybylski, "Chemical composition, antioxidant and antimicrobial activities of basil (*Ocimum basilicum*) essential oils depends on seasonal variations," *Food Chemistry*, vol. 108, no. 3, pp. 986–995, 2008.

[41] Y. Rajashekar, A. Raghavendra, and N. Bakthavatsalam, "Acetylcholinesterase inhibition by biofumigant (Coumaran) from leaves of *Lantana camara* in stored grain and household insect pests," *BioMed Research International*, vol. 2014, Article ID 187019, 6 pages, 2014.

[42] A. Othman, N. Abdullah, S. Ahmad, I. Ismail, and M. Zakaria, "Elucidation of in-vitro anti-inflammatory bioactive compounds isolated from *Jatropha curcas* L. plant root," *BMC Complementary and Alternative Medicine*, vol. 15, no. 1, p. 11, 2015.

6

Effects of *Cordyceps sinensis* on the Expressions of NF-κB and TGF-β1 in Myocardium of Diabetic Rats

You-you Gu,[1] Huan Wang,[2,3] Su Wang,[1] Hua Gao,[4] and Ming-cai Qiu[4]

[1]*Department of Endocrinology, The Fifth Central Hospital of Tianjin, Tianjin 300450, China*
[2]*Community Health Service Center of Hu Jiayuan Street, Binhai New District, Tianjin 300454, China*
[3]*Graduate School of Tianjin Medical University, Tianjin 300070, China*
[4]*Department of Endocrinology, General Hospital of Tianjin Medical University, Tianjin 300052, China*

Correspondence should be addressed to Su Wang; wsrealm@126.com

Academic Editor: Ken Yasukawa

Objective. To investigate the effect of *Cordyceps sinensis* (CS) on the expressions of NF-κB and TGF-β1 in myocardium of streptozotocin-induced diabetic rats. *Methods.* A total of 53 healthy male SD rats, mice age of 8 weeks and weight of 220 ± 20 g, were randomly divided into five groups by randomized block design: normal control group ($n = 10$), diabetic group ($n = 10$), low dose of CS group ($n = 12$; CS $0.6 \, \text{g·kg}^{-1}\text{·d}^{-1}$), middle dose of CS group ($n = 11$; CS $2.5 \, \text{g·kg}^{-1}\text{·d}^{-1}$), and high dose of CS group ($n = 10$; CS $5 \, \text{g·kg}^{-1}\text{·d}^{-1}$). The diabetic models with tail intravenous injection by streptozotocin ($45 \, \text{mg·kg}^{-1}$). Diabetic rats were sacrificed after 8 weeks; the expressions of NF-κB and TGF-β1 proteins and mRNA in the cardiac muscle were determined by using immunohistochemistry staining and reverse transcription polymerase chain reaction (RT-PCR) method. The data were analyzed using one factor analysis of variance. *Result.* The expressions of NF-κB and TGF-β1 proteins and mRNA in the cardiac muscle of diabetic rats were significantly raised ($P < 0.05$), which could be decreased by CS ($P < 0.05$). *Conclusions.* The changes on the expressions of NF-κB and TGF-β1 in myocardium may be involved in the occurrence of diabetic cardiomyopathy (DC). CS may play its role on myocardial protection by regulating the expressions of NF-κB and TGF-β1 in myocardium.

1. Introduction

Chronic complications of diabetes mellitus (DM) can drag in whole body organs. DC is the specific lesions of the diabetic cardiac injury, and the primary pathological features are cardiomyocyte hypertrophy, dissolution and destruction of muscle fibers, loss of muscle horizontal stripes, hyaline degeneration, interstitial fibrosis, and inflammatory cell infiltration; however, its mechanism is still unclear. Recent studies showed that immune response and low-grade inflammation was closely associated with DM and DC, and the generation of inflammatory factor was the result of immune response. Recent research has found that the abnormal expressions of NF-κB and TGF-β1 may participate in the occurrence of DC [1, 2]. Previous evidence suggested that streptozotocin induced diabetic rats had multiorgan immune damage, and immunosuppressive therapy can reduce the immune organ damage [3]. Immunosuppressant has many side effects, such as hepatic and renal toxicity and elevated blood pressure, so we should actively seek an effective therapeutic schedule which has smaller side effects. CS, also called Dong Chong Xia Cao (winter worm summer grass) in Chinese, is one of the most valued herbs in traditional Chinese medicine [4]. Yang et al. [5] consider that CS have strong inhibitory effect to immune function on body. In our research, we used CS to intervene in streptozotocin-induced diabetic rats and observed the effects of CS on the expressions of NF-κB and TGF-β1 in myocardium of diabetic rats, and whether CS have myocardial protection of diabetic rats was evaluated.

2. Materials and Methods

2.1. Experimental Material. A total of 53 healthy male SD rats, mice age of 8 weeks and weight of 220 ± 20 g, were purchased from Beijing Experimental Animal Center of

Chinese Academy of Sciences (China). CS was provided by Jiangxi Jimin Trusted Pharmaceutical Co., Ltd. (China). CS was dissolved in distilled water, with concentration of 0.5 g/mL solution. Streptozotocin was purchased from Sigma company in the United States. Rabbit anti-rat NF-κB, TGF-β1, and PV-6001 immunohistochemical detection kit were bought from Wuhan Boster Biological Engineering Co., Ltd. (China). Reverse transcription-polymerase chain reaction (RT-PCR) primer was compounded by Nanjing Genscript Biotechnology Co., Ltd. (China). NF-κB primer: sense 5′-CTGC GACA GATG GGCT ACAC-3′; antisense 5′-GGAA CGAT ATGA TGGC CTTTC-3′; product length 361 bp. TGF-β1 primer: Sense 5′-ACCC TTCC TGCT CCTC ATGG-3′; antisense 5′-AGCG CACG ATCA TGTT GGAC-3′; product length 392 bp. β-actin primer: sense 5′-TAAA GGGC ATCC TGGG CTAC ACTG-3′; antisense 5′-TTAC TCCT TGGA GGCC ATGT AGG-3′; product length 199 bp.

2.2. Rat Diabetes Model. All rats were randomly divided into five groups by randomized block design: normal control group ($n = 10$), diabetic group ($n = 10$), low dose of CS group ($n = 12$; CS 0.6 g·kg^{-1}·d^{-1}), middle dose of CS group ($n = 11$; CS 2.5 g·kg^{-1}·d^{-1}), and high dose of CS group ($n = 10$; CS 5 g·kg^{-1}·d^{-1}). The diabetic models with tail intravenous injection by streptozotocin (45 mg·kg^{-1}), and normal control rats were injected with 0.1 M sodium citrate buffer. Blood samples were taken 7 days after the injection of streptozotocin or sodium citrate buffer, and rats with glucose level >16.7 mmol/L were considered diabetic. Normal control group and diabetic group used gavage with equivalent drinking water every day, and three CS groups used gavage with CS solution of different concentration. All rats were sacrificed after 8 weeks. The myocardium was separated and cut into two sections: the first section was fixed in 10% buffered formalin for hematoxylin eosin (HE) staining, Masson's trichome staining, and immunohistochemistry staining; the second section was stored at −80°C for RT-PCR.

2.3. HE Staining, Masson's Trichome Staining, and Immunohistochemistry Staining. HE staining, Masson's trichome staining, and immunohistochemistry staining used conventional paraffin embedding tissue and 5 μm thick serial section. The ABC method was adopted to detect expressions of NF-κB and TGF-β1 protein in myocardium. The dilute concentration of NF-κB and TGF-β1 was 1 : 100 and 1 : 50. The position of positive reaction in image was analyzed with accumulative optical density value by the Image-Pro Plus 6.0.

2.4. RT-PCR. Tatal RNA 1 ug was prepared, and RNA was reverse transcribed into cDNA. NF-κB reaction conditions were 94°C degeneration for 30 s, 67°C annealing for 30 s, 72°C extension for 40 s, and 35 cycles. TGF-β1 reaction conditions were 94°C degeneration for 30 s, 67°C annealing for 30 s, 72°C extension for 40 s, and 35 cycles. β-actin reaction conditions were 94°C degeneration for 40 s, 50°C annealing for 40 s, 72°C extension for 40 s, and 35 cycles. Amplification products were sequenced, and the images of agarose electrophoresis gel were acquired. The relative expression level of mRNA was

calculated, and the calculating formula was as follows: the relative expression level of mRNA = absorbance values of objective stripe/absorbance values of β-actin.

2.5. Statistical Analysis. The data was represented in mean ± standard deviation. The data were analyzed using one factor analysis of variance by SPSS17.0. The P value < 0.05 was statistically significant.

3. Result

3.1. Pathological Features of Myocardium in Diabetic Rats. The results of HE staining showed us that myocardial of normal control group rats had no obvious abnormalities. However, cardiomyocyte hypertrophy, myofiber dissolution and damage, loss of muscle horizontal stripes, and inflammatory cell infiltration were observed in myocardial of diabetic group (Figure 1). Masson's trichome staining revealed an increased collagen accumulation in myocardial intercellular substance and around blood vessels of streptozotocin-induced diabetic rats compared with normal control rats (Figure 1). Compared with diabetes group, quantification of inflammatory cell and collagen accumulation in the CS treatment groups were decreased ($P < 0.05$) (Figure 1).

3.2. NF-κB and TGF-β1 Protein Expressions by Immunohistochemistry. There was a little expression of the NF-κB and TGF-β1 protein in myocardial cell of normal control group rats. The expressions of NF-κB and TGF-β1 in myocardial cell of diabetic rats were significantly increased ($P < 0.05$) compared with normal control group rats. Compared with diabetes group, the expressions of NF-κB and TGF-β1 in the CS treatment groups were decreased ($P < 0.05$), and the expressions of NF-κB and TGF-β1 were reduced gradually with the increase of CS dose (Figure 2).

3.3. NF-κB and TGF-β1 mRNA Expressions by RT-PCR. The amplification products of NF-κB and TGF-β1 conformed to the gene sequence by sequencing analysis. In normal control group, a little expression of the NF-κB and TGF-β1 mRNA was shown in cardiac muscle cell. Compared with normal control group, the expressions of NF-κB and TGF-β1 were significantly increased in myocardial cell of diabetic rats ($P < 0.05$). The expressions of NF-κB and TGF-β1 in the CS treatment groups were decreased compared with diabetes group ($P < 0.05$), and the expressions of NF-κB and TGF-β1 were reduced gradually with the increase of CS dose (Figure 3).

4. Discussion

DC is the specific lesions of the diabetic cardiac injury, and the primary pathological features are cardiomyocyte hypertrophy, dissolution and destruction of muscle fibers, loss of muscle horizontal stripes, hyaline degeneration, interstitial fibrosis, and inflammatory cell infiltration. So far, DC pathogenesis has not been fully elucidated. Glucose and lipid metabolism disorder, insulin resistance, oxidative

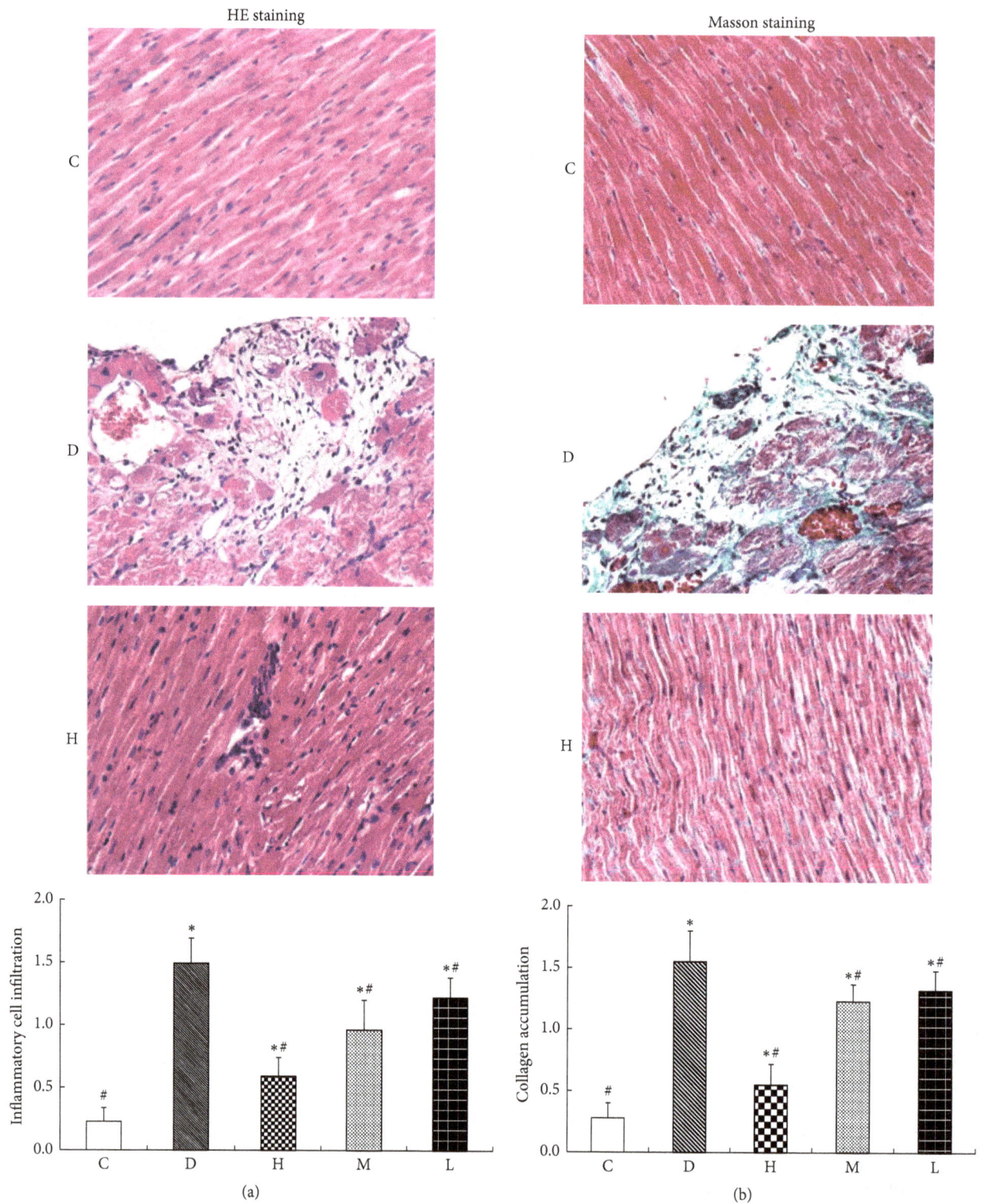

FIGURE 1: Pathological features of myocardium in diabetic rats. (a) HE staining; (b) Masson staining; C: normal control group; D: diabetic group; H: high dose of CS group; M: middle dose of CS; L: low dose of CS group. Compared with group C, $^{*}P < 0.05$; compared with group D, $^{#}P < 0.05$.

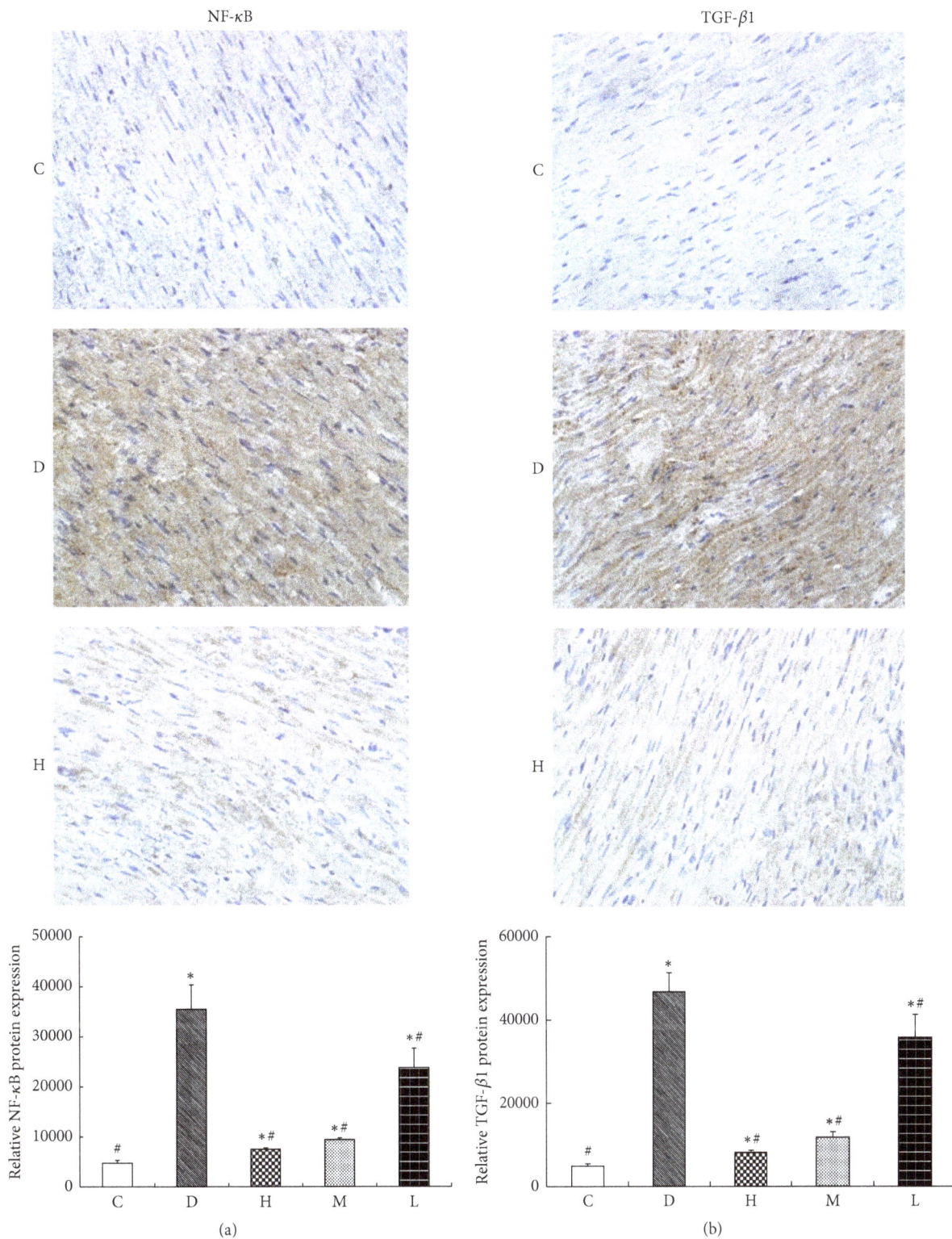

FIGURE 2: NF-κB and TGF-β1 protein expressions by immunohistochemistry. (a) NF-κB protein expression; (b) TGF-β1 protein expression; C: normal control group; D: diabetic group; H: high dose of CS group; M: middle dose of CS; L: low dose of CS group. Compared with group C, $^*P < 0.05$; compared with group D, $^\#P < 0.05$.

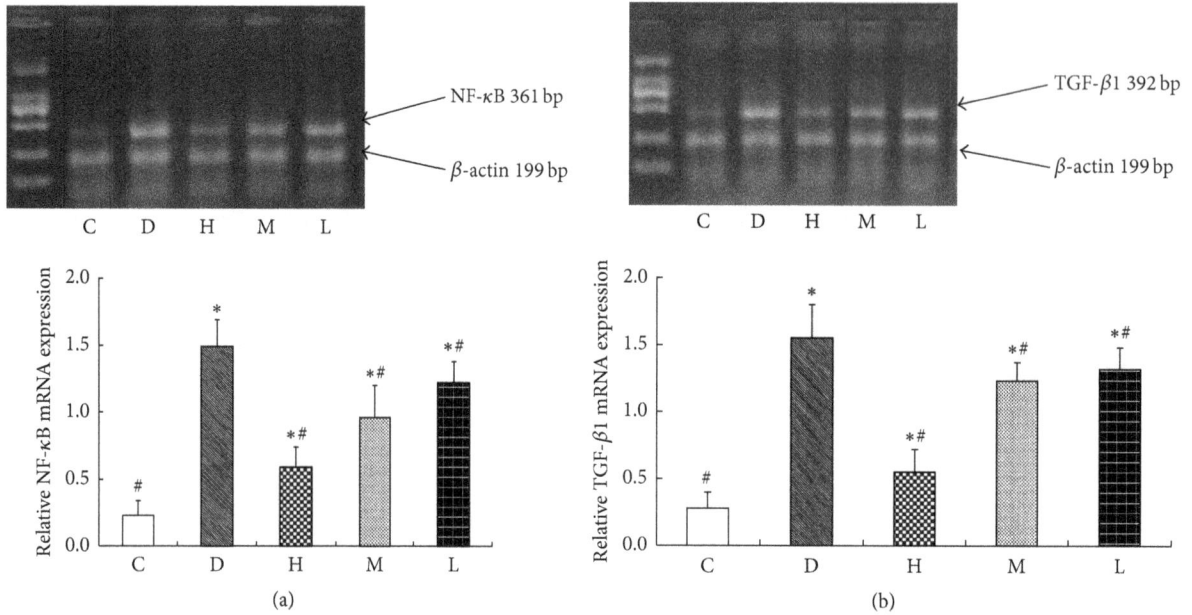

FIGURE 3: NF-κB and TGF-β1 mRNA expressions by RT-PCR. (a) NF-κB mRNA expression; (b) TGF-β1 mRNA expression; C: normal control group; D: diabetic group; H: high dose of CS group; M: middle dose of CS; L: low dose of CS group. Compared with group C, $^*P < 0.05$; compared with group D, $^\#P < 0.05$.

stress, apoptosis, microangiopathy, and myocardial fibrosis are involved in the occurrence and development of DC [6]. Recent studies showed that immune response and low-grade inflammation was closely associated with DM and DC, and the abnormal expressions of NF-κB and TGF-β1 may participate in the occurrence of DC [1].

NF-κB is a key transcription factor which was first found in B lymphocyte. NF-κB can participate in many pathological and physiological processes by specific binding with enhancer sequence of immunoglobulin kappa light chain gene, such as immune response, cell apoptosis, and effect that cause cancer and inflammation. The NF-κB almost exists in all types of tissues and cells and participate in a variety of signal transduction of inflammatory reaction [7]. The advanced glycation end products increased in diabetes patient's body, which combined with specific receptors on the cell membrane. Then they can release a large number of reactive oxygen species, prompt the NF-κB, enter into the nucleus, start inflammation factors transcription, lead to the proliferation of vascular endothelial cells and smooth muscle cells, and promote the occurrence of DC. Animal experiments found that the activation of the NF-κB can lead to increased oxidative stress, mitochondrial dysfunction and cardiac insufficiency in diabetic rats [8]. Studies from Wu et al. [9] showed that estrogen can inhibit fibroblast differentiation and proliferation which induced by angiotensin Π through mitogen activated protein kinase (MAPK)/NF-κB pathway, thus inhibiting myocardial fibrosis. These studies have indicated that the NF-κB pathway was involved in the occurrence and progress of myocardial fibrosis.

TGF-β1, composed of two polypeptide chains, is a kind of growth factor which has a variety of biological activities.

Studies have shown that abnormal expression and activity of TGF-β1 may be involved in the occurrence and development of DC. Hyperglycemia can induce increased synthesis of diacylglycerol pyrophosphate, activate protein kinase C, and result in the expression of TGF-β1 and significantly increased activity [10]. TGF-β1 may stimulate increased synthesis of cardiac fibroblasts I and III type collagen fiber and fibronectin and cause extracellular matrix obviously increased and extracellular matrix degradation reduced. Sun et al. [11] report that TGF-β1 may promote fibroblasts hyperplasia of differentiation and increase collagen synthesis and inhibition of collagen enzyme release in vitro cultures, and the expression of TGF-β1 increased significantly in fibrosis area with increased muscle fibroblast cells and macrophages.

In this study, immunohistochemistry and RT-PCR analysis indicated that expressions of NF-κB and TGF-β1 increased in diabetic rats myocardial cells and suggest that the expression level changes of NF-κB and TGF-β1 may be involved in the occurrence and development of DC.

CS is a kind of valuable Chinese traditional medicine which is rich in polysaccharides, amino acids, fatty acid, mannitol, and trace element. CS presents irreplaceable advantages from modern chemical synthetic drug, along with the further discussion of microscopic mechanism of prevention and treatment of diabetes. CS may play the role of myocardial protection by inhibiting aldose reductase and reducing inflammatory reaction and relieving immune complex deposition, resisting oxidation, and adjusting the immune function [8]. Different studies have different results for the influence of CS on the expressions of NF-κB and TGF-β1. Wang et al. [12] reported that *Cordyceps sinensis* polysaccharide CPS-2 could inhibit PDGF-BB-induced human mesangial cells proliferation in a dose-dependent manner and return expression of PDGFRβ and TGF-β1. Meng et al. [13] found that UM01, QH11, BNQM, GNCC, and DCXC are *Cordyceps* aqueous extracts, and UM01 significantly increased the expression of p-NF-κB-p65 in a concentration dependent manner, while DCXC, GNCC, QH11, and BNQM had no obvious effects on expression of p-NF-κB-p65 in RAW 264.7 macrophages. Yan et al. [14] considered that an acid polysaccharide fraction from *Cordyceps sinensis* fungus could increase the expressions of TNF-α and IL-12 and reduce the expression of IL-10 of Ana-1 cells and convert M2 macrophages to M1 phenotype by activating NF-κB pathway.

In our topic, we observed cardiac protection of CS in diabetic rats, and used CS of low dose ($0.6\,\mathrm{g\cdot kg^{-1}\cdot d^{-1}}$), middle dose ($2.5\,\mathrm{g\cdot kg^{-1}\cdot d^{-1}}$), and high dose ($5\,\mathrm{g\cdot kg^{-1}\cdot d^{-1}}$) to intervene in the treatment of the diabetic rats induced by streptozotocin. Results showed that myocardial expressions of NF-κB and TGF-β1 were decreased after CS treatment, and all three kinds of CS dose can reduce expressions of NF-κB and TGF-β1. And the expressions of mRNA and protein showed a trend of gradual decline, along with the increase of CS dosage. Large dose of CS intervention can significantly reduce expressions of NF-κB and TGF-β1 in myocardium of diabetic rats. We found that larger doses of CS intervention were likely to have more significant treatment effect in a relatively safe dose range. The occurrence of DC was the result of a variety of factors; the increased expressions level of NF-κB and TGF-β1 may be only one of the taches. As a consequence, we will test the expressions of inflammatory and fibrogenesis related cytokines such as TNF-α, IL-1, IL-6, and type I Collagens I and III by experiment in our future, in order to further clarify the damage mechanism of DC and whether CS have an effect on its intervention.

In conclusion, CS intervention treatment can obviously reduce the myocardial injury of streptozotocin-induced diabetic rats. CS may play its role on myocardial protection by decreasing the expressions of NF-κB and TGF-β1 in the myocardium, but the specific mechanism needs further study.

Ethical Approval

The study was approved by the ethics committee.

Conflict of Interests

The authors have no conflict of interests or other disclosures to report.

Authors' Contribution

You-you Gu and Huan Wang contributed equally to this work.

References

[1] C. M. Thomas, Q. C. Yong, R. M. Rosa et al., "Cardiac-specific suppression of NF-κB signaling prevents diabetic cardiomyopathy via inhibition of the renin-angiotensin system," *American Journal of Physiology: Heart and Circulatory Physiology*, vol. 307, no. 7, pp. H1036–H1045, 2014.

[2] Y. F. Chen, C. Y. Wang, W. M. Li et al., "Effect of Huangqi gegen decoction (HGD) on TGF-beta1/Smad3 pathway in diabetic cardiomyopathy rats," *Zhong Yao Cai*, vol. 35, no. 11, pp. 1809–1813, 2012.

[3] J. Cui, M.-C. Qiu, D.-Q. Li, X. Zhang, J.-S. Zhang, and P. Zhang, "The protective effects of cyclosporine A on aortic immunological injuries in STZ-induced diabetic rats," *Zhonghua Xin Xue Guan Bing Za Zhi*, vol. 38, no. 5, pp. 440–444, 2010.

[4] W. C. Kan, H. Y. Wang, C. C. Chien et al., "Effects of extract from solid-state fermented *Cordyceps sinensis* on type 2 diabetes mellitus," *Evidence-Based Complementary and Alternative Medicine*, vol. 2012, Article ID 743107, 10 pages, 2012.

[5] M.-L. Yang, P.-C. Kuo, T.-L. Hwang, and T.-S. Wu, "Anti-inflammatory principles from *Cordyceps sinensis*," *Journal of Natural Products*, vol. 74, no. 9, pp. 1996–2000, 2011.

[6] Y. Wang, W. Sun, B. Du et al., "Therapeutic effect of MG-132 on diabetic cardiomyopathy is associated with its suppression of proteasomal activities: roles of Nrf2 and NF-κB," *American Journal of Physiology—Heart and Circulatory Physiology*, vol. 304, no. 4, pp. H567–H578, 2013.

[7] H. Cheng, Y. Bo, W. Shen et al., "Leonurine ameliorates kidney fibrosis via suppressing TGF-β and NF-κB signaling pathway in UUO mice," *International Immunopharmacology*, vol. 25, no. 2, pp. 406–415, 2015.

[8] N. Mariappan, C. M. Elks, S. Sriramula et al., "NF-κB-induced oxidative stress contributes to mitochondrial and cardiac dysfunction in type II diabetes," *Cardiovascular Research*, vol. 85, no. 3, pp. 473–483, 2010.

[9] M. Wu, M. Han, J. Li et al., "17β-estradiol inhibits angiotensin II-induced cardiac myofibroblast differentiation," *European Journal of Pharmacology*, vol. 616, no. 1–3, pp. 155–159, 2009.

[10] J. T. Bazzaz, M. M. Amoli, Z. Taheri, B. Larijani, V. Pravica, and I. V. Hutchinson, "TGF-β1 and IGF-I gene variations in type 1 diabetes microangiopathic complications," *Journal of Diabetes and Metabolic Disorders*, vol. 13, article 45, 2014.

[11] Y. Sun, J. Zhang, J. Q. Zhang, and F. J. A. Ramires, "Local angiotensin II and transforming growth factor-beta1 in renal fibrosis of rats," *Hypertension*, vol. 35, no. 5, pp. 1078–1084, 2000.

[12] Y. Wang, D. Liu, H. Zhao et al., "Cordyceps sinensis polysaccharide CPS-2 protects human mesangial cells from PDGF-BB-induced proliferation through the PDGF/ERK and TGF-β1/Smad pathways," *Molecular and Cellular Endocrinology*, vol. 382, no. 2, pp. 979–988, 2014.

[13] L.-Z. Meng, B.-Q. Lin, B. Wang et al., "Mycelia extracts of fungal strains isolated from *Cordyceps sinensis* differently enhance the function of RAW 264.7 macrophages," *Journal of Ethnopharmacology*, vol. 148, no. 3, pp. 818–825, 2013.

[14] J.-K. Yan, W.-Q. Wang, and J.-Y. Wu, "Recent advances in *Cordyceps sinensis* polysaccharides: mycelial fermentation, isolation, structure, and bioactivities: a review," *Journal of Functional Foods*, vol. 6, no. 1, pp. 33–47, 2014.

7

Phytochemical Profile and Biological Activity of *Nelumbo nucifera*

Keshav Raj Paudel and Nisha Panth

Department of Pharmacy, School of Health and Allied Science, Pokhara University, P.O. Box 427, Dhungepatan, Kaski, Nepal

Correspondence should be addressed to Keshav Raj Paudel; keshav_krp20@yahoo.com

Academic Editor: Hyunsu Bae

Nelumbo nucifera Gaertn. (Nymphaeaceae) is a potential aquatic crop grown and consumed throughout Asia. All parts of *N. nucifera* have been used for various medicinal purposes in various systems of medicine including folk medicines, Ayurveda, Chinese traditional medicine, and oriental medicine. Many chemical constituents have been isolated till the date. However, the bioactive constituents of lotus are mainly alkaloids and flavonoids. Traditionally, the whole plant of lotus was used as astringent, emollient, and diuretic. It was used in the treatment of diarrhea, tissue inflammation, and homeostasis. The rhizome extract was used as antidiabetic and anti-inflammatory properties due to the presence of asteroidal triterpenoid. Leaves were used as an effective drug for hematemesis, epistaxis, hemoptysis, hematuria, and metrorrhagia. Flowers were used to treat diarrhea, cholera, fever, and hyperdipsia. In traditional medicine practice, seeds are used in the treatment of tissue inflammation, cancer and skin diseases, leprosy, and poison antidote. Embryo of lotus seeds is used in traditional Chinese medicine as Lian Zi Xin, which primarily helps to overcome nervous disorders, insomnia, and cardiovascular diseases (hypertension and arrhythmia). Nutritional value of lotus is as important as pharmaceutical value. These days' different parts of lotus have been consumed as functional foods. Thus, lotus can be regarded as a potential nutraceutical source.

1. Introduction

Traditional medicine or indigenous medicine denotes medical practice developed by local ethnic people via use of natural herbs and mineral. Different place of world has its own history of traditional medicine, for example, ayurvedic medicine originated from Southeast Asia, unani medicine originated in Arab countries/middle east, and acupuncture and traditional Chinese medicine (TCM) originated in China [1–3]. Herbal plants contain secondary metabolite like alkaloids, glycosides, terpene, steroids, flavonoids, tannins, and so forth. Some chemical substances are phenols or their oxygen-substituted derivatives such as tannins while some may contain nitrogen or sulphur that are biologically active and useful for the prevention of disease and treatment of ailment and preserve well-being in humans and animals. Polyphenols exhibit antioxidant activity which lead to many health benefits [4, 5]. Apart from biological activity in human, these chemicals function as plant defense mechanisms against their predator. For human, many of these herbal products and spices serve as useful medicinal source since antiquity [6].

2. History

Nelumbo nucifera comes under the family Nelumbonaceae, which has various local tribal names (Indian lotus, bean of India, Chinese water lily, and sacred lotus) and several botanical names (*Nelumbium nelumbo, N. speciosa, N. speciosum,* and *Nymphaea nelumbo*). As far as the history is concerned, this beautiful flowering aquatic plant has been honored in the history by three countries: China, India, and Egypt [7–9]. Pictorial representation of the flower can be seen in the art of all of these countries' cultures, symbolizing perfection, purity, and beauty. On the dietary aspect, almost all parts of the plant are used in preparing diverse cuisines depending upon cultures of that place. History reveals that sacred blue lotus (*Nymphaea caerulea*) was distributed and widespread along the Nile river banks [9, 10]. In ancient period, Egyptians worshipped different parts of lotus, widely depicted in their architectural design. Initiation of lotus horticulture in western Europe was introduced by Sir Joseph Banks during 1787 in the form of stove-house water lily whereas these days it is widespread almost everywhere in modern herbal garden. Mostly, lotus plants are popular in Australia pacific, China, India, Korea, and Japan [9, 11].

3. Physical Characteristics and Description

Nelumbo nucifera is a large aquatic rhizomatous herb consisting of slender, elongated, creeping stem with nodal roots. Lotus is perennial plant with both aerial and floating orbicular leaves. Aerial leaves are cup shaped and floating leaves have flat shape. Its petioles are considerably long and rough with distinct prickles. Flowers vary in color from white to rosy and are pleasantly sweet-scented, solitary, and hermaphrodite. Flower average diameter is 10–25 cm, and it is ovoid and glabrous. Fruit which contain seeds, are black in color, and are hard and ovoid are arranged in whorls; seeds ripened and were released as a result of bending down of pod to the water. Tuberous roots are 8 inches long and 2 inches in diameter. Smooth outer skin of the lotus root is green in color; however, the inner part possesses numerous big air pockets running throughout the length of the tuber assisting for floating in the aquatic system [12, 13].

4. Phytochemicals and Constituents

The reported chemical constituents in the different parts of Nelumbo nucifera are as shown in the following.

(1) Embryo. The phytochemicals reported in embryo of Nelumbo nucifera are shown in Figure 1 [14, 15].

(2) Stamen. The phytochemicals reported in stamen of Nelumbo nucifera are shown in Figure 2 [12, 16–18].

(3) Flower. The phytochemicals reported in flower of Nelumbo nucifera are shown in Figure 3 [16, 19].

(4) Leaf. The phytochemicals reported in leaf of Nelumbo nucifera are shown in Figure 4 [12, 16, 19, 20].

(5) Seed. The phytochemicals reported in seed of Nelumbo nucifera are shown in Figure 5 [12, 16].

5. Reported Pharmacological Activity of Nelumbo nucifera

5.1. Antioxidants. Hydroalcoholic extract of Nelumbo nucifera (HANN) seeds was investigated for antioxidant potency using in vitro and in vivo models. In vitro results showed that HANN exhibited significant DPPH (1,1-diphenyl-2-picrylhydrazyl) free radical scavenging activity with IC_{50} values of 6.12 ± 0.41 $\mu g/mL$ and nitric oxide (NO) scavenging activity with IC_{50} value of 84.86 ± 3.56 $\mu g/mL$. These results were even better than rutin used as standard. In in vivo model, HANN administration to Wistar strain rats at a dose

of 100 and 200 mg/kg body weight for a time period of 4 days prior to carbon tetrachloride (CCl_4) administration resulted in a significant dose-dependent raise of superoxide dismutase (SOD) and catalase enzyme level and significant fall in the level of thiobarbituric acid reactive substances (TBARS), as compared to CCl_4 treated alone (control group) in both liver and kidney. The changes observed at 100 mg/kg body weight treatment were comparable to those observed for tocopherol (50 mg/kg) treatment. Nelumbo nucifera seeds contain variety of phytochemical-like saponins, alkaloids, polyphenolics, and carbohydrates supporting significant antioxidant activity of HANN [21]. Lee et al., 2005, studied the antioxidant effect of Korean Traditional Lotus Liquor (Yunyupju) which was made from lotus blossom and leaves. The antioxidant effects were dose-dependent and reached a peak (about 80% inhibition) at a concentration of more than 25 μg of lotus liquor. The liquor exhibited significant DPPH scavenging activities (IC_{50} = 17.9 μg) [22]. Yen et al., 2006, reported the reactive nitrogen species scavenging activity of lotus seed extracts. The potency of lotus seed extracts, namely, water extract (LSWE), ethyl acetate (LSEAE), and hexane (LSHE), to inhibit reactive nitrogen species in macrophage RAW 264.7 cells was investigated. In results, all the extracts of lotus suppress NO production in lipopolysaccharide stimulated RAW 264.7 cells. There was a dose-dependent inhibition of the accumulation of NO upon decomposition of sodium nitroprusside (SNP). In comparison, the potency order was LSEAE > LSWE > LSHE. Further supportive role of lotus extracts to protect DNA breakage in macrophage RAW 264.7 cells promoted by SNP was shown in comet assay. LSWE, LSEAE, and LSHE, at a dose of 0.2 mg/mL, showed 63%, 59%, and 38% inhibition of DNA damage induced by peroxynitrite, respectively. All extracts were found to be peroxynitrite scavengers and thus capable of preventing tyrosine nitration [23]. Ling et al., 2005, extracted the procyanidins from lotus seedpod with Me_2CO/H_2O. Among the monomers, dimers, and tetramers of procyanidins, the extract contained high amounts of dimers whereas catechin and epicatechin were the base units. These procyanidins were also investigated for lipid peroxidation, lipoxygenase enzyme activity, and reactive free radical scavenging activity. The superoxide radical scavenging potency of lotus pod procyanidin shows the IC_{50} value of 17.6 mg/L (4-fold less potent as compared to IC_{50} 4.1 mg/L of ascorbic acid). The study also revealed that 0.1% of procyanidins have a significant antioxidant activity in a system of soybean oil, even better than butylated hydroxytoluene (BHT) at a similar concentration [24]. Kim et al., 2014, showed that 80% methanol extract of Nelumbo nucifera seed's embryo decreases in ROS production in mouse hippocampal HT22 cells and scavenges DPPH free radical (IC_{50} value as 240.51 $\mu g/mL$) and H_2O_2 (IC_{50} value as 1769.01 $\mu g/mL$) [25].

5.2. Antisteroids. The antisteroidogenic activity of N. nucifera seed extract in the ovary and testis of the rat was studied by Gupta et al., 1996. In this study, petroleum ether extract fraction was orally given to sexually immature female rats and mature male rats up to 15 days at alternative day. There was a marked delay in sexual maturation in prepubertal

	R_1	R_2	R_3
Liensinine	CH_3	H	H
Isoliensinine	H	H	CH_3
Neferine	CH_3	CH_3	H

Nuciferine

Lotusine

Pronuciferine

Rutin

Hyperin

Demethylcoclaurine

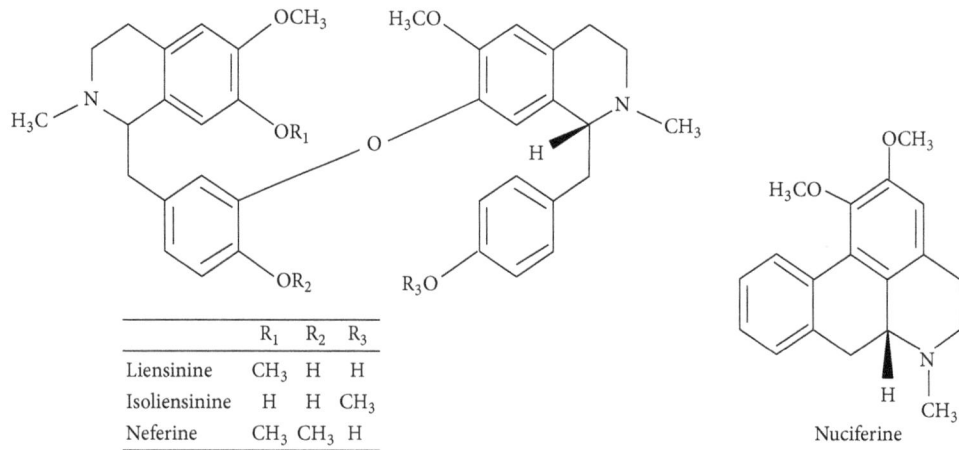

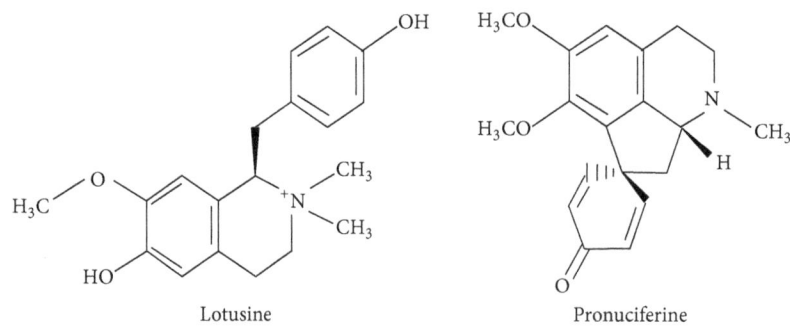

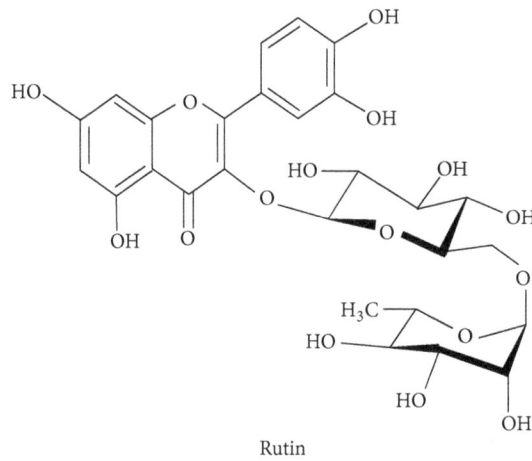

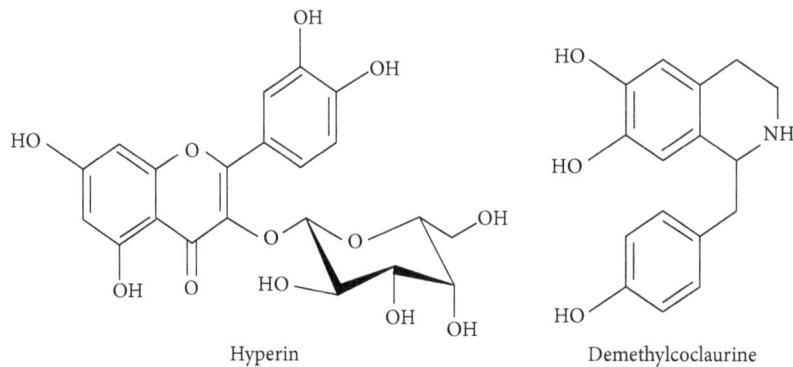

FIGURE 1: Major chemical constituents present in *Nelumbo nucifera* embryo.

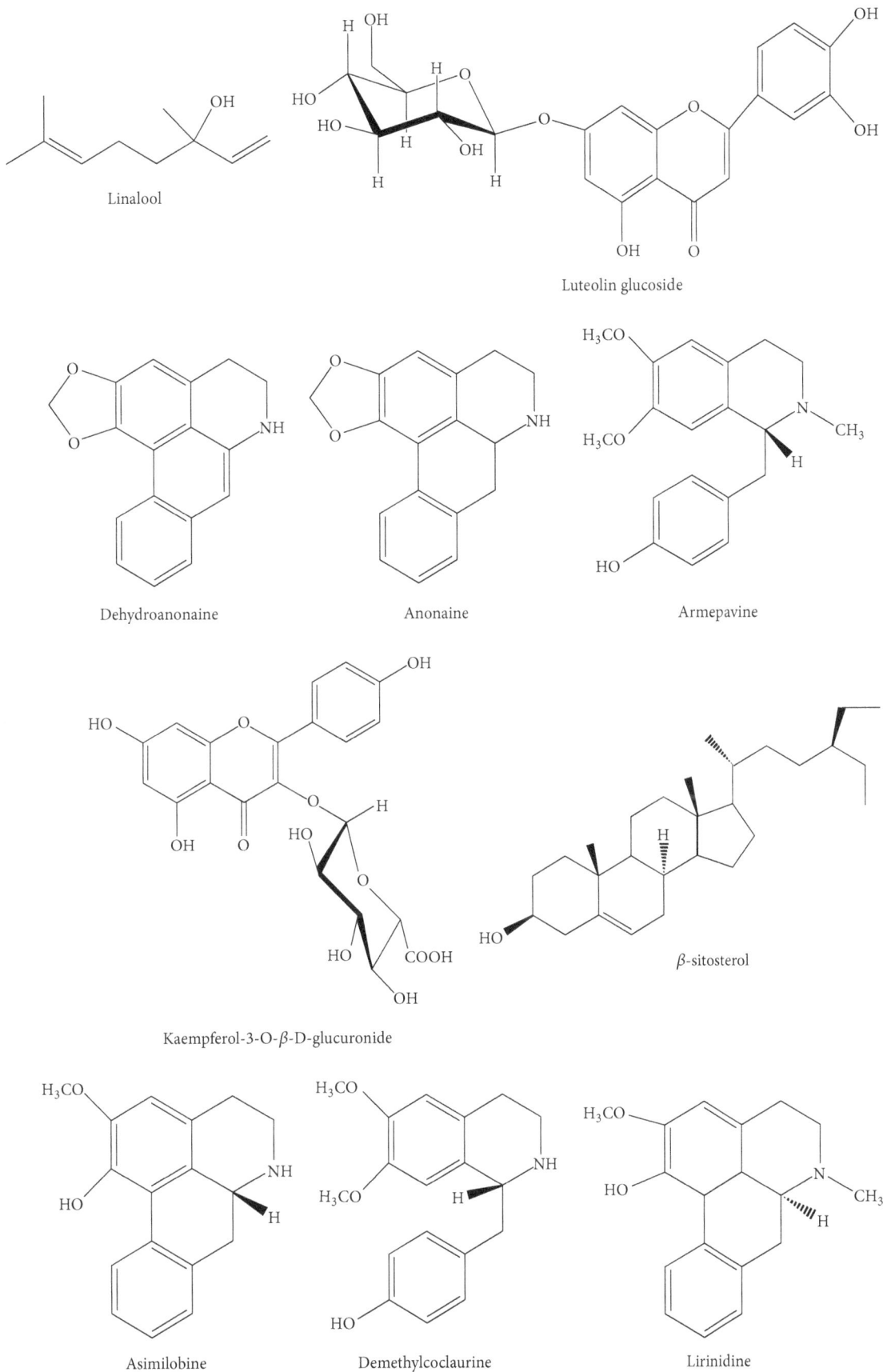

Linalool

Luteolin glucoside

Dehydroanonaine

Anonaine

Armepavine

Kaempferol-3-O-β-D-glucuronide

β-sitosterol

Asimilobine

Demethylcoclaurine

Lirinidine

FIGURE 2: Continued.

Dehydronuciferine

	R_1	R_2	R_3
Isoliensinine	H	H	CH_3
Liensinine	CH_3	H	H

Quercetin

Liriodenine

Dehydroemerine

Isoquercitrin (Hirsutrin)

Nornuciferine

N-methylasimilobine

N-methylcoclaurine

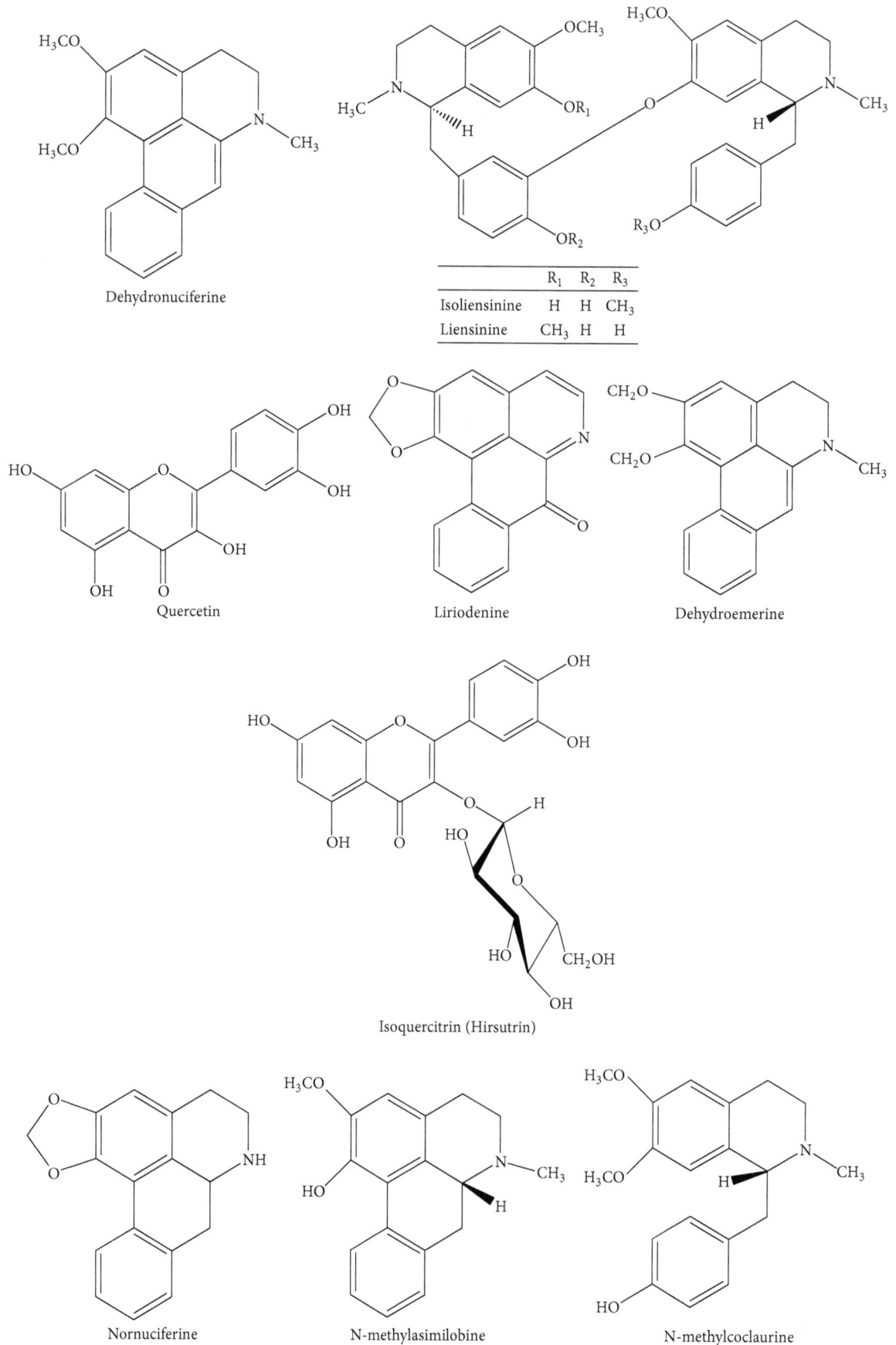

FIGURE 2: Continued.

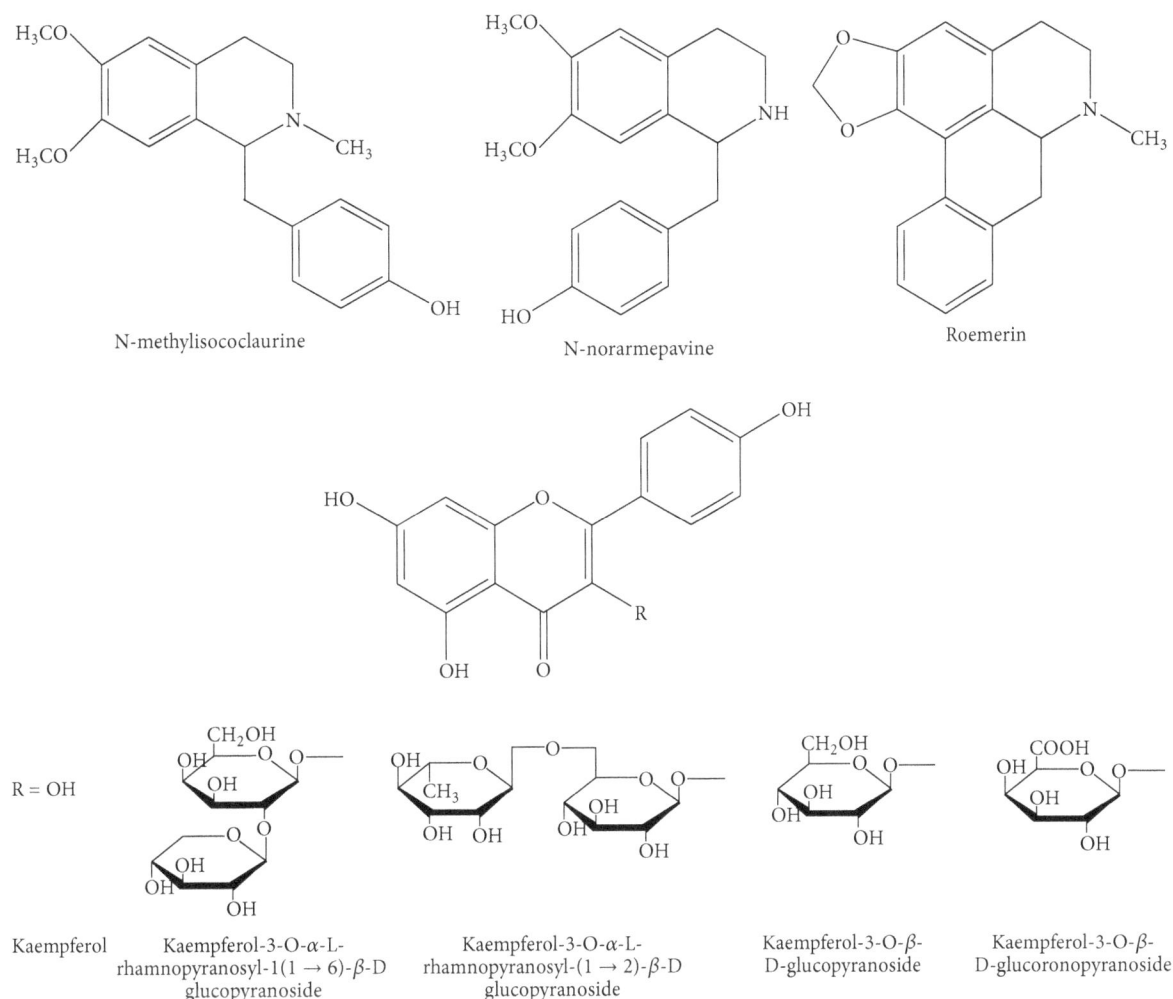

FIGURE 2: Major chemical constituents present in *Nelumbo nucifera* stamen.

female rats as revealed from age of vaginal opening and first estrus (cornified smear) whereas there was reduction in sperm motility and sperm count in male rats. Furthermore, the application of extract resulted in accumulation of ascorbic acid and cholesterol and reduction in δ-5-3-β-hydroxysteroid dehydrogenase and glucose-6-phosphate dehydrogenase activity in the ovary and testis. Thus, this research explores that the petroleum ether extract can suppress the genesis of steroids in reproductive organs of rats [26]. Similarly, Wethangkaboworn and Munglue, 2014, purpose the 3 hypotheses for inhibitory effect of *N. nucifera* seed extract on male rat sexual behavior to support its antifertility activity: (1) suppression of hypothalamic gonadotropin releasing hormone production, (2) pituitary gonadotropic hormone production, including follicle stimulating hormone (FSH) and luteinizing hormone (LH), or (3) testosterone production [27]. Mutreju et al., 2008, showed that administration of *N. nucifera* to female rats caused estrogen inhibition due to its antiestrogenic nature [28].

5.3. Antipyretic Activity. Sinha et al., 2000, reported the antipyretic potential of ethanol extract of lotus stalks on normal body temperature as well as yeast-induced pyrexia using rat as *in vivo* model. Lotus extract, at a dose of 200 mg/kg, markedly decreases the body temperature for a period of 3 hr after administration, while at 400 mg/kg dose it decreases for up to 6 hr. In this yeast model, elevation of body temperature was dose dependently lowered up to 4 hr at both doses by lotus extract and these results were comparable to standard medicine for fever: paracetamol at 150 mg/kg [29]. Similar result was reported by Mukherjee et al., 1996, in yeast-induced pyrexia using rat model [30].

5.4. Antiviral Activity. Kashiwada et al., 2005, isolated quercetin 3-O-β-D-glucuronide, (+)-1(R)-coclaurine, and (−)-1(S)-norcoclaurine from *Nelumbo nucifera* leaves. The latter two compounds possessed therapeutic activity against HIV with EC_{50} values of 0.8 and <0.8 μg/mL and therapeutic index (TI) values of >125 and >25, respectively, while the first compound was less potent (EC_{50}, 2 μg/mL). Other active principles like aporphine, benzylisoquinoline, and bis-benzylisoquinoline alkaloids (liensinine, isoliensinine, and neferine) isolated from leaves and embryo of lotus exhibited potent anti-HIV activities (EC_{50}, <0.81 μg/mL; TI of >9.9,

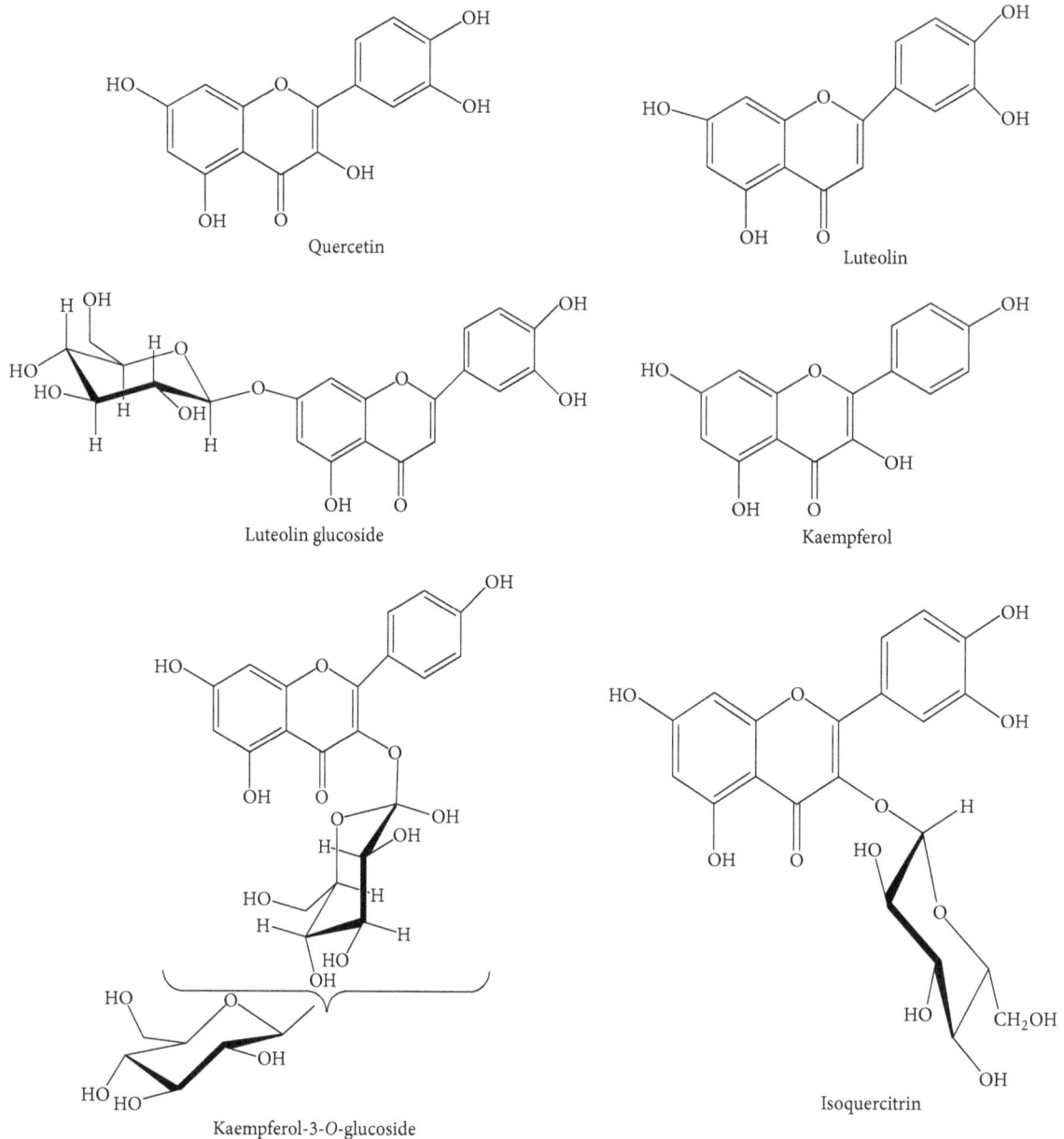

FIGURE 3: Major chemical constituents present in *Nelumbo nucifera* flower.

>8.6, and >6.5, resp.). An aporphine alkaloid, nuciferine also showed EC$_{50}$, 0.8 μg/mL, and TI of 36 μg/mL [31]. Kuo et al., 2005, reported the antiviral activity of lotus seed ethyl alcohol extract on herpes simplex type 1 (HSV-1). At a dose of 100 μg/mL, ethyl alcohol extract of lotus markedly inhibited HSV-1 replication with IC$_{50}$ of 50.0 μg/mL for replication. Various subfractions of *Nelumbo nucifera* seeds butanol (NN-B) extract were investigated for the HSV-1 inhibitory effects indicating that NN-B-5 out of major nine fractions, NN-B-1 to NN-B-9, had the highest suppresser activity. However, ethyl alcohol extracts obtained from fresh lotus seeds showed anti-HSV-1 activity with IC$_{50}$ 62.0 ± 8.9 μg/mL. Furthermore, to get deeper insight of NN-B-5 potency to suppress the acyclovir-resistant HSV-1 replication, the TK HSV-1 strain was targeted and plaque reduction assay was carried out.

Results showed 85.9% inhibition of TK HSV-1 replication in HeLa cells by 50 μg/mL of NN-B-5. These results provide evidence that NN-B-5 inhibit the acyclovir-resistant HSV-1 replication [32].

5.5. *Immunity.* Liu et al., 2004, study the effect of ethyl alcohol extracts of lotus in primary human peripheral blood mononuclear cells (PBMC) stimulated by phytohemagglutinin (PHA: a specific mitogen for T lymphocytes) to inhibit the cell proliferation and cytokines production [33]. Liu et al., 2006, also studied the effects of (S)-armepavine from *Nelumbo nucifera* to suppress T cells proliferation. The therapeutic benefit of (S)-armepavine on immune disease, systemic lupus erythematosus (SLE), was investigated on MRL/MpJ-lpr/lpr mice as an *in vivo* model having disease

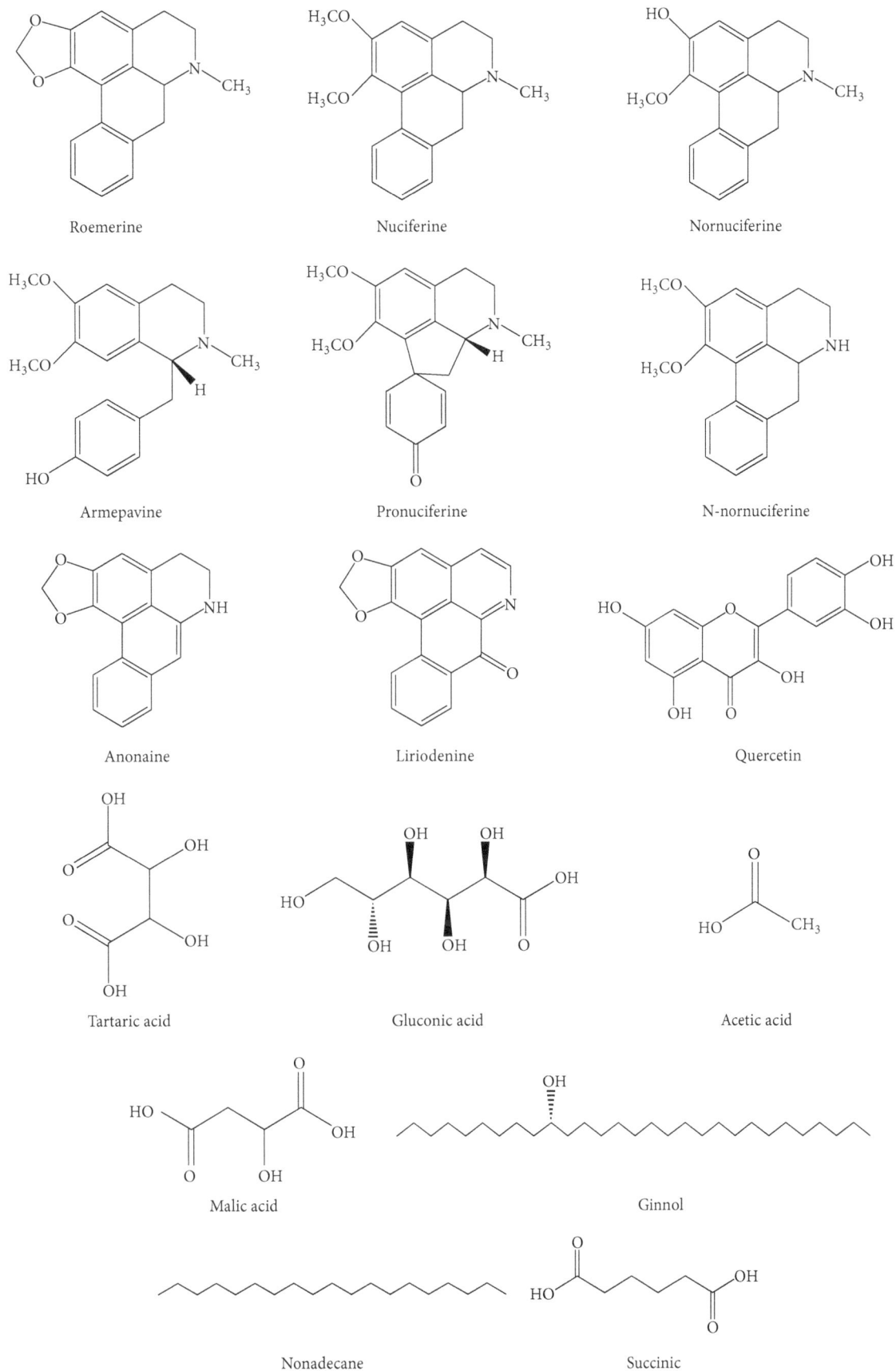

Roemerine

Nuciferine

Nornuciferine

Armepavine

Pronuciferine

N-nornuciferine

Anonaine

Liriodenine

Quercetin

Tartaric acid

Gluconic acid

Acetic acid

Malic acid

Ginnol

Nonadecane

Succinic

Figure 4: Continued.

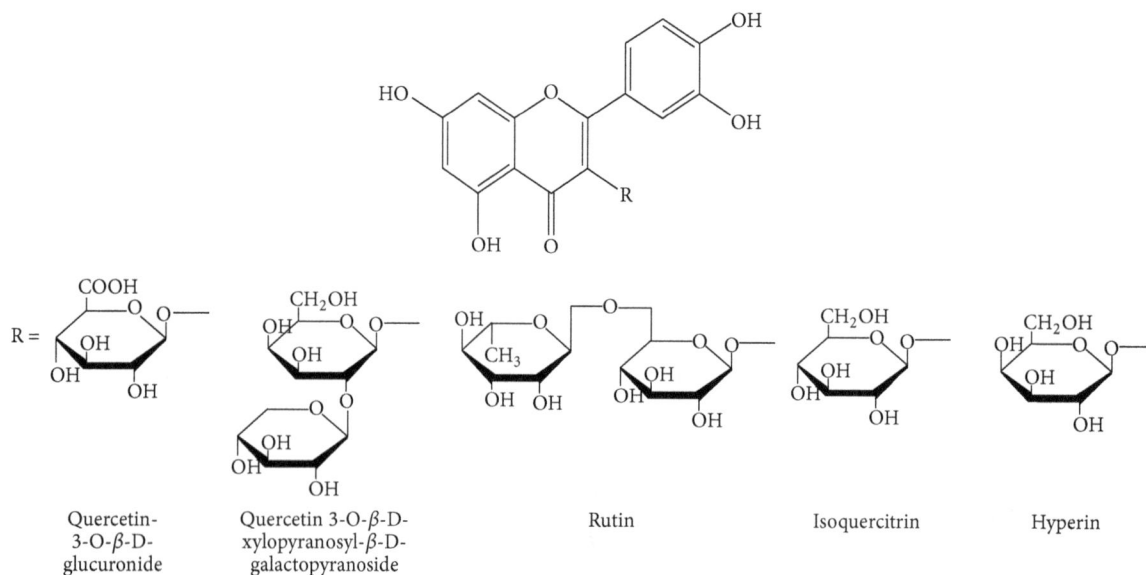

FIGURE 4: Major chemical constituents present in *Nelumbo nucifera* leaf.

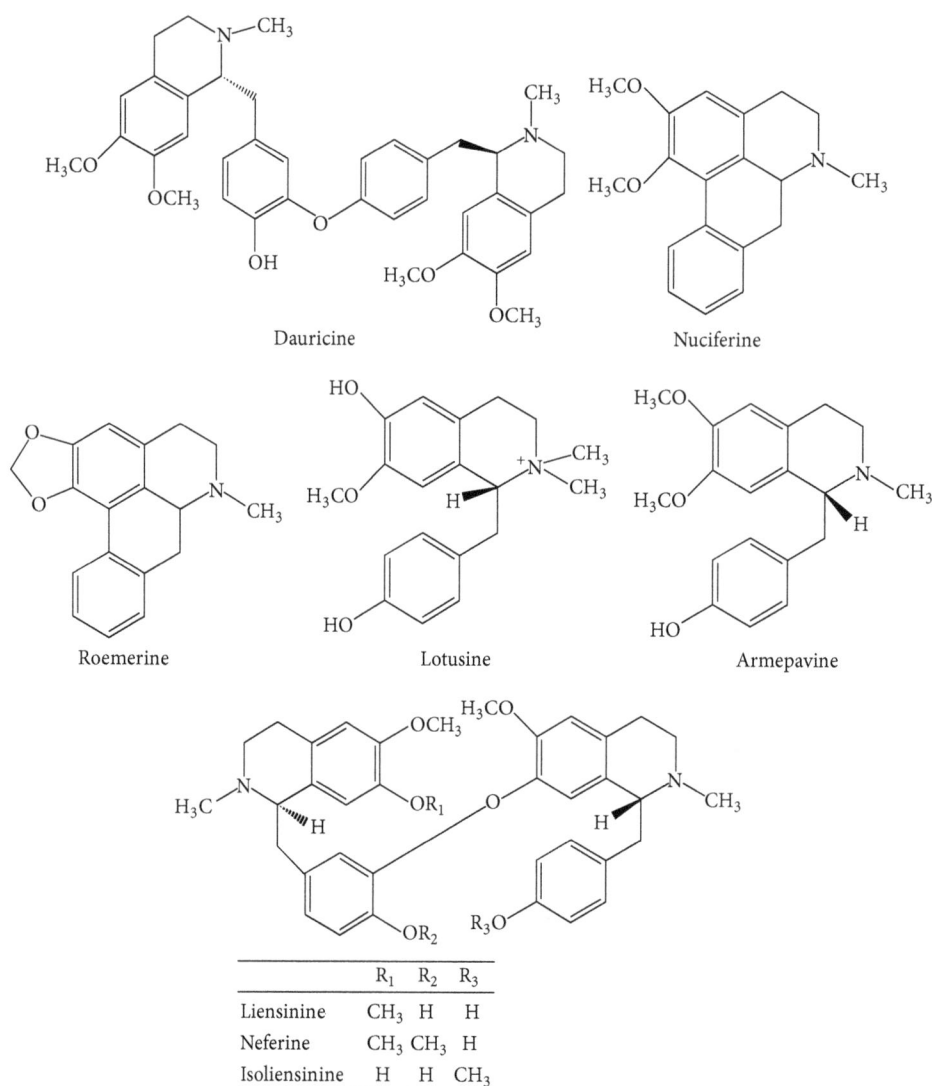

FIGURE 5: Major chemical constituents present in *Nelumbo nucifera* seeds.

feature similar to human SLE. For this study, (S)-armepavine was treated orally for 6 weeks to MRL/MpJ-lpr/lpr mice and their SLE features were evaluated. The results showed that (S)-armepavine was successful to prevent lymphadenopathy as well as extend the life span of mice. Also, (S)-armepavine treatment resulted in significant decrease of T lymphocyte-mediated cytokines production in dose-dependent manner. Likewise, (S)-armepavine impaired interleukin-2 (IL-2) and interferon (IFN-γ) transcripts in human PBMC. This study concluded that (S)-armepavine could be potential therapeutic option as an immunomodulator for the management of SLE [34]. In another study, Liu et al., 2007, revealed the suppressive action on PHA-induced PBMC proliferation and genes expression of IL-2 and IFN-γ by (S)-armepavine without direct cytotoxicity [35].

5.6. Anti-Inflammatory Activity. Tissue inflammation is harmful response that produces tissue injury and may cause serious diseases such as asthma, atopic dermatitis, and rheumatoid arthritis [36]. There is now convincing evidence that cytokines secreted by T cells such as IL-4, IL-10, and INF-γ in response to antigen stimulation play a role in atopic dermatitis, lung inflammation, and asthma [37]. Phytochemical (NN-B-4) identified by a bioassay-based screening procedure from ethanol extract of *Nelumbo nucifera* extracts significantly attenuated proliferation of PMBC induced by phytohemagglutinin, expression of IL-4, IL-10, and INF-γ, and cdk-4 gene. NN-B-4 arrest progression of cell cycle of activated PBMC by blocking PBMC from the G1 transition to S phase [32]. Triterpenoid betulinic acid isolated from methanol extract of *Nelumbo nucifera* rhizome was evaluated for the marked anti-inflammatory activity against edema in rat paw caused by carrageenan and serotonin. Methanol extract showed anti-inflammatory activity at doses of 200 and 400 mg/kg p.o. Similarly betulinic acid demonstrated significant anti-inflammatory effect in inflammatory experimental models at doses of 50 mg/kg and 100 mg/kg p.o. Extract and betulinic acid produce similar effect as compared to two potent anti-inflammatory drugs, phenylbutazone and dexamethasone [38].

5.7. Diabetes and Complications. The effect of ethanolic extract of *N. nucifera* rhizome was studied in glucose-fed hyperglycemic and streptozotocin-induced diabetic rats. The extract showed improved tolerance action of glucose. Similarly, the potentiating action of extract on the exogenous insulin was seen. The antidiabetic potential of the extract was compared and found to be similar with that of tolbutamide in normal and diseased rat [39]. Such effect could be due to, in part, attenuated absorption of glucose from intestine, as noted, for example, when plant fiber is given orally with glucose [40]. Key enzyme aldose reductase of the polyol pathway has been suggested to play central role in the diabetes and its complications. A methanol extract from *Nelumbo nucifera* stamens revealed inhibitory activity against rat lens aldose reductase. Out of 13 isolated flavonoids from the extract, compounds having 3-O-alpha-1-rhamnopyranosyl-1(1 → 6)-beta-d-glucopyranoside groups in their carbon ring, including kaempferol 3-O-alpha-1-rhamnopyranosyl-1(1 →

6)-beta-d-glucopyranoside and isorhamnetin 3-O-alpha-1-rhamnopyranosyl-1(1 → 6)-beta-d-glucopyranoside, demonstrate highest inhibitory effect of rat lens aldose reductase *in vitro* [41].

5.8. Treatment for Erectile Dysfunction. Chen et al. in 2008 investigated the effects of extract neferine on basal concentration of the cyclic adenosine monophosphate and cyclic guanosine monophosphate. Neferine potentiated the cAMP concentration dose dependently; however, this effect was not suppressed by inhibitor of adenylyl cyclase in rabbit corpus cavernosum *in vitro*. Neferine dose dependently increased cAMP accumulation catalyzed by a stimulator of cAMP production, namely, prostaglandin E1 (PGE1). The level of cGMP was not affected by guanylyl cyclase inhibitor and sodium nitroprusside. Neferine enhances the concentration of cAMP in tissue of rabbit corpus cavernosum notably by suppressing activity of phosphodiesterase [42]. In another study, Chen et al. further highlighted treatment of erectile dysfunction of the *in vitro* relaxation mechanisms of neferine on the rabbit corpus cavernosum tissue [43] and *in vitro* effects of neferine on cytosolic free calcium concentration in corpus cavernosum smooth muscle cells of rabbits [44].

5.9. Restenosis and Atherosclerosis. Proliferation and expression of matrix metalloproteinase 2 (MMP-2) by smooth muscle cells after percutaneous transluminal coronary angioplasty (PTCA) are responsible for degradation of extracellular matrix (ECM) and migration of smooth muscle cells from tunica media to tunica intima, thereby narrowing the luminal area. Administration of leaf and root extract of *N. nucifera* for 4 weeks significantly suppressed the narrowing of luminal area and stenosis rate in rat model. Similarly, proliferation of vascular smooth muscle cell (VSMC) and expression of MMP-2 in VSMC was dose dependently inhibited by different parts of *N. nucifera* extracts [8]. Similarly, in rabbit model of atherosclerosis induced by high cholesterol diet, leaf extract of *N. nucifera* showed potent antiatherosclerotic activity via inhibition of VSMC proliferation and migration [45] and improved plasma cholesterol level [46]. The active principle of *N. nucifera*, neferine, inhibits angiotensin II-stimulated proliferation in VSMC through heme oxygenase-1 [47] as well as downregulating fractalkine gene expression [48].

5.10. Antiaging. Sacred lotus (*Nelumbo nucifera*) seed extract contains antiaging agent that has beneficial effect to reduce symptoms like loss of elasticity, acne, pores, wrinkles, fine lines, blemishes, and so forth. A suitable vehicle possesses the formulations which has potent antiaging agent. It promotes younger looking skin [49]. Mahmood and Akhtar, 2013, study the efficacy of green tea and lotus extract cosmetic formulations for the treatment of facial wrinkles in healthy Asian using a noninvasive device, the Visioscan VC, along with software for surface evaluation of living skin [50] and a noninvasive photometric device (Sebumeter) for the measurement of casual sebum secretions on both sides of the face [51]. Result showed that green tea and lotus combined in multiple emulsions demonstrated a synergistic antiaging effect. The active constituents having antioxidant activity in both herbal plants may possess a beneficial effect on skin surface, thus recommending these plants as the future of new antiaging products.

5.11. Antiarrythmia. Phytochemicals, dauricine and neferine, obtained from *N. nucifera* seed have cardiovascular pharmacological effect. Phytochemicals of *N. nucifera* blocked the Na^+K^+ and Ca^{+2} cardiac transmembrane current. Notable compound neferine has antiarrhythmic effect and also significantly inhibits aggregation of platelet in rabbits [52]. The antiarrhythmic potency of principle alkaloid from *N. nucifera*, neferine, has been demonstrated in several *in vivo* experimental studies [53]. In a guinea pig papillary muscles and atria, the activity of neferine was investigated on the electrical and mechanical activity. Neferine, at a dose of 0.1 mmol/L, decreased the force of contraction, lowered the amplitude and also V_{max} of action potential (AP), and prolonged the action potential duration at 50% (APD50), action potential duration at 90% (APD90), and effective refractory period (ERP). Furthermore, neferine (30 μmol/L) partly antagonized the effect of acetylcholine 10 μmol/L [54]. In guinea pig atria, automaticity inducing effect of adrenaline was attenuated by neferine 30 μmol/L. Similarly, neferine at dose of 30 μmol/L inhibited and shifted dose-effect curve of isoprenaline, an action varied from propranolol action. Also, neferine effect on the Ca^{2+} dose response curve in guinea pigs left atria was studied. Neferine, similar to verapamil, revealed dualistic action in antagonism of Ca^{2+} [55]. Neferine (8 mg/kg, i.v.) electrophysiological effects on ischemic ventricular tachyarrhythmias were studied in both normal and ischemic myocardium by using programmed electrical stimulation (PES) in open chest during 5–8 days after acute myocardial infarction. Neferine was effective in preventing ventricular tachycardias and sudden cardiac death after damage due to myocardial ischemia [56].

5.12. Hepatoprotective Activity. Sohn et al., 2003, reported *Nelumbo nucifera* hepatoprotective effect. The protective effects of the ethanol extract of seeds of *Nelumbo nucifera* (ENN) against cytotoxicity induced by CCl_4 in primary cultured rat hepatocytes were evaluated by the cellular leakage of aspartate transaminase (AST) and cell survival rate. The cellular leakage of AST and the cell death caused by CCl_4 were significantly inhibited in dose-dependent manners by ENN concentrations between 10 and 500 μg/mL. Similarly, the hepatoprotective effect of ENN against hepatotoxin Aflatoxin B1 (AFB1) was also tested. ENN showed significant hepatoprotective activity at concentrations of both 250 and 500 μg/mL by 74.5% and 94.6%, respectively, as compared with AFB1 controls (48.9%) [57]. Je and Lee investigated the *in vitro* hepatoprotective effect of *Nelumbo nucifera* leaves butanol extract (NNBE) on hepatic damage in cultured hepatocytes induced by H_2O_2. The hepatoprotective effect of NNBE was related to the upregulation of various enzymes: superoxide dismutase-1 (SOD-1) by 0.62-fold, catalase (CAT) by 0.42-fold, and heme oxygenase-1 (HO-1) by 2.4-fold. Likewise, pretreatment of NNBE increased the accumulation of nuclear factor erythroid 2-related factor 2 (Nrf2) in nucleus by 8.1-fold signifying that increased SOD-1, CAT, and HO-1 expressions

are mediated by Nrf2 [58]. In another study by Yuan et al., ethyl acetate (NUEA) and *n*-butanol (NUBU) extracts of *N. nucifera* leaves were evaluated for hepatoprotective effect on CCl_4 induced acute liver injury in mice. Except for NUEA group, the levels of aspartate aminotransferase (AST/GOT) and alanine aminotransferase (ALT/GPT) in each treatment group significantly decreased. Moreover, the contents of malondialdehyde (MDA) and the level of SOD in liver of each group were significantly decreased [59]. Likewise, Tang et al. evaluated the mechanisms of hepatoprotective effect of *Nelumbo nucifera* leaves extract (NLE) in *in vivo* model of experimental alcoholic steatohepatitis. The result showed the inhibitory action of NLE on lipid accumulation by altering the levels of triglycerides (TG) and cholesterol (TC) in both plasma and hepatic content analysis. Furthermore, NLE increased the expression of the 5′ adenosine monophosphate-activated protein kinase (p-AMPK/AMPK) ratio and peroxisome proliferator-activated receptor- (PPAR-) α responsible for fatty acid oxidation and transport via carnitine palmitoyltransferase-1 (CPT1) and microsomal triglyceride transfer protein (MTP). These results clarify that the NLE can prevent alcoholic steatohepatitis by multiple pathways [60].

5.13. Pulmonary Fibrosis. Xiao et al. evaluated the effect of bisbenzylisoquinoline alkaloid isoliensinine isolated from the seed embryo of *Nelumbo nucifera*, on pulmonary fibrosis induced by bleomycin in mice. This study demonstrated that isoliensinine significantly inhibited the hydroxyproline content. Also, isoliensinine subsided histological injury in lungs due to enhancing superoxide dismutase (SOD) activity and malondialdehyde (MDA) level by bleomycin. Moreover, it also inhibits, tumor necrosis factor- (TNF-) α and TGF-β1 overexpression [61]. Similarly evidence was provided by Zhao et al., 2010, on antifibrosis property of neferine by reversing the decrease in SOD activity, increased in MDA levels and myeloperoxidase activity. Neferine also alleviated bleomycin-induced increase of TNF-α, interleukin- (IL-) 6, and endothelin-1 in plasma or in tissue [62]. Niu et al., 2013, showed inhibitory effect of neferine on amiodarone-induced pulmonary fibrosis, due to its potency of anti-inflammation, inhibition of surfactant protein-D (SP-D), and balancing of the increased $CD4^+CD25^+$ regulatory T cells (Tregs) which may modulate Th1/Th2 imbalance by suppressing Th2 response [63].

5.14. Antiobesity Activity. Ohkoshi et al., 2007, reported the antiobesity efficacy of active constituents isolated from the leaves of *Nelumbo nucifera* via stimulated lipolysis in mice adipose tissue. Constituent obtained showed antiobesity activity via beta-adrenergic receptor pathway. *Nelumbo nucifera* leaves reduced body weight in A/J mice given high fat diet significantly. Several flavonoids were identified and isolated from NN by fractionation and chromatography. Flavonoids like quercetin, isoquercitrin, catechin, hyperoside, and astragalin showed lipolytic activity in visceral adipose tissue [64]. Ono et al., 2006, outlined the potential pharmacological mechanism of extract isolated from leaves of *N. nucifera* (NNE) in diabetic mice and rats. NNE demonstrated concentration dependent suppression of α-amylase, lipase activity, lipid metabolism, and expression of UCP3 mRNA in C2C12 myotubes in mice administrated extract for five weeks. The NNE also exhibited inhibitory activity of α-amylase and lipase *in vitro*. Lipase inhibitory activity by NNE (IC$_{50}$, 0.46 mg/mL) was shown to be stronger when compared with α-amylase (IC$_{50}$, 0.82 mg/mL). The extract revealed significant suppression in weight gain of body and parametrial adipose tissue. Also extract suppresses concentration of liver triacylglycerol in high fat diet induced obese mice and inhibits UCP3 mRNA expression in skeletal muscle [65]. Similarly, Velusami et al., 2013, study the antiobesity efficacy of methyl alcohol and successive aqueous extracts of *N. nucifera* petals. Parameter studied was effect of those extracts on adipogenesis, adipolysis, lipase, serotonin (5-HT2C), cannabinoid (CNR2), melanocyte concentrating hormone (MCHR1), and melanocortin (MC4R) receptors. Both methyl alcohol and successive aqueous extracts of *N. nucifera* petals inhibited lipid storage in adipocytes and increased lipolysis. Also, *N. nucifera* petal's methyl alcohol extract showed dose-dependent inhibition of lipase activity (IC$_{50}$ value: 47 μg/mL). Furthermore, *N. nucifera* petal extracts possess antagonist and agonist activity on CNR2 and 5-HT2C receptors, respectively. However, it does not show any effect on MCHR1 and MC4R receptors. Overall result summarizes that methyl alcohol extract of *N. nucifera* petals showed better promising activity than successive aqueous extract to control obesity [66].

5.15. Anticancer Activity. Various extracts and isolated compound from different parts of *N. nucifera* possess anticancer activity both *in vitro* and *in vivo*. Among the three major alkaloids, isoliensinine possesses the most potent cytotoxic effect, primarily by inducing apoptosis on triple-negative breast cancer cells through ROS generation and p38 MAPK/JNK activation [67]. *N. nucifera* markedly suppressed the proliferation of non-small-cell lungs cancer (NSCLC) cells in the presence of nicotine, inhibited Wnt/β-catenin signaling activity, promoted the stabilization of Axin, and induced apoptosis. *N. nucifera* decreased the levels of β-catenin and its downstream targets including c-myc, cyclin D, and vascular endothelial growth factor- (VEGF-) A. *N. nucifera* also decreased the ratio of B-cell lymphoma 2/Bcl-2-associated X protein (Bcl-2/Bax), which may explain the proapoptosis effect of nuciferine [68]. Out of 15 compounds isolated from leaves from *Nelumbo nucifera*, 7-hydroxydehydronuciferine significantly inhibited the proliferation of melanoma, prostate, and gastric cancer cells [69]. Reversal effect of neferine on multidrug resistance human gastric carcinoma cell line (SGC7901) was studied by Cao et al. SGC7901 and its vincristine- (VCR-) resistant variant (SGC7901/VCR) were treated in the presence or absence of neferine and/or VCR. Neferine reverses multidrug resistance of human gastric carcinoma SGC7901/VCR cells by inhibiting permeability glycoprotein (P-gp) and multidrug resistance-associated protein (MRP) expression in SGC701/VCR cells [70]. In another study, apoptosis inducing effect of neferine was proposed in lung cancer cells (A549 cells). Neferine treatment leads apoptosis by downregulation of nuclear factor kappaB and B-cell lymphoma 2 (Bcl2), upregulation of Bcl-2-associated X protein

(Bax) and Bcl-2-associated death promoter (BAD), release of cytochrome C, activation of apoptosis regulator caspase cascade, and DNA fragmentation. Furthermore, neferine caused G1 cell cycle arrest by inducing p53 and its effector protein p21 as well as downregulation of cell cycle regulatory protein cyclin D1 [71]. In addition, neferine possessed growth-inhibitory effect due to cell cycle arrest at G1 on human osteosarcoma cells. It was observed that G1 arrest induction was dependent on p21(WAF1/CIP1); however, it was independent of p53 or RB (retinoblastoma-associated protein). Neferine caused upregulation of p21 due to rise in p21 protein half-life. Researchers examined four kinases that are supposed to affect the stabilization of p21 and found that neferine activated p38 MAPK and JNK. They demonstrated that inhibitor of p38 (SB203580), but not the inhibitor of JNK (SP600125), could decrease p21 upregulation of p21 in response to neferine. Neferine increased phosphorylation of p21 at Ser130 dependent on p38. These results highlighted a direct antitumor action of neferine revealing that neferine possesses cancer-preventive and cancer-therapeutic potential [72].

5.16. Nutritional Value. Rhizomes consist of 1.7% protein, 0.1% fat, 9.7% carbohydrate, and 1.1% ash [73]. The taste of rhizome is like beet and exhibits moderate flavor and is used in Chinese cooking [74, 75]. Ogle et al., 2001, reported the use of lotus stem containing 6, 2.4, and 0.2 mg/100 g of calcium, iron, and zinc, respectively, in Vietnamese salad recipes [76]. Lotus leaves are beneficial as natural home remedy for summer heat syndrome and obesity treatment in Asian countries Japan and China [65]. Petals of this plant are sometimes used for garnish and the stamens are used as flavoring agent in the tea [77]. Ibrahim and El-Eraqy in 1996 reported that Egyptian lotus seeds consist of 14.8% crude protein [78]. The green embryos present in the seeds are bitter in taste so they are often eliminated before selling food product to the markets. The seeds can be eaten after popping and can be grounded into flour and eaten raw or used in homemade bread making. Roasted seeds are common substitute of coffee and constitute saponins, phenolics, and carbohydrates in reasonable amount [11, 24]. *N. nucifera* seed contains 348.45 cal/100 g energy, 10.6–15.9% protein, 1.93–2.8% crude fat, 2.7% crude fibre, 3.9–4.5% ash, 70–72.17% carbohydrate, and 10.5% moisture [73, 79]. Minerals of lotus seeds contain iron (0.199%), manganese (0.356%), zinc (0.084%), copper (0.0463%), magnesium (9.2%), calcium (22.1%), potassium (28.5%), chromium (0.0042%), and sodium (1%).

5.17. Traditional Uses. Traditional knowledge on medicinal uses of lotus plant is demonstrated by many scientific investigations. The whole plant is used as antifungal, antipyretic, emollient, sudorific, diuretic, and cardiotonic. Uses of various parts of the lotus plant are common in tissue inflammation diarrhea treatment and haemostasis [80]. The rhizomes are traditionally used for pectoralgia, leucoderma, pharyngopathy, dysentery, spermatorrhoea, cough, small pox, and diarrhea. In ayurveda, the stem is used as diuretic and anthelmintic and to treat nervous exhaustion, strangury, leprosy, skin disease, and vomiting. Young leaves are mixed with sugar for rectal prolapse therapy. Leaves boiled with goat's milk and *Mimosa pudica* are used as antidiarrheal. Natural remedies obtained from leaf paste are effective in fever and inflammatory skin. Leaves can be used for treatment of metrorrhagia, hematemesis, hemoptysis, hematuria, and epistaxis [81]. Experiment reported treatment of hyperlipidaemia in rodents with lotus leaves [82, 83]. Astringent properties is attributed in leaves to treat strangury, fever, and sweating and as styptic [84]. The flowers and leaves are of importance in treating bleeding disorders. Flowers consumption can promote conception and also are important to treat fever, diarrhea, hyperdipsia, cholera, and hepatopathy. In traditional folk medicines, seeds are used for the treatment of poison antidote and disease of skin and usually prescribed as refrigerant and as diuretic to children [85]. The seeds and fruits are also astringent in nature and can be used for the treatment of various skin diseases, hyperdipsia, halitosis, and menorrhagia [86]. Mixed honey and seed powder is useful in treating cough. Ghee and roots, milk, and gold potentiate strength and virility. Lotus seeds have been used as antimicrobial due to its antimicrobial properties [87, 88]. Lian Zi Xin, Chinese drug, is prepared by using embryo of lotus seed which is useful in insomnia, various cardiovascular diseases (e.g., hypertension and arrhythmia), nervous disorders, and high fevers (with restlessness) [89].

6. Conclusions

The perennial aquatic herb, *Nelumbo nucifera*, belonging to family Nymphaeaceae, is gaining its popularity because of its nutraceutical and historical importance. It was used in the treatment of tissue inflammation, cancer, diabetes, skin diseases, bleeding disorders, and cardiovascular diseases as mentioned in the traditional system of medicines. Conducting and documenting the evidence based researches to reveal the possible mechanism of action regarding those effects are today's necessity. Moreover, it will be of economic value if it can be developed as functional food.

Conflict of Interests

The authors declare that there is no conflict of interests regarding the publication of this paper.

Authors' Contribution

Both authors contributed equally to this paper.

References

[1] H.-H. Lee, K. R. Paudel, and D.-W. Kim, "Terminalia chebula fructus inhibits migration and proliferation of vascular smooth muscle cells and production of inflammatory mediators in RAW 264.7," *Evidence-Based Complementary and Alternative Medicine*, vol. 2015, Article ID 502182, 10 pages, 2015.

[2] C. Kessler, M. Wischnewsky, A. Michalsen, C. Eisenmann, and J. Melzer, "Ayurveda: between religion, spirituality, and medicine," *Evidence-Based Complementary and Alternative Medicine*, vol. 2013, Article ID 952432, 11 pages, 2013.

[3] H. Bae, H. Bae, B.-I. Min, and S. Cho, "Efficacy of acupuncture in reducing preoperative anxiety: a meta-analysis," *Evidence-Based Complementary and Alternative Medicine*, vol. 2014, Article ID 850367, 12 pages, 2014.

[4] S. R. Devkota, K. R. Paudel, K. Sharma et al., "Investigation of antioxidant and anti-inflammatory activity of roots of *Rumex nepalensis*," *World Journal of Pharmacy and Pharmaceutical Sciences*, vol. 4, no. 3, pp. 582–594, 2015.

[5] H. Lee, Y. Kim, H. J. Kim et al., "Herbal formula, PM014, attenuates lung inflammation in a murine model of chronic obstructive pulmonary disease," *Evidence-Based Complementary and Alternative Medicine*, vol. 2012, Article ID 769830, 10 pages, 2012.

[6] M. S. Khan, S. Khanam, M. Deepak, and B. G. Shivanda, "Antioxidant activity of a new diarylheptanoid from *Zingiber officinale*," *Pharmacognosy Magazine*, vol. 2, no. 8, pp. 254–257, 2006.

[7] R. Karki, M.-A. Jung, K.-J. Kim, and D.-W. Kim, "Inhibitory effect of *Nelumbo nucifera* (Gaertn.) on the development of atopic dermatitis-like skin lesions in NC/Nga mice," *Evidence-Based Complementary and Alternative Medicine*, vol. 2012, Article ID 153568, 7 pages, 2012.

[8] R. Karki, E.-R. Jeon, and D.-W. Kim, "Nelumbo nucifera leaf extract inhibits neointimal hyperplasia through modulation of smooth muscle cell proliferation and migration," *Nutrition*, vol. 29, no. 1, pp. 268–275, 2013.

[9] W. B. Harer, "Pharmacological and biological properties of the Egyptian lotus," *Journal of the American Research Center in Egypt*, vol. 22, pp. 49–54, 1985.

[10] *The Wealth of India—A Dictionary of Indian Raw Materials*, vol. 7, Council of Scientific Industrial Research, New Delhi, India, 1966.

[11] *The Wealth of India*, vol. 3, Council of Scientific Industrial Research, New Delhi, India, 1992.

[12] P. K. Mukherjee, D. Mukherjee, A. K. Maji, S. Rai, and M. Heinrich, "The sacred lotus (Nelumbo nucifera)—phytochemical and therapeutic profile," *Journal of Pharmacy and Pharmacology*, vol. 61, no. 4, pp. 407–422, 2009.

[13] P. K. Mukherjee, R. Balasubramanian, K. Saha, B. P. Saha, and M. Pal, "A review on *Nelumbo nucifera* gaertn," *Ancient Science of Life*, vol. 15, no. 4, pp. 268–276, 1996.

[14] J. Wang, X. Hu, W. Yin, and H. Cai, "Alkaloids of plumula Nelumbinis," *Zhongguo Zhong Yao Za Zhi*, vol. 16, no. 11, pp. 673–675, 1991.

[15] H. Koshiyama, H. Ohkuma, H. Kawaguchi, H. Hsu, and Y. Chen, "Isolation of 1-(p-Hydroxybenzyl)-6,7-dihydroxy-1,2,3,4-tetrahydroisoquinoline (demethylcoclaurine), an active alkaloid from *Nelumbo nucifera*," *Chemical and Pharmaceutical Bulletin*, vol. 18, no. 12, pp. 2564–2568, 1970.

[16] N. R. Mehta, E. P. Patel, P. V. Patani, and B. Shah, "Nelumbo nucifera (Lotus): a review on ethanobotany, phytochemistry and pharmacology," *Indian Journal of Pharmrmaceutical and Biological Research*, vol. 1, no. 4, pp. 152–167, 2013.

[17] H. A. Jung, J. E. Kim, H. Y. Chung, and J. S. Choi, "Antioxidant principles of *Nelumbo nucifera* stamens," *Archives of Pharmacal Research*, vol. 26, no. 4, pp. 279–285, 2003.

[18] A. Omata, K. Yomogida, S. Nakamura, T. Ohta, Y. Izawa, and S. Watanabe, "The scent of lotus flowers," *Journal of Essential Oil Research*, vol. 3, no. 4, pp. 221–227, 1991.

[19] S. Chen, L. Fang, H. Xi et al., "Simultaneous qualitative assessment and quantitative analysis of flavonoids in various tissues

of lotus (*Nelumbo nucifera*) using high performance liquid chromatography coupled with triple quad mass spectrometry," *Analytica Chimica Acta*, vol. 724, pp. 127–135, 2012.

[20] C. Ma, J. Wang, H. Chu et al., "Purification and characterization of aporphine alkaloids from leaves of *Nelumbo nucifera* gaertn and their effects on glucose consumption in 3T3-L1 adipocytes," *International Journal of Molecular Sciences*, vol. 15, no. 3, pp. 3481–3494, 2014.

[21] S. Rai, A. Wahile, K. Mukherjee, B. P. Saha, and P. K. Mukherjee, "Antioxidant activity of *Nelumbo nucifera* (sacred lotus) seeds," *Journal of Ethnopharmacology*, vol. 104, no. 3, pp. 322–327, 2006.

[22] H. K. Lee, Y. M. Choi, D. O. Noh, and H. J. Suh, "Antioxidant effect of Korean traditional lotus liquor (Yunyupju)," *International Journal of Food Science and Technology*, vol. 40, no. 7, pp. 709–715, 2005.

[23] G.-C. Yen, P.-D. Duh, H.-J. Su, C.-T. Yeh, and C.-H. Wu, "Scavenging effects of lotus seed extracts on reactive nitrogen species," *Food Chemistry*, vol. 94, no. 4, pp. 596–602, 2006.

[24] Z.-Q. Ling, B.-J. Xie, and E.-L. Yang, "Isolation, characterization, and determination of antioxidative activity of oligomeric procyanidins from the seedpod of *Nelumbo nucifera* Gaertn," *Journal of Agricultural and Food Chemistry*, vol. 53, no. 7, pp. 2441–2445, 2005.

[25] E. S. Kim, J. B. Weon, B.-R. Yun et al., "Cognitive enhancing and neuroprotective effect of the embryo of the *Nelumbo nucifera* seed," *Evidence-Based Complementary and Alternative Medicine*, vol. 2014, Article ID 869831, 9 pages, 2014.

[26] M. Gupta, U. K. Mazumder, R. K. Mukhopadhyay, and S. Sarkar, "Antisteroidogenic effect of the seed extract of *Nelumbo nucifera* in the testis and the ovary of the rat," *Indian Journal of Pharmaceutical Sciences*, vol. 58, no. 6, pp. 236–242, 1996.

[27] Y. Wethangkaboworn and P. Munglue, "Effect of ethanolic seed extract of *Nelumbo nucifera* on male rat sexual behavior," *KKU Research Journal*, vol. 19, supplement, pp. 156–161, 2014.

[28] A. Mutreju, M. Agarwal, S. Kushwaha, and A. Chauhan, "Effect of *Nelumbo nucifera* seeds on the reproductive organs of female rats," *Iranian Journal of Reproductive Medicine*, vol. 6, no. 1, pp. 7–11, 2008.

[29] S. Sinha, P. K. Mukherjee, K. Mukherjee, M. Pal, S. C. Mandal, and B. P. Saha, "Evaluation of antipyretic potential of *Nelumbo nucifera* stalk extract," *Phytotherapy Research*, vol. 14, no. 4, pp. 272–274, 2000.

[30] P. K. Mukherjee, J. Das, K. Saha, S. N. Giri, M. Pal, and B. P. Saha, "Antipyretic activity of *Nelumbo nucifera* rhizome extract," *Indian Journal of Experimental Biology*, vol. 34, no. 3, pp. 275–276, 1996.

[31] Y. Kashiwada, A. Aoshima, Y. Ikeshiro et al., "Anti-HIV benzylisoquinoline alkaloids and flavonoids from the leaves of *Nelumbo nucifera* and structure-activity correlations with related alkaloids," *Bioorganic and Medicinal Chemistry*, vol. 13, no. 2, pp. 443–448, 2005.

[32] Y.-C. Kuo, Y.-L. Lin, C.-P. Liu, and W.-J. Tsai, "Herpes simplex virus type 1 propagation in HeLa cells interrupted by Nelumbo nucifera," *Journal of Biomedical Science*, vol. 12, no. 6, pp. 1021–1034, 2005.

[33] C.-P. Liu, W.-J. Tsai, Y.-L. Lin, J.-F. Liao, C.-F. Chen, and Y.-C. Kuo, "The extracts from *Nelumbo nucifera* suppress cell cycle progression, cytokine genes expression, and cell proliferation in human peripheral blood mononuclear cells," *Life Sciences*, vol. 75, no. 6, pp. 699–716, 2004.

[34] C.-P. Liu, W.-J. Tsai, C.-C. Shen et al., "Inhibition of (S)-armepavine from Nelumbo nucifera on autoimmune disease

of MRL/MpJ-lpr/lpr mice," *European Journal of Pharmacology*, vol. 531, no. 1–3, pp. 270–279, 2006.

[35] C.-P. Liu, Y.-C. Kuo, C.-C. Shen et al., "(S)-Armepavine inhibits human peripheral blood mononuclear cell activation by regulating Itk and PLCγ activation in a PI-3K-dependent manner," *Journal of Leukocyte Biology*, vol. 81, no. 5, pp. 1276–1286, 2007.

[36] T. Hanada and A. Yoshimura, "Regulation of cytokine signaling and inflammation," *Cytokine and Growth Factor Reviews*, vol. 13, no. 4-5, pp. 413–421, 2002.

[37] R. B. Goodman, R. M. Strieter, D. P. Martin et al., "Inflammatory cytokines in patients with persistence of the acute respiratory distress syndrome," *American Journal of Respiratory and Critical Care Medicine*, vol. 154, no. 3, pp. 602–611, 1996.

[38] P. K. Mukherjee, K. Saha, J. Das, M. Pal, and B. P. Saha, "Studies on the anti-inflammatory activity of rhizomes of *Nelumbo nucifera*," *Planta Medica*, vol. 63, no. 4, pp. 367–369, 1997.

[39] P. K. Mukherjee, K. Saha, M. Pal, and B. P. Saha, "Effect of Nelumbo nucifera rhizome extract on blood sugar level in rats," *Journal of Ethnopharmacology*, vol. 58, no. 3, pp. 207–213, 1997.

[40] C. Day, T. Cartwright, J. Provost, and C. J. Bailey, "Hypoglycaemic effect of *Momordica charantia* extracts," *Planta Medica*, vol. 56, no. 5, pp. 426–429, 1990.

[41] S. S. Lim, Y. J. Jung, S. K. Hyun, Y. S. Lee, and J. S. Choi, "Rat lens aldose reductase inhibitory constituents of *Nelumbo nucifera* stamens," *Phytotherapy Research*, vol. 20, no. 10, pp. 825–830, 2006.

[42] J. Chen, J.-H. Liu, T. Wang, H.-J. Xiao, C.-P. Yin, and J. Yang, "Effects of plant extract neferine on cyclic adenosine monophosphate and cyclic guanosine monophosphate levels in rabbit corpus cavernosum in vitro," *Asian Journal of Andrology*, vol. 10, no. 2, pp. 307–312, 2008.

[43] J. Chen, J. Qi, F. Chen et al., "Relaxation mechanisms of neferine on the rabbit corpus cavernosum tissue in vitro," *Asian Journal of Andrology*, vol. 9, no. 6, pp. 795–800, 2007.

[44] J. Chen, J. H. Liu, Z. J. Jiang et al., "Effects of neferine on cytosolic free calcium concentration in corpus cavernosum smooth muscle cells of rabbits," *Andrologia*, vol. 39, no. 4, pp. 141–145, 2007.

[45] H.-H. Ho, L.-S. Hsu, K.-C. Chan, H.-M. Chen, C.-H. Wu, and C.-J. Wang, "Extract from the leaf of nucifera reduced the development of atherosclerosis via inhibition of vascular smooth muscle cell proliferation and migration," *Food and Chemical Toxicology*, vol. 48, no. 1, pp. 159–168, 2010.

[46] H.-J. Lee, C.-C. Chen, F.-P. Chou et al., "Water extracts from nelumbo nucifera leaf reduced plasma lipids and atherosclerosis in cholesterol-fed rabbits," *Journal of Food Biochemistry*, vol. 34, no. 4, pp. 779–795, 2010.

[47] X.-C. Li, G.-X. Tong, Y. Zhang et al., "Neferine inhibits angiotensin II-stimulated proliferation in vascular smooth muscle cells through heme oxygenase-1," *Acta Pharmacologica Sinica*, vol. 31, no. 6, pp. 679–686, 2010.

[48] L. Zheng, Y. Cao, S. Liu, Z. Peng, and S. Zhang, "Neferine inhibits angiotensin II-induced rat aortic smooth muscle cell proliferation predominantly by downregulating fractalkine gene expression," *Experimental and Therapeutic Medicine*, vol. 8, no. 5, pp. 1545–1550, 2014.

[49] P. A. Riley and T. Babcock, "Methods utilizing compositions containing sacred lotus (methyltransferase) to treat aging skin," US Patent 5925348, 1999.

[50] T. Mahmood and N. Akhtar, "Combined topical application of lotus and green tea improves facial skin surface parameters," *Rejuvenation Research*, vol. 16, no. 2, pp. 91–97, 2013.

[51] T. Mahmood, N. Akhtar, and C. Moldovan, "A comparison of the effects of topical green tea and lotus on facial sebum control in healthy humans," *Hippokratia*, vol. 17, no. 1, pp. 64–67, 2013.

[52] J.-Q. Qian, "Cardiovascular pharmacological effects of bis-benzylisoquinoline alkaloid derivatives," *Acta Pharmacologica Sinica*, vol. 23, no. 12, pp. 1086–1092, 2002.

[53] Q. R. Li, J. Q. Qian, and F. H. Lue, "Anti-experimental arrhythmias of neferine and quinidine," *Chinese Traditional and Herbal Drugs*, vol. 19, pp. 25–28, 1988.

[54] G. R. Li, X. G. Li, J. Q. Qian, and F. H. Lu, "Effects of neferine on electrical and mechanical activity in isolated guinea pig myocardium," *Chinese Journal of Pharmacology and Toxicology*, vol. 1, no. 4, pp. 268–271, 1987.

[55] G. R. Li, F. H. Lue, and J. Q. Qian, "Effects of neferine on physiologic properties and dose-effect response of isoprenaline and Ca^{2+} in guinea pig atria," *Acta Pharmacologica Sinica*, vol. 23, no. 4, pp. 241–245, 1988.

[56] Z. Guo, "Electrophysiological effects of neferine against ischemic ventricular tachyarrhythmias," *Zhonghua Xin Xue Guan Bing Za Zhi*, vol. 20, no. 2, pp. 119–134, 1992.

[57] D.-H. Sohn, Y.-C. Kim, S.-H. Oh, E.-J. Park, X. Li, and B.-H. Lee, "Hepatoprotective and free radical scavenging effects of *Nelumbo nucifera*," *Phytomedicine*, vol. 10, no. 2-3, pp. 165–169, 2003.

[58] J. Y. Je and D. B. Lee, "Nelumbo nucifera leaves protect hydrogen peroxide-induced hepatic damage via antioxidant enzymes and HO-1/Nrf2 activation," *Food and Function*, vol. 6, no. 6, pp. 1911–1918, 2015.

[59] L. Yuan, X. Gu, Z. Yin, and W. Kang, "Antioxidant activities in vitro and hepatoprotective effects of *Nelumbo nucifera* leaves in vivo," *African Journal of Traditional, Complementary and Alternative Medicines*, vol. 11, no. 3, pp. 85–91, 2014.

[60] C.-C. Tang, W.-L. Lin, Y.-J. Lee, Y.-C. Tang, and C.-J. Wang, "Polyphenol-rich extract of *Nelumbo nucifera* leaves inhibits alcohol-induced steatohepatitis via reducing hepatic lipid accumulation and anti-inflammation in C57BL/6J mice," *Food and Function*, vol. 5, no. 4, pp. 678–687, 2014.

[61] J.-H. Xiao, J.-H. Zhang, H.-L. Chen, X.-L. Feng, and J.-L. Wang, "Inhibitory effects of isoliensinine on bleomycin-induced pulmonary fibrosis in mice," *Planta Medica*, vol. 71, no. 3, pp. 225–230, 2005.

[62] L. Zhao, X. Wang, Q. Chang et al., "Neferine, a bisbenzyliso-quinline alkaloid attenuates bleomycin-induced pulmonary fibrosis," *European Journal of Pharmacology*, vol. 627, no. 1–3, pp. 304–312, 2010.

[63] C.-H. Niu, Y. Wang, J.-D. Liu, J.-L. Wang, and J.-H. Xiao, "Protective effects of neferine on amiodarone-induced pulmonary fibrosis in mice," *European Journal of Pharmacology*, vol. 714, no. 1–3, pp. 112–119, 2013.

[64] E. Ohkoshi, H. Miyazaki, K. Shindo, H. Watanabe, A. Yoshida, and H. Yajima, "Constituents from the leaves of *Nelumbo nucifera* stimulate lipolysis in the white adipose tissue of mice," *Planta Medica*, vol. 73, no. 12, pp. 1255–1259, 2007.

[65] Y. Ono, E. Hattori, Y. Fukaya, S. Imai, and Y. Ohizumi, "Anti-obesity effect of *Nelumbo nucifera* leaves extract in mice and rats," *Journal of Ethnopharmacology*, vol. 106, no. 2, pp. 238–244, 2006.

[66] C. C. Velusami, A. Agarwal, and V. Mookambeswaran, "Effect of *Nelumbo nucifera* petal extracts on lipase, adipogenesis, adipolysis, and central receptors of obesity," *Evidence-Based Complementary and Alternative Medicine*, vol. 2013, Article ID 145925, 7 pages, 2013.

[67] X. Zhang, X. Wang, T. Wu et al., "Isoliensinine induces apoptosis in triple-negative human breast cancer cells through ROS generation and p38 MAPK/JNK activation," *Scientific Reports*, vol. 29, no. 5, pp. 1–13, 2015.

[68] W. Liu, D. D. Yi, J. L. Guo, Z. X. Xiang, L. F. Deng, and L. He, "Nuciferine, extracted from *Nelumbo nucifera* Gaertn, inhibits tumor-promoting effect of nicotine involving Wnt/β-catenin signaling in non-small cell lung cancer," *Journal of Ethnopharmacology*, vol. 165, pp. 83–93, 2015.

[69] C.-M. Liu, C.-L. Kao, H.-M. Wu et al., "Antioxidant and anticancer aporphine alkaloids from the leaves of Nelumbo nucifera Gaertn. cv. Rosa-plena," *Molecules*, vol. 19, no. 11, pp. 17829–17838, 2014.

[70] J.-G. Cao, X.-Q. Tang, and S.-H. Shi, "Multidrug resistance reversal in human gastric carcinoma cells by neferine," *World Journal of Gastroenterology*, vol. 10, no. 20, pp. 3062–3064, 2004.

[71] P. Poornima, C. F. Weng, and V. V. Padma, "Neferine, an alkaloid from lotus seed embryo, inhibits human lung cancer cell growth by MAPK activation and cell cycle arrest," *BioFactors*, vol. 40, no. 1, pp. 121–131, 2014.

[72] X. Zhang, Z. Liu, B. Xu, Z. Sun, Y. Gong, and C. Shao, "Neferine, an alkaloid ingredient in lotus seed embryo, inhibits proliferation of human osteosarcoma cells by promoting p38 MAPK-mediated p21 stabilization," *European Journal of Pharmacology*, vol. 677, no. 1–3, pp. 47–54, 2012.

[73] B. E. Reid, *Famine Foods of the Chiu-Huang Pen-Ts'ao*, Southern Materials Centre, Taipei, Taiwan, 1977.

[74] U. P. Hedrick, *Sturtevant's Edible Plants of the World*, Dover Publications, New York, NY, USA, 1972.

[75] T. Tanaka, *Tanaka's Cyclopedia of Edible Plants of the World*, Keigaku Publishing, Tokyo, Japan, 1976.

[76] B. M. Ogle, H. T. A. Dao, G. Mulokozi, and L. Hambraeus, "Micronutrient composition and nutritional importance of gathered vegetables in Vietnam," *International Journal of Food Sciences and Nutrition*, vol. 52, no. 6, pp. 485–499, 2001.

[77] S. Facciola, *Cornucopia: A Source Book of Edible Plants*, Kampong Publications, Vista, Calif, USA, 1990.

[78] N. Ibrahim and W. El-Eraqy, "Protein content and amino acid composition of *Nelumbo nucifera* seeds and its evaluation as hypoglycaemic agent," *Egyptian Journal of Pharmaceutical Sciences*, vol. 37, no. 1–6, pp. 635–641, 1996.

[79] A. K. Indrayan, S. Sharma, D. Durgapal, N. Kumar, and M. Kumar, "Determination of nutritive value and analysis of mineral elements for some medicinally valued plants from Uttaranchal," *Current Science*, vol. 89, no. 7, pp. 1252–1255, 2005.

[80] J. Yu and W. S. Hu, "Effects of neferine on platelet aggregation in rabbits," *Yaoxue Xuebao*, vol. 32, no. 1, pp. 1–4, 1997.

[81] M. Ou, *Chinese-English Manual of Common-Used in Traditional Chinese Medicine*, Joint Publishing Company, Hong Kong, 1989.

[82] B. La Cour, P. Mølgaard, and Z. Yi, "Traditional Chinese medicine in treatment of hyperlipidaemia," *Journal of Ethnopharmacology*, vol. 46, no. 2, pp. 125–129, 1995.

[83] E. Onishi, K. Yamada, T. Yamada et al., "Comparative effects of crude drugs on serum lipids," *Chemical & Pharmaceutical Bulletin*, vol. 32, no. 2, pp. 646–650, 1984.

[84] *Chinese Materia Medica*, Jiangsu New Medical College, Peoples Publishing House, Shanghai, China, 1997.

[85] R. N. Chopra, S. L. Nayar, and I. C. Chopra, *Glossary of Indian Medicinal Plants*, Council of Scientific Industrial Research, New Delhi, India, 1956.

[86] A. K. Nadkarni, *The Indian Materia Medica*, vol. 1, Popular Prakashan Pvt, Bombay, India, 1982.

[87] P. K. Mukherjee, S. N. Giri, K. Saha, M. Pal, and B. P. Saha, "Antifungal screening of *Nelumbo nucifera* (Nymphaeaceae) rhizome extract," *Indian Journal of Microbiology*, vol. 35, pp. 327–330, 1995.

[88] P. K. Mukherjee, *Quality Control of Herbal Drugs: An Approach to Evaluation of Botanicals*, Business Horizons, New Delhi, India, 1st edition, 2002.

[89] Y. Chen, G. Fan, H. Wu, Y. Wu, and A. Mitchell, "Separation, identification and rapid determination of liensine, isoliensinine and neferine from embryo of the seed of *Nelumbo nucifera* GAERTN. by liquid chromatography coupled to diode array detector and tandem mass spectrometry," *Journal of Pharmaceutical and Biomedical Analysis*, vol. 43, no. 1, pp. 99–104, 2007.

8

Luoyutong Treatment Promotes Functional Recovery and Neuronal Plasticity after Cerebral Ischemia-Reperfusion Injury in Rats

Ning-qun Wang,[1,2] Li-ye Wang,[3] Hai-ping Zhao,[1,4] Ping Liu,[1,5] Rong-liang Wang,[1,4] Jue-xian Song,[5] Li Gao,[5] Xun-ming Ji,[4] and Yu-min Luo[1,4]

[1]Cerebrovascular Diseases Research Institute, Xuanwu Hospital, Capital Medical University, Ministry of Education, 45 Changchun Street, Beijing 100053, China
[2]Department of Traditional Chinese Medicine, Xuanwu Hospital, Capital Medical University, Ministry of Education, 45 Changchun Street, Beijing 100053, China
[3]Dongfang Hospital, Beijing University of Chinese Medicine, Beijing 100078, China
[4]Key Laboratory of Neurodegenerative Diseases (Capital Medical University), Ministry of Education, 45 Changchun Street, Beijing 100053, China
[5]Department of Neurology, Xuanwu Hospital, Capital Medical University, Ministry of Education, 45 Changchun Street, Beijing 100053, China

Correspondence should be addressed to Yu-min Luo; yumin111@ccmu.edu.cn

Academic Editor: Shan-Yu Su

Luoyutong (LYT) capsule has been used to treat cerebrovascular diseases clinically in China and is now patented and approved by the State Food and Drug Administration. In this retrospective validation study we investigated the ability of LYT to protect against cerebral ischemia-reperfusion injury in rats. Cerebral ischemia-reperfusion injury was induced by middle cerebral artery occlusion followed by reperfusion. Capsule containing LYT (high dose and medium dose) as treatment group and Citicoline Sodium as positive control treatment group were administered daily to rats 30 min after reperfusion. Treatment was continued for either 3 days or 14 days. A saline solution was administered to control animals. Behavior tests were performed after 3 and 14 days of treatment. Our findings revealed that LYT treatment improved the neurological outcome, decreased cerebral infarction volume, and reduced apoptosis. Additionally, LYT improved neural plasticity, as the expression of synaptophysin, microtubule associated protein, and myelin basic protein was upregulated by LYT treatment, while neurofilament 200 expression was reduced. Moreover, levels of brain derived neurotrophic factor and basic fibroblast growth factor were increased. Our results suggest that LYT treatment may protect against ischemic injury and improve neural plasticity.

1. Introduction

Stroke is one of the leading causes of death worldwide and causes long-term disability. It has a significant impact upon health, well-being, and social interactions. Despite this, the available treatments remain limited and unsatisfactory and there is a considerable demand for novel therapies [1–3]. The use of Traditional Chinese Medicines (TCMs) in treating cerebral ischemia injury has increased in recent years and the regulatory pathways targeted by these medicines have been investigated [4–6]. A special group of medicinal plants and animals used in TCMs have been widely administered as patented Chinese medications to manage the symptoms of stroke, such as spasticity, altered muscle tone, and motor neuron excitability [7–10].

Neuronal plasticity involves changes in intracerebral structure and function in both gray matter and white matter. Gray matter consists mainly of neuronal cell bodies and unmyelinated axons. Within the gray matter, synaptic distribution and density can be measured by expression of the

TABLE 1: LYT ingredients.

Ingredients (Latin name)	Family	Part used	Processing	Amount used %
Plants				
Astragalus membranaceus (Fisch.) Bge.	Leguminosae	Dried root	Extraction	18.159
Ligusticum chuanxiong Hort.	Umbelliferae	Root and rhizome	Extraction	9.079
Spatholobus suberectus Dunn	Papilionaceae	Rattan and stem	Extraction	13.681
Insects				
Pheretima vulgaris Chen	Guaibasauridae	Dried body	Farina	27.238
Whitmania pigra Whitman	Hirundinidae	Dried body	Farina	13.681
Buthus martensii Karsch	Buthidae	Dried body	Farina	5.472
Scolopendra subspinipes mutilans L. Koch	Psittacidae	Dried body	Farina	4.477
Bombyx mori Linnaeus	Bombycidae	Dried body	Farina	8.208

synaptic vesicle protein synaptophysin, while dendrites can be visualized using microtubule associated protein (MAP-2) as a marker. White matter is composed mainly of myelinated axons and myelin-producing oligodendrocytes as well as other glial cells. Myelin basic protein (MBP) is a marker of myelin and neurofilament 200 (NF200) is expressed in myelinated axons. The effect of stroke on gray matter has been well studied in the past, but more attention has been paid recently to white matter injury following stroke [11].

Luoyutong (LYT) capsule contains eight active TCM ingredients (Table 1) and is patented and approved by the State Food and Drug Administration in China. It has been used clinically for the treatment of acute and chronic cerebrovascular diseases. Previous studies showed it has a therapeutic effect of stroke [12, 13]. Our preliminary results suggest LYT plays a protective role in cerebral ischemia-reperfusion injury of rats [14]; however, the mechanism underlying the therapeutic effects of LYT in cerebrovascular diseases remains undefined. To address this, in this retrospective validation study, we investigated the protective effect and underlying mechanisms of LYT treatment in a rat model of cerebral ischemia-reperfusion injury.

2. Methods

2.1. Drug and Preparation. LYT (505 Pharmaceutical Co. Ltd., Lot number: 960815, Xianyang, Shanxi, China) was in the form of a dried superfine powder ($\leq 10\,\mu m$) composed of eight ingredients (Table 1), which were ground using a micronizer. LYT powder was prepared as a capsule, which was authenticated and standardized based on marker compounds in the Chinese Pharmacopoeia (Committee, 2005). The ingredients of the LYT capsule were carefully analyzed and quality-controlled. One gram of capsule is equivalent to 2.68 g of crude drug. The powder was dissolved in saline (0.08 g/mL) and stored at 4°C until subsequent use. Citicoline Sodium (CS) capsule (QILU Pharmaceutical Group Co. Ltd., Lot number: H20020220, Jinan, Shandong, China) was used clinically for cerebral ischemia, cerebral hemorrhage, and dementia because of its repair effect in recovery phase. Citicoline Sodium (CS) capsules were diluted in saline to a final concentration of 2 mg/mL as a positive control treatment group.

2.2. Animals. Male Sprague-Dawley rats weighing 280–300 g were purchased from Vital River Laboratory Animal Technology Co. Ltd. (Beijing, China). Animals were housed in an environmentally controlled room at $22 \pm 2°C$, with a 12 h/12 h light/dark cycle and were allowed free access to food and water throughout the entire study. The study was approved by the Institutional Animal Care and Use Committee of Capital Medical University and was in accordance with the principles outlined in the National Institutes of Health Guide for the Care and Use of Laboratory Animals.

2.3. Rat Model of Cerebral Ischemia-Reperfusion. Focal cerebral ischemia was induced in rats as previously described [15]. Briefly, rats were anesthetized with enflurane, and the right common carotid artery, the external carotid artery (ECA), and the internal carotid artery (ICA) were exposed. A 4-0 suture (diameter, 0.26 mm) with a blunted tip coated with poly-L-lysine was gently advanced into the ICA through the ECA. The suture was advanced 18–20 mm (reaching the origin of the right middle cerebral artery) beyond the carotid artery bifurcation. To allow reperfusion, the suture was slowly withdrawn after 1.5 h of middle cerebral artery occlusion (MCAO). Regional cerebral blood flow (0.5 mm anterior and 5.0 mm lateral to bregma) was monitored using laser Doppler flowmetry (PeriFlux System 5000, Perimed, Stockholm, Sweden) to ensure the occurrence of ischemia by MCAO. Rectal temperature was maintained at 37.0°C during and after surgery with a temperature-controlled heating pad (CMA 150 Carnegie Medicine, Sweden). Operations in the sham group were performed using the same surgical procedures, excepting the occlusion of the carotid arteries. All animals were housed in an air-conditioned room at $22 \pm 2°C$ after recovering from anesthesia.

2.4. Grouping and Treatment. In total, 90 rats were randomly divided into five groups: sham group, MCAO group, medium dose (0.4 g/kg) of LYT (LYTM), high dose (0.8 g/kg) of LYT (LYTH), and CS (0.1 g/kg). Each group was divided into two subgroups, one treated for 3 days and the other for 14 days. Each subgroup contained nine animals; six were used for 2,3,5-triphenyltetrazolium chloride (TTC) staining to evaluate brain infarct and swelling volume and three rats were allocated for histological and Western blot analyses.

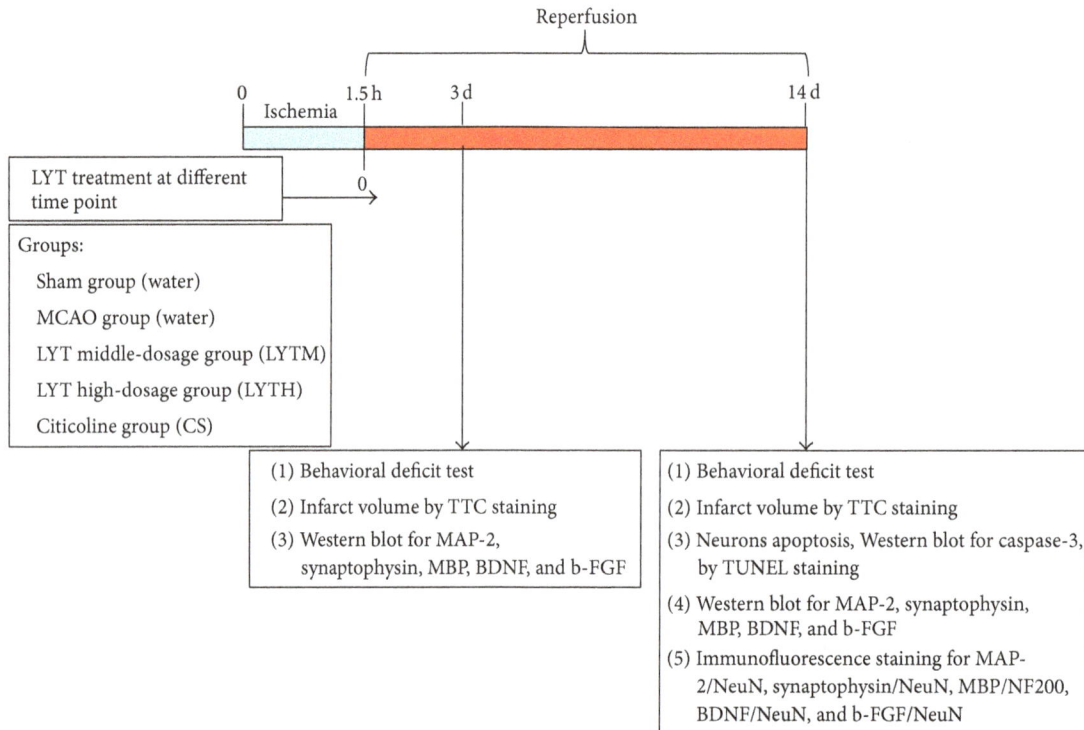

FIGURE 1: Schematic representation of the experimental procedures. (Luoyutong: LYT; middle cerebral artery occlusion: MCAO; 2,3,5-triphenyltetrazolium chloride: TTC; microtubule associated protein: MAP-2; myelin basic protein: MBP; brain derived neurotrophic factor: BDNF; basic fibroblast growth factor: b-FGF; neuron-specific nuclear protein: NeuN; neurofilament 200: NF200).

A drug solution (2 mL) was administered by gavage and was calculated according to the body surface area based on the daily clinical dosage recommended for humans. Treatment started 30 min after reperfusion and was administered once a day for 3 or 14 days. Animals in the sham and MCAO groups received 2 mL 0.9% NaCl in the same manner. The experimental design is illustrated in Figure 1.

2.5. Evaluation of Motor Performance.

Behavioral tests were performed blindly by a trained investigator to eliminate bias. Three tests were carried out to evaluate various aspects of neurological function. (1) The first one is Longa's score test [15], where a normal score is 0 and the maximum score is 5. (2) The second one is the 0–12 neurological score test, which included the postural reflex and forelimb placing test, graded on a scale of 0 to 12. The postural reflex test examined the upper body posture while the animal was suspended by the tail and the forelimb placing test evaluated the response of the forelimb to visual, tactile, and proprioceptive stimuli. (3) The third one is the modified foot fault test [16, 17] which recorded the number of times the forelimb was misplaced, causing the rat to fall through the grid.

2.6. Measurement of Infarct Volume.

The animals were sacrificed 3 or 14 days after reperfusion in a carbon dioxide chamber and the brains were quickly removed and sectioned into six consecutive coronal slices of 2 mm thickness. The slices were stained by immersing in 2% TTC for 30 min at 37°C, followed by fixation in 8% formalin. The border between infarcted and noninfarcted tissues was outlined with an image analysis system. The area of infarction was measured by subtracting the area of the nonlesioned ipsilateral hemisphere from that of the contralateral hemisphere based on Swanson's method [18]. The infarct volume was calculated as follows: 100% × (contralateral hemisphere volume − nonlesioned ipsilateral hemisphere volume)/contralateral hemisphere volume. The swelling volume was calculated as follows: 100% × (ipsilateral hemisphere volume − contralateral hemisphere volume)/contralateral hemisphere volume.

2.7. Terminal Deoxynucleotidyl Transferase dUTP Nick End Labeling (TUNEL).

Rats were euthanized 14 days after reperfusion with intraperitoneal injections of chloral hydrate (300 mg/kg) and were perfused transcardially with 4% w/v paraformaldehyde in phosphate-buffered saline (PBS). The brains were dehydrated in 30% sucrose in 4% formaldehyde in PBS. Frozen brains were sectioned coronally. Apoptotic cell death was detected using the In Situ Cell Death Detection Kit, POD (Roche, San Francisco, CA, USA), according to the manufacturer's instructions.

2.8. Western Blotting Analysis.

The forward fontanelle, cut at a coronal slice thickness of 2 mm from the optic chiasma, was harvested 3 or 14 days after reperfusion. Samples were homogenized in lysis buffer (50 mM Tris-HCl, pH 7.5, 100 mM NaCl, and 1% Triton X-100) containing protease inhibitors (aprotinin, leupeptin, phenylmethylsulfonyl

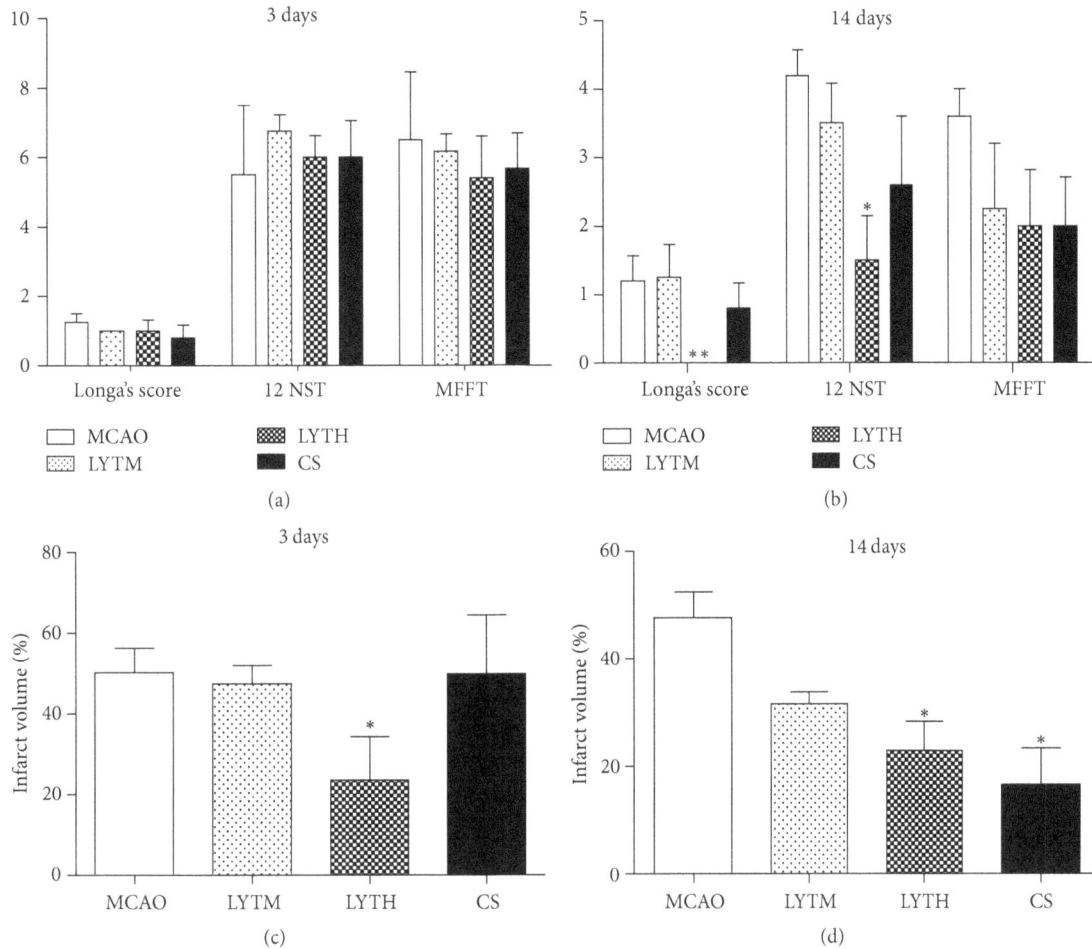

FIGURE 2: LYT (Luoyutong) decreases infarct volume and improves neurological function in rats following ischemic reperfusion. (a) Longa's score, 0–12 neurological score test, and modified foot fault test of MCAO (middle cerebral artery occlusion), LYTM (medium dose (0.4 g/kg) of LYT), LYTH (high dose (0.8 g/kg) of LYT), and CS (Citicoline Sodium) 3 days after MCAO. (b) Longa's score, 0–12 neurological score test, and modified foot fault test of MCAO, LYTM, LYTH, and CS 14 days after MCAO. (c) Infarct volume (%) of MCAO, LYTM, LYTH, and CS 3 days after MCAO. (d) Infarct volume (%) of MCAO, LYTM, LYTH, and CS 14 days after MCAO; $^*P < 0.05$ versus $MCAO$ and $^{**}P < 0.01$ versus $MCAO$.

fluoride, and pepstatin) and phosphatase inhibitors (Sigma cocktail, Sigma-Aldrich, St. Louis, MO, USA). For each sample, 100 μg total protein was resolved by sodium dodecyl sulfate polyacrylamide gel electrophoresis, followed by electrophoretic transfer to polyvinylidene difluoride membranes. Membranes were incubated overnight at 4°C in a 1:1000 dilution of primary antibodies against caspase-3 (Abcam, Cambridge, UK), synaptophysin (Abcam), MAP-2 (Cell Signaling Technology, Boston, MA, USA), MBP (Abcam), brain derived neurotrophic factor (BDNF) (Abcam), or basic fibroblast growth factor (b-FGF) (Abcam). Chemiluminescent detection of antigens was performed following incubation with horseradish peroxidase-conjugated secondary antibodies (Santa Cruz Biotechnology, Santa Cruz, CA, USA) for 60 min at room temperature using an enhanced luminescence kit (Millipore, Billerica, MA, USA).

2.9. Immunofluorescence.
Rats were euthanized 14 days after reperfusion with intraperitoneal injections of chloral hydrate

(300 mg/kg) and perfusion with cold saline. The brains were dehydrated in 30% sucrose and 4% formaldehyde in PBS. Frozen brains were sectioned coronally for immunohistochemistry. Following incubation for 2 h in a blocking solution containing 1% bovine serum albumin, 2% normal goat serum, 0.3% Triton X-100, and 5% nonfat dry milk in PBS, sections were labelled using primary antibodies against synaptophysin (Abcam), MAP-2 (Cell Signaling Technology), MBP (Abcam), NF200 (Abcam), BDNF (Abcam), b-FGF (Abcam), or neuron-specific nuclear protein (NeuN) (Millipore) at a dilution of 1:50. Sections were then incubated in fluorescently conjugated secondary antibodies (Alexa 488/Alexa 594-conjugated anti-mouse/anti-rabbit IgG) and fluorescence was detected using a fluorescence microscope (Carl Zeiss, Jena, Germany).

2.10. Statistical Analysis.
Statistical analysis was performed using SPSS 11.0 (SPSS, Chicago, IL, USA). Data were expressed as means ± SEM and were statistically analyzed by

(a)

(b)

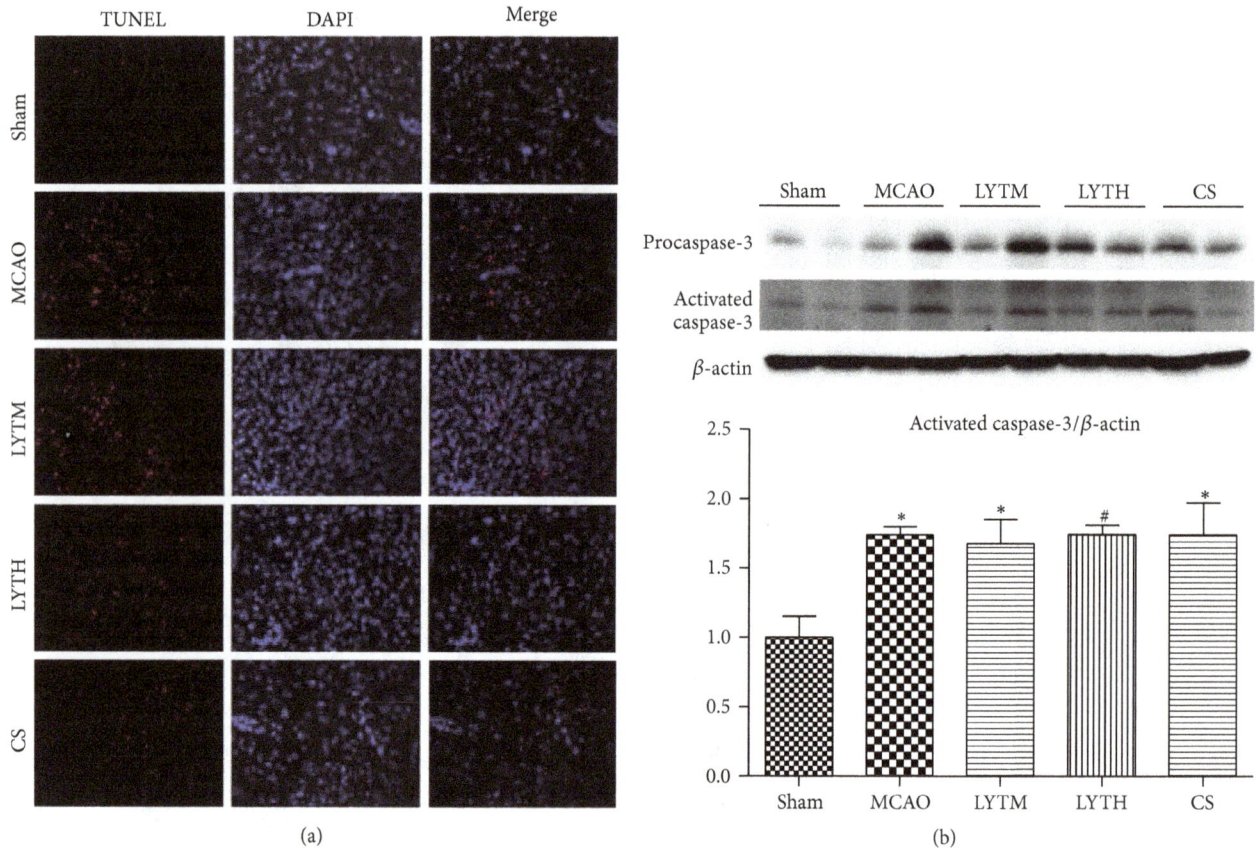

FIGURE 3: LYT (Luoyutong) reduces neuronal apoptosis and decreases the level of caspase-3. (a) Neuronal apoptosis in the ipsilateral cortex was detected by terminal deoxynucleotidyl transferase dUTP nick end labeling and $4'$ 6-diamidino-2-phenylindole double staining 14 days after ischemic reperfusion. (b) Expression of activated caspase-3 was detected by Western blot 14 days after ischemic reperfusion. $n = 3$. $^{*}P < 0.05$ versus *Sham* and $^{#}P < 0.05$ versus *MCAO*.

one-way analysis of variance (ANOVA) followed by LSD post hoc test. *P* values less than 0.05 were considered statistically significant.

3. Results

3.1. LYT Decreases Infarct Volume and Improves Neurological Function following Cerebral Ischemia-Reperfusion Injury in Rats.
Behavioral tests and measurements of the infarct volume were used to evaluate the neurological outcome. The scores in all behavioral tests performed 3 days after reperfusion were not significantly different among groups (Figure 2(a)). There was a significant reduction in Longa's score test and the 0–12 neurological score test performance on day 14 in the LYTH group compared to the MCAO group (Longa's, $P < 0.01$; 0–12 neurological score test, $P < 0.05$), but the effect was not obvious in LYTM group and CS group, indicating improved neurological function in the LYTH group. Scores in the modified foot fault test were lower following all treatments (Figure 2(b)).

Cerebral infarct volume was measured by TTC staining (Figures 2(c) and 2(d)). The infarct volume in the LYTH group was significantly reduced compared to the MCAO group 3 and 14 days after ischemia-reperfusion

injury (Figures 2(c) and 2(d), $P < 0.05$). LYTM did not impact infarct volume as significantly as LYTH. CS treatment only decreased infarct volume after 14 days of treatment (Figure 2(d), $P < 0.05$).

3.2. LYT Reduces Apoptosis in Neurons and Decreases the Level of Caspase-3.
To measure apoptosis, TUNEL staining was performed in the cortex of ipsilateral cerebral tissue 14 days after reperfusion (Figure 3(a)). The number of apoptotic neurons in the MCAO group was significantly higher than that in the sham group. LYTH, LYTM, and CS treatment significantly decreased the number of TUNEL-positive cells compared to the MCAO group (Figure 3(a)). We also quantified the expression of activated caspase-3 in cerebral tissue 14 days after reperfusion (Figure 3(b)). Activated caspase-3 expression in the MCAO group was significantly higher than that in the sham group (Figure 3(b), $P < 0.05$). The expression of activated caspase-3 was reduced by LYTH, LTYM, and CS treatment, but a significant reduction was only observed in the LYTH group (Figure 3(b), $P < 0.05$).

3.3. LYT Protects against Ischemia-Reperfusion Injury by Enhancing Neural Plasticity.
To investigate the effect of LYT on neural plasticity following ischemia-reperfusion injury

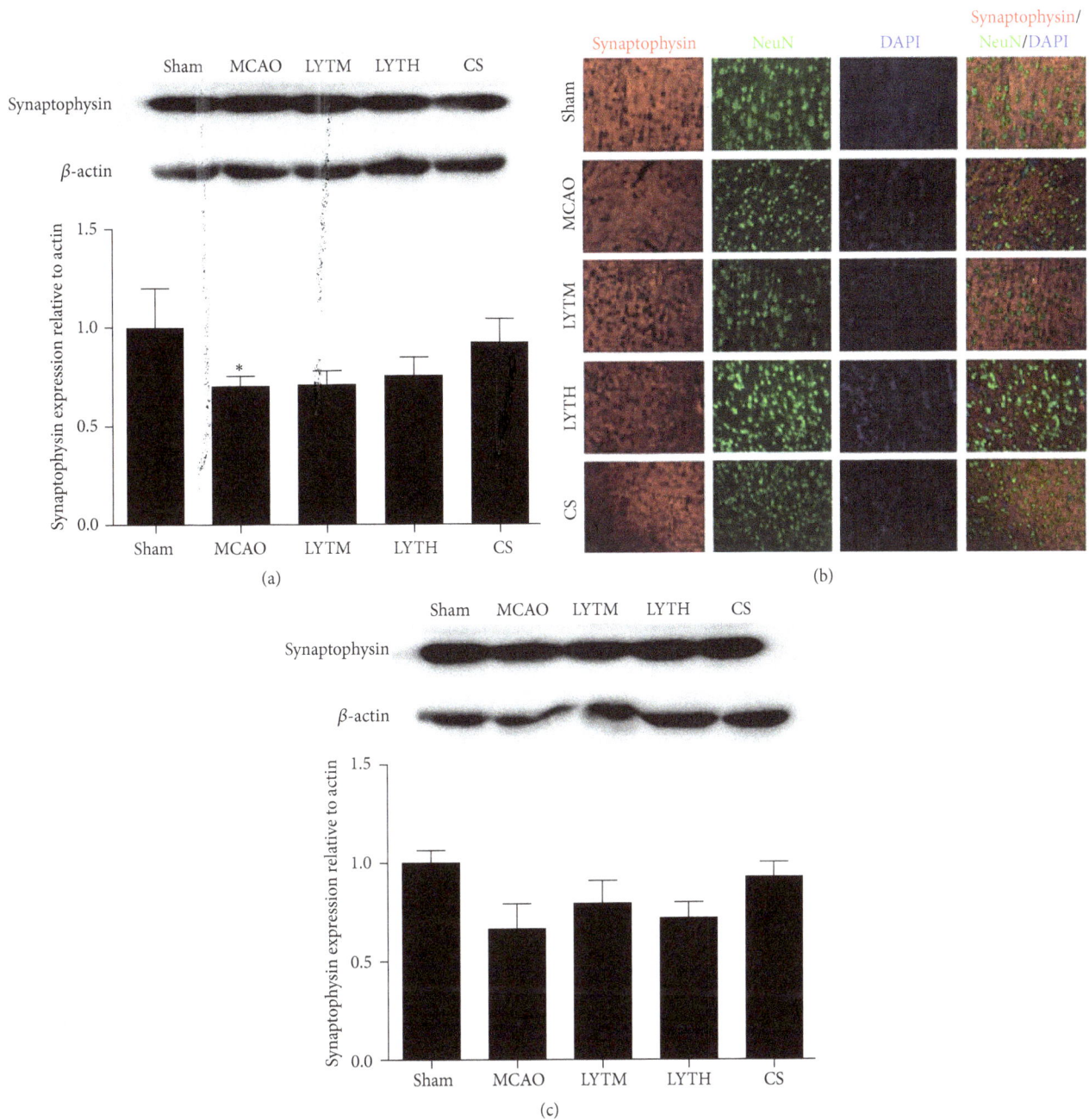

FIGURE 4: LYT (Luoyutong) induced upregulation of synaptophysin expression after MCAO (middle cerebral artery occlusion). Western blot detection and quantitative analysis of (a) synaptophysin expression 3 days after MCAO and (c) synaptophysin expression 14 days after MCAO. (b) Representative immunofluorescence images showing colocalization of synaptophysin (red) and NeuN (neuron-specific nuclear protein) (green) in the cortex. Blue DAPI staining indicates the nuclei. $n = 3$. $^*P < 0.05$ versus Sham.

in rats, we measured the levels of synaptophysin, MAP-2, and MBP by Western blotting. We also analyzed the colocalization of synaptophysin and MAP-2 with NeuN in the cortex and MBP with NF 200 in the corpus callosum by immunofluorescence.

Synaptophysin expression was decreased in the MCAO group compared with the sham group 3 days after reperfusion (Figure 4(a), $P < 0.05$). Both of LYT and CS had no obvious effect on it (Figure 4(a), $P < 0.05$). After 14

days, there were no significant differences between sham, MCAO, and treatment groups (Figure 4(c)). Immunofluorescence revealed that synaptophysin staining appeared as punctate-like or bouton-like distribution pattern with high immunofluorescence signal; staining of NeuN was shiny and sparkly. MCAO disrupted the localization of synaptophysin and dampened brightness of NeuN in the cortex, and this effect was reversed after 14 days of LYT and CS treatment (Figure 4(b)).

(a)

(b)

(c)

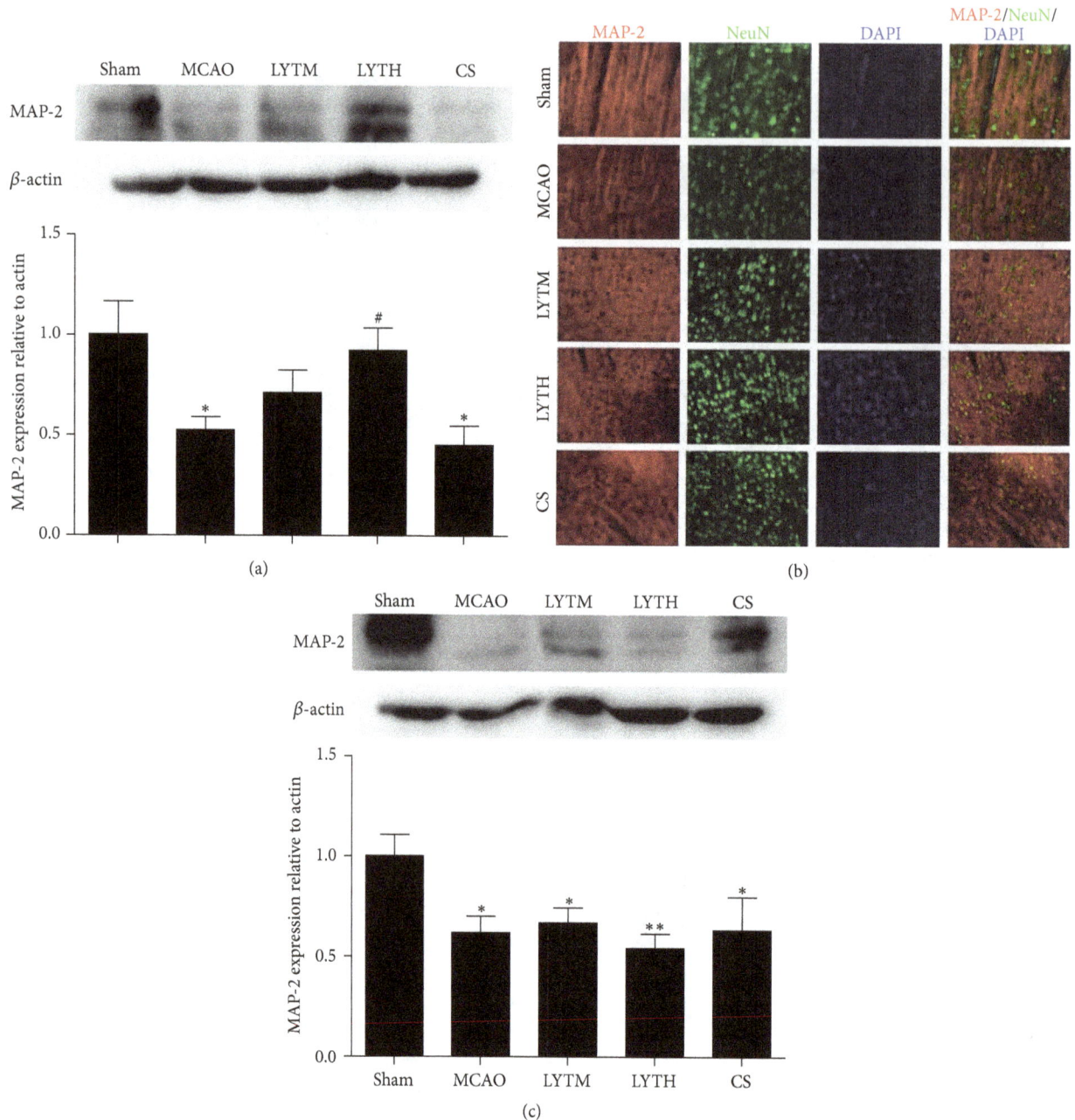

FIGURE 5: LYT (Luoyutong) induced upregulation of MAP-2 (microtubule associated protein) expression after MCAO (middle cerebral artery occlusion). Western blot detection and quantitative analysis of (a) MAP-2 expression 3 days after MCAO and (c) MAP-2 expression 14 days after MCAO. (b) Representative immunofluorescence images showing colocalization of MAP-2 (red) and NeuN (neuron-specific nuclear protein) (green) in the cortex. Blue DAPI staining indicates the nuclei. $n = 3$. $^*P < 0.05$ versus *Sham*, $^{**}P < 0.01$ versus *Sham*, and $^#P < 0.05$ versus *MCAO*.

Western blot analysis showed a reduced expression of MAP-2 in the MCAO group compared with the sham group 3 and 14 days after reperfusion (Figures 5(a) and 5(c), $P < 0.05$). MAP-2 levels were increased by 3 days of LYTH treatment after reperfusion (Figure 5(a), $P < 0.05$), whereas administration of LYTM and CA did not rescue MAP-2 expression. After 14 days, there was no difference between MCAO and treatment groups (Figure 5(c)). As shown in immunofluorescence, the expression of MAP-2 in sham group was shown in

dendrites; it became irregular, discontinuous, and weaker in MCAO and it was improved by LYTH and LYTM treatment but not CS treatment (Figure 5(b)).

The expression of MBP was lower in the MCAO group compared to the sham group 3 and 14 days after reperfusion, but this was only statistically significant after 14 days (Figures 6(a) and 6(c), $P < 0.01$). We observed an increased MBP expression after 3 and 14 days of treatment with LYT and CS (Figures 6(a) and 6(c)); similarly the significant

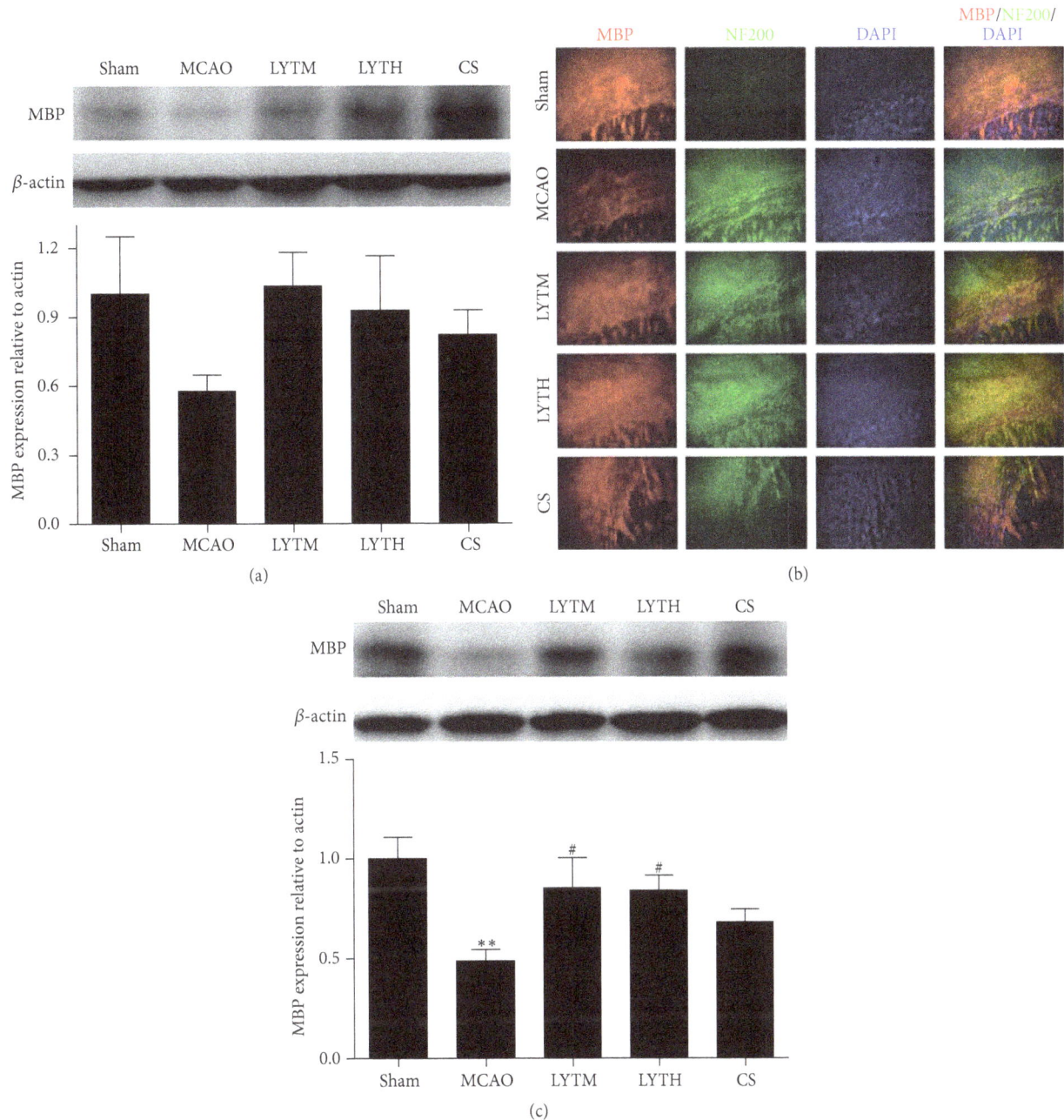

FIGURE 6: LYT (Luoyutong) induced upregulation of MBP (myelin basic protein) expression after MCAO (middle cerebral artery occlusion). Western blot detection and quantitative analysis of (a) MBP expression 3 days after MCAO and (c) MBP expression 14 days after MCAO. (b) Representative immunofluorescence images showing colocalization of MBP (red) and NF200 (neurofilament 200) (green) in the cortex. Blue DAPI staining indicates the nuclei. $n = 3$. $^{**}P < 0.01$ versus *Sham* and $^{#}P < 0.05$ versus *MCAO*.

difference was only significant after 14 days of LYT treatment (Figure 6(c), $P < 0.05$). MBP immunoreactivity was affected mostly by myelin sheaths in the sham group. However, low immunoreactivity was detected for MBP after MCAO, while NF200 staining increased in intensity in the MCAO group. These effects were reversed by all treatments (Figure 6(b)).

Taken together, these findings demonstrated that the different treatments protected neural plasticity following ischemia-reperfusion injury, particularly the high dose of LYT.

3.4. LYT Treatment Upregulated BDNF and b-FGF after Ischemia-Reperfusion Injury. To investigate the effect of LYT treatment on the expression of growth factors, we measured BDNF and b-FGF expressions by Western blot 3 and 14 days after reperfusion. BDNF expression was significantly lower in the MCAO group compared to the sham group 3 days after reperfusion (Figure 7(a), $P < 0.05$). LYT and CS treatment dramatically increased BDNF expression 3 days after reperfusion and it was even higher than that in the sham group (Figure 7(a), $P < 0.05$). After 14 days, no

(a)

(b)

(c)

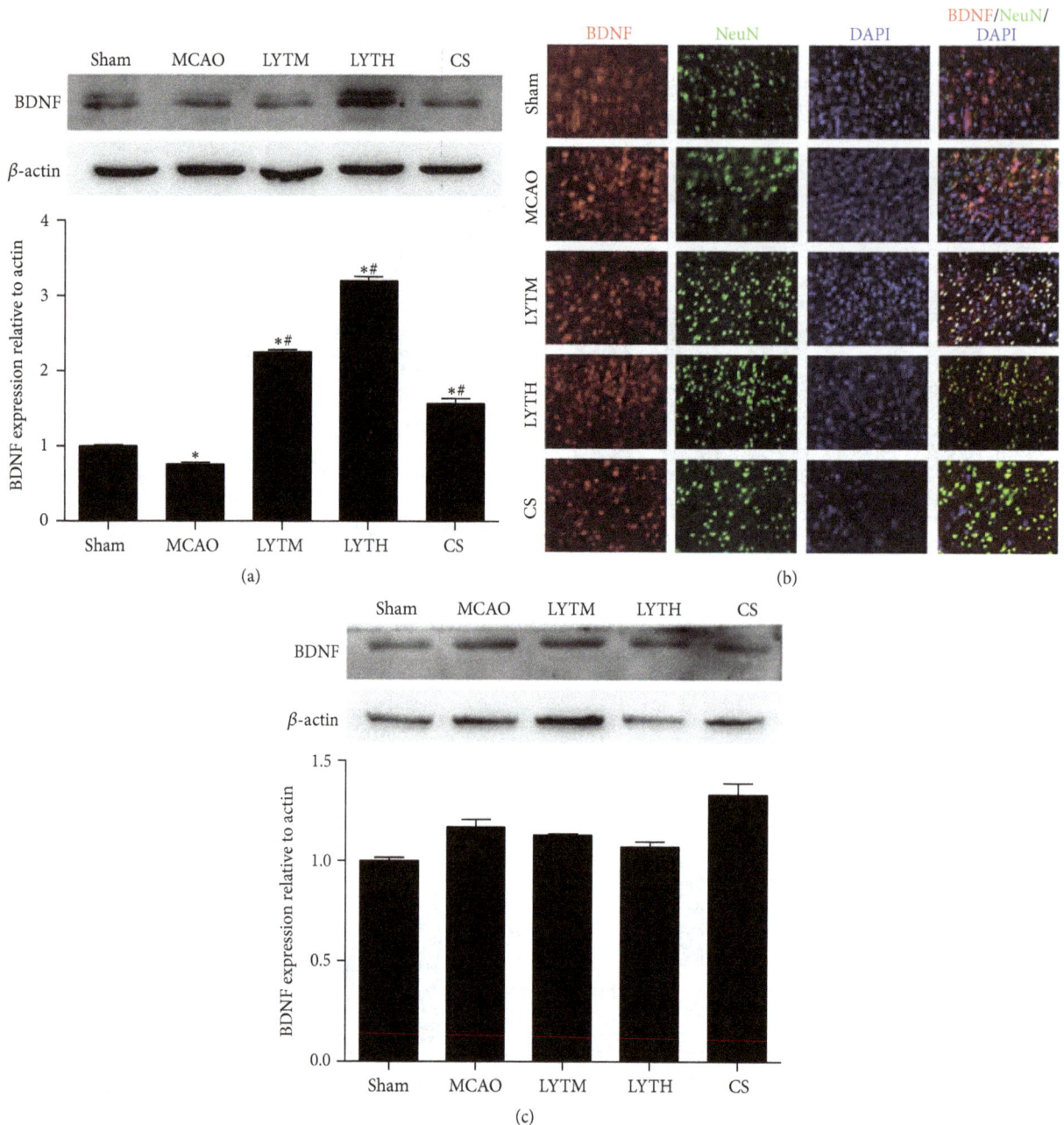

FIGURE 7: LYT (Luoyutong) induced upregulation of BDNF (brain derived neurotrophic factor) expression after MCAO (middle cerebral artery occlusion). Western blot detection and quantitative analysis of (a) BDNF expression 3 days after MCAO and (c) BDNF expression 14 days after MCAO. (b) Representative immunofluorescence images showing colocalization of BDNF (red) and NeuN (neuron-specific nuclear protein) (green) in the cortex. Blue DAPI staining indicates the nuclei. $n = 3$. $^{**}P < 0.01$ versus *Sham* and $^{#}P < 0.05$ versus *MCAO*.

significant differences were observed in BDNF expression between the groups (Figure 7(c)). BDNF positive cells partly colocalized with NeuN as demonstrated by immunofluorescence; the staining of BDNF was not different among groups (Figure 7(b)).

b-FGF expression was also lower in the MCAO group compared to the sham group 3 days after reperfusion (Figure 8(a), $P < 0.05$) and only treatment with LYTH could reverse this effect. No difference in b-FGF expression was

observed 14 days after reperfusion (Figure 8(c)). Immunofluorescence revealed that a portion of b-FGF showed colocalization with NeuN in the cortex; MCAO and treatment had no effect on its expression (Figure 8(b)).

4. Discussion

Clinical research showed that LYT has a therapeutic effect of stroke [12, 13]; however, the mechanism underlying the

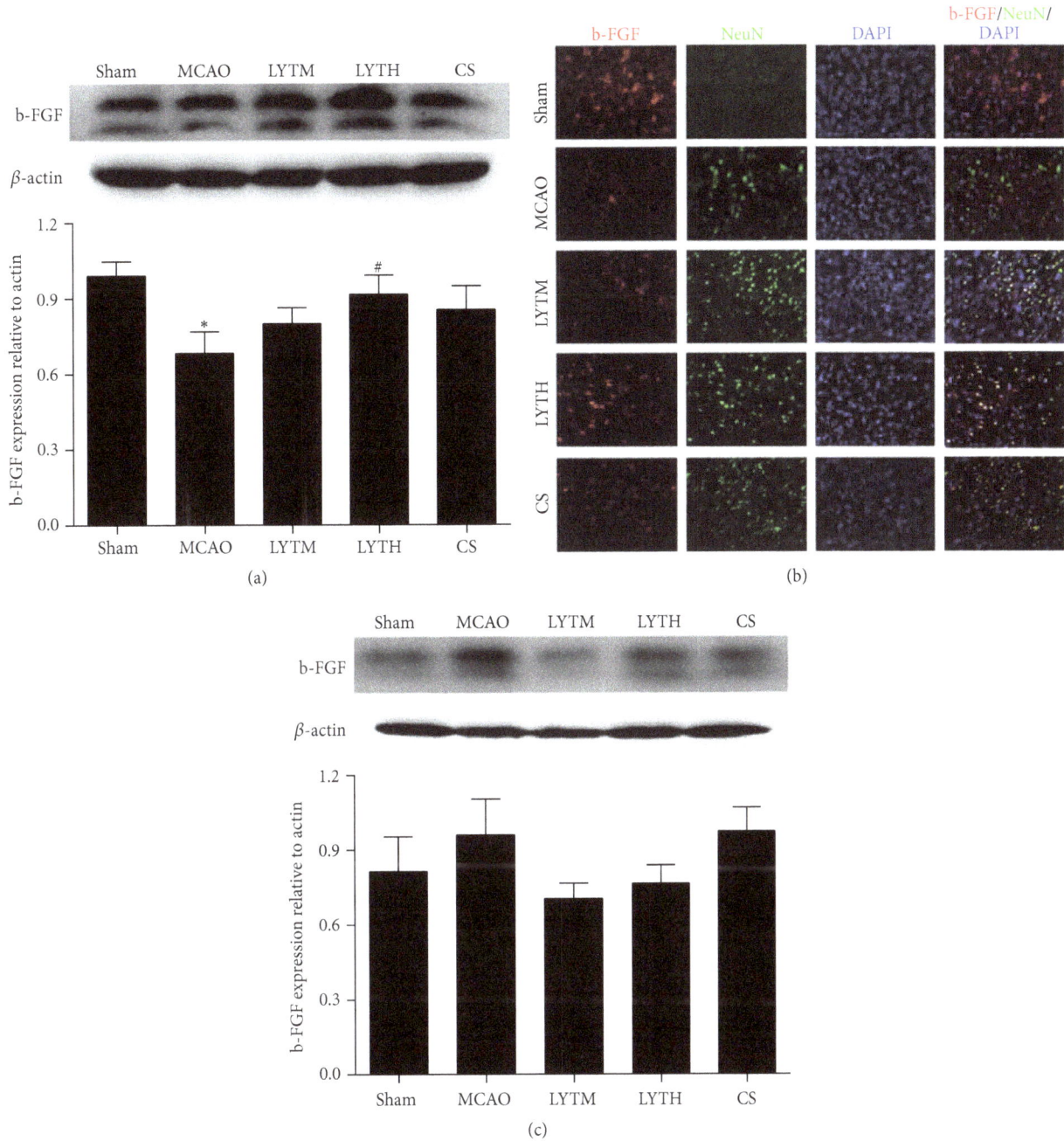

FIGURE 8: LYT (Luoyutong) induced upregulation of b-FGF (basic fibroblast growth factor) expression after MCAO (middle cerebral artery occlusion). Western blot detection and quantitative analysis of (a) b-FGF expression 3 days after MCAO and (c) b-FGF expression 14 days after MCAO. (b) Representative immunofluorescence images showing colocalization of b-FGF (red) and NeuN (neuron-specific nuclear protein) (green) in the cortex. Blue DAPI staining indicates the nuclei. $n = 3$. $^{**}P < 0.01$ versus *Sham* and $^{#}P < 0.05$ versus *MCAO*.

therapeutic effects remains undefined. To address this, LYT was applied to rat model of cerebral ischemia-reperfusion injury. As expected, LYTH treatment could improve neurologic function and reduce infarction volume, which is more significant than CS treatment group. Further studies revealed that the protective effect of LYT is potentially related to the improvement of neural plasticity and upregulation of BDNF and b-FGF. The measurement of infarction volume showed that LYT reduces infarct volume significantly in both acute stage (3 d) and restoration stage (14 d). It is noteworthy that CS has no effect on it in acute stage (3 d). Although CS is widely used in clinic, its treatment still has limitations. Moreover, LYT showed the improvement effect of neurological function at 14 days after ischemia-reperfusion injury in accord with clinical research [12, 13]. We speculate that early inhibition of infarction volume is more advantageous to the late reply of neurological function.

In order to make clear whether the therapeutic effect of LYT depends on antiapoptosis function, we measured apoptosis by TUNEL and quantified the expression of activated caspase-3 in cerebral tissue 14 days after reperfusion. Both CS and LYTH have pronounced influence on apoptosis, but only LYTH could reduce the expression of activated caspase-3. Since caspase-3 is not only a known regulator of apoptosis, it can also influence neural plasticity [19]. Therefore, the downregulation of caspase-3 in response to LYT treatment not only may influence apoptosis exclusively but also can promote neural plasticity.

Neural plasticity is important for neurological function recovery after reperfusion, and neural plasticity has different performance at different time points. Neural plasticity plays a vital role in ischemic injury [20], depression, and memory [21, 22]. MAP-2 is dendritic marker and synaptophysin is synaptic marker. Synaptophysin regulates activity-dependent synapse formation [23]. MAP-2 nucleates and stabilizes microtubules, regulates organelle transport, and anchors regulatory proteins within neurons to regulate process outgrowth, synaptic plasticity, and apoptosis [24]. In present study, our results demonstrated that synaptophysin and MAP-2 levels decrease after MCAO, in agreement with previous findings [25, 26]. Meanwhile MCAO disorganized the arrangement structure of MAP-2, but the arrangement structure is the foundation of its function. The result showed that only LYTH could increase the level of MAP-2, and this function only embodied in 3 days. CS and LYTM do not have obvious effect on it. But all of the treatments have no effect on synaptophysin. These findings suggest that LYTH can enhance neural plasticity through regulating the expression of MAP-2 following ischemia-reperfusion injury in gray matter. Cerebral white matter is also highly vulnerable to ischemia, and white matter is subject to a novel form of neural plasticity which is termed "myelin plasticity" [27]. Changes in MBP and NF200 expression can be indicative of white matter injury following MCAO [28]. The present study is consistent with previous reports on MBP and NF200 expression changes after ischemia-reperfusion injury. After 14 days, the change is more prominent. LYT treatment can reverse these effects and the improvement of LYT is more remarkable after 14 days. However, the effect of CS is not obvious. Our results revealed a regulatory role of LYT in white matter plasticity following cerebral ischemia-reperfusion injury, while CS treatment could not improve white matter injury.

In addition, LYT treatment upregulates the expression of BDNF and b-FGF following ischemia-reperfusion injury, both of which are critical mediators of neural plasticity and survival [19, 29–35]. The influence of MCAO and the intervention effect of treatment only reflect on the third day. The results from the expression of BNDF and b-FGF indicate that LYT is stronger than CS in regulating growth factors, especially LYTH.

In summary, we have provided evidence that LYT has a protective effect after ischemia-reperfusion injury in rats by suppressing neuronal apoptosis and repairing neural plasticity of both gray matter and white matter. These effects may be mediated by regulating caspase-3, BDNF, and b-FGF expressions. Further elucidation of the signaling pathways involved is required. It is likely that the herbal ingredients of LYT act synergistically, but the relative contribution of each herb to the beneficial outcome has not yet been defined.

Disclosure

Ning-qun Wang and Li-ye Wang are co-first authors.

Conflict of Interests

The authors declare that there is no conflict of interests regarding the publication of this paper.

Acknowledgments

This work was supported by Projects of Beijing Nova Program (Grant no. Z151100000315065) and Chinese Natural Science Foundation grants (Grant nos. 81271461, 81571280, and 81325007).

References

[1] R. S. Pandya, L. Mao, H. Zhou et al., "Central nervous system agents for ischemic stroke: neuroprotection mechanisms," *Central Nervous System Agents in Medicinal Chemistry*, vol. 11, no. 2, pp. 81–97, 2011.

[2] K. Sun, Q. Hu, C. M. Zhou et al., "Cerebralcare Granule, a Chinese herb compound preparation, improves cerebral microcirculatory disorder and hippocampal CA1 neuron injury in gerbils after ischemia-reperfusion," *Journal of Ethnopharmacology*, vol. 130, no. 2, pp. 398–406, 2010.

[3] Z.-J. Zhang, P. Li, Z. Wang et al., "A comparative study on the individual and combined effects of baicalin and jasminoidin on focal cerebral ischemia-reperfusion injury," *Brain Research*, vol. 1123, no. 1, pp. 188–195, 2006.

[4] Y. He, H. Wan, Y. Du et al., "Protective effect of Danhong injection on cerebral ischemia-reperfusion injury in rats," *Journal of Ethnopharmacology*, vol. 144, no. 2, pp. 387–394, 2012.

[5] Z. H. Lin, D. N. Zhu, Y. Q. Yan, and B. Yu, "Herbal formula FBD extracts prevented brain injury and inflammation induced by cerebral ischemia-reperfusion," *Journal of Ethnopharmacology*, vol. 118, no. 1, pp. 140–147, 2008.

[6] L.-D. Zhao, J.-H. Wang, G.-R. Jin, Y. Zhao, and H.-J. Zhang, "Neuroprotective effect of Buyang Huanwu decoction against focal cerebral ischemia/reperfusion injury in rats—time window and mechanism," *Journal of Ethnopharmacology*, vol. 140, no. 2, pp. 339–344, 2012.

[7] M. H. Cohen and K. J. Kemper, "Complementary therapies in pediatrics: a legal perspective," *Pediatrics*, vol. 115, no. 3, pp. 774–780, 2005.

[8] C.-C. Shih, C.-C. Liao, Y.-C. Su, C.-C. Tsai, and J.-G. Lin, "Gender differences in traditional chinese medicine use among adults in Taiwan," *PLoS ONE*, vol. 7, no. 4, Article ID e32540, 2012.

[9] V. Chung, E. Wong, J. Woo, S. V. Lo, and S. Griffiths, "Use of traditional Chinese medicine in the Hong Kong special

administrative region of China," *Journal of Alternative and Complementary Medicine*, vol. 13, no. 3, pp. 361–367, 2007.

[10] Z. Junhua, F. Menniti-Ippolito, G. Xiumei et al., "Complex traditional Chinese medicine for poststroke motor dysfunction: a systematic review," *Stroke*, vol. 40, no. 8, pp. 2797–2804, 2009.

[11] C. Matute, M. Domercq, A. Pérez-Samartín, and B. R. Ransom, "Protecting white matter from stroke injury," *Stroke*, vol. 44, no. 4, pp. 1204–1211, 2013.

[12] J. F. Wan, X. N. Zhang, J. Q. Guo, and C. F. Wang, "Clinical efficacy and safety evaluation of Luoyutong capsule treating on stroke," *Asia-Pacific Traditional Medicine*, vol. 10, no. 7, pp. 106–107, 2014.

[13] T. S. Liu, S. Zhou, D. H. Wu et al., "Summary of 99 patients used Luoyutong capsule to treating stroke (cerebral thrombosis)," *Geriatrics Health Care*, vol. 10, no. 4, p. 243, 2004.

[14] L.-Y. Wang, H.-P. Zhao, R.-H. Wang et al., "Effect of Luoyutong capsule on focal cerebral ischemia-reperfusion injury in rats," *Chinese Journal of Cerebrovascular Diseases*, vol. 11, no. 12, pp. 650–655, 2014.

[15] E. Z. Longa, P. R. Weinstein, S. Carlson, and R. Cummins, "Reversible middle cerebral artery occlusion without craniectomy in rats," *Stroke*, vol. 20, no. 1, pp. 84–91, 1989.

[16] S. J. Kim, B. K. Kim, Y. J. Ko, M. S. Bang, M. H. Kim, and T. R. Han, "Functional and histologic changes after repeated transcranial direct current stimulation in rat stroke model," *Journal of Korean Medical Science*, vol. 25, no. 10, pp. 1499–1505, 2010.

[17] D. C. Rogers, C. A. Campbell, J. L. Stretton, and K. B. Mackay, "Correlation between motor impairment and infarct volume after permanent and transient middle cerebral artery occlusion in the rat," *Stroke*, vol. 28, no. 10, pp. 2060–2066, 1997.

[18] J. M. Mountz, "Measuring brain infarct volume," *Journal of Cerebral Blood Flow & Metabolism*, vol. 11, no. 1, p. 168, 1991.

[19] Z. Li, J. Jo, J.-M. Jia et al., "Caspase-3 activation via mitochondria is required for long-term depression and AMPA receptor internalization," *Cell*, vol. 141, no. 5, pp. 859–871, 2010.

[20] T. H. Murphy, "Two-photon imaging of neuronal structural plasticity in mice during and after ischemia," *Cold Spring Harb Protoc*, no. 6, pp. 548–557, 2015.

[21] C. L. Busceti, P. D. Pietro, B. Riozzi et al., "5-HT$_{2C}$ serotonin receptor blockade prevents tau protein hyperphosphorylation and corrects the defect in hippocampal synaptic plasticity caused by a combination of environmental stressors in mice," *Pharmacological Research*, vol. 99, pp. 258–268, 2015.

[22] E. Castrén and R. Hen, "Neuronal plasticity and antidepressant actions," *Trends in Neurosciences*, vol. 36, no. 5, pp. 259–267, 2013.

[23] L. Tarsa and Y. Goda, "Synaptophysin regulates activity-dependent synapse formation in cultured hippocampal neurons," *Proceedings of the National Academy of Sciences of the United States of America*, vol. 99, no. 2, pp. 1012–1016, 2002.

[24] C. Sánchez, J. Díaz-Nido, and J. Avila, "Phosphorylation of microtubule-associated protein 2 (MAP2) and its relevance for the regulation of the neuronal cytoskeleton function," *Progress in Neurobiology*, vol. 61, no. 2, pp. 133–168, 2000.

[25] F. D. Pinheiro Fernandes, A. P. Fontenele Menezes, J. C. de Sousa Neves et al., "Caffeic acid protects mice from memory deficits induced by focal cerebral ischemia," *Behavioural Pharmacology*, vol. 25, no. 7, pp. 637–647, 2014.

[26] L. C. Yang, J. Li, S. F. Xu et al., "L-3-n-butylphthalide promotes neurogenesis and neuroplasticity in cerebral ischemic rats,"

CNS Neuroscience & Therapeutics, vol. 21, no. 9, pp. 733–741, 2015.

[27] S. Rosenzweig and S. T. Carmichael, "Age-dependent exacerbation of white matter stroke outcomes: a role for oxidative damage and inflammatory mediators," *Stroke*, vol. 44, no. 9, pp. 2579–2586, 2013.

[28] J. Suenaga, X. Hu, H. Pu et al., "White matter injury and microglia/macrophage polarization are strongly linked with age-related long-term deficits in neurological function after stroke," *Experimental Neurology*, vol. 272, pp. 109–119, 2015.

[29] M.-M. Poo, "Neurotrophins as synaptic modulators," *Nature Reviews Neuroscience*, vol. 2, no. 1, pp. 24–32, 2001.

[30] R. S. Duman and B. Voleti, "Signaling pathways underlying the pathophysiology and treatment of depression: novel mechanisms for rapid-acting agents," *Trends in Neurosciences*, vol. 35, no. 1, pp. 47–56, 2012.

[31] V. Duric, M. Banasr, P. Licznerski et al., "A negative regulator of MAP kinase causes depressive behavior," *Nature Medicine*, vol. 16, no. 11, pp. 1328–1332, 2010.

[32] G. L. Collingridge, S. Peineau, J. G. Howland, and Y. T. Wang, "Long-term depression in the CNS," *Nature Reviews Neuroscience*, vol. 11, no. 7, pp. 459–473, 2010.

[33] B. Lu, "BDNF and activity-dependent synaptic modulation," *Learning and Memory*, vol. 10, no. 2, pp. 86–98, 2003.

[34] S. Yang and J. Cui, "Study on the value of exogenous bFGF in the treatment of brain injury," *Chinese Journal of Traumatology*, vol. 3, no. 3, pp. 131–135, 2000.

[35] K. Chaiyasate, A. Schaffner, I. T. Jackson, and V. Mittal, "Comparing FK-506 with basic fibroblast growth factor (b-FGF) on the repair of a peripheral nerve defect using an autogenous vein bridge model," *Journal of Investigative Surgery*, vol. 22, no. 6, pp. 401–405, 2009.

The Consumption of Bicarbonate-Rich Mineral Water Improves Glycemic Control

Shinnosuke Murakami,[1,2] Yasuaki Goto,[3] Kyo Ito,[4] Shinya Hayasaka,[3,5] Shigeo Kurihara,[3] Tomoyoshi Soga,[1,2] Masaru Tomita,[1,2] and Shinji Fukuda[1,2]

[1]Systems Biology Program, Graduate School of Media and Governance, Keio University, 5322 Endo, Fujisawa, Kanagawa 252-0882, Japan
[2]Institute for Advanced Biosciences, Keio University, 246-2 Mizukami, Kakuganji, Tsuruoka, Yamagata 997-0052, Japan
[3]Onsen Medical Science Research Center, Japan Health and Research Institute, 1-29-4 Kakigaracho, Nihonbashi, Chuo-ku, Tokyo 103-0014, Japan
[4]Ito Medical Office, 7985-5, Nagayu, Naoirimachi, Taketa, Oita 878-0402, Japan
[5]Faculty of Human Life Sciences, Tokyo City University, 8-9-18 Todoroki, Setagaya-ku, Tokyo 158-8586, Japan

Correspondence should be addressed to Shinnosuke Murakami; mushin@sfc.keio.ac.jp
and Shinji Fukuda; sfukuda@sfc.keio.ac.jp

Academic Editor: Jenny M. Wilkinson

Hot spring water and natural mineral water have been therapeutically used to prevent or improve various diseases. Specifically, consumption of bicarbonate-rich mineral water (BMW) has been reported to prevent or improve type 2 diabetes (T2D) in humans. However, the molecular mechanisms of the beneficial effects behind mineral water consumption remain unclear. To elucidate the molecular level effects of BMW consumption on glycemic control, blood metabolome analysis and fecal microbiome analysis were applied to the BMW consumption test. During the study, 19 healthy volunteers drank 500 mL of commercially available tap water (TW) or BMW daily. TW consumption periods and BMW consumption periods lasted for a week each and this cycle was repeated twice. Biochemical tests indicated that serum glycoalbumin levels, one of the indexes of glycemic controls, decreased significantly after BMW consumption. Metabolome analysis of blood samples revealed that 19 metabolites including glycolysis-related metabolites and 3 amino acids were significantly different between TW and BMW consumption periods. Additionally, microbiome analysis demonstrated that composition of lean-inducible bacteria was increased after BMW consumption. Our results suggested that consumption of BMW has the possible potential to prevent and/or improve T2D through the alterations of host metabolism and gut microbiota composition.

1. Introduction

Self-medication is an important approach to maintain and promote human health. There are many strategies of self-medication such as improving one's lifestyle and/or dietary habits, consumption of functional foods/beverages, and getting adequate exercise [1, 2]. Hot spring water and natural mineral water are traditionally used in public baths and balneotherapy in many countries. Balneotherapy is the use of thermal and/or mineral water derived from natural springs or drilled wells for treatment of human health by employing various methods such as bathing, drinking, mud therapy, and inhalation [3]. According to previous studies, it has been reported that balneotherapy has beneficial effects for various diseases such as type 2 diabetes (T2D) [4–6], rheumatism [7], low back pain [3], and cardiovascular disease [8, 9]. Particularly, consumption of bicarbonate-rich mineral water (BMW) has been reported to prevent or improve T2D [4, 6]. However, as the reported benefits of BMW were determined epidemiologically and clinically, the molecular mechanisms of the beneficial effects behind BMW remain unclear.

Metabolomics is a method of comprehensive measurement of metabolites and it has been known to be a powerful tool to gain new insights into various research fields such as metabolic syndrome [10], cancer [11, 12], chronic kidney disease [13], and biomarker screening [14]. A recent study has reported that plasma metabolome profiles were altered between healthy people and T2D patients [15]. Moreover, it has been also reported that gut microbial composition and function in T2D patients are different from that of healthy subjects [16–18]. Therefore, preventive and/or therapeutic effects for T2D derived from BMW consumption are expected via influencing blood metabolites concentrations and gut microbial compositions.

For this reason, blood metabolome analysis and gut microbiome analysis were included in our study to elucidate the molecular level effects of BMW consumption on glycemic control. In this study, BMW consumption test was conducted amongst 19 healthy volunteers. Here we show that serum glycoalbumin levels were decreased and 19 metabolites including glycolysis-related metabolites and 3 amino acids were changed after consumption of BMW. Additionally, microbiome analysis demonstrated that composition of lean-inducible bacteria, family Christensenellaceae, was increased after BMW consumption. This current study is an important study reporting the molecular level effects derived from consumption of BMW.

2. Materials and Methods

2.1. Sample Preparation. This study was approved by the Ethical Committees of Japan Health and Research Institute and Keio University Shonan Fujisawa Campus. All subjects were informed of the purpose of this study, and written consent was obtained from all subjects.

In this study, BMW consumption test was conducted amongst 19 healthy subjects (7 men and 12 women, ages from 26 to 59, 47 years old on the average). Initially, individual identification numbers were randomly assigned to 26 volunteers from N01 to N26; however N12 and N25 dropped out due to personal reasons. Additionally, N01, N02, N14, N18, and N21 were excluded from analysis because they forgot to drink TW and/or BMW at least once. BMW was obtained from Nagayu hot spring (Taketa, Oita, Japan) as it contains one of the highest bicarbonate concentrations in Japan. TW was purchased from Nishikawa water treatment plant (Yamagata, Japan). Mineral contents and pH of the TW and BMW used in this study were measured by the Hot Spring Research Center (Tokyo, Japan) and are as shown in Table 1. BMW were collected in 500 mL plastic bottles and stored in refrigerator until consumption. All BMW were consumed within 10 days from bottling. TW bottles were also similarly stored in refrigerator until consumption. During the test, volunteers opened 1 plastic bottle of TW or BMW every day and drank the 500 mL of TW or BMW divided into thrice daily (30–60 minutes before breakfast, lunch, and dinner). TW consumption periods and BMW consumption periods lasted for a week each and this cycle was repeated twice. Volunteers were instructed to keep to their normal dietary habits

TABLE 1: Mineral contents and pH of TW and BMW used in this study.

Minerals	Formula	Conc. (mg/kg) TW	BMW
Bicarbonate ion	HCO_3^-	28	2485
Chlorine ion	Cl^-	11	182
Sulfate ion	SO_4^{2-}	6.9	355
Carbonate ion	CO_3^{2-}	<0.1	1.2
Nitrate ion	NO_3^-	0.7	1.2
Fluoride ion	F^-	<0.1	0.3
Hydrogen sulfide ion	HS^-	<0.1	<0.1
Iodide ion	I^-	<0.1	<0.1
Bromide ion	Br^-	<0.1	<0.1
Sodium ion	Na^+	10	412
Magnesium ion	Mg^{2+}	1.9	291
Calcium ion	Ca^{2+}	6.1	177
Potassium ion	K^+	<0.1	80
Aluminum ion	Al^{3+}	0.2	0.6
Manganese ion	Mn^{2+}	<0.1	0.4
Ferrous ion	Fe^{2+}	<0.1	2.3
Ferric ion	Fe^{3+}	<0.1	<0.1
Metasilicic acid	H_2SiO_3	10	207
Metaboric acid	HBO_2	0.8	6.2
Carbon dioxide	CO_2	0.9	161
Hydrogen sulfide	H_2S	<0.1	<0.1
Mercury	Hg	<0.0005	<0.0005
Arsenic	As	<0.005	0.005
Copper	Cu	<0.05	<0.05
Zinc	Zn	<0.1	<0.1
Lead	Pb	<0.05	<0.05
Cadmium	Cd	<0.01	<0.01
pH		7.58	7.07

during the test, but consumption of medicinal drugs was prohibited.

Blood and fecal samples were collected on the first day of the test and last days of every week. Blood samplings that were collected from the same subject were performed at approximately the same time during the test. Body weight, body mass index (BMI), height, abdominal circumference, and blood pressure were measured on the first day of the test (see Table S1 of the Supplementary Material available online at http://dx.doi.org/10.1155/2015/824395). A schematic representation of the experimental design is as shown in Figure S1 of Supplementary Material.

2.2. Clinical Blood Tests. Clinical blood tests were performed at each sampling point, including measurement of fasting plasma glucose, serum glucose, glycoalbumin, insulin, total cholesterol, HDL cholesterol, LDL cholesterol, triglyceride, urate, sodium, chlorine, calcium, magnesium, and cortisol. The measurement of the concentrations of these parameters was outsourced to RINTEC Co., Ltd. (Fukuoka, Japan).

Plasma glucose measurement was performed using morning fasting blood samples obtained from only 8 volunteers. For these samples, the homeostasis model assessment ratio (HOMA-R) was calculated from plasma glucose and insulin levels.

2.3. Metabolome Analysis.

Metabolome analysis was conducted as described previously with some modifications [13]. In brief, to extract metabolites from blood, 400 μL of methanol including the internal standards (20 μM each of methionine sulfone and D-camphor-10-sulfonic acid (CSA)) was added to the 40 μL of blood samples. Next, this mixture was then mixed with 120 μL of ultrapure water and 400 μL of chloroform before centrifuging at 10,000 $\times$g for 3 min at 4°C. Subsequently, the aqueous layer was transferred to a centrifugal filter tube (UltrafreeMC-PLHCC 250/pk for Metabolome Analysis, Human Metabolome Technologies) to remove protein and lipid molecules. The filtrate was centrifugally concentrated and dissolved in 20 μL of ultrapure water that contained reference compounds (200 μM each of 3-aminopyrrolidine and trimesic acid) immediately before capillary electrophoresis with electrospray ionization time-of-flight mass spectrometry (CE-TOFMS) analysis.

The measurement of extracted metabolites in both positive and negative modes was performed by CE-TOFMS. All CE-TOFMS experiments were performed using the Agilent CE capillary electrophoresis system (Agilent Technologies). Annotation tables were produced from measurement of standard compounds and were aligned with the datasets according to similar m/z value and normalized migration time. Then, peak areas were normalized against those of the internal standards methionine sulfone or CSA for cationic and anionic metabolites, respectively. Concentrations of each metabolite were calculated based on their relative peak areas and concentrations of standard compounds.

After statistical analysis, metabolite set enrichment analysis (MSEA) [19] was performed using the metabolites that were significantly different between TW and BMW consumption periods.

2.4. DNA Isolation.

Fecal DNA isolation was performed as described previously with some modifications [20]. Briefly, fecal samples were initially lyophilized by using VD-800R lyophilizer (TAITEC) for at least 18 hours. Freeze-dried feces were disrupted with 3.0 mm Zirconia Beads by vigorous shaking (1,500 r.p.m. for 10 min) using Shake Master (Biomedical Science). Fecal samples (10 mg) were suspended with DNA extraction buffer containing 200 μL of 10% (w/v) SDS/TE (10 mM Tris-HCl, 1 mM EDTA, and pH 8.0) solution, 400 μL of phenol/chloroform/isoamyl alcohol (25 : 24 : 1), and 200 μL of 3 M sodium acetate. Feces in mixture buffer were further disrupted with 0.1 mm zirconia/silica beads by vigorous shaking (1,500 r.p.m. for 5 min) using Shake Master. After centrifugation at 17,800 $\times$g for 5 min at room temperature, bacterial genomic DNA was purified by the standard phenol/chloroform/isoamyl alcohol protocol. RNAs were removed from the sample by RNase A treatment and

then DNA samples were purified once more by the standard phenol/chloroform/isoamyl alcohol protocol.

2.5. 16S rRNA Gene Sequencing.

16S rRNA genes in the fecal DNA samples were analyzed using the MiSeq sequencer (Illumina). The V1-V2 region of the 16S rRNA genes was amplified from the DNA isolated from feces using bacterial universal primer set 27Fmod (5′-AGRGTTTGATYMTGG-CTCAG-3′) and 338R (5′-TGCTGCCTCCCGTAGGAGT-3′) [21]. PCR was performed with Tks Gflex DNA Polymerase (Takara Bio Inc.) and amplification proceeded with one denaturation step at 98°C for 1 min, followed by 20 cycles of 98°C for 10 s, 55°C for 15 s, and 68°C for 30 s, with a final extension step at 68°C for 3 min. The amplified products were purified using Agencourt AMPure XP (Beckman Coulter) and then further amplified using forward primer (5′-AATGATACGGCGACCACCGAGATCTAC-AC-NNNNNNNN-TATGGTAATTGT-AGRGTTTGATY-MTGGCTCAG-3′) containing the P5 sequence, a unique 8 bp barcode sequence for each sample (indicated in N), Rd1 SP sequence and 27Fmod primer and reverse primer (5′-CAAGCAGAAGACGGCATACGAGAT-NNNNNNNN-AGTCAGTCAGCC-TGCTGCCTCCCGAGGAGT-3′) containing the P7 sequence, a unique 8-bp barcode sequence for each sample (indicated in N), Rd2 SP sequence, and 338R primer. After purification using Agencourt AMPure XP, mixed sample was prepared by pooling approximately equal amounts of PCR amplicons from each sample. Finally, MiSeq sequencing was performed according to the manufacturer's instructions. In this study, 2 × 300 bp paired-end sequencing was employed.

2.6. Analysis of 16S rRNA Gene Sequences.

Initially, to assemble the paired-end reads, fast length adjustment of short reads (FLASH) (v1.2.11) [22] was used. Assembled reads with an average Q-value < 25 were filtered out using in-house script. 5,000 filter-passed reads were randomly selected from each sample and used for further analysis. Reads were then processed using quantitative insights into microbial ecology (QIIME) (v1.8.0) pipeline [23]. Sequences were clustered into operational taxonomic units (OTUs) using 97% sequence similarity and OTUs were assigned to taxonomy using RDP classifier.

2.7. Statistical Analysis.

To analyze the intraindividual alterations, statistical evaluation between two groups was performed by Wilcoxon signed-rank test (nonparametric paired test) using the R package exactRankTests (available at https://cran.r-project.org/web/packages/exactRankTests/index.html) or XLSTAT (v2014.6.04) (Addinsoft). For multiple comparisons, the data were analyzed using Friedman's test and post hoc Nemenyi test using XLSTAT. All statements indicating significant differences show at least a 5% level of probability.

2.8. Nucleotide Sequence Accession Number.

The microbiome analysis data have been deposited at the DDBJ Sequence Read Archive (http://trace.ddbj.nig.ac.jp/dra/) under accession number DRA004008.

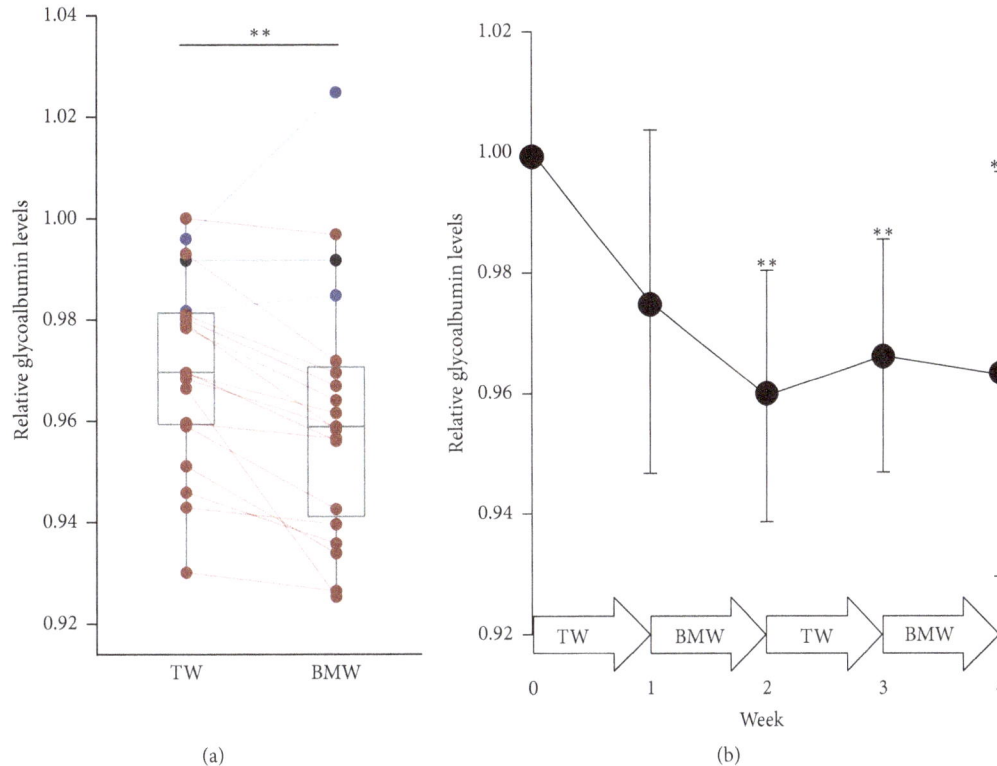

FIGURE 1: Comparisons of relative serum glycoalbumin levels between TW and BMW consumption periods. Glycoalbumin levels were expressed as a relative value to week 0. (a) Individual data of mean relative glycoalbumin levels of weeks 1 and 3 (TW) and weeks 2 and 4 (BMW) were shown in dot plots overlaid on box plots. Plots corresponding to the same individuals were connected with red, blue, or gray lines when the values were decreased, increased, or not changed in BMW consumption periods as compared with TW consumption periods, respectively. Plots were also colored in the same color as their lines. (b) Records of weekly glycoalbumin levels. Data were expressed as mean ± standard deviation (SD). Significances between week 0 and each week were shown at top of the graph. $^{**}P < 0.005$.

3. Results

3.1. Serum Glycoalbumin Levels Were Decreased after BMW Consumption. Firstly, intraindividual alterations of clinical parameters were analyzed. Serum glycoalbumin levels, one of the indexes of glycemic controls, were significantly decreased during BMW consumption periods as compared with TW consumption periods (Figure 1(a)). Serum glucose levels were not decreased significantly but tended to be lowered (P value = 0.092). Other parameters related to glycemic controls, like plasma glucose levels, insulin concentrations, and HOMA-R, were not different between TW and BMW consumption periods. In this study, other biochemical parameters involved with hypercholesterolemia, hyperuricemia, mineral consumption, and stress were also measured, but consumption of BMW did not have any impact on the above-mentioned parameters apart from blood calcium levels (Table 2). These results suggested that BMW consumption has the possible potential to prevent and/or improve T2D without changing insulin secretion and insulin resistance.

Although the serum glycoalbumin levels were significantly decreased during BMW consumption periods as compared with TW consumption periods, reduction of serum glycoalbumin levels was also observed after TW consumption periods as compared with before the test (week 0)

(Figure 1(b)). Relative serum glycoalbumin levels decreased after the first TW consumption period (week 1) and further decreased after first BMW consumption period (week 2). Subsequently, it slightly increased after second TW consumption period (week 3) and then decreased again after second BMW consumption period (week 4). Taken together, these results suggest that the habit of water consumption before every meal has the possible potential to decrease serum glycoalbumin levels, but BMW consumption is more effective.

3.2. BMW Consumption-Related Changes of Physiological Metabolism. To evaluate the molecular level effects of BMW consumption, blood metabolome analysis was performed using CE-TOFMS. A total of 152 metabolites were detected from blood samples at least from 1 subject and 1 time point and concentrations of these metabolites were compared within subject. Over 85% of metabolites were not significantly changed after BMW consumption periods and it was expected that the concentrations of most metabolites remained consistent due to physiological homeostasis (Figure 2(a)). However, the concentrations of 19 metabolites were significantly different between TW and BMW consumption periods (Figures 2(a) and 2(b)). These effects were expected to be derived from BMW

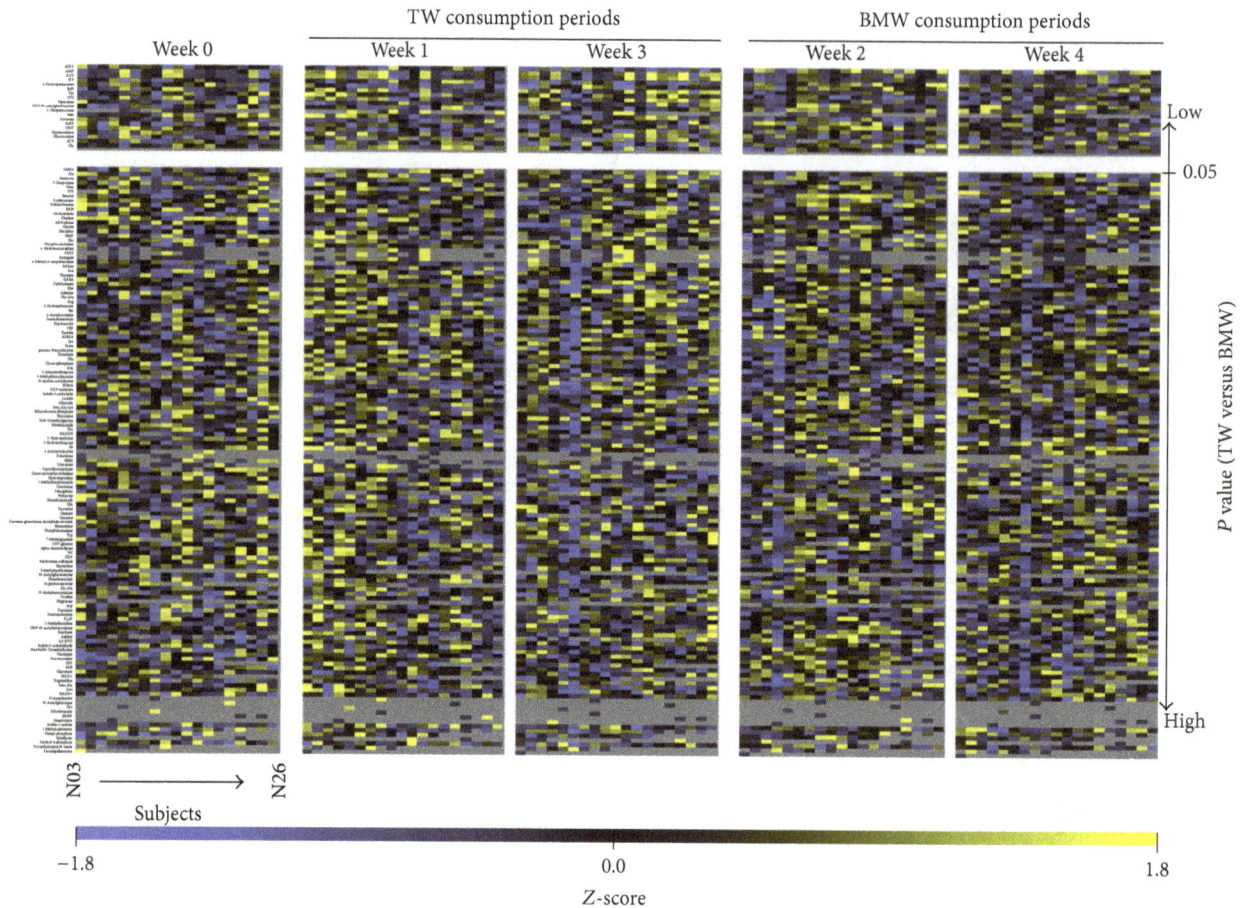

(a)

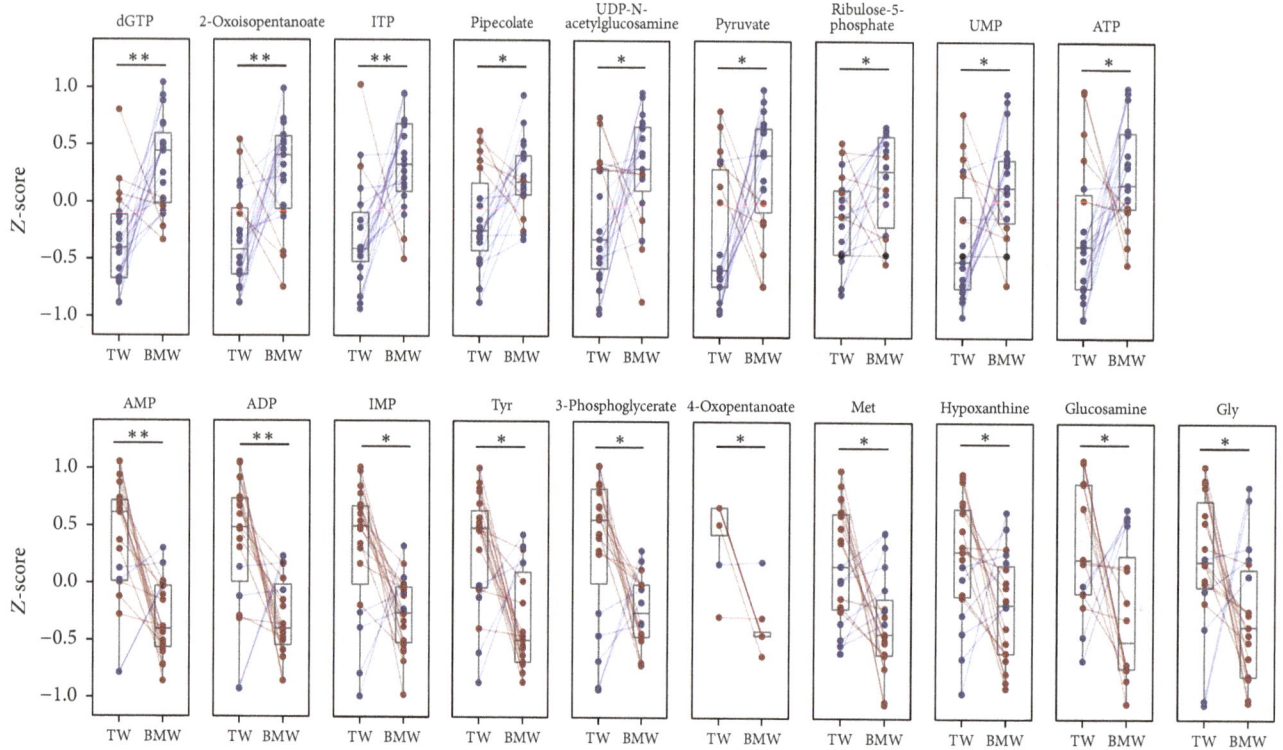

(b)

FIGURE 2: Continued.

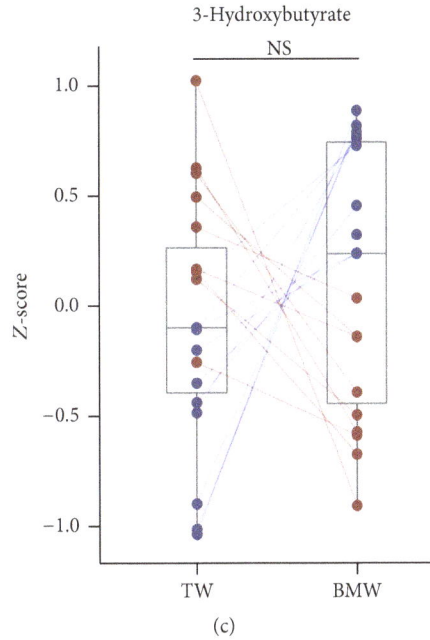

3-Hydroxybutyrate

(c)

FIGURE 2: Comparisons of blood metabolites between TW and BMW consumption periods. (a) Relative concentrations of each metabolite in blood were transformed to Z-score by subjects and shown as heat maps using blue-black-yellow scheme. Gray color indicates that the metabolites were not detected in the sample. A total of 152 metabolites were arranged in increasing order of P value that was calculated by Wilcoxon signed-rank test between TW and BMW consumption periods. (b) Mean relative concentrations of each metabolite (Z-score) of weeks 1 and 3 (TW) and weeks 2 and 4 (BMW) were shown in dot plots overlaid on box plots in the same manner as in Figure 1(a). Only 19 metabolites that their concentrations were significantly increased (upper 9 metabolites) or decreased (lower 10 metabolites) after BMW consumption (shown in upper block of panel (a)) were demonstrated. (c) Relative concentrations of 3-hydroxybutyrate in blood were shown in dot plots overlaid on box plots in the same manner as in Figure 1(a). NS: not significant; $^{*}P < 0.05$; $^{**}P < 0.005$.

TABLE 2: Results of clinical blood test.

Tests	TW		BMW		P value
	Average	SD	Average	SD	
Fasting blood glucose (plasma) (mg/dL)	91.2	4.3	88.6	4.7	0.156
Blood glucose (serum) (mg/dL)	93.5	23.7	91.4	29.0	0.092
Glycoalbumin (% of total albumin)	14.4	1.7	14.2	1.7	0.002**
Insulin (μU/mL)	19.3	28.0	18.8	31.0	0.294
HOMA-R	1.2	0.5	1.2	0.4	1.000
Total cholesterol (mg/dL)	200.6	26.0	202.4	30.3	0.914
HDL cholesterol (mg/dL)	60.9	14.9	60.1	14.1	0.685
LDL cholesterol (mg/dL)	112.0	22.5	112.3	24.1	1.000
Triglycerides (mg/dL)	151.2	142.1	180.7	159.0	0.123
Urate (mg/dL)	5.2	1.2	5.2	1.2	0.396
Na (mEq/L)	139.8	1.3	140.3	1.2	0.172
Cl (mEq/L)	102.6	1.7	102.9	1.9	0.457
Ca (mg/dL)	9.3	0.2	9.4	0.2	0.021*
Mg (mg/dL)	2.3	0.1	2.3	0.1	0.518
Cortisol (μg/dL)	10.1	4.0	10.0	3.6	0.623

$^{*}P$ value is under 0.05; $^{**}P$ value is under 0.005.

consumption. As compared with TW consumption periods, 9 metabolites were significantly increased and 10 metabolites were significantly decreased in BMW consumption periods (Figure 2(b)). Metabolites that may be related to T2D such

as glycolysis-related metabolites (pyruvate, ATP, and ADP), amino acids (tyrosine, methionine, and glycine), and UDP-N-acetylglucosamine were included in significantly changed metabolites. In addition, 3 amino acids were significantly

TABLE 3: Results of MSEA: list of metabolite sets/pathways that are significantly different between TW and BMW consumption periods.

Pathway	Total[*1]	Hits[*2]	Expect[*3]	Fold change (hits/expect)	P value	FDR[*4]
Purine metabolism	45	7	0.98	7.1	<0.001	0.001
Ammonia recycling	18	4	0.39	10.2	<0.001	0.014
Urea cycle	20	4	0.44	9.2	<0.001	0.014
RNA transcription	9	3	0.20	15.3	<0.001	0.014
Intracellular signaling through prostacyclin receptor and prostacyclin	6	2	0.13	15.3	0.006	0.103
Glycolysis	21	3	0.46	6.6	0.009	0.121
Citric acid cycle	23	3	0.50	6.0	0.012	0.133
Methionine metabolism	24	3	0.52	5.7	0.013	0.133
Gluconeogenesis	27	3	0.59	5.1	0.018	0.163
Amino sugar metabolism	15	2	0.33	6.1	0.040	0.290
Mitochondrial electron transport chain	15	2	0.33	6.1	0.040	0.290

[*1]Total numbers of metabolites that corresponded in each pathway.
[*2]Observed numbers of metabolites that derived from given dataset in each pathway.
[*3]Expected observed numbers of metabolites that are calculated by given dataset in each pathway.
[*4]False discovery rate (FDR) according to the Benjamini and Hochberg method that was provided by MSEA software.

decreased, but almost all amino acids were also lowered after BMW consumption periods (see Figure S2 of Supplementary Material).

Additionally, MSEA was performed using the 19 significantly changed metabolites (Table 3). These metabolites were involved with central metabolic pathways (glycolysis, gluconeogenesis, and citric acid cycle) and nitrogen metabolism pathways such as ammonia recycling, urea cycle, and methionine metabolism. These results suggested that physiological metabolism was modified by consumption of BMW.

On the other hand, it was observed that 3-hydroxybutyrate, one of the indexes of diabetic ketoacidosis, was not altered by BMW consumption (Figure 2(c)).

3.3. BMW Consumption-Related Changes of Microbiota Compositions.
Microbiome analysis was conducted using fecal samples that were collected weekly during the study. A total of 7,075 OTUs were constructed from 16S rRNA gene sequences derived from 19 subjects. These OTUs corresponded to 62 families and whole structures of fecal microbiota are shown (Figure 3(a)). To investigate the intraindividual changes of gut microbiota during the test, relative abundances of each microbial taxon were compared between TW and BMW consumption periods within subjects. From the results, it was observed that over 85% of families were not altered similarly to blood metabolites, but relative proportions of 8 families especially Christensenellaceae were significantly different between TW and BMW consumption periods (Figure 3(b)). These results suggested that consumption of BMW has a potential to change some gut microbial compositions.

4. Discussion

In the present study, it was shown that serum glycoalbumin levels were significantly decreased after BMW consumption as compared with TW consumption. Although glycoalbumin levels have been known to reflect blood glucose levels during

the last 14 days of the experiment [24], the mean blood glucose levels were not decreased significantly but tended to be lowered by BMW consumption as observed in our data. This might be attributed to the fact that blood glucose levels are influenced by external factors such as food intake and exercise [25]. Although insulin is one of the major factors involved in blood glucose control, the reduction of glycoalbumin level that was observed in this study was not expected to be related to the changing of insulin secretion and/or insulin resistance because insulin concentrations and HOMA-R were not significantly changed after BMW consumption. Previous studies have also reported the reduction of blood glucose levels by consumption of BMW or sulfate containing water [4, 5], but this study is the first evidence of reduction of serum glycoalbumin levels by consumption of BMW. Additionally, relative glycoalbumin levels were partly decreased even after TW consumption period. Although it has been previously reported that body weights of the volunteers were decreased by consumption of TW before every meal during 12 weeks [26], the reduction in serum glycoalbumin levels is a novel result.

Clinical tests also indicated significant increments in blood calcium levels. This phenomenon was expected to be attributed to BMW consumption because BMW used in this study contains calcium (177 mg/kg). According to the previous report, calcium deficiency may apparently lead to insulin resistance [27]. Therefore, calcium supplementation by drinking mineral water that includes calcium may be important as well as BMW consumption to better manage glycemic control.

According to the metabolome analysis of blood samples, ATP and pyruvate were significantly increased whereas ADP was decreased. This result suggested that glycolysis was upregulated after consumption of BMW. Since blood glucose levels were not decreased significantly but tended to be lowered as observed in our results, the effects of glycolysis enhancement were expected. On the other hand, concentrations of 3 amino acids (tyrosine, methionine, and

(a)

(b)

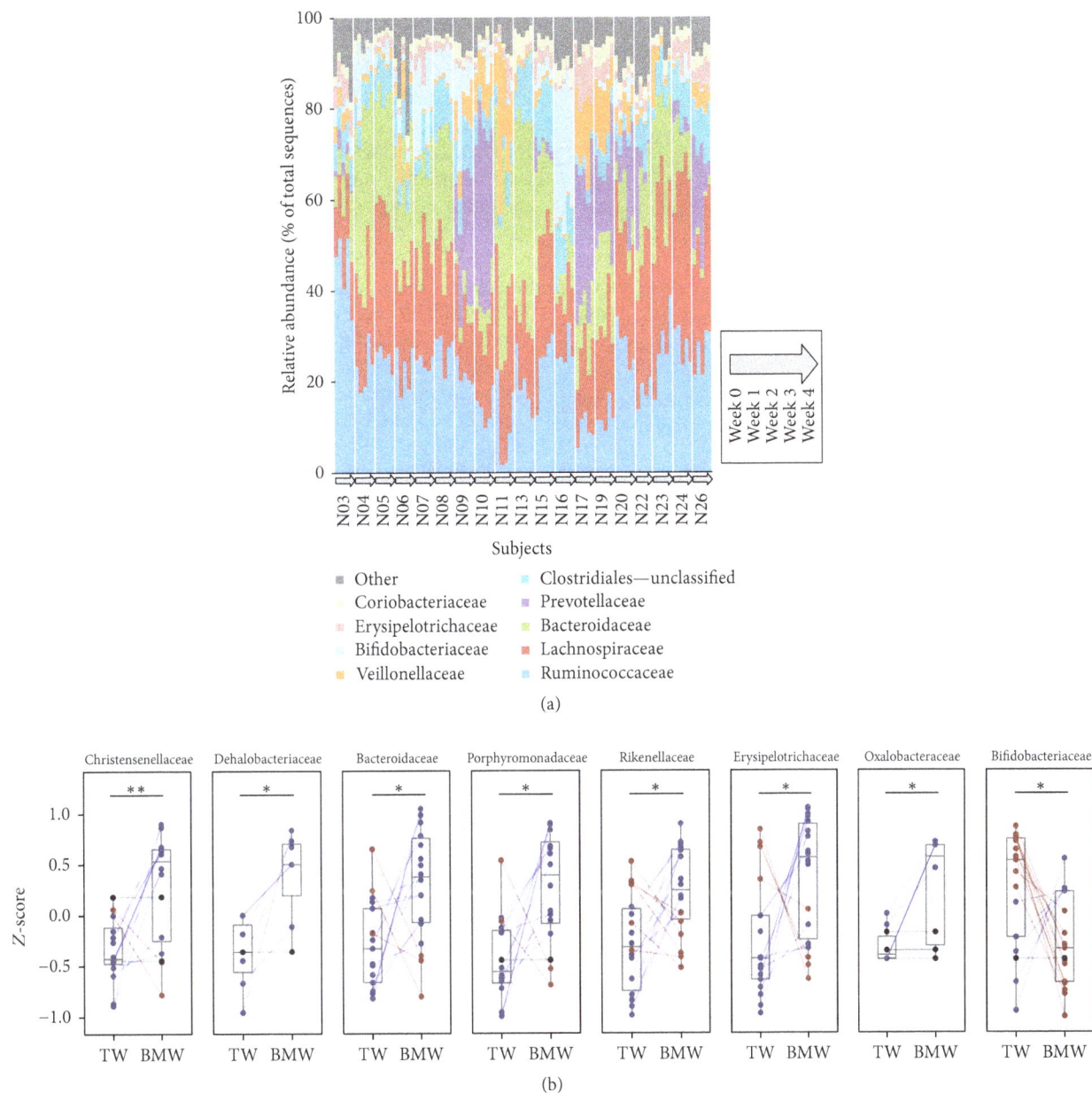

FIGURE 3: Comparisons of fecal microbiota compositions between TW and BMW consumption periods. (a) Family level compositions of fecal microbiota during the test. (b) Mean relative abundances of each taxa (Z-score) of weeks 1 and 3 (TW) and weeks 2 and 4 (BMW) were shown in dot plots overlaid on box plots in the same manner as in Figure 1(a). Only 8 families that their compositions were significantly different between TW and BMW consumption periods were demonstrated. $^*P < 0.05$; $^{**}P < 0.005$.

glycine) were significantly lowered after consumption of BMW. A previous study reported that high concentrations of various amino acids especially tyrosine in blood are one of the risk factors of T2D [28]. Additionally, it has been also reported that plasma concentrations of several amino acids including tyrosine and methionine were significantly high in hyperinsulinemia (it is often observed in early stage of T2D) patients as compared to healthy subjects [29]. Our results demonstrated that concentrations of 3 amino acids including tyrosine and methionine in blood were significantly decreased and that those of other standard amino acids

were tended to be lowered after consumption of BMW. As such, it can be suggested that the BMW consumption has a possible potential to prevent and/or improve T2D through the alterations of metabolism in the body.

After insulin resistance was increased, it can be expected that proteolysis and ketogenesis would be enhanced [30]. As a result, the increment of blood concentrations of amino acids or ketone bodies is expected. Since metabolome analysis indicated that the concentrations of 3-hydroxybutyrate, a type of ketone body, between TW and BMW consumption periods were not changed, consumption of BMW may not affect generation of energy from free fatty acids. As our results demonstrated that concentrations of almost of all amino acids especially tyrosine, methionine, and glycine were decreased, but that of 3-hydroxybutyrate was not changed, BMW consumption may influence energy metabolism through proteolysis but not ketogenesis.

UDP-N-acetylglucosamine is the substrate of O-linked N-acetylglucosamine transferase and the relationship between O-linked N-acetylglucosamine transferase and insulin resistance has been previously reported [31]. However, it was also reported that concentration of UDP-N-acetylglucosamine in muscle tissue was increased after reaching euglycemia by insulin treatment in obese subjects [32]. These reports suggested that UDP-N-acetylglucosamine is related to glucose control and/or insulin resistance, but the details are still unclear. In the current study, metabolome analysis indicated that blood concentrations of UDP-N-acetylglucosamine were significantly increased after BMW consumption, but future studies are required to understand the meaning of this phenomenon.

Since recent studies reported the relationships between gut microbiota and T2D and/or obesity [33–35], we hypothesized that beneficial effect for glycemic control derived from BMW consumption might involve gut microbiota. As expected, alterations of gut microbiota compositions derived from BMW consumption were observed. In this study, family Christensenellaceae was the most significantly increased taxon. Previous study reported that Christensenellaceae was enriched in lean group (BMI < 25) as compared with obese group (BMI > 30) [36]. Additionally, it was also reported that transplantation of *Christensenella minuta* to germ-free mice reduced weight gain. Moreover, abundance of the family Dehalobacteriaceae that was also increased after BMW consumption has been reported to be positively correlated with Christensenellaceae. Therefore, our results suggested that consumption of BMW has a possible potential to prevent getting obese via increments of the abundance of lean-inducible bacteria, Christensenellaceae and Dehalobacteriaceae.

5. Conclusions

In this study, we have shown that serum glycoalbumin levels were significantly decreased after BMW consumption as compared with TW consumption. It was also observed that 19 blood metabolites were significantly changed and lean-inducible bacteria were significantly increased after BMW consumption (see Figure S3 of Supplementary Material). The current study is expected to become important evidence detailing the molecular level effects of BMW consumption. Finally, we believe that the molecular level elucidation of the beneficial effects derived from balneotherapy is vital for further progress and understanding of balneology and our study is the first step towards this approach.

Conflict of Interests

The authors declare that there is no conflict of interests regarding the publication of this paper.

Acknowledgments

The authors would like to thank Ms. Chiharu Ishii, Ms. Yuka Ohara, and Mr. Yuki Yoshida for their experimental and/or analytical support. They also wish to thank Dr. Wanping Aw for critical reading and editing of the paper. As performing blood sampling, they really thank Ms. Mitsuyo Matsuo and members of Ito Medical Office. They would like to offer their gratitude to officials, Ms. Ryoko Washitsukasa, Ms. Kyoko Nakashita, Ms. Nozomi Mai, Mr. Toru Miyazaki, Mr. Yasuyuki Morita, Mr. Takahiro Kudo, Mr. Teiji Shimizu, Mr. Toshinori Hayashi, Mr. Hironori Shin, and Mayor Katsuji Shuto from Taketa for their governmental support. This study was supported in part by research grants from the Ministry of Education, Culture, Sports, Science and Technology, Japan (26117725 and 15H01522 to Shinji Fukuda), Japan Society for the Promotion of Science (254930 to Shinnosuke Murakami and 24380072 to Shinji Fukuda), the Yamagata Prefectural Government and the city of Tsuruoka, and the Japan Health and Research Institute (Shinji Fukuda).

References

[1] K. Z. Walker, K. O'Dea, M. Gomez, S. Girgis, and R. Colagiuri, "Diet and exercise in the prevention of diabetes," *Journal of Human Nutrition and Dietetics*, vol. 23, no. 4, pp. 344–352, 2010.

[2] J. Salas-Salvadó, M. Martinez-González, M. Bulló, and E. Ros, "The role of diet in the prevention of type 2 diabetes," *Nutrition, Metabolism and Cardiovascular Diseases*, vol. 21, supplement 2, pp. B32–B48, 2011.

[3] M. Karagülle and M. Z. Karagülle, "Effectiveness of balneotherapy and spa therapy for the treatment of chronic low back pain: a review on latest evidence," *Clinical Rheumatology*, vol. 34, no. 2, pp. 207–214, 2015.

[4] C. Gutenbrunner, "Kontrollierte Studie über die Wirkung einer Haustrinkkur mit einem Natrium-Hydrogencarbonat-Säuerling auf die Blutzuckerregulation bei gesunden Versuchspersonen," *Physikalische Medizin, Rehabilitationsmedizin, Kurortmedizin*, vol. 3, no. 4, pp. 108–110, 1993.

[5] Y. Ohtsuka, J. Nakaya, K. Nishikawa, and N. Takahashi, "Effect of hot spring water drinking on glucose metabolism," *The Journal of the Japanese Society of Balneology, Climatology and Physical Medicine*, vol. 66, no. 4, pp. 227–230, 2003.

[6] S. Schoppen, F. J. Sánchez-Muniz, A. M. Pérez-Granados et al., "Does bicarbonated mineral water rich in sodium change insulin sensitivity of postmenopausal women?" *Nutricion Hospitalaria*, vol. 22, no. 5, pp. 538–544, 2007.

[7] F. Annegret and F. Thomas, "Long-term benefits of radon spa therapy in rheumatic diseases: results of the randomised, multicentre IMuRa trial," *Rheumatology International*, vol. 33, no. 11, pp. 2839–2850, 2013.

[8] A. M. Pérez-Granados, S. Navas-Carretero, S. Schoppen, and M. P. Vaquero, "Reduction in cardiovascular risk by sodium-bicarbonated mineral water in moderately hypercholesterolemic young adults," *Journal of Nutritional Biochemistry*, vol. 21, no. 10, pp. 948–953, 2010.

[9] E. D. Pagourelias, P. G. Zorou, M. Tsaligopoulos, V. G. Athyros, A. Karagiannis, and G. K. Efthimiadis, "Carbon dioxide balneotherapy and cardiovascular disease," *International Journal of Biometeorology*, vol. 55, no. 5, pp. 657–663, 2011.

[10] S. Samino, M. Vinaixa, M. Díaz et al., "Metabolomics reveals impaired maturation of HDL particles in adolescents with hyperinsulinaemic androgen excess," *Scientific Reports*, vol. 5, article 11496, 2015.

[11] A. Sreekumar, L. M. Poisson, T. M. Rajendiran et al., "Metabolomic profiles delineate potential role for sarcosine in prostate cancer progression," *Nature*, vol. 457, no. 7231, pp. 910–914, 2009.

[12] M. Uetaki, S. Tabata, F. Nakasuka, T. Soga, and M. Tomita, "Metabolomic alterations in human cancer cells by vitamin C-induced oxidative stress," *Scientific Reports*, vol. 5, Article ID 13896, 2015.

[13] E. Mishima, S. Fukuda, H. Shima et al., "Alteration of the intestinal environment by lubiprostone is associated with amelioration of adenine-induced CKD," *Journal of the American Society of Nephrology*, vol. 26, no. 8, pp. 1787–1794, 2015.

[14] M. Sugimoto, D. T. Wong, A. Hirayama, T. Soga, and M. Tomita, "Capillary electrophoresis mass spectrometry-based saliva metabolomics identified oral, breast and pancreatic cancer-specific profiles," *Metabolomics*, vol. 6, no. 1, pp. 78–95, 2010.

[15] P. Kaur, N. Rizk, S. Ibrahim et al., "Quantitative metabolomic and lipidomic profiling reveals aberrant amino acid metabolism in type 2 diabetes," *Molecular BioSystems*, vol. 9, no. 2, pp. 307–317, 2013.

[16] N. Larsen, F. K. Vogensen, F. W. J. van den Berg et al., "Gut microbiota in human adults with type 2 diabetes differs from non-diabetic adults," *PLoS ONE*, vol. 5, no. 2, Article ID e9085, 2010.

[17] J. Qin, Y. Li, Z. Cai, and et al, "A metagenome-wide association study of gut microbiota in type 2 diabetes," *Nature*, vol. 490, no. 7418, pp. 55–60, 2012.

[18] F. H. Karlsson, V. Tremaroli, I. Nookaew et al., "Gut metagenome in European women with normal, impaired and diabetic glucose control," *Nature*, vol. 498, no. 7452, pp. 99–103, 2013.

[19] J. Xia and D. S. Wishart, "MSEA: a web-based tool to identify biologically meaningful patterns in quantitative metabolomic data," *Nucleic Acids Research*, vol. 38, no. 2, pp. W71–W77, 2010.

[20] Y. Furusawa, Y. Obata, S. Fukuda et al., "Commensal microbe-derived butyrate induces the differentiation of colonic regulatory T cells," *Nature*, vol. 504, no. 7480, pp. 446–450, 2013.

[21] S.-W. Kim, W. Suda, S. Kim et al., "Robustness of gut microbiota of healthy adults in response to probiotic intervention revealed by high-throughput pyrosequencing," *DNA Research*, vol. 20, no. 3, pp. 241–253, 2013.

[22] T. Magoč and S. L. Salzberg, "FLASH: fast length adjustment of short reads to improve genome assemblies," *Bioinformatics*, vol. 27, no. 21, pp. 2957–2963, 2011.

[23] J. G. Caporaso, J. Kuczynski, J. Stombaugh et al., "QIIME allows analysis of high-throughput community sequencing data," *Nature Methods*, vol. 7, no. 5, pp. 335–336, 2010.

[24] M. Koga and S. Kasayama, "Clinical impact of glycated albumin as another glycemic control marker," *Endocrine Journal*, vol. 57, no. 9, pp. 751–762, 2010.

[25] S. Moebus, L. Göres, C. Lösch, and K.-H. Jöckel, "Impact of time since last caloric intake on blood glucose levels," *European Journal of Epidemiology*, vol. 26, no. 9, pp. 719–728, 2011.

[26] E. A. Dennis, A. L. Dengo, D. L. Comber et al., "Water consumption increases weight loss during a hypocaloric diet intervention in middle-aged and older adults," *Obesity*, vol. 18, no. 2, pp. 300–307, 2010.

[27] T. Fujita, "Calcium paradox: consequences of calcium deficiency manifested by a wide variety of diseases," *Journal of Bone and Mineral Metabolism*, vol. 18, no. 4, pp. 234–236, 2000.

[28] T. J. Wang, M. G. Larson, R. S. Vasan et al., "Metabolite profiles and the risk of developing diabetes," *Nature Medicine*, vol. 17, no. 4, pp. 448–453, 2011.

[29] H. Nakamura, H. Jinzu, K. Nagao et al., "Plasma amino acid profiles are associated with insulin, C-peptide and adiponectin levels in type 2 diabetic patients," *Nutrition & Diabetes*, vol. 4, p. e133, 2014.

[30] P. Sonksen and J. Sonksen, "Insulin: understanding its action in health and disease," *British Journal of Anaesthesia*, vol. 85, no. 1, pp. 69–79, 2000.

[31] X. Yang, P. P. Ongusaha, P. D. Miles et al., "Phosphoinositide signalling links O-GlcNAc transferase to insulin resistance," *Nature*, vol. 451, no. 7181, pp. 964–969, 2008.

[32] M.-J. J. Pouwels, P. N. Span, C. J. Tack et al., "Muscle uridine diphosphate-hexosamines do not decrease despite correction of hyperglycemia-induced insulin resistance in type 2 diabetes," *The Journal of Clinical Endocrinology & Metabolism*, vol. 87, no. 11, pp. 5179–5184, 2002.

[33] P. J. Turnbaugh, R. E. Ley, M. A. Mahowald, V. Magrini, E. R. Mardis, and J. I. Gordon, "An obesity-associated gut microbiome with increased capacity for energy harvest," *Nature*, vol. 444, no. 7122, pp. 1027–1031, 2006.

[34] G. Musso, R. Gambino, and M. Cassader, "Obesity, diabetes, and gut microbiota: the hygiene hypothesis expanded?" *Diabetes Care*, vol. 33, no. 10, pp. 2277–2284, 2010.

[35] V. K. Ridaura, J. J. Faith, F. E. Rey et al., "Gut microbiota from twins discordant for obesity modulate metabolism in mice," *Science*, vol. 341, no. 6150, Article ID 1241214, 2013.

[36] J. K. Goodrich, J. L. Waters, A. C. Poole et al., "Human genetics shape the gut microbiome," *Cell*, vol. 159, no. 4, pp. 789–799, 2014.

Fuyuan Decoction Enhances SOX9 and COL2A1 Expression and Smad2/3 Phosphorylation in IL-1β-Activated Chondrocytes

Yudi Zhang,[1,2] Rongheng Li,[1] Yu Zhong,[1] Sihan Zhang,[1,3] Lingyun Zhou,[1] and Shike Shang[1]

[1]*Department of Combination of Chinese and Western Medicine, The First Affiliated Hospital of Chongqing Medical University, Chongqing 400016, China*
[2]*College of Laboratory Medicine, Chongqing Medical University, Yuzhong District, Chongqing 400016, China*
[3]*Longgang District People's Hospital of Shenzhen, Longgang District, Shenzhen, Guangdong 518172, China*

Correspondence should be addressed to Yu Zhong; yuyumou@sina.com

Academic Editor: Youn C. Kim

Fuyuan Decoction (FYD), a herbal formula in China, has been widely used for osteoarthritis (OA) treatment. Herein, we determined the effects of FYD on the expression of transcription factor SOX9 and its target gene collagen type II, alpha 1 (COL2A1) as well as the activation of Smad2/3 in interleukin- (IL-) 1β-stimulated SW1353 chondrosarcoma cells. Serum-derived FYD (FYD-CS) was prepared to treat SW1353 cells with or without SB431542, a TGF-β1 receptor inhibitor. Cell cycle progression was tested by flow cytometry. The expression of SOX9 and COL2A1 and the activation of Smad2/3 (p-Smad2/3) were analyzed by quantitative reverse transcription polymerase chain reaction (qRT-PCR) and/or western blot. The results showed that, after treatment, FYD-CS, while inducing S-phase cell cycle arrest, enhanced cell proliferation and protected the cells against IL-1β- and/or SB431542-induced cell growth inhibition. Furthermore, FYD-CS reversed the decreased expression of COL2A1 and SOX9 induced by IL-1β and SB431542 and blocked the decreased phosphorylation of Smad2/3 induced by IL-1β alone or in combination with SB431542. Our results suggest that FYD promotes COL2A1 and SOX9 expression as well as Smad2/3 activation in IL-1β-induced chondrocytes, thus benefiting cell survival.

1. Introduction

Fuyuan Decoction (FYD) is an empirical formula used to treat Bi Zheng in clinical practice and has been proven effective in the treatment of osteoarthritis (OA). FYD can inhibit the development of OA [1]. To date, several bioactive components of FYD have been identified, including icariin and arasaponin R1, which exhibit a number of biological activities, including inhibiting inflammation and oxidative damage [2] as well as the development and progression of OA [3]. In addition, pilose antler, another component of FYD, has been found to increase the expression of Smad2/3 in OA cartilage [4].

In the early stages of OA, the inflammatory response is an important contributing factor that initiates and promotes the disease. Several inflammatory mediators have been identified to be responsible for the inflammatory pathology of OA [5–7]; among them, interleukin-1 beta (IL-1β) plays a key role

in amplifying the inflammatory response and, in combination with dysregulated other factors including transforming growth factor-β (TGF-β) [8], exacerbates the pathogenesis of OA [9]. TGF-β is a multifunctional growth factor that plays an important role in the formation, homeostasis, and repair of cartilage [10–12]. TGF-β stimulates the formation of cartilage, including chondrogenic condensation [13, 14] and chondroprogenitor cell proliferation and differentiation [15, 16]. It also inhibits the terminal differentiation of chondrocytes into the hypertrophic phenotype by intercepting the calcification of cartilage matrix, differentiation, and ossification of osteoblasts [12, 17], resulting in the formation of articular cartilage at the end of long bones [18].

Of the current treatment options for OA, nonsteroidal anti-inflammatory drugs and selective cyclooxygenase-2 inhibitors are widely used. However, due to the potential side effects and concerned effectiveness of these agents [19–21], it is necessary to develop more safe and effective alternative drugs for the treatment of OA. In the context of traditional Chinese medicine, OA belongs to the category Bi Zheng, which is defined as a syndrome marked by arthralgia and dyskinesia of the joints and limbs due to the meridians of the limbs being attacked by wind, dampness, and heat or cold pathogens. FYD is an empirical formula used to treat Bi Zheng in clinical practice and has been proven effective in the treatment of OA. Now, Fuyuan capsule made from FYD has been confirmed to have a better effect on the treatment of experimental OA than the positive control western medicine glucosamine hydrochloride [2]. The purpose of this study was to investigate the effects and mechanisms of FYD in chondrocytes in the OA microenvironment. In particular, the expression levels of SOX9 and COL2A1 as well as the phosphorylation of Smad2/3 were analyzed.

2. Materials and Methods

2.1. Materials and Reagents. Notoginsenoside R1, icariin, and digoxin were purchased from the National Institute for the Control of Pharmaceutical and Biological Products (Beijing, China). SB431542, a TGF-β1 receptor inhibitor, was obtained from Selleckchem (Houston, TX, USA). IL-1β was purchased from PeproTech (Rocky Hill, NJ, USA). Cell Counting Kit-8 (CCK-8) was obtained from Beyotime Biotechnology (Shanghai, China). The mRNA primers were synthesized by Sangon Biotech (Shanghai, China). TRIzol reagent was obtained from Ambion (Grand Island, NY, USA). The RevertAid First Strand cDNA Synthesis Kit was obtained from Thermo Fisher Scientific Inc. (Waltham, MA, USA). The SYBR Green PCR Master Mix Kit was provided by the College of Laboratory Medicine, CWBIO (Beijing, China). Rabbit anti-GAPDH antibody was obtained from Zhongding (Nanjing, China). Rabbit anti-P-Smad2/Smad3 antibodies were obtained from Cell Signaling Technology (Danvers, MA, USA). COL2A1 and SOX9 antibodies were obtained from Bioworld Technology (Minneapolis, MN, USA). Horseradish peroxidase- (HRP-) conjugated goat anti-rabbit secondary antibody was obtained from ABGENT (San Diego, CA, USA). Western blot Chemiluminescent HRP was provided by the College of Laboratory Medicine (Immobilon Western, USA).

2.2. Herbal Preparation. FYD was prepared from nine dried powdered plant species as follows: 15 g of *Epimedium brevicornum*, 15 g of *Astragalus membranaceus*, 15 g of *Davallia formosana*, 15 g of *Psoralea corylifolia*, 10 g of *Angelica sinensis*, 10 g of *Panax ginseng*, 5 g of *Panax pseudoginseng* var. *notoginseng*, 10 g of *Salvia miltiorrhiza*, and 5 g of *Glycyrrhiza uralensis*. These plant materials were from Chongqing Tongjunge Pharmacy (Chongqing, China) and identified by Professor Rongheng Li, The First Affiliated Hospital of Chongqing Medical University (Chongqing, China). Currently, these dried powdered plant species are being stored in the Department of Pharmacy of The First Affiliated Hospital of Chongqing Medical University. FYD was extracted according to the standard methods recommended by the Chinese Pharmacopoeia (2010). In short, the herbal

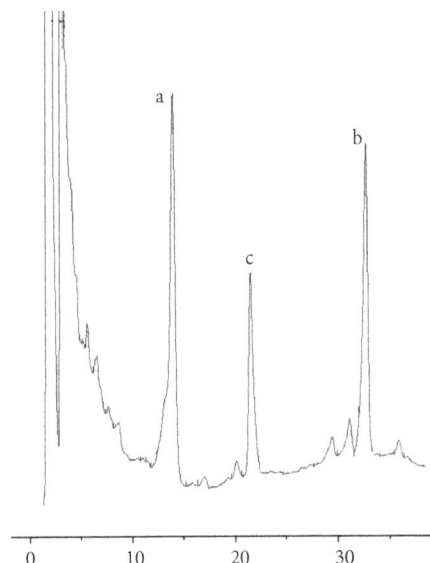

FIGURE 1: HPLC chromatograms of notoginsenoside R1 and icariin in FYD. a: notoginsenoside R1; b: icariin; and c: digoxin as an internal standard.

mixture was extracted twice in boiling water for 2 h each, and the final residues were filtered using a 0.45 μm microfilter, concentrated, and then made into a freeze-dried powder (1). The extraction yield of FYD was 13.67% (w/w), containing 12.18 mg of notoginsenoside R1 and 54.65 mg of icariin per g of freeze-dried powder, according to a high-performance liquid chromatography (HPLC) method (Figure 1). The resultant powder was subsequently dissolved in sterile water at the desired concentrations for the animal studies.

2.3. Preparation of FYD-Containing Serum (FYD-CS). Four-month-old New Zealand rabbits weighing 1800–2000 g were purchased from the Chongqing Medical Laboratory Animal Center (License, SYXK (yu) 2012-0001). Animal care and all experimental procedures were approved by the Ethics Committee of Animal Research of Chongqing University of Medical Sciences (CUMS11-66). Rabbits were randomly assigned to two groups containing two animals each. One group was orally administered with 4.07 g/kg/d FYD (5.8 mL/rabbit) twice daily for 7 consecutive days, while the other group was gavaged with an equal volume of physiological saline. This dose and regimen were picked based on extrapolation of the dosage for humans used in our clinical practice. Approximately 2 h after the last administration on day 7, the rabbits were euthanized by injection of pentobarbital sodium at a dose of 40 mg/kg in the marginal ear vein, and blood was retrieved from the carotid artery. Serum from both groups (FYD-CS and Con-s) was collected by centrifugation at 3000 ×g for 20 min at 4°C, then filtered through a 0.22 μm filter, and stored in −20°C in aliquots.

2.4. SW1353 Cell Culture and Treatment. Human chondrosarcoma cells (SW1353) have a similar phenotype as chondrocytes [22, 23]; therefore, they were used instead of

(a)

(b)

(c)

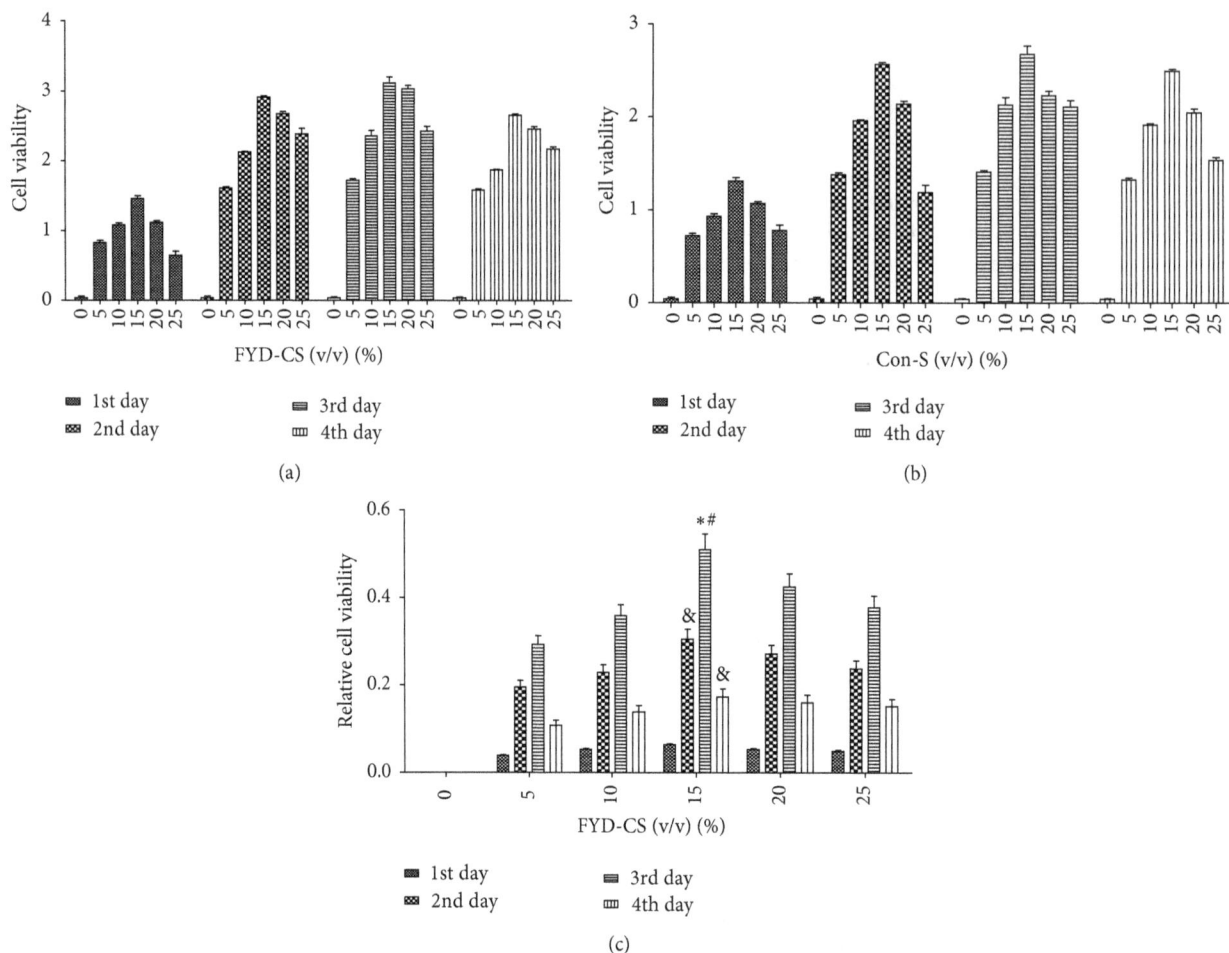

FIGURE 2: Effect of FYD-CS on cell viability in IL-1β-activated SW1353 cells. The cells were treated with different concentrations of FYD-CS or Con-s for 24–96 h; then cell viability was assayed by a colorimetric kit. The data are expressed as the mean ± SD (n = 3). (a) Cells treated with different concentrations of FYD-CS. (b) Cells treated with the corresponding concentration of blank serum as used in the FYD-CS treatments. (c) The effect of FYD alone, which was obtained by subtracting the blank serum results from the FYD-CS results. $^{*}P < 0.05$ versus 10% FYD-CS, $^{\#}P < 0.05$ versus 15% FYD-CS, and $^{\&}P < 0.05$ versus 15% FYD-CS on day 3.

cartilage cells to evaluate the regulatory effects of FYD in this study. The SW1353 cells were obtained from the Institute of Biochemistry and Cell Biology (Shanghai, China). The cells were grown in Dulbecco's modified Eagle's medium supplemented with 10% (v/v) fetal bovine serum, 100 IU/mL penicillin, 100 μg/mL streptomycin, and 2 mM glutamine at 37°C in a 5% CO_2 incubator. When the cells reached 85% confluence, different concentrations of FYD-CS (5–25% (v/v)) and/or 10 μM SB431542 were added. One hour later, 10 ng/mL IL-1β was added to stimulate the cells. The cells were further incubated for 24–96 h before assaying cell viability, gene expression, and protein expression.

2.5. Cell Viability.

SW1353 cells were incubated in 96-well plates (0.5×10^4 cells/well) in the presence or absence of the indicated concentrations of FYD-CS, Con-s, SB431542, and/or IL-1β for 24–96 h. Next, 20 μL of CCK-8 was added to each well, and the plates continued to be incubated at 37°C for

an additional 4 h. The optical density values were measured at 450 nm on a microplate reader.

2.6. Cell Cycle Assay.

SW1353 cells were grown in 6-well plates (2×10^5 cells per well) in the presence or absence of the indicated concentrations of FYD-CS, Con-s, SB431542, and/ or IL-1β. After treatment for 72 h, the cells were harvested and washed three times with cold phosphate-buffered saline (PBS) and then fixed in cold 75% ethanol for at least 8 h at 4°C. After fixation, the cells were treated with PI/RNase staining followed by fluorescence-activated cell sorting analysis.

2.7. Quantitative Reverse Transcription Polymerase Chain Reaction (RT-qPCR).

Total RNA was extracted using TRIzol reagent as recommended by the manufacturer. First-strand cDNA synthesis was performed using the Thermo Scientific RevertAid First Strand cDNA Synthesis Kit. The SYBR Green PCR Master Mix Kit was used for real-time PCR to determine the relative quantification of mRNA. β-actin was used as an internal control. The following primer pairs were used: β-actin (XM_006715764.1), 5′-AAAGACCTGTACGCCAAC-AC-3′ (forward) and 5′-GTCATACTCCTGCTTGCTGAT-3′ (reverse); COL2A1 (XM_006719242.1), 5′-AACCAGATT-GAGAGCATCCG-3′ (forward) and 5′-AACGTTTGCTGG-ATTGGGGT-3′ (reverse); and SOX9 (NM_000346.3), 5′-GCTCTGGAGACTTCTGAACGA-3′ (forward) and 5′-CCGTTCTTCACCGACTTCCT-3′ (reverse). The PCR primers were designed by Invitrogen Biotechnology (Shang-hai, China). Quantitative (real-time) PCR was performed using a Bio-Rad CFX96 Real-Time PCR System (Hercules, CA, USA) with 40 cycles of 95°C for 10 min, 95°C for 10 s, and 58°C for 30 s; measurements were made at the end of a 58°C annealing step. Data were analyzed using Bio-Rad CFX Manager software (version 2.0). The $2^{-\Delta\Delta CT}$ method was used to calculate the relative fold changes of the COL2A1 and SOX9 mRNA expression.

2.8. Western Blot Analysis.

The SW1353 cells were washed three times with ice-cold PBS and lysed with cell lysis buffer (20 mM Tris-HCl (pH 7.5), 150 mM NaCl, 1% EDTA, 1% TritonX-100, and 2.5 mM sodium pyrophosphate) sup-plemented with 1 mM phenylmethylsulfonyl fluoride, 1 mM NaF, and 1 mM sodium orthovanadate. Equal amounts of cellular protein (40 μg per well) were separated on a 12% sodium dodecyl sulfate-polyacrylamide gel and elec-trophoretically transferred to a nitrocellulose membrane. After blocking with 5% fat-free milk and 0.1% Tween 20 in PBS, the membrane was incubated with a primary antibody (anti-GAPDH (1:1000), anti-p-Smad2/Smad3 (1:1000), anti-COL2A1 (1:500), or anti-SOX9 (1:500)) overnight at 4°C and then a HRP-conjugated goat anti-rabbit secondary antibody for 2 h at room temperature. The immunocomplexes were visualized using a chemiluminescent HRP substrate, and band intensities were quantitated using densitometry and normalized to the density of GAPDH from the same treat-ment group.

2.9. Statistical Analysis.

All experiments were performed in triplicate using independent samples. The data were pre-sented as means ± standard deviation (SD) and analyzed using SPSS (version 19.0, SPSS Inc., Chicago, IL, USA). Differences between groups were analyzed by analysis of variance, and $P < 0.05$ was considered statistically significant.

3. Results

3.1. FYD-CS Enhances Cell Viability.

To determine the cytotoxicity and optimal dose of FYD-CS, IL-1β-activated SW1353 cells were treated with different concentrations of FYD-CS for different periods of time. As shown in Figure 2, 5–15% FYD-CS stimulated cell proliferation in a concentration-dependent manner. However, higher concentrations of FYD-CS reduced cell viability when compared to 15% FYD-CS, suggesting that 15% FYD-CS achieved the maximal enhancing effect of cell viability in IL-1β-induced SW1353 cells, especially at 72 h after treatment.

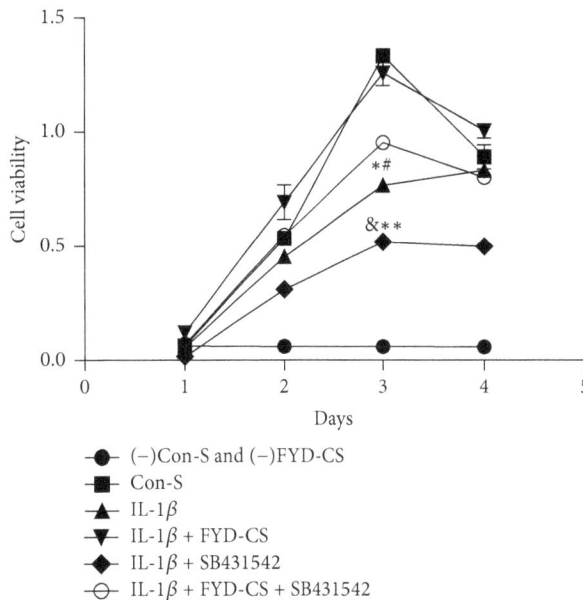

FIGURE 3: Effect of FYD-CS on cell viability in IL-1β- and/or SB431542-treated SW1353 cells. The cells were treated with 15% FYD-CS, 10 μM SB431542, and/or 10 ng/mL IL-1β for 24–96 h, and then the cell viability was assayed. The data are expressed as the mean ± SD ($n = 3$). We found that cell growth peaked at 72 h. $^*P < 0.05$ versus the control; $^{\#}P < 0.05$ versus the group treated with both IL-1β and FYD-CS; $^{\&}P < 0.05$ versus the group treated with IL-1β alone; $^{**}P < 0.05$ versus the group treated with IL-1β, FYD-CS, and SB431542.

Therefore, this concentration was used in the subsequent experiments.

In another set of experiments, the involvement of TGF-1β signaling in the FYD-CS regulation of cell growth was evaluated. As shown in Figures 3 and 4, IL-1β induction reduced SW1353 cell proliferation, inducing cell cycle G0/G1 arrest, compared to the Con-s control. When IL-1β-activated cells were treated with 15% FYD-CS and/or 10 μM SB431542 for 72 h, FYD-CS completely reversed the IL-1β-mediated inhibition of cell viability, inducing cell cycle arrest at the S phase, while the ALK5 inhibitor enhanced the IL-1β-mediated inhibition. Interestingly, FYD-CS completely abol-ished the inhibitory effect of the ALK5 inhibitor, indicating that chondrocyte growth needs the help of the TGF-1β receptor and TGF-1β signaling and that FYD-CS protects SW1353 cells against ALK5 inhibitor-induced inhibition of IL-1β-activated cells.

3.2. FYD-CS Upregulates the Gene Levels of COL2A1 and SOX9.

To further understand the underlying mechanisms of FYD-CS in the regulation of IL-1β- and SB431542-induced cell proliferation inhibition, the mRNA expression levels of COL2A1 and SOX9 were detected in IL-1β-activated cells treated with 15% FYD-CS and/or SB431542 by qRT-PCR (Figure 5). The results showed that FYD-CS significantly recovered the IL-1β-induced decrease in the gene expression of COL2A1 and SOX9. Moreover, SB431542 and IL-1β showed

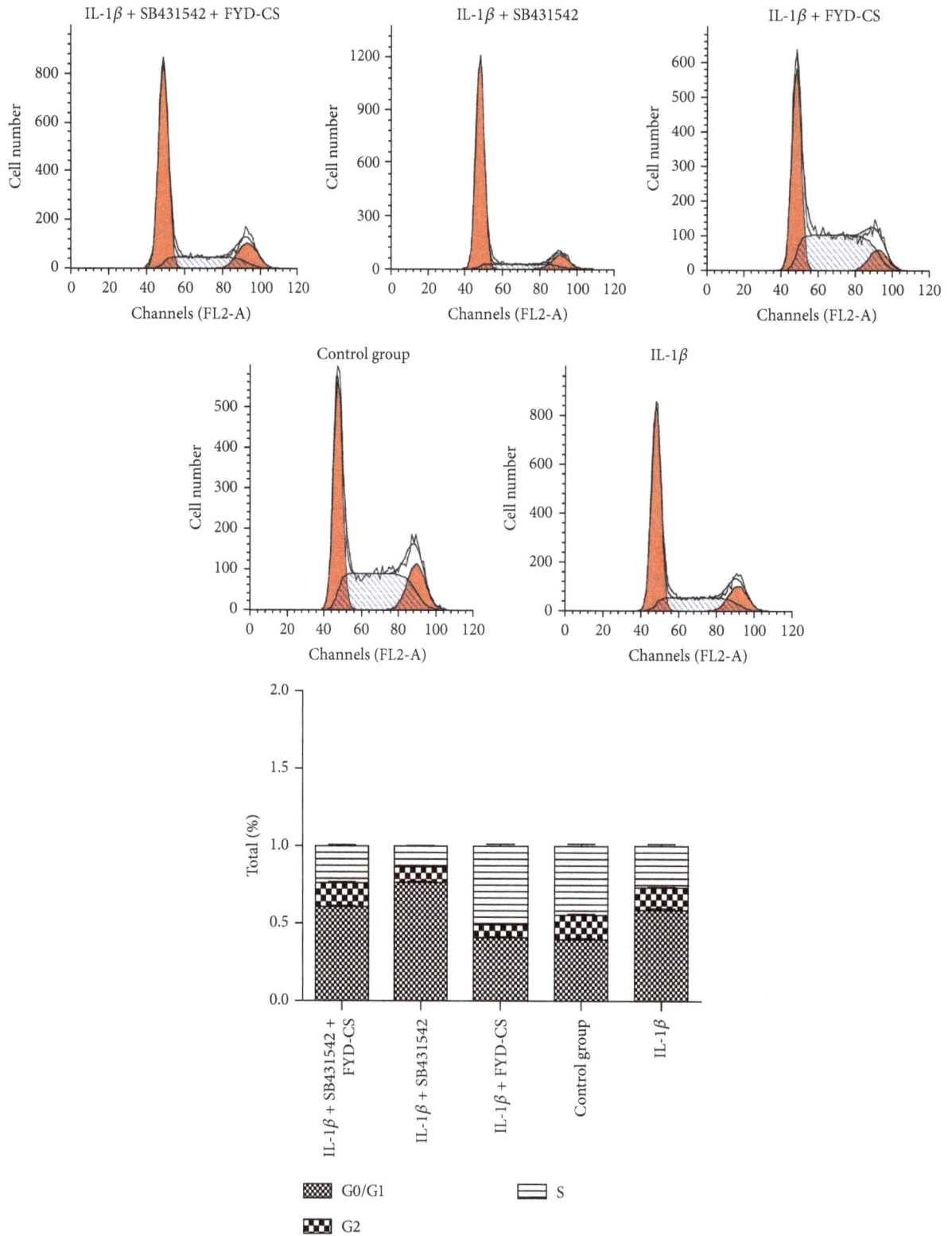

FIGURE 4: Effect of FYD-CS on cell cycle progression in IL-1β- and/or SB431542-treated SW1353 cells. The cells were treated with 15% FYD-CS, 10 μM SB431542, and/or 10 ng/mL IL-1β for 72 h, and then cell cycle progression was assayed.

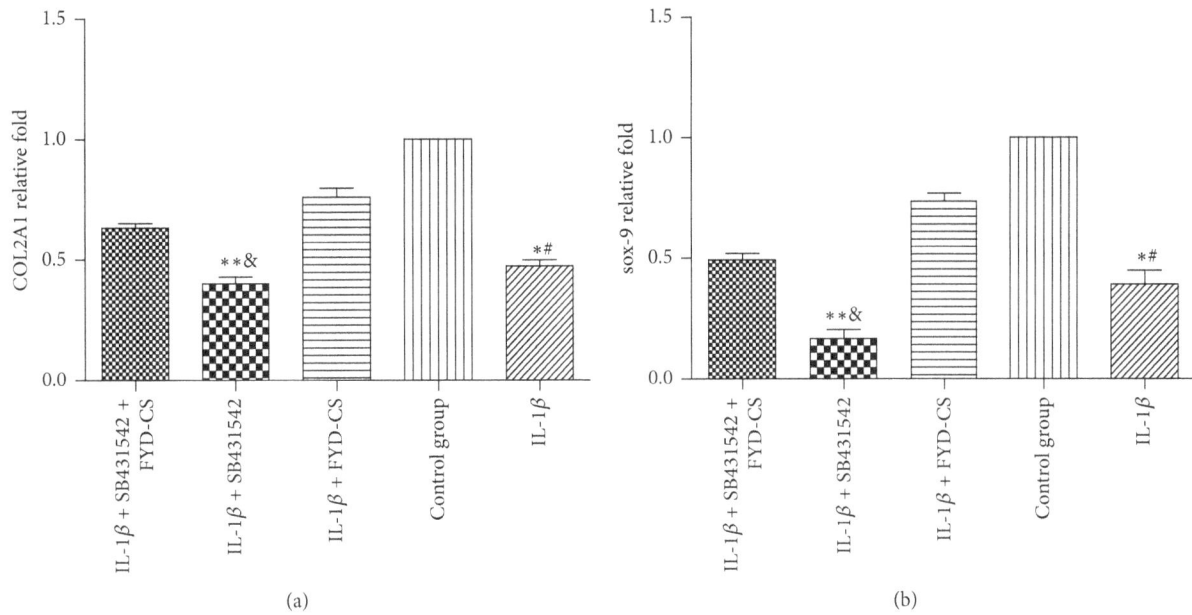

Figure 5: Quantitative RT-PCR assay of COL2A1 and SOX9 in IL-1β-activated SW1353 cells pretreated with 15% FYD-CS and/or 10 μM SB431542. The data are expressed as the mean ± SD (n = 3). *P < 0.05 versus the control. #P < 0.05 versus the group treated with IL-1β and FYD-CS; **P < 0.05 versus the group treated with IL-1β; &P < 0.05 versus the group treated with IL-1β, FYD-CS, and SB431542.

a synergistic inhibitory effect on the expression of the two genes, but this inhibition was partially blocked by FYD-CS. These data suggest that FYD-CS promotes collagen type II expression in IL-1β-activated SW1353 cells, partially through the classical TGF-β signaling pathway.

3.3. FYD-CS Enhances Smad2/Smad3 Phosphorylation as well as COL2A1 and SOX9 Protein Expression.
To examine the effects of FYD-CS on the protein expression of COL2A1 and SOX9 as well as the activation of TGF-1β signaling, IL-1β-activated cells were treated with 15% FYD-CS and/or SB431542 for 72 h, and the expression levels of COL2A1, SOX9, and p-Smad2/Smad3 were analyzed by western blot (Figure 6). It was found that the expression levels of p-Smad2/Smad3, COL2A1, and SOX9 were significantly decreased in IL-1β-treated cells when compared to the baseline SW1353 cells (P < 0.05); however, FYD-CS cotreatment abrogated the effect of IL-1β (P < 0.05). Moreover, SB431542 further decreased the IL-1β-induced inhibition of COL2A1 and SOX9 protein expression and Smad2/Smad3 phosphorylation, but this synergistic effect on TGF-1β signaling and collagen type II synthesis was significantly suppressed by FYD-CS (P < 0.05). These data further confirmed that FYD-CS regulates IL-1β-mediated Smad2/3 phosphorylation as well as COL2A1 and SOX9 expression, which were partially dependent on the classical TGF-β signaling pathway.

4. Discussion

OA is a common chronic degenerative joint disease in the elderly. The typical pathological changes of OA include

articular cartilage impairment, bone sclerosis, osteophytes, and subchondral synovial tissue fibrosis. Although the pathogenesis of OA remains obscure, it is generally attributable to the interactions of multiple factors including mechanical and biological factors that cause an imbalance between tissue damage and repair and resultant degradation of joint tissues, especially articular cartilage.

Chondrocytes are the only cells found in cartilage and are embedded in an extensive extracellular matrix (ECM) [24]. Collagens and proteoglycans are the main components of the ECM [24]. The majority of the collagen in articular cartilage is type II collagen, which provides the tissue with tensile strength [25, 26]. The major proteoglycan of articular cartilage is aggrecan, which provides structural support by retaining water in the matrix [27]. SOX9 is a transcription factor essential for regulating the expression of many cartilage ECM genes, including COL2A1 [28].

TGF-β signaling functions through cell surface heterogenic receptor complexes containing type II and type I (ALK5 or ALK1) receptors to phosphorylate two receptor-regulated Smad proteins, Smad2 and Smad3. Smad2/3 phosphorylation mediates anabolic signaling in chondrocytes essential for articular cartilage matrix turnover and homeostasis [10, 12]. The TGF-β/Smad2/3 signaling pathway is truncated by using a powerful combination of competitive ALK5 receptor inhibitors. Therefore, these inhibitors can affect the synthesis of downstream target genes. This combination is very strong, so the use of these inhibitors can simulate the reduced expression of TGF-β receptors to the maximum limit in vitro [29].

In normal chondrocytes, TGF-β signals the phosphorylation of Smad2/3 predominantly via ALK5, resulting in

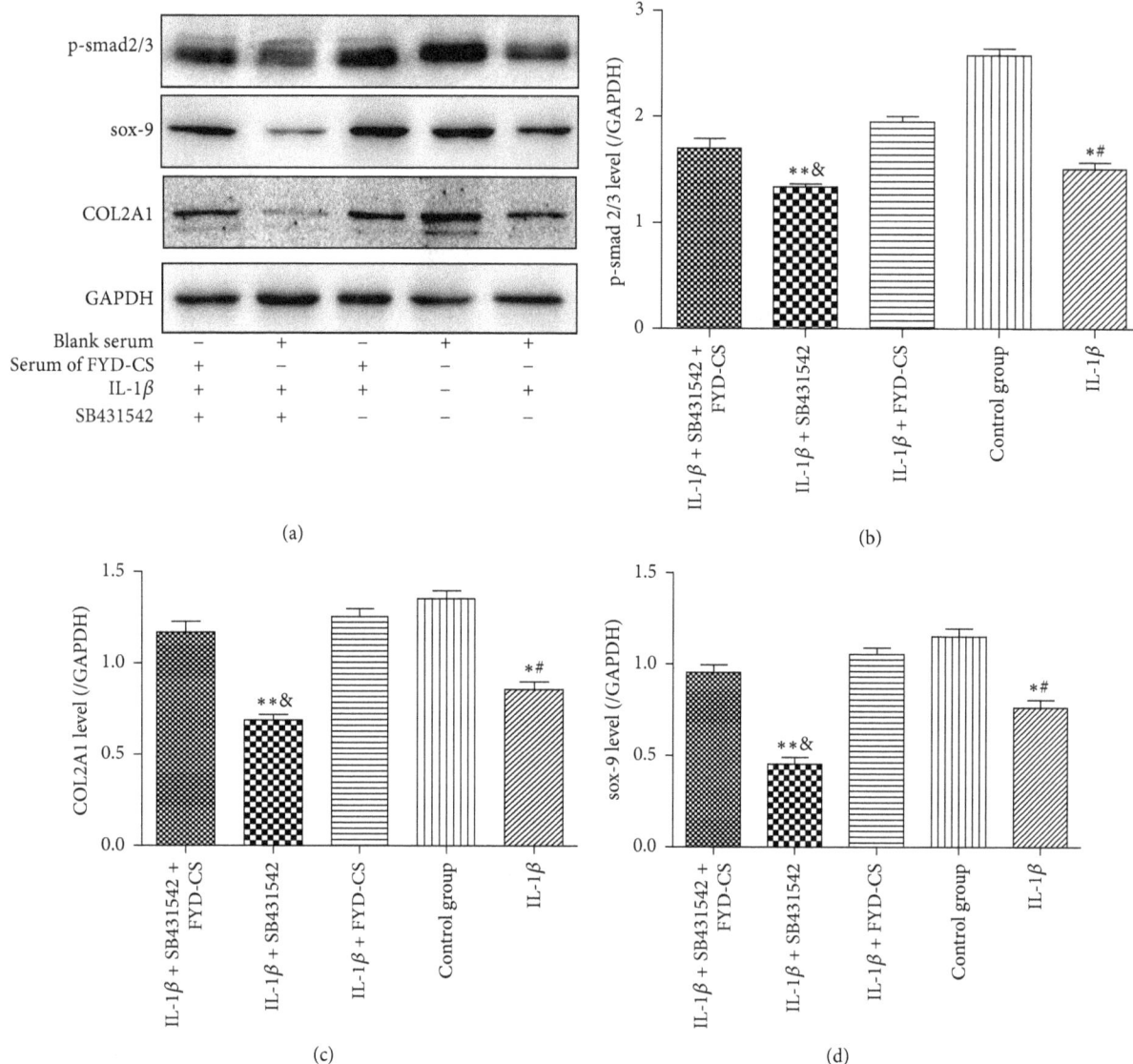

(a)

(b)

(c)

(d)

FIGURE 6: Western blot assay of COL2A1, SOX9, and p-Smad2/3 in IL-1β-activated SW1353 cells pretreated with 15% FYD-CS and/or 10 μM SB431542. Representative bands are shown. The band intensities were compared to that of the corresponding GAPDH band with the same treatment. The data are expressed as the mean ± SD ($n = 3$). $^*P < 0.05$ versus the control; $^\#P < 0.05$ versus the group treated with IL-1β and FYD-CS; $^{**}P < 0.05$ versus the group treated with IL-1β; $^\&P < 0.05$ versus the group treated with IL-1β, FYD-CS, and SB431542.

the formation of a complex with Smad4 and translocation into the nucleus, where it regulates the expression of target genes such as type II collagen and aggrecan. However, in OA, TGF-β may phosphorylate Smad1 and Smad5 preferentially via ALK1, leading to increased expression of matrix metalloproteinase 13 and decreased expression of type II collagen and aggrecan. It has been shown that the phosphorylated Smad2 level is reduced in cartilage during the progression of OA in both spontaneous and collagenase-induced OA mouse models [30]. Also, Smad2 phosphorylation in cartilage of old mice is lower than that of young mice [31]. Another study has reported that the decreased levels of phosphorylated Smad3 in Smurf-2 transgenic mice cause the development of an OA-like phenotype [32]. Additionally, Smad3 knockout mice develop a degenerative joint disease resembling human

OA [18] and intervertebral disc degeneration [33]. Moreover, some genetic studies have shown that Smad3 gene mutations are a risk factor for the susceptibility to OA. Therefore, the expression levels of TGF-β receptors and their downstream proteins Smad2/3 are intimately associated with OA pathogenesis.

In the present study, we used serum-derived FYD as the drug source to mirror the *in vivo* biotransformation and pharmacological effects of FYD and to minimize other uncertain confounding factors [34, 35]. We focused on TGF-β signaling and SOX9 expression because they have a pivotal role in the pathophysiology of joint cartilage. One of the aims of this study was to simulate the TGF-β receptor expression level decrease by using receptor inhibitors. When the receptors were completely inhibited, the expression of phosphorylated

Smad2/3 in chondrocytes was further downregulated, thus achieving the purposes of the experimental modelling. FYD could still activate certain Smad2/3 protein phosphorylation in the presence of SB431542, but the level was lower than that in the no SB431542 inhibitor group. These results indicated that FYD could activate Smad2/3 protein phosphorylation through the TGF-β receptor as well as by other means.

We demonstrated that the water-soluble active components of FYD-CS increase Smad2/3 phosphorylation and promote COL2A1 and SOX9 expression, leading to increased cell proliferation in IL-1β-induced SW1353 cells. This regulatory process may partly depend on the classical TGF-β signaling pathway.

Healthy articular cartilage depends on the balance between anabolic and catabolic cytokines and growth factors. Accumulated evidence supports the association of OA with reduced TGF-β/ALK5/Smad2/3 signaling. IL-1β, a proinflammatory cytokine and a critical catabolic factor, has been found recently to induce MMP production, reduce Smad2/3 phosphorylation, and inhibit Smad3/4 activity and DNA binding [9]. In the current study, IL-1β was used to establish a cellular OA model in SW1353 cells [36]. We found a rapid decrease in the expression levels of p-Smad2/3, COL2A1, and SOX9 in response to IL-1β; however, FYD-CS effectively abolished the inhibitory effects of IL-1β in SW1353 cells. To the best of our knowledge, this is the first study to determine that FYD-CS is a potent activator of Smad2/3 activity. Moreover, we found that SB431542, an inhibitor of the TGF-β1 receptor, not only reduced the levels of phosphorylated Smad2/3 but also reduced the expression levels of COL2A1 and SOX9. In addition, FYD-CS antagonized the effects of the inhibitor, further confirming the role of FYD-CS in the TGF-β signaling pathway.

FYD-CS is clinically effective in the treatment of OA. In this study, we explored the mechanism of FYD-CS in regulating the expression of COL2A1 and SOX9 in IL-1β-induced SW1353 cells. The results suggest that FYD-CS increases the levels of phosphorylated Smad2/3 as well as the expression of COL2A1 and SOX9 in IL-1β-induced SW1353 cells.

5. Conclusion

In summary, our data support FYD as a beneficial agent in the treatment of OA; it stimulates cell proliferation, possibly through the positive regulation of TGF-β signaling and its target genes that participate in the structure and function of articular cartilage. These noteworthy findings will help to treat OA by repairing the ECM. However, further studies are needed to confirm the regulation of the TGF-β/Smad2/Smad3 signaling pathway by FYD in animal models.

Conflict of Interests

The authors declare that there is no conflict of interests.

Acknowledgments

This work was supported by the Grants of Chinese Medicine of the Health Bureau in Chongqing City (no. 2008-2-35). The authors wish to thank Professor Qin Zhou for providing an experimental platform and his team for their technical assistance.

References

[1] P. Jia, G. Chen, G. Zhou, Y. Zhong, and R. Li, "Fuyuan Decoction inhibits nitric oxide production via inactivation of nuclear factor-κB in SW1353 chondrosarcoma cells," *Journal of Ethnopharmacology*, vol. 146, no. 3, pp. 853–858, 2013.

[2] W. Zhang, R. Li, S. Wang, X. Zhou, and Y. Zhong, "Study of molecular mechanisms of fuyuan capsule, icariin and arasaponin R1 in treatment of osteoarthritis," *Zhongguo Zhong Yao Za Zhi*, vol. 36, no. 15, pp. 2113–2117, 2011.

[3] L. Zeng, W. Wang, X.-F. Rong et al., "Chondroprotective effects and multi-target mechanisms of Icariin in IL-1 β-induced human SW 1353 chondrosarcoma cells and a rat osteoarthritis model," *International Immunopharmacology*, vol. 18, no. 1, pp. 175–181, 2014.

[4] W. Niu, Z.-T. Sun, X.-W. Cao et al., "Regulation of single herb pilose antler on the expression of Smad2 and Smad3 in the cartilage of OA rats: an experimental research," *Zhongguo Zhong Xi Yi Jie He Za Zhi*, vol. 34, no. 2, pp. 209–213, 2014.

[5] H. J. Salminen, A.-M. K. Säämänen, M. N. Vankemmelbeke, P. K. Auho, M. P. Perälä, and E. I. Vuorio, "Differential expression patterns of matrix metalloproteinases and their inhibitors during development of osteoarthritis in a transgenic mouse model," *Annals of the Rheumatic Diseases*, vol. 61, no. 7, pp. 591–597, 2002.

[6] J. Martel-Pelletier, "Pathophysiology of osteoarthritis," *Osteoarthritis and Cartilage*, vol. 6, no. 6, pp. 374–376, 1998.

[7] P. Wang, F. Zhu, N. H. Lee, and K. Konstantopoulos, "Shear-induced interleukin-6 synthesis in chondrocytes: roles of E prostanoid (EP) 2 and EP3 in cAMP/protein kinase A- and PI3-K/Akt-dependent NF-κB activation," *The Journal of Biological Chemistry*, vol. 285, no. 32, pp. 24793–24804, 2010.

[8] C. Chen, J. Xie, R. Rajappa, L. Deng, and J. Fredberg, "Interleukin-1β and tumor necrosis factor-α increase stiffness and impair contractile function of articular chondrocytes," *Acta Biochimica et Biophysica Sinica*, vol. 47, no. 2, pp. 121–129, 2015.

[9] J. A. Roman-Blas, D. G. Stokes, and S. A. Jimenez, "Modulation of TGF-β signaling by proinflammatory cytokines in articular chondrocytes," *Osteoarthritis and Cartilage*, vol. 15, no. 12, pp. 1367–1377, 2007.

[10] E. N. B. Davidson, P. M. van der Kraan, and W. B. van den Berg, "TGF-β and osteoarthritis," *Osteoarthritis and Cartilage*, vol. 15, no. 6, pp. 597–604, 2007.

[11] B. Song, K. D. Estrada, and K. M. Lyons, "Smad signaling in skeletal development and regeneration," *Cytokine and Growth Factor Reviews*, vol. 20, no. 5-6, pp. 379–388, 2009.

[12] P. M. van der Kraan, E. N. Blaney Davidson, A. Blom, and W. B. van den Berg, "TGF-beta signaling in chondrocyte terminal differentiation and osteoarthritis: modulation and integration of signaling pathways through receptor-Smads," *Osteoarthritis and Cartilage*, vol. 17, no. 12, pp. 1539–1545, 2009.

[13] M. B. Goldring, K. Tsuchimochi, and K. Ijiri, "The control of chondrogenesis," *Journal of Cellular Biochemistry*, vol. 97, no. 1, pp. 33–44, 2006.

[14] I. Onyekwelu, M. B. Goldring, and C. Hidaka, "Chondrogenesis, joint formation, and articular cartilage regeneration," *Journal of Cellular Biochemistry*, vol. 107, no. 3, pp. 383–392, 2009.

[15] Y. Kawakami, J. Rodriguez-León, and J. C. I. Belmonte, "The role of TGFβs and Sox9 during limb chondrogenesis," *Current Opinion in Cell Biology*, vol. 18, no. 6, pp. 723–729, 2006.

[16] L. Quintana, N. I. Zur Nieden, and C. E. Semino, "Morphogenetic and regulatory mechanisms during developmental chondrogenesis: new paradigms for cartilage tissue engineering," *Tissue Engineering B: Reviews*, vol. 15, no. 1, pp. 29–41, 2009.

[17] P. M. van der Kraan, E. N. Blaney Davidson, and W. B. van den Berg, "A role for age-related changes in TGFβ signaling in aberrant chondrocyte differentiation and osteoarthritis," *Arthritis Research and Therapy*, vol. 12, no. 1, article 201, 2010.

[18] X. Yang, L. Chen, X. Xu, C. Li, C. Huang, and C.-X. Deng, "TGF-beta/Smad3 signals repress chondrocyte hypertrophic differentiation and are required for maintaining articular cartilage," *The Journal of Cell Biology*, vol. 153, no. 1, pp. 35–46, 2001.

[19] B. Palmieri, D. Lodi, and S. Capone, "Osteoarthritis and degenerative joint disease: local treatment options update," *Acta Biomedica*, vol. 81, no. 2, pp. 94–100, 2010.

[20] R. Cheung, T.-T. Cheng, Y. Dong et al., "Incidence of gastroduodenal ulcers during treatment with celecoxib or diclofenac: pooled results from three 12-week trials in Chinese patients with osteoarthritis or rheumatoid arthritis," *International Journal of Rheumatic Diseases*, vol. 13, no. 2, pp. 151–157, 2010.

[21] R. Singh, N. Akhtar, and T. M. Haqqi, "Green tea polyphenol epigallocatechin-3-gallate: inflammation and arthritis. [corrected]," *Life Sciences*, vol. 86, no. 25-26, pp. 907–918, 2010.

[22] S. E. Campbell, D. Bennett, L. Nasir, E. A. Gault, and D. J. Argyle, "Disease- and cell-type-specific transcriptional targeting of vectors for osteoarthritis gene therapy: further development of a clinical canine model," *Rheumatology*, vol. 44, no. 6, pp. 735–743, 2005.

[23] A. Ketola, A.-M. Määttä, T. Pasanen, K. Tulimäki, and J. Wahlfors, "Osteosarcoma and chondrosarcoma as targets for virus vectors and herpes simplex virus thymidine kinase/ganciclovir gene therapy," *International Journal of Molecular Medicine*, vol. 13, no. 5, pp. 705–710, 2004.

[24] A. M. Bhosale and J. B. Richardson, "Articular cartilage: structure, injuries and review of management," *British Medical Bulletin*, vol. 87, no. 1, pp. 77–95, 2008.

[25] D. R. Eyre, "Collagens and cartilage matrix homeostasis," *Clinical Orthopaedics and Related Research*, no. 427, supplement, pp. S118–S122, 2004.

[26] D. R. Eyre, M. A. Weis, and J.-J. Wu, "Articular cartilage collagen: an irreplaceable framework?" *European Cells and Materials*, vol. 12, pp. 57–63, 2006.

[27] D. Heinegård, "Proteoglycans and more—from molecules to biology," *International Journal of Experimental Pathology*, vol. 90, no. 6, pp. 575–586, 2009.

[28] D. M. Bell, K. K. H. Leung, S. C. Wheatley et al., "SOX9 directly regulates the type-II collagen gene," *Nature Genetics*, vol. 16, no. 2, pp. 174–178, 1997.

[29] G. J. Inman, F. J. Nicolás, J. F. Callahan et al., "SB-431542 is a potent and specific inhibitor of transforming growth factor-β superfamily type I activin receptor-like kinase (ALK) receptors ALK4, ALK5, and ALK7," *Molecular Pharmacology*, vol. 62, no. 1, pp. 65–74, 2002.

[30] E. N. Blaney Davidson, E. L. Vitters, P. M. van der Kraan, and W. B. van den Berg, "Expression of transforming growth factor-β (TGFβ) and the TGFβ signalling molecule SMAD-2P in spontaneous and instability-induced osteoarthritis: Role in cartilage degradation, chondrogenesis and osteophyte formation," *Annals of the Rheumatic Diseases*, vol. 65, no. 11, pp. 1414–1421, 2006.

[31] E. N. Blaney Davidson, A. Scharstuhl, E. L. Vitters, P. M. van der Kraan, and W. B. van den Berg, "Reduced transforming growth factor-beta signaling in cartilage of old mice: role in impaired repair capacity," *Arthritis Research & Therapy*, vol. 7, no. 6, pp. R1338–1347, 2005.

[32] Q. Wu, J. H. Huang, E. R. Sampson et al., "Smurf2 induces degradation of GSK-3β and upregulates β-catenin in chondrocytes: a potential mechanism for Smurf2-induced degeneration of articular cartilage," *Experimental Cell Research*, vol. 315, no. 14, pp. 2386–2398, 2009.

[33] C.-G. Li, Q.-Q. Liang, Q. Zhou et al., "A continuous observation of the degenerative process in the intervertebral disc of Smad3 gene knock-out mice," *Spine*, vol. 34, no. 13, pp. 1363–1369, 2009.

[34] I. Hiroko, A. Sakae, and O. Yukio, "Effect of shosaikoto, a Japanese and Chinese traditional herbal medicinal mixture, on the mitogenic activity of lipopolysaccharide: a new pharmacological testing method," *Journal of Ethnopharmacology*, vol. 21, no. 1, pp. 45–53, 1987.

[35] W. Bochu, Z. Liancai, and C. Qi, "Primary study on the application of Serum Pharmacology in Chinese traditional medicine," *Colloids and Surfaces B: Biointerfaces*, vol. 43, no. 3-4, pp. 194–197, 2005.

[36] J. A. Roman-Blas, M. A. Contreras-Blasco, R. Largo, M. A. Álvarez-Soria, S. Castañeda, and G. Herrero-Beaumont, "Differential effects of the antioxidant n-acetylcysteine on the production of catabolic mediators in IL-1β-stimulated human osteoarthritic synoviocytes and chondrocytes," *European Journal of Pharmacology*, vol. 623, no. 1-3, pp. 125–131, 2009.

Strong Manual Acupuncture Stimulation of "Huantiao" (GB 30) Reduces Pain-Induced Anxiety and p-ERK in the Anterior Cingulate Cortex in a Rat Model of Neuropathic Pain

Xiao-mei Shao, Zui Shen, Jing Sun, Fang Fang, Jun-fan Fang, Yuan-yuan Wu, and Jian-qiao Fang

Department of Neurobiology & Acupuncture Research, The Third Clinical College, Zhejiang Chinese Medical University, Hangzhou 310053, China

Correspondence should be addressed to Jian-qiao Fang; fangjianqiao7532@163.com

Academic Editor: Ayikoé Guy Mensah-Nyagan

Persistent neuropathic pain is associated with anxiety. The phosphorylation of extracellular signal-regulated kinase (p-ERK) in the anterior cingulate cortex (ACC) plays an important role in pain-induced anxiety. Acupuncture is widely used for pain and anxiety. However, little is known about which acupuncture technique is optimal on pain-induced anxiety and the relationship between acupuncture effect and p-ERK. The rat model was induced by L5 spinal nerve ligation (SNL). Male adult SD rats were randomly divided into control, SNL, strong manual acupuncture (sMA), mild manual acupuncture (mMA), and electroacupuncture (EA) group. Bilateral "Huantiao" (GB 30) were stimulated by sMA, mMA, and EA, respectively. The pain withdrawal thresholds (PWTs) and anxiety behavior were measured, and p-ERK protein expression and immunoreactivity cells in ACC were detected. PWTs increased significantly in both sMA and EA groups. Meanwhile, anxiety-like behavior was improved significantly in the sMA and mMA groups. Furthermore, the overexpression of p-ERK induced by SNL was downregulated by strong and mild manual acupuncture. Therefore, strong manual acupuncture on bilateral "Huantiao" (GB 30) could be a proper therapy relieving both pain and pain-induced anxiety. The effect of different acupuncture techniques on pain-induced anxiety may arise from the regulation of p-ERK in ACC.

1. Introduction

Anxiety and depression often coexist with persistent pain [1–4]. In humans, patients with persistent pain frequently suffer from a series of aversive emotions including anxiety, fear, depression, loneliness, and misanthropy, which can be more distressing than the pain itself [5].

In clinical studies, Chinese acupuncture has been practiced in many cultures and is nowadays widely used to relieve pain all over the world [6–9]. In 1996, the World Health Organization conference in Milan suggested 64 indications for acupuncture, including many psychiatric disorders such as cardiac neurosis, depression, and schizophrenia. Manual acupuncture (needling using manual stimulation) and electroacupuncture (EA, needling with electrical stimulation) are two common methods of acupoint stimulation. Both are applied clinically for the treatment of chronic pain and various mental disorders [10, 11]. Furthermore, manual acupunctures were divided into mild manual acupuncture (mMA) and strong manual acupuncture (sMA) on the basis of strength for needling manipulation, defined as reinforcing and reducing methods, respectively, in traditional Chinese medicine. But studies on the distinct effects of the three methods (EA, mMA, and sMA) are lacking. In last decades, preclinical and clinical researches have demonstrated that MA and EA are, respectively, effective for neuropathic pain [12–15] and anxiety [16–18]; however, it is unknown whether they have an effective role for neuropathic pain-induced negative mood.

Several studies have reported that persistent pain in humans is associated with changes in brain anatomy [19] and suggest that activation of the ACC has been found to be

TABLE 1: The comparison of three different acupuncture stimulation groups.

Stimulation patterns	Stimulation parameters	Acupoints	Time of treatment
EA	Constant square wave current output (pulse width: 0.6 ms at 2 Hz, 0.2 ms at 100 Hz); remaining intensities at 1 ± 0.5 mA (causing the slight vibration of muscles around acupoints); alternating frequencies of 2 Hz and 100 Hz (automatically shifting between 2 Hz and 100 Hz stimulation for three seconds each).		
sMA	Sterilized disposable stainless steel needles (0.3 mm in diameter) on bilateral GB 30 were inserted to a depth of 10 mm and then twisted manually clockwise and counterclockwise (360°) for 2 min at a rate of 180 times per min, followed by an interval of 13 min with needles retained and then another 2 min twisting stimulation. Finally the needles were retained in place for 13 min before removal. The bilateral GB 34 simply retained the needles for 30 min without any twirling and rotating manipulation.	The main point is GB 30 and the additional point is GB 34.	30 min
mMA	Sterilized disposable stainless steel needles (0.22 mm in diameter) on bilateral GB 30 were inserted to a depth of 10 mm and then twisted manually clockwise and counterclockwise (180°) for 2 min at a rate of 60 times per min, followed by an interval of 13 min with needles retained and then another 2 min twisting stimulation. Finally the needles were retained in place for 13 min before removal. The bilateral GB 34 simply retained the needles for 30 min without any twirling and rotating manipulation.		

associated with the affective dimension of pain [20–23]. No part of the cingulate cortex is activated only by noxious stimulation, although there may be small aggregates of purely nociceptive neurons [24]. Therefore, it is important to determine the functional significance of changes in the ACC when studying persistent pain-induced anxiety and other mood disorders.

Accumulating evidence has shown that extracellular signal-regulated kinase (ERK), a family member of mitogen-activated protein kinases (MAPKs), in the ACC is activated in the chemical inflammatory pain or neuropathic pain model [25, 26] and suggested that pain-induced anxiety is regulated by the ERK activation in the ACC after incision [27]. Moreover, inhibition of ERK1/2 activation in ACC after acetic acid injection by subcutaneous injection of the mitogen-activating extracellular kinase (MEK) inhibitor, SL327, attenuates visceral pain-induced anxiety-like behavior [28]. All of these data demonstrate that ERK activity in the ACC may be an important hub for various types of pain-induced anxiety and thus constitutes a critical target for revealing the underlying mechanism.

In the present work, we hypothesized that mMA, sMA, and EA have differential effects on pain-induced anxiety and that the cellular mechanism underlying such anxiety involves ERK phosphorylation in the ACC. To test these hypotheses, we used the L5 spinal nerve ligation (SNL) rat model of persistent pain to assess the changes in pain-induced anxiety and phosphorylated- (p-) ERK levels in the ACC and to investigate the effect of mMA, sMA, and EA on these measures (Table 1).

2. Methods

2.1. Subject. Male adult Sprague-Dawley rats, about 70 days old (220–250 g), were obtained from the Experimental Animal Center of Zhejiang Chinese Medical University.

The animals were housed in groups of five in plastic cages with soft bedding at the University Animal Care facility, with an artificial 12/12 h light-dark cycle (lights on at 8 a.m.). Animals received food and water ad libitum with a constant room temperature of 23–25°C and a relative humidity of 40–70%. Before experimental manipulations, the rats were given 1 week to adjust to their new surroundings. All animal procedures performed in this work followed guidelines in accordance with the Regulations for the Administration of Affairs Concerning Experimental Animals and were approved by the Animal Care and Welfare Committee of Zhejiang Chinese Medical University, Zhejiang, China.

2.2. Surgery for Neuropathic Pain Model. The rats were anesthetized with 7% (w/v) choral hydrate (5 mL/kg, intraperitoneally). Each rat was placed on a heated surgical platform at a constant temperature at 37°C in the prone position, and the right paraspinal muscles were separated from the spinous processes at the L4-S2 levels. The L6 transverse process was carefully removed with a small rongeur to identify the L4-L5 spinal nerves visually. Once enough length of the L5 spinal nerve was freed from the adjacent structure, a piece of 6/0 silk thread was placed around the L5 spinal nerve and pulled tightly to interrupt all axons in the nerve. On completion of the operation, hemostasis was confirmed and the muscles were sutured in layers using silk thread. Finally, animals were placed in a new cage with warm bedding until complete recovery from anesthesia. After the operation, the rats showed no motor deficits except a mild inversion of the ipsilateral hind paw with slightly ventroflexed toes.

2.3. EA, sMA, and mMA Procedures. EA, sMA, and mMA treatments were applied, respectively, to bilateral acupoints "Huantiao" (GB 30, located at the junction of the lateral 1/3 and medial 2/3 of the distance between the great trochanter of the femur and the last sacral vertebrae) and "Yanglingquan"

(GB 34, located in the depression anterior and inferior to the small head of the fibula) (Figure 5) every other day from 3 to 11 days after SNL. In the EA stimulation group, inserted needles (0.3 mm in diameter and 10 mm in depth) on bilateral "Huantiao" and "Yanglingquan" were attached to the output terminals of the Hans Acupoint Nerve Stimulator (HANS 200E, Huawei Co., Ltd., Beijing, China). The EA parameters were set as follows: constant square wave current output (pulse width: 0.6 ms at 2 Hz, 0.2 ms at 100 Hz); remaining intensities at 1 ± 0.5 mA (causing the slight vibration of muscles around acupoints); alternating frequencies of 2 Hz and 100 Hz (automatically shifting between 2 Hz and 100 Hz stimulation for three seconds each). In the sMA stimulation group, sterilized disposable stainless steel needles (0.3 mm in diameter) on bilateral "Huantiao" were inserted to a depth of 10 mm and then twisted manually clockwise and counterclockwise (360°) for 2 min at a rate of 180 times per min, followed by an interval of 13 min with needles retained and then another 2 min twisting stimulation. Finally the needles were retained in place for 13 min before removal. In the MA stimulation group, sterilized disposable stainless steel needles (0.22 mm in diameter) on bilateral "Huantiao" were inserted to a depth of 10 mm and then twisted manually clockwise and counterclockwise (180°) for 2 min at a rate of 60 times per min, followed by an interval of 13 min with needles retained and then another 2 min twisting stimulation. Finally the needles were retained in place for 13 min before removal. The total time including twisting and retaining the needles is 30 min. In two MA groups, bilateral "Yanglingquan" simply retained the needles for 30 min without any twirling and rotating manipulation. In the whole procedure, all rats maintained relatively comfortable states without any struggling and screaming.

2.4. Nociceptive Behavioral Testing.
Mechanical hyperalgesia confirmed the success of the SNL. The PWT was automatically measured with a dynamic plantar aesthesiometer (model 37450; Ugo Basile, Comerio, Italy). Animals were habituated to the testing surroundings daily for two consecutive days (between 9 a.m. and 12 p.m.) before baseline testing. The room temperature and humidity remained stable with a low noise level (<40 dB) during testing. Bilateral PWTs were measured before SNL and 3, 7, and 12 days after SNL. Each rat was allowed to move freely in a transparent plastic compartment of a six-compartment box with a wire mesh floor and acclimatize for 20 min before the test session. A paw-flick response was elicited by applying an increasing vertical force (increase steadily from 0 to 50 grams in 20 sec) produced by a stainless steel probe (a straight 0.5 mm diameter) which was placed underneath the mesh floor and focused on the middle of the plantar surface of the bilateral hind paws. The hind paws of each rat were measured five times with at least 1 min intervals and then averaged. All manipulations were taken by the same operator. The whole test was performed by an investigator blind to the experimental groups.

2.5. Anxiety-Like Behavioral Testing.
Repeated exposure to test conditions may significantly decrease anxiety-like behaviors. Therefore, in the present study, anxiety-like behavior was tested only once, 12 days after SNL. Spontaneous exploratory activity was monitored using an automatic video tracking system (SMART, Panlab, Spain) and all parameters were analyzed by SMART software (version 3.0, Panlab). Test apparatus were cleaned with 70% ethanol and dried after each testing session.

The elevated zero maze consisted of two open (stressful) and two enclosed (protecting) sections opposite to each other, forming a black plastic annular platform (100 cm diameter, 25 cm width, and 50 cm above the ground). The enclosed sections had walls (30 cm high) on the inner and outer edges. At the beginning of the 5 min testing session, each rat was placed in the same closed section. Time spent in and entries into the open sections and transitions of open/closed arm were taken as primary parameters.

2.6. Western Blotting.
Animals were rapidly sacrificed after anesthesia with chloral hydrate, and the spinal dorsal horn and brains were rapidly removed and frozen on ice. The ACC was identified according to the atlas of Paxinos and Watson [29] and dissected out and quickly frozen in liquid nitrogen. Frozen samples were homogenized with lysis buffer containing a cocktail of phosphatase and proteinase inhibitors and PMSF (Beyotime, Shanghai, China). After denaturation, the lysates were separated on 10% SDS-PAGE gel and transferred to polyvinylidene difluoride PVDF membranes (Bio-Rad, Hercules, CA, USA). The membranes were blocked with 5% nonfat powdered milk in TBST (Tris-buffered saline containing 0.1% Tween 20) for 1 h at room temperature (RT) and then incubated overnight at 4°C with monoclonal rabbit anti-phospho-ERK primary antibody (p-ERK1/2, anti-rabbit, 1 : 2000, in 5% w/v BSA, Cell Signaling, Beverly, MA, USA). After washing in TBST, the membrane was incubated for 1 h at RT with HRP-conjugated goat anti-rabbit antibody (1 : 7500; Bio-Rad), and protein bands were visualized using the Immun-Star HRP Chemiluminescence Kit (Bio-Rad). Images of bands were recorded by the ImageQuant LAS 4000 system (GE Healthcare, Hino, Japan) and the band intensities were quantified using ImageQuant TL software (version 7.0, GE Healthcare). The membranes were then incubated in stripping buffer (0.5 M Tris-HCl [pH 6.8], 10%SDS, and 14.4 mol/L β-mercaptoethanol) for 30 min at 50°C and reprobed with monoclonal anti-ERK antibody (total ERK1/2, 1 : 1000; Cell Signaling) as loading controls.

2.7. Immunofluorescence.
Animals were terminally anesthetized with chloral hydrate and perfused through the ascending aorta with saline followed by 4% paraformaldehyde with 0.01 M PBS (pH 7.2–7.4, 4°C). After perfusion, brains were removed and postfixed in the same fixative for 4–6 h, which was then replaced with 15% and 30% sucrose successively overnight. Brain sections (30 μm) were cut in a cryostat and processed for immunofluorescence. All sections were blocked with 5% goat serum in TBST for 1 h at 37°C and incubated overnight at 4°C with anti-phospho-ERK antibody (p-ERK1/2, rabbit anti-rat, 1 : 400; Cell Signaling). The sections were then incubated for 1 h at 37°C with Cy3-conjugated secondary antibody (1 : 1000; Jackson Immunolabs, West Grove, PA, USA). For p-ERK/NeuN/GFAP/OX-42 double

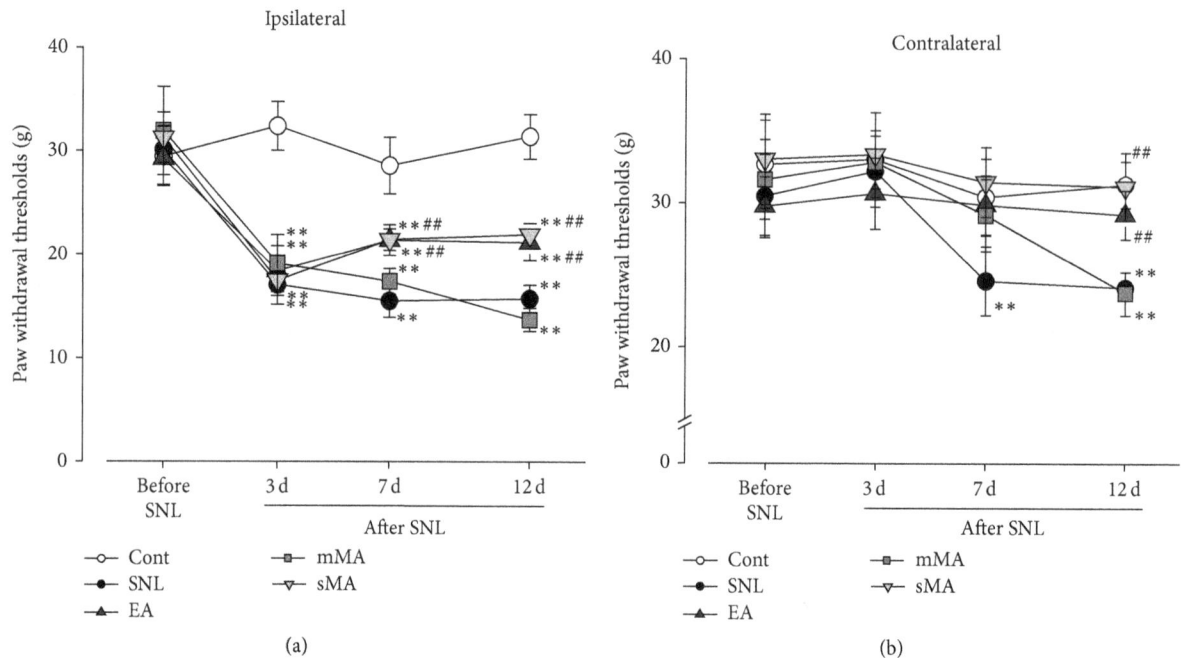

FIGURE 1: Bilateral changes in nociceptive behaviors after L5 spinal nerve ligation (SNL) in control (non-SNL control, Cont), SNL alone (SNL control, SNL), SNL+ EA stimulation (EA), SNL+ mMA stimulation (mMA), and SNL+ sMA stimulation (sMA) groups. Pain hypersensitivity is measured by ipsilateral and contralateral hind paw withdrawal thresholds (PWTs, g) in response to mechanical stimulation. $^{**}P < 0.01$ versus control group at each time-point; $^{##}P < 0.01$ versus SNL group at each time-point.

immunofluorescence, sections were incubated with mixture of rabbit anti-p-ERK and mouse anti-NeuN (neuronal marker, 1:1000; Abcam, USA), GFAP (astrocytic marker, 1:100, Abcam, USA), or OX-42 (microglial marker, 1:100, Serotec, Oxford, UK) separately for 16 h at 4°C, followed by a mixture of CY3- and FITC-conjugated (1:100, Jackson Immunolabs) secondary antibodies for 1 h at 4°C.

The stained sections were visualized with a Nikon Eclipse Ti confocal microscope (Nikon, Japan) and images were captured with NIS Elements D3.22 software (Nikon).

2.8. Statistical Analysis.
All data are expressed as mean ± SEM, and statistical analyses were performed using analysis of variance (ANOVA) followed by the least significant difference (LSD) post hoc test with $P < 0.05$ considered significant.

3. Results

3.1. Pain Hypersensitivity.
Five groups of rats (non-SNL control (control) and four SNL groups: SNL control (SNL), sMA, mMA, and EA) were tested before surgery and 3, 7, and 12 days afterwards. At 3 d after surgery, the withdrawal threshold of the ipsilateral hind paw showed a profound decrease with control group (Figure 1(a), $P < 0.01$); this had not recovered until 12 d, while sMA and EA intervention, administered at 3 d after surgery and for continuous 4 treatments with 2 d interval, increased the threshold at days 7 and 12 compared with the SNL rats (Figure 1(a), $P < 0.01$). On the contralateral hind paw, PWTs in the SNL rats decreased at 7 d and 12 d compared with the control group (Figure 1(b), $P < 0.01$). At the same time, PWTs did not decreased in the sMA and EA

groups on days 7 and 12 compared with SNL rats (Figure 1(b), $P < 0.01$), with no significant difference between these two groups. PWTs in the mMA group rats decreased at 12 d with control rats (Figure 1(b), $P < 0.01$).

3.2. Pain-Induced Anxiety.
The elevated zero maze (EZM) is widely used to assess anxiety-like behavior in rodents. It is a modification of the elevated plus maze and has the advantage of lacking the ambiguous central area of the plus maze, resulting in greater sensitivity and reliability. There were no significant difference on total distance in the five groups (Figure 2(a), $F_{(4,28)} = 1.039, P = 0.405$). Distance in open arm in SNL rats decreased compared with control rats, and the same happened with EA group (Figure 2(b), $P < 0.01$), while mMA and sMA intervention increased the distance in open arms compared with SNL rats (Figure 2(b), $P < 0.01$). SNL rats spent less total time and resting time in the open sections compared with control rats and so did EA rats (Figures 2(c) and 2(d), $P < 0.05$). Compared with the SNL group, rats in the mMA and sMA groups spent notably more exploratory and resting time in the open sections (Figures 2(c) and 2(d), $P < 0.05$).

3.3. Expression of p-ERK in the ACC.
Our immunofluorescence assay revealed an overexpression of p-ERK1/2-positive cells in the ACC of rats on day 12 after surgery, and western blots showed a higher level of p-ERK1/2 protein expression in the SNL group than in non-SNL controls (Figures 3(a), 3(b), and 3(f)–3(h), $P < 0.01$). Interestingly, p-ERK1/2-immunoreactive cell number and protein expression were

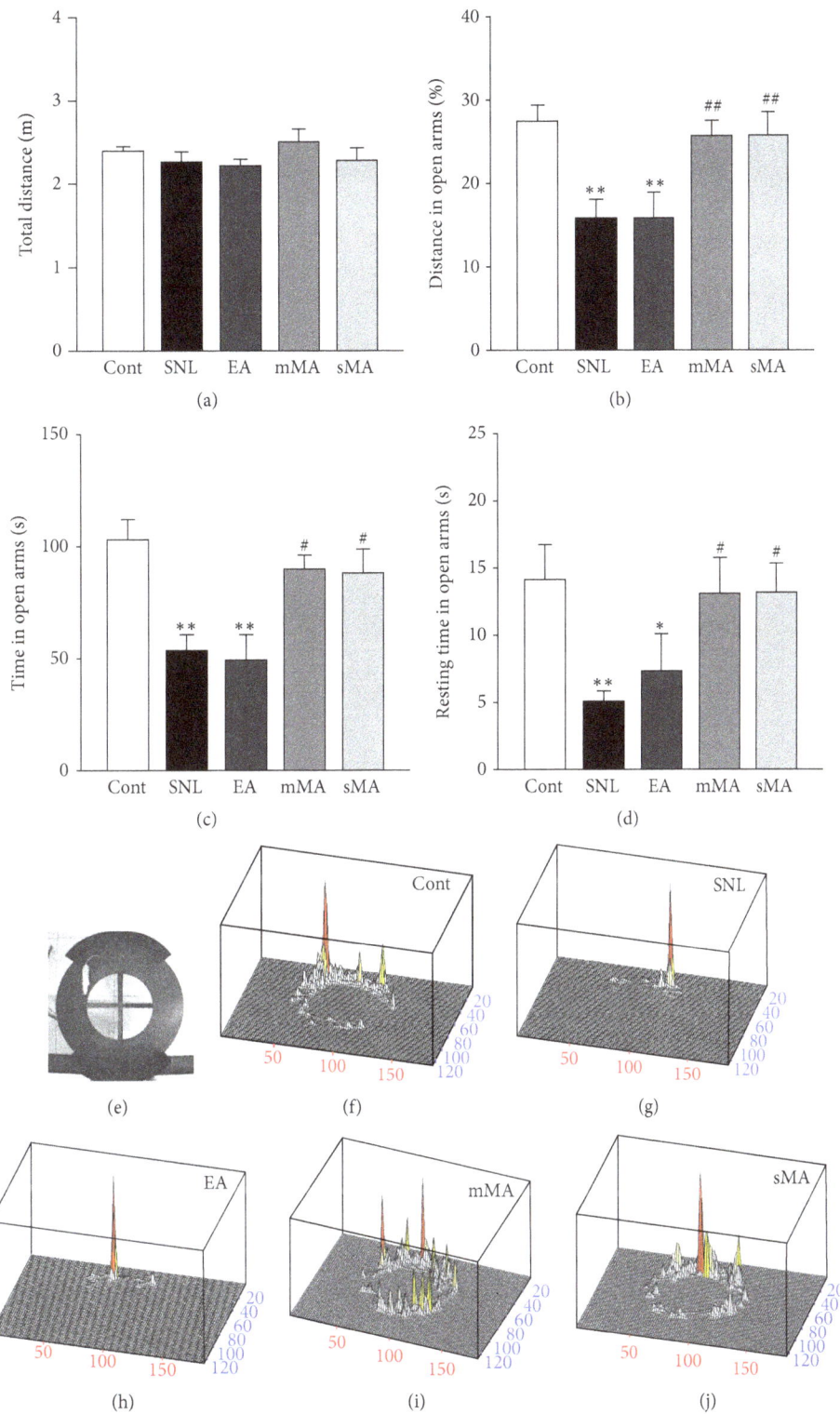

FIGURE 2: Anxiety-like behaviors in the elevated zero maze during a 5 min test session on day 12 after L5 spinal nerve ligation. (a) Total distance ($F_{(4,28)}$ = 1.039, P = 0.405); (b) distance in open arms ($F_{(4,28)}$ = 5.751, P = 0.002); (c) time in open arms ($F_{(4,28)}$ = 6.973, P = 0.001); (d) resting time in open arms ($F_{(4,28)}$ = 3.199, P = 0.028); (e) image of detection; ((f)-(g)) analysis graphics of trace. Each column represents the mean ± SEM of six animals per group. $^{*}P < 0.05$, $^{**}P < 0.01$ versus control group; $^{#}P < 0.05$, $^{##}P < 0.01$ versus SNL group.

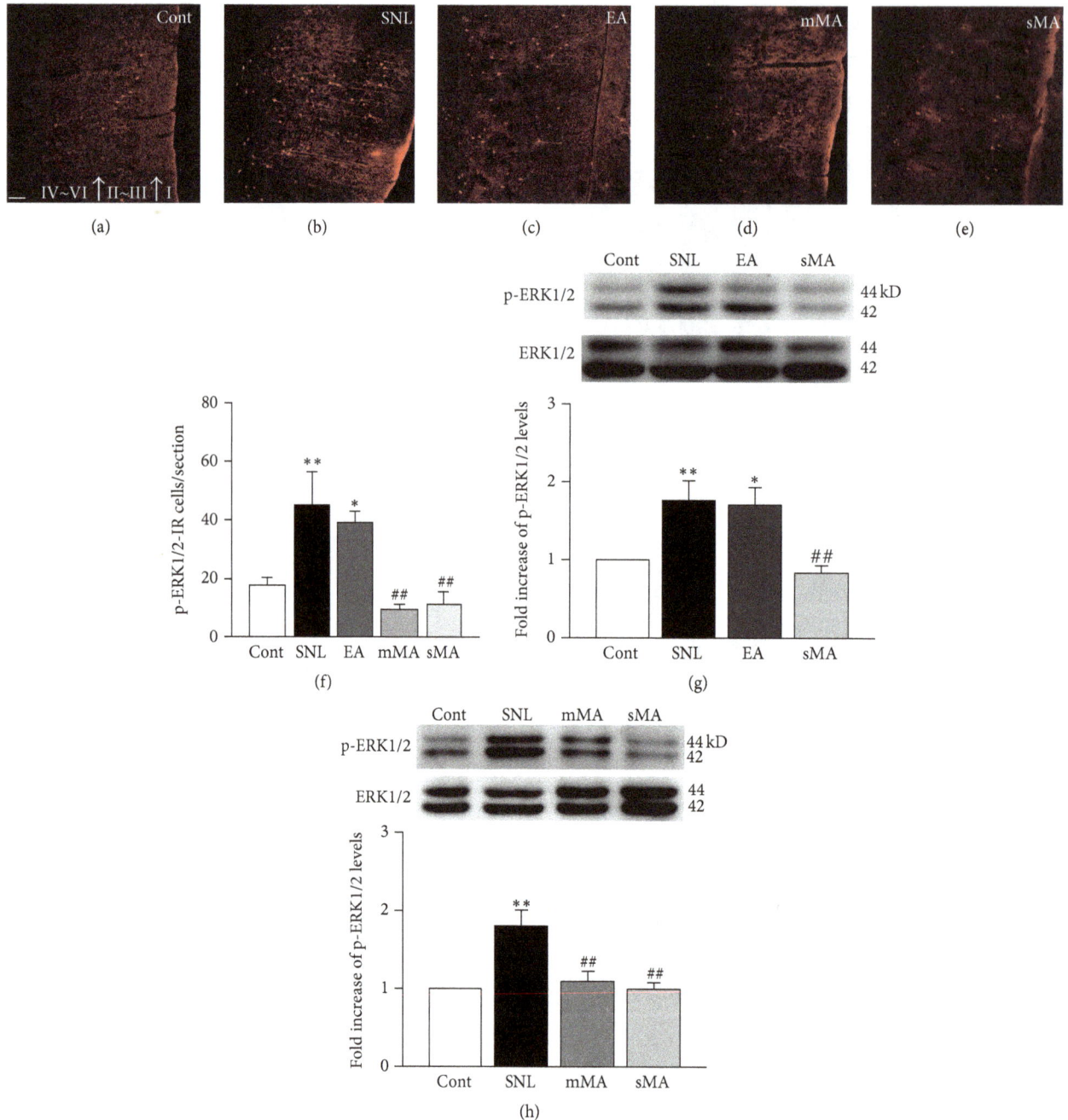

FIGURE 3: Immunohistochemical ((a)–(f)) and immunoblot ((g)-(h)) analysis of the effect of EA, mMA, and sMA stimulation on p-ERK1/2 protein expression in the anterior cingulate cortex (ACC) after L5 spinal nerve ligation. ((a)–(e)) Expression of p-ERK in the ACC (scale bar = 50 μm; cortical laminae represented by roman numerals); (f) quantification of p-ERK-immunoreactive (IR) cells in the ACC ($F_{(4,10)}$ = 8.325, P = 0.003); ((g)-(h)) representative blots from ACC homogenates and p-ERK quantification (equal loading was verified by assaying ERK1/2) ($F_{(3,12)}$ = 7.418, P = 0.005, $F_{(3,12)}$ = 9.372, and P = 0.002, resp.). Histogram bars represent the mean ± SEM of 5 animals per group. $^{*}P$ < 0.05, $^{**}P$ < 0.01 versus control group; $^{##}P$ < 0.01 versus SNL group.

significantly lower in rats that underwent mMA and sMA stimulation than in SNL rats (Figures 3(b) and 3(d)–3(h), P < 0.01). There was no significant difference in p-ERK1/2-immunoreactive cells or protein expression between the EA and SNL groups (Figures 3(b), 3(c), 3(f), and 3(g), P > 0.05).

3.4. Distribution and Location of p-ERK in ACC Neurons, Macrophages, and Astrocytes. In the control group, p-ERK was expressed largely in laminae II-III (Figure 3(a)), whereas SNL resulted in a wide distribution of p-ERK-immunoreactive cells throughout laminae II–VI (Figure 3(b)).

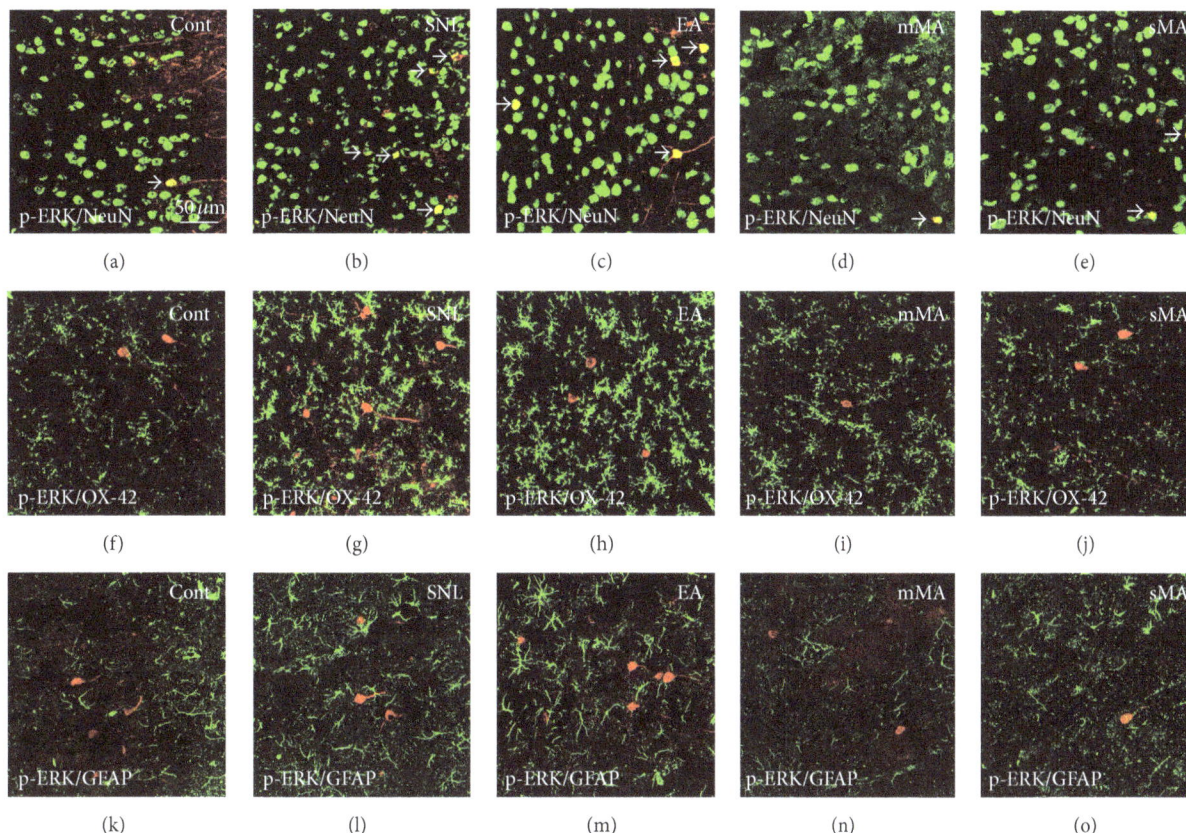

FIGURE 4: Double immunofluorescence localizing p-ERK in ACC neurons, macrophages, and astrocytes in the ACC after L5 spinal nerve ligation. ((a)–(e)) p-ERK (red) colocalizes with NeuN (green); ((f)–(j)) p-ERK (red) does not colocalize with OX-42 (green); ((k)–(o)) p-ERK (red) does not colocalize with GFAP (green).

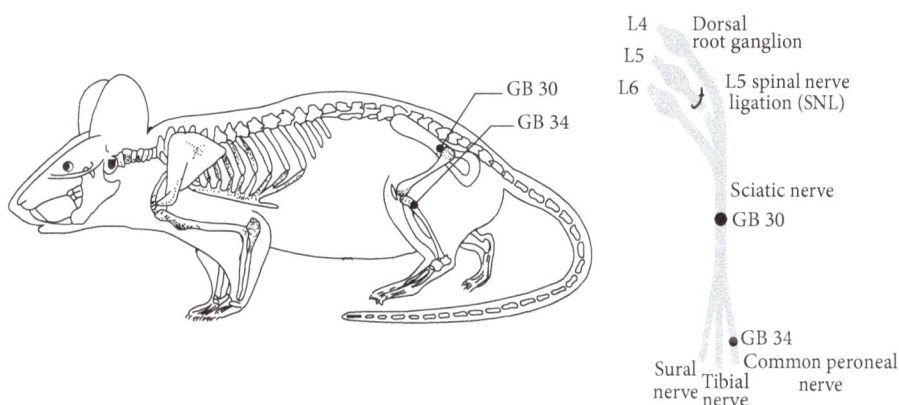

FIGURE 5: Schematic representation of the GB 30 and GB 34 in the rat.

The number of p-ERK1/2-positive cells in the ACC was substantially decreased by mMA and sMA intervention, but their distribution in laminae II–VI was not changed (Figures 3(d) and 3(e)). In comparison with SNL rats, animals that received EA stimulation showed no difference in p-ERK-immunoreactive cell numbers (Figure 3(c)).

Very few p-ERK-immunoreactive neurons were found in the ACC in non-SNL control rats (Figure 4(a)). SNL induced an immediate activation of ERK in ACC neurons (Figure 4(b)). No visual difference in p-ERK/NeuN double-labeled neurons was observed in the ACC of rats that received EA compared with SNL (Figures 4(b) and 4(c)). Compared with SNL, mMA, and sMA stimulation decreased p-ERK/NeuN double-labeled neurons (Figures 4(b), 4(d), and 4(e)). We found no p-ERK/OX-42 or p-ERK/GFAP double-labeled macrophages or astrocytes (Figures 4(f)–4(o)).

4. Discussion

The present study is the first to show that both sMA and EA stimulation significantly relieve mechanical hypersensitivity in a rat model of neuropathic pain, and both sMA and mMA stimulation significantly reduce anxiety-like behavior. The changes in anxiety-like behavior correlate with ERK activation in ACC neurons. These results extend our previous data showing that p-ERK in the bilateral spinal horn is involved in sMA inhibition of SNL-induced bilateral mechanical hyperalgesia [30]. Hence, sMA might be the treatment of choice in cases of neuropathic pain accompanied by anxiety.

The International Association for the Study of Pain (IASP) defines pain as "an unpleasant sensory and emotional experience associated with actual or potential tissue damage or described in terms of such damage" [31]. It denotes that the experience of pain comprises a sensory dimension and an affective dimension. Pain-induced negative sequelae can be more disabling than the pain itself, severely affecting the daily activities of patients with persistent pain [5]. Many studies on persistent pain have paid considerable attention to its effects on anxiety-like behavior [32, 33]. It is necessary to distinguish the sensory and affective changes in pain treatment. SNL is a common model for mechanical hyperalgesia and pain-induced anxiety [34, 35]. Animals with SNL have enhanced escape/avoidance behavior 3 days following the lesion [36]. Anxiogenic-like behaviors have also been observed in the light/dark test up to 4 weeks after SNL [37, 38].

Acupuncture is an important component of traditional Chinese medicine (TCM) and a practical science of preventing and treating diseases. Needling technique means the methods through stimulating certain parts of human body (acupoints) by means of different kinds of needles or non-needle methods with certain manipulation techniques [39]. Manual acupuncture (MA) is the insertion of an acupuncture needle into acupoints followed by the twisting of the needle with different manual strength, and electroacupuncture (EA), a stimulating current via the inserted needle, is delivered to acupoints [40]. As a clinical acupuncturist, it is a key factor to select optimal needling techniques based on the disease condition of patient.

In clinical application of acupuncture, GB 30 is always the main point or the basic point in the low back pain and GB 34 is used as an additional point when low back pain is associated with the numbness and pain of lower extremities [39, 41]. The L5 spinal nerve ligation-induced neuropathic pain is similar to the low back pain in clinical. Moreover, in anatomy, L4, L5, and L6 spinal nerve were combined into the sciatic nerve, which is divided into common peroneal nerve, tibial nerve, and sural nerve. GB 30 locates on the sciatic nerve path and GB 34 situates on the common peroneal nerve. Therefore, in this study we select GB 30 (main point) and GB 34 (additional point) to alleviate SNL-induced neuropathic pain.

Analgesia with manual acupuncture or EA is essentially a manifestation of integrative processes at the dorsal root ganglion and central nervous systems between the afferent impulses from the pain regions and acupoints [42–45]. Researchers and clinicians have increasingly focused on EA analgesia [46, 47], for its feasibility in developing a standardized treatment protocol for analgesia; this approach is supported by our results, in which sMA and EA treatments had equivalent effects on pain. However, clinical evidence has not been conclusive on the effects of manual acupuncture or EA on anxiety [18], despite the fact that both are increasingly used for the treatment of anxiety. In basic research, a few studies examining the effects of manual acupuncture and EA on anxiety have indicated that the technique might reduce anxiety-like behavior in adult rats [48–50]. Our early results indicated that sMA, but not mMA, could alleviate SNL-induced bilateral pain which is closely related to its effect in downregulating the expression of p-ERK in the bilateral spinal dorsal horn regions [30]. In the present study, we observed that the sensory dimension of neuropathic pain, measured by PWTs, decreased consistently from day 3 after surgery. The rat's bilateral mechanical hypersensitivity was significantly inhibited by either sMA or EA stimulation on 12 days after SNL, but not mMA. We also explored the affective dimension with EZM tests. Twelve days after SNL, rats displayed increased anxiety behavior. Interestingly, sMA and mMA stimulation alleviated pain-induced anxiety in the EZM test, whereas EA stimulation was without effect. These results indicate that sMA is considerably more effective than mMA and EA in relieving both mechanical hypersensitivity and concomitant anxiety. The differential effects may reflect a difference in afferent activation in the supraspinal pathway, especially in cerebral nuclei.

To examine this possible mechanism underlying the effects of sMA stimulation on pain-induced anxiety, we explored p-ERK expression in the ACC. Peripheral nerve injury has been reported to induce neuroplastic changes in different regions including the insular cortex, amygdala, and ACC, which have been associated with pain-like aversive behaviors and depressive-like symptoms [34, 51, 52]. Results from numerous human and animal studies indicated that the ACC, which forms one of the largest parts of the limbic system, plays an important role in the affective component of pain [20, 43, 53]. Extensive studies supported the notion that the ACC is a pivotal region for emotion [22]. Another study reported that electrical stimulation of the ACC attenuates the aversive quality of noxious cutaneous hind paw stimulation without producing an antiallodynia effect in rats with SNL [54]. These suggested that the ACC regulates affective pain processing.

ERK activation in the ACC was required for the expression of pain-induced anxiety [27]. Another study hypothesized that attenuation of p-ERK1/2 overactivity in the ACC represented a potentially valuable therapeutic strategy for the relief of pain-induced anxiety [28]. A previous report suggested that ERK cascades in the ACC are involved in pain-induced negative emotion in the rat [55]. ERK also played a crucial role in persistent pain-enhanced temporal synaptic plasticity [56]. In our study, ERK1/2 activation in the ACC of rats after SNL was significantly stronger than in non-SNL control rats, and this coincided with changes in anxiety-like behavior. Accordingly, sMA and mMA stimulation downregulated ERK1/2 activation in ACC neurons and also improved anxiety-like behavior, suggesting a mechanism behind the effect of sMA and mMA on pain-induced anxiety.

Differences in stimulation strength and method may lead to differences in treatment results; the parameters used in manual acupuncture and EA when treating anxiety are not yet clear and are worthy of further study. It is also important to evaluate the present findings in a clinical setting.

In summary, sMA stimulation may relieve both mechanical hyperalgesia and pain-induced anxiety in a rat model of neuropathic pain, while mMA only reduces anxiety and EA only alleviates mechanical hypersensitivity. We propose that sMA could be a two-dimensional Chinese medicine therapy on the sensory and affective dimension of pain. The effect of different acupuncture stimulation on anxiety-like behavior may arise from the regulation of p-ERK in ACC neurons.

Conflict of Interests

The authors declare that there is no conflict of interests regarding the publication of this paper.

Authors' Contribution

Xiao-mei Shao and Zui Shen contributed equally to this work as co-first authors. Jian-qiao Fang and Xiao-mei Shao designed and performed experimental protocols described in this paper and wrote the initial draft of the paper. Xiao-mei Shao and Zui Shen performed immunofluorescence, western blotting, tissue fractionation, and associated analyses. Fang Fang and Yuan-yuan Wu supervised behavioral monitoring, data analysis, study direction, image acquisition, paper design, and revisions. Jing Sun and Jun-fan Fang performed experiments and contributed to the design, data analysis, and writing of the paper. All of the authors have read and approved the final paper.

Acknowledgments

The authors sincerely thank all the volunteers for their participation in this study. This study was supported by the Key Science and Technology Innovation Team of Zhejiang Province (2013TD15), the National Nature Science Foundation of China (81574056), Traditional Chinese Medicine of Zhejiang Province Outstanding Young Talent Fund Plan (no. 2013ZQ017), Zhejiang Provincial Natural Science Found of China (no. LY15H270009), and Young and Middle-Aged Discipline Leaders of Institutions of Higher Learning in Zhejiang Province (no. 2013203); the project was supported by Zhejiang Province Top Key Discipline of Chinese Medicine-Acupuncture & Tuina.

References

[1] K. Demyttenaere, R. Bruffaerts, S. Lee et al., "Mental disorders among persons with chronic back or neck pain: results from the world mental health surveys," *Pain*, vol. 129, no. 3, pp. 332–342, 2007.

[2] M. Tegethoff, A. Belardi, E. Stalujanis, and G. Meinlschmidt, "Comorbidity of mental disorders and chronic pain: chronology of onset in adolescents of a national representative cohort," *The Journal of Pain*, vol. 16, no. 10, pp. 1054–1064, 2015.

[3] J. Wang, X. Tang, Y. Shen et al., "The correlations between health-related quality of life changes and pain and anxiety in orthodontic patients in the initial stage of treatment," *BioMed Research International*, vol. 2015, Article ID 725913, 7 pages, 2015.

[4] S. Bozkurt Zincir, M. Sunbul, E. Aydin Sunbul et al., "Evaluation of alexithymia, somatosensory sensitivity, and health anxiety levels in patients with noncardiac chest pain," *BioMed Research International*, vol. 2014, Article ID 896183, 6 pages, 2014.

[5] G. Crombez, J. W. S. Vlaeyen, P. H. T. G. Heuts, and R. Lysens, "Pain-related fear is more disabling than pain itself: evidence on the role of pain-related fear in chronic back pain disability," *Pain*, vol. 80, no. 1-2, pp. 329–339, 1999.

[6] Y.-L. Hsieh, C.-C. Yang, S.-Y. Liu, L.-W. Chou, and C.-Z. Hong, "Remote dose-dependent effects of dry needling at distant myofascial trigger spots of rabbit skeletal muscles on reduction of substance P levels of proximal muscle and spinal cords," *BioMed Research International*, vol. 2014, Article ID 982121, 11 pages, 2014.

[7] E. Skorupska, M. Rychlik, and W. Samborski, "Validation and test-retest reliability of new thermographic technique called thermovision technique of dry needling for gluteus minimus trigger points in sciatica subjects and TrPs-negative healthy volunteers," *BioMed Research International*, vol. 2015, Article ID 546497, 11 pages, 2015.

[8] R. Zhang, L. Lao, K. Ren, and B. M. Berman, "Mechanisms of acupuncture-electroacupuncture on persistent pain," *Anesthesiology*, vol. 120, no. 2, pp. 482–503, 2014.

[9] A. J. Vickers and K. Linde, "Acupuncture for chronic pain," *The Journal of the American Medical Association*, vol. 311, no. 9, pp. 955–956, 2014.

[10] Y. Chae, M. Yeom, J.-H. Han et al., "Effect of acupuncture on anxiety-like behavior during nicotine withdrawal and relevant mechanisms," *Neuroscience Letters*, vol. 430, no. 2, pp. 98–102, 2008.

[11] H. U. Zeilhofer, "Loss of glycinergic and GABAergic inhibition in chronic pain—contributions of inflammation and microglia," *International Immunopharmacology*, vol. 8, no. 2, pp. 182–187, 2008.

[12] F. J. Cidral-Filho, M. D. da Silva, A. O. O. Moré, M. M. Córdova, M. F. Werner, and A. R. S. Santos, "Manual acupuncture inhibits mechanical hypersensitivity induced by spinal nerve ligation in rats," *Neuroscience*, vol. 193, pp. 370–376, 2011.

[13] M. H. Cha, J. S. Choi, S. J. Bai et al., "Antiallodynic effects of acupuncture in neuropathic rats," *Yonsei Medical Journal*, vol. 47, no. 3, pp. 359–366, 2006.

[14] Y. Dai, E. Kondo, T. Fukuoka, A. Tokunaga, K. Miki, and K. Noguchi, "The effect of electroacupuncture on pain behaviors and noxious stimulus-evoked fos expression in a rat model of neuropathic pain," *The Journal of Pain*, vol. 2, no. 3, pp. 151–159, 2001.

[15] J. H. Kim, B.-I. Min, H. S. Na, and D. S. Park, "Relieving effects of electroacupuncture on mechanical allodynia in neuropathic pain model of inferior caudal trunk injury in rat: mediation by spinal opioid receptors," *Brain Research*, vol. 998, no. 2, pp. 230–236, 2004.

[16] Z. L. Zhao, G. W. Zhao, H. Z. Li et al., "Acupuncture attenuates anxiety-like behavior by normalizing amygdaloid catecholamines during ethanol withdrawal in rats," *Evidence-Based Complementary and Alternative Medicine*, vol. 2011, Article ID 429843, 8 pages, 2011.

[17] N. Errington-Evans, "Acupuncture for anxiety," *CNS Neuroscience & Therapeutics*, vol. 18, no. 4, pp. 277–284, 2012.

[18] K. Pilkington, "Anxiety, depression and acupuncture: a review of the clinical research," *Autonomic Neuroscience: Basic & Clinical*, vol. 157, no. 1-2, pp. 91–95, 2010.

[19] D. A. Seminowicz, A. L. Laferriere, M. Millecamps, J. S. C. Yu, T. J. Coderre, and M. C. Bushnell, "MRI structural brain changes associated with sensory and emotional function in a rat model of long-term neuropathic pain," *NeuroImage*, vol. 47, no. 3, pp. 1007–1014, 2009.

[20] P. Rainville, G. H. Duncan, D. D. Price, B. Carrier, and M. C. Bushnell, "Pain affect encoded in human anterior cingulate but not somatosensory cortex," *Science*, vol. 277, no. 5328, pp. 968–971, 1997.

[21] M. Minami, "Neuronal mechanisms for pain-induced aversion behavioral studies using a conditioned place aversion test," *International Review of Neurobiology*, vol. 85, pp. 135–144, 2009.

[22] B. A. Vogt, "Pain and emotion interactions in subregions of the cingulate gyrus," *Nature Reviews Neuroscience*, vol. 6, no. 7, pp. 533–544, 2005.

[23] D. D. Price, "Psychological and neural mechanisms of the affective dimension of pain," *Science*, vol. 288, no. 5472, pp. 1769–1772, 2000.

[24] R. W. Sikes and B. A. Vogt, "Nociceptive neurons in area 24 of rabbit cingulate cortex," *Journal of Neurophysiology*, vol. 68, no. 5, pp. 1720–1732, 1992.

[25] H. Cao, Y.-J. Gao, W.-H. Ren et al., "Activation of extracellular signal-regulated kinase in the anterior cingulate cortex contributes to the induction and expression of affective pain," *The Journal of Neuroscience*, vol. 29, no. 10, pp. 3307–3321, 2009.

[26] F. Wei and M. Zhuo, "Activation of Erk in the anterior cingulate cortex during the induction and expression of chronic pain," *Molecular Pain*, vol. 4, article 28, 2008.

[27] R.-P. Dai, C.-Q. Li, J.-W. Zhang et al., "Biphasic activation of extracellular signal-regulated kinase in anterior cingulate cortex distinctly regulates the development of pain-related anxiety and mechanical hypersensitivity in rats after incision," *Anesthesiology*, vol. 115, no. 3, pp. 604–613, 2011.

[28] X.-L. Zhong, R. Wei, P. Zhou et al., "Activation of anterior cingulate cortex extracellular signal-regulated kinase-1 and -2 (ERK1/2) regulates acetic acid-induced, pain-related anxiety in adult female mice," *Acta Histochemica et Cytochemica*, vol. 45, no. 4, pp. 219–225, 2012.

[29] G. Paxinos and C. Watson, *The Rat Brain in Stereotaxic Coordinates*, Academic Press, 6th edition, 2007.

[30] Z. Shen, X. M. Shao, F. Fang, J. Sun, J. F. Fang, and J. Q. Fang, "Effect of mild and strong manual acupuncture stimulation of 'Huantiao' (GB 30) on mechanical pain thresholds and extracellular signal-regulated kinase protein expression in spinal dorsal horns in rats with neuropathic mirror-image pain," *Acupuncture Research*, vol. 39, no. 2, pp. 106–111, 2014.

[31] J. D. Loeser and R.-D. Treede, "The Kyoto protocl of IASP basic pain terminology," *Pain*, vol. 137, no. 3, pp. 473–477, 2008.

[32] L. Caes, E. Fisher, J. Clinch, J. H. Tobias, and C. Eccleston, "The role of pain-related anxiety in adolescents' disability and social impairment: ALSPAC data," *European Journal of Pain*, vol. 19, no. 6, pp. 842–851, 2015.

[33] F. Kouya, Z. Iqbal, D. Charen, M. Shah, and R. K. Banik, "Evaluation of anxiety-like behaviour in a rat model of acute postoperative pain," *European Journal of Anaesthesiology*, vol. 32, no. 4, pp. 242–247, 2015.

[34] H. Jiang, D. Fang, L. Y. Kong et al., "Sensitization of neurons in the central nucleus of the amygdala via the decreased GABAergic inhibition contributes to the development of neuropathic pain-related anxiety-like behaviors in rats," *Molecular Brain*, vol. 7, p. 72, 2014.

[35] H. Leite-Almeida, J. J. Cerqueira, H. Wei et al., "Differential effects of left/right neuropathy on rats' anxiety and cognitive behavior," *Pain*, vol. 153, no. 11, pp. 2218–2225, 2012.

[36] S. C. LaGraize, C. J. Labuda, M. A. Rutledge, R. L. Jackson, and P. N. Fuchs, "Differential effect of anterior cingulate cortex lesion on mechanical hypersensitivity and escape/avoidance behavior in an animal model of neuropathic pain," *Experimental Neurology*, vol. 188, no. 1, pp. 139–148, 2004.

[37] M. Narita, N. Kuzumaki, M. Narita et al., "Chronic pain-induced emotional dysfunction is associated with astrogliosis due to cortical δ-opioid receptor dysfunction," *Journal of Neurochemistry*, vol. 97, no. 5, pp. 1369–1378, 2006.

[38] K. Matsuzawa-Yanagida, M. Narita, M. Nakajima et al., "Usefulness of antidepressants for improving the neuropathic pain-like state and pain-induced anxiety through actions at different brain sites," *Neuropsychopharmacology*, vol. 33, no. 8, pp. 1952–1965, 2008.

[39] J. Q. Fang, *Science of Acupuncture and Moxibustion*, vol. 155, China Press of Traditional Chinese Medicine, 2014.

[40] Z.-Q. Zhao, "Neural mechanism underlying acupuncture analgesia," *Progress in Neurobiology*, vol. 85, no. 4, pp. 355–375, 2008.

[41] W.-B. Zhang, A. Wu, G. Litscher, and Y. Chae, "Effects and mechanism of acupuncture based on the principle of meridians," *Evidence-Based Complementary and Alternative Medicine*, vol. 2013, Article ID 684027, 2 pages, 2013.

[42] J.-Q. Fang, J.-Y. Du, Y. Liang, and J.-F. Fang, "Intervention of electroacupuncture on spinal p38 MAPK/ATF-2/VR-1 pathway in treating inflammatory pain induced by CFA in rats," *Molecular Pain*, vol. 9, p. 13, 2013.

[43] S.-M. Wang, R. E. Harris, Y.-C. Lin, and T.-J. Gan, "Acupuncture in 21st century anesthesia: is there a needle in the haystack?" *Anesthesia and Analgesia*, vol. 116, no. 6, pp. 1356–1359, 2013.

[44] Y.-L. Jiang, X.-H. Yin, Y.-F. Shen, X.-F. He, and J.-Q. Fang, "Low frequency electroacupuncture alleviated spinal nerve ligation induced mechanical allodynia by inhibiting TRPV1 upregulation in ipsilateral undamaged dorsal root ganglia in rats," *Evidence-Based Complementary and Alternative Medicine*, vol. 2013, Article ID 170910, 9 pages, 2013.

[45] C. Men, J. Wang, B. Deng, X.-L. Wei, Y.-Q. Che, and C.-X. Han, "Decoding acupuncture electrical signals in spinal dorsal root ganglion," *Neurocomputing*, vol. 79, pp. 12–17, 2012.

[46] W. K. Lau, Y. M. Lau, H. Q. Zhang, S. C. Wong, and Z. X. Bian, "Electroacupuncture versus celecoxib for neuropathic pain in rat SNL model," *Neuroscience*, vol. 170, no. 2, pp. 655–661, 2010.

[47] J. R. T. Silva, M. L. Silva, and W. A. Prado, "Analgesia induced by 2- or 100-Hz electroacupuncture in the rat tail-flick test depends on the activation of different descending pain inhibitory mechanisms," *The Journal of Pain*, vol. 12, no. 1, pp. 51–60, 2011.

[48] H.-J. Park, Y. Chae, J. Jang, I. Shim, H. Lee, and S. Lim, "The effect of acupuncture on anxiety and neuropeptide Y expression in the basolateral amygdala of maternally separated rats," *Neuroscience Letters*, vol. 377, no. 3, pp. 179–184, 2005.

[49] Z. Zhao, X. Jin, Y. Wu et al., "Amygdaloid corticotropin-releasing factor is involved in the anxiolytic effect of acupuncture during ethanol withdrawal in rats," *Journal of Acupuncture and Meridian Studies*, vol. 6, no. 5, pp. 234–240, 2013.

[50] Q. Li, N. Yue, S.-B. Liu et al., "Effects of chronic electroacupuncture on depression- and anxiety-like behaviors in rats with chronic neuropathic pain," *Evidence-Based Complementary and Alternative Medicine*, vol. 2014, Article ID 158987, 10 pages, 2014.

[51] Y. Terasawa, M. Shibata, Y. Moriguchi, and S. Umeda, "Anterior insular cortex mediates bodily sensibility and social anxiety," *Social Cognitive and Affective Neuroscience*, vol. 8, no. 3, Article ID nss108, pp. 259–266, 2013.

[52] F. Barthas, J. Sellmeijer, S. Hugel, E. Waltisperger, M. Barrot, and I. Yalcin, "The anterior cingulate cortex is a critical hub for pain-induced depression," *Biological Psychiatry*, vol. 77, no. 3, pp. 236–245, 2015.

[53] C. Berna, S. Leknes, E. A. Holmes, R. R. Edwards, G. M. Goodwin, and I. Tracey, "Induction of depressed mood disrupts emotion regulation neurocircuitry and enhances pain unpleasantness," *Biological Psychiatry*, vol. 67, no. 11, pp. 1083–1090, 2010.

[54] C. J. LaBuda and P. N. Fuchs, "Attenuation of negative pain affect produced by unilateral spinal nerve injury in the rat following anterior cingulate cortex activation," *Neuroscience*, vol. 136, no. 1, pp. 311–322, 2005.

[55] H. Cao, "Involvement of ERK cascades in the anterior cingulate cortex in pain-related negative emotion in rat," *Neuroscience Research*, vol. 58, supplement 1, S49 pages, 2007.

[56] M.-G. Liu, R.-R. Wang, X.-F. Chen, F.-K. Zhang, X.-Y. Cui, and J. Chen, "Differential roles of ERK, JNK and p38 MAPK in pain-related spatial and temporal enhancement of synaptic responses in the hippocampal formation of rats: multi-electrode array recordings," *Brain Research*, vol. 1382, pp. 57–69, 2011.

Acupuncture for Lateral Epicondylitis: A Systematic Review

Hongzhi Tang,[1] **Huaying Fan,**[2] **Jiao Chen,**[2] **Mingxiao Yang,**[2] **Xuebing Yi,**[1] **Guogang Dai,**[1] **Junrong Chen,**[1] **Liugang Tang,**[1] **Haibo Rong,**[1] **Junhua Wu,**[1] **and Fanrong Liang**[2]

[1]*Sichuan Orthopaedic Hospital, Chengdu, Sichuan 610041, China*
[2]*Chengdu University of Traditional Chinese Medicine, Chengdu, Sichuan 610075, China*

Correspondence should be addressed to Fanrong Liang; acuresearch@126.com

Academic Editor: Christopher Zaslawski

Objective. This systematic review aimed to assess the effectiveness and safety of acupuncture for lateral epicondylitis (LE). *Methods.* Seven databases and the WHO International Clinical Trials Registry Platform Search Portal were searched to identify relevant studies. The data were extracted and assessed by two independent authors, and Review Manager Software (V.5.3) was used for data synthesis with effect estimate presented as standard mean difference (SMD) and mean difference (MD) with a 95% confidence interval. The Grading of Recommendations Assessment, Development, and Evaluation (GRADE) was used to assess the level of evidence. *Results.* Four RCTs with 309 participants were included with poor methodological quality. Participants who received acupuncture and acupuncture plus moxibustion with material insulation were likely to have an improvement in elbow functional status and/or myodynamia. The overall quality rated by GRADE was from very low to low. Two studies reported that the needle pain would be the main reason for the dropout. *Conclusion.* For the small number of included studies with poor methodological quality, no firm conclusion can be drawn regarding the effect of acupuncture of elbow functional status and myodynamia for LE. This trial is registered with CRD42015016199.

1. Introduction

Lateral epicondylitis (LE), also known as tennis elbow, is upper limbs associated musculoskeletal disorder and can be responsible for loss of function of the affected limb and substantial pain, which can have a major impact on patient's social and professional life [1]. It is estimated that the prevalence of LE ranges from 1% to 3% in the overall population [2], mainly occurring in those aged 45–54 years [3]. Activities that involve excessive and repetitive use of the forearm extensor, such as typing, tennis, badminton, and manual work, may cause LE [4]. The principal cause of LE is the degeneration of the proximal wrist extensor tendons [5].

LE not only is a major problem that causes prolonged recovery of functional disability and long-time pain that impact patient's daily life, but also produces a heavy economic burden as lost workdays and, in some patients, inability to work may last for several weeks [6, 7]. While a number of treatment methods, such as nonsteroidal anti-inflammatory drugs (NSAIDs), corticosteroid injections, exercise and mobilization, extracorporeal shock wave therapy, orthoses, and surgery, are used for LE, the lines of evidence of the effectiveness and safety of these therapy methods still remain uncertain [8–13].

As acupuncture is a green, simple, inexpensive, and helpful treatment which has been widely practiced in China and increasingly used in some Western countries, such as the Unite States, it has been accepted for treating musculoskeletal disease, especially for the functional disability and pain symptoms [14]. In recent years, a number of clinical trials have been conducted to assess the effectiveness and safety of acupuncture therapy for LE.

There were five systematic reviews that have been published during the last few years for assessing the effectiveness and safety of acupuncture for LE by evaluating the pain changes, but none of them draw a definitive conclusion on whether acupuncture is effective for LE or not. The systematic review published in 2002 by Green et al. [15] on lateral epicondylitis did not draw a conclusion on whether the acupuncture is effective for LE or not because of the small number of included trials and problems with methodology of the included trials, and the systematic review published in 2008 by Buchbinder et al. [16] also did not draw a specific conclusion because they thought there is conflicting evidence about the value of acupuncture for LE. However, the systematic review published in 2004 by Trinh et al. [17] suggested that acupuncture is effective for short-term pain relief for LE pain, and another systematic review published in 2005 by Bisset et al. [18] suggested that acupuncture is effective over placebo as treatment for LE in short-term outcomes, and the systematic review published by Gadau et al. in 2014 [19] also showed that acupuncture may be effective in the relief of LE pain up to a period of six months. Besides, although the systematic reviews published by Buchbinder et al. [16] and Gadau et al. [19] have also assessed the functional improvement or arm strength of LE, the conclusion still remains unclear because there was only one RCT included by assessing the functional improvement in review published by Buchbinder et al. and the author did not pool-analyze the included studies in the review published by Gadau et al.

Therefore, we can see in these systematic reviews that acupuncture has some effect on treating LE pain, but what remains unclear is whether acupuncture is effective and safe in improving the functional disability and changing the myodynamia, which seems to be important to improving patient's quality of life, or not. Thus, we decided to conduct the latest systematic review by evaluating the elbow functional status and myodynamia changes of the included trials to assess the effectiveness and safety of acupuncture for LE.

2. Method and Analysis

2.1. Search Method.
The following 7 databases were electronically searched from their inception to 2015: EMBASE, PubMed, the Cochrane Library, China National Knowledge Infrastructure (CNKI), Chinese Scientific Journal Database (VIP database), Wanfang Database, and Chinese Biomedical Literature Database (Sinomed). For the last four Chinese databases, we only included the researches published on core journals, such as Chinese Acupuncture and Moxibustion. The search terms consisted of four parts: acupuncture (acupuncture, electroacupuncture, warm acupuncture, needle acupuncture, and manual acupuncture), LE (lateral epicondylitis, tennis elbow, lateral epicondyle, external humeral epicondylitis, and lateral humeral epicondylitis), and randomized controlled trial. The detailed search strategies are presented in the Appendix.

Besides, we also searched the WHO International Clinical Trials Registry Platform Search Portal that contains Current Controlled Trials, ClinicalTrials.gov, and Chinese Clinical Trial Register for ongoing or recently completed studies by using simple search combining acupuncture and LE.

2.2. Inclusion Criteria

2.2.1. Type of Studies.
All randomized controlled trials (RCTs) involving acupuncture for treating LE were included. Completed or ongoing trials were included in this review, as well as trials using only the two parallel designs.

2.2.2. Type of Participants.
Adult participants (≥18 years old) presenting with LE were included regardless of sex, race, or educational and economic status.

2.2.3. Types of Interventions.
Interventions in the treatment group included acupuncture, electroacupuncture, warm acupuncture, needle acupuncture, and manual acupuncture. Controlled interventions with sham acupuncture, placebo control, no treatment/waiting list control, or active treatment (e.g., nonsteroidal anti-inflammatory drugs and/or local injection of corticosteroids) were included. RCTs evaluating acupuncture combined with another treatment compared with that other treatment alone will also be included.

2.2.4. Types of Outcome Measures.
Studies that reported at least one clinical outcome related to LE were included. Studies reporting only physiological or laboratory parameters were excluded. The primary outcome was the elbow functional status. The secondary outcome was the myodynamia and adverse events.

2.3. Exclusion Criteria

2.3.1. Other Types of Studies.
Nonrandomized controlled trials, randomized crossover trials, retrospective studies, case studies, and review studies were excluded.

2.3.2. Other Participants.
Participants with severe physical or mental disease were excluded.

2.3.3. Other Types of Interventions.
We did not include trials in which points were stimulated without needle insertion (such as via laser stimulation, acupressure, or transcutaneous electrical nerve stimulation). Besides, RCTs that compare different forms of acupuncture or herbal medicine were excluded.

2.4. Study Identification and Data Extraction.
Two reviewers (Hongzhi Tang and Huaying Fan) independently assessed the eligibility of the searched studies. The full-text articles that met the inclusion criteria were obtained, and the relevant references were retrieved according to predefined eligibility criteria. The data has been extracted by two reviewers (Jiao Chen and Huaying Fan) independently using a specially designed extraction form developed according to the Cochrane Handbook. The following factors were included in the data extraction form: participants' characteristics, study methods, interventions, and outcomes. We resolved any disagreements of study identification and data extraction by discussion and adjudication with a third reviewer (Hongzhi Tang). If any data were insufficient or unclear, the first or corresponding author for the study concerned would be contacted via E-mail or telephone to provide additional information.

2.5. Risk of Bias of the Included Studies.
Two reviewers (Hongzhi Tang and Jiao Chen) assessed the included studies for bias risk according to the Cochrane Collaboration Risk of Bias Tool based on the following six separate domains:

random sequence generation (selection bias), allocation concealment (selection bias), blinding of participants and personnel (performance bias), blinding of outcome assessment (detection bias), incomplete outcome data (attrition bias), and selective reporting (reporting bias). The assessments were categorized into three levels of bias: low risk, high risk, or unclear risk.

2.6. Data Synthesis.

Meta-analysis was done by using Review Manager Software (V.5.3) developed by the Cochrane Collaboration. Trials are combined according to the type of intervention, type of outcome measure, and control. For the continuous data, the mean difference (MD) with 95% confidence intervals was used with random-effects model. For different studies assessed the elbow functional status and myodynamia in a variety of ways, according to the Cochrane Handbook, the standardized mean difference (SMD) was used to standardize the results of the studies to a uniform scale before they were combined. Heterogeneity among the included studies was assessed using chi-square and I^2 test. I^2 values indicate the degree of statistical heterogeneity. When $P > 0.1$, it was considered that there was no statistical heterogeneity among studies; if $P \leq 0.1$, it was inverse. I^2 values less than 50% were accepted as homogeneous. If substantial heterogeneity was detected, we explored the reason for heterogeneity.

2.7. Quality of Evidence.

We used the Grading of Recommendations Assessment, Development, and Evaluation (GRADE), which is a method of grading the level of evidence and is developed by the GRADE Working Group [24, 25], to assess the quality of evidence, and the GRADEpro software (version 3.6 for Windows, Grade Working Group) was used.

3. Results

3.1. Study Identification.

The flow of the literature search and selection process is shown in Figure 1. A total of 344 records and two registered trials were identified from the included databases. 75 duplicate records were excluded, among which 74 records were excluded by reading the title and abstract, and one record was excluded by reading the full article. 264 articles were excluded (including one registered trial) because they did not meet the inclusion criteria; one article was further excluded because the data of the study cannot be collected from the article and there was no response from the corresponding author. Two studies about acupuncture of LE are ongoing. Finally, four studies [20–23] were included and two ongoing trials [26, 27] were described in this systematic review.

3.2. Characteristics of the Included Studies.

Characteristics of the methods, participants, intervention, and outcome measures of all included studies and ongoing studies were shown in Tables 1 and 2 separately. Among the four included studies, there were two conducted in China [22, 23], and two were conducted in Germany [20, 21]. In total, there were 309 patients who participated in the included studies, among

which there were 155 patients in the acupuncture group and 154 patients in the controlled group. Their age ranged from 18 years to 70 years, and the duration of the LE was varied from one month to 15 months. All studies included both men and women. Two trials [20, 21] compared acupuncture with sham acupuncture, one trial [22] compared electroacupuncture plus moxibustion with material insulation with blockage therapy, and one trial [23] compared electroacupuncture plus blockage therapy with blockage therapy. In these trials, frequency of acupuncture was at least 20 min per treatment and 3 treatments. Four studies [20–23] reported outcomes including the functional status and pain change; three studies [20, 21, 23] reported the myodynamia change as outcome.

3.3. Methodological Quality of Included Studies.

The methodological quality of included studies was assessed by risk of bias, presented in Figures 2 and 3. All of the included studies reported randomization allocation. One study [20] described the method of random sequence generation which was a list random number prepared by the Department of Biostatistics of Hannover Medical School. One study [23] reported the randomization allocation by using Microsoft Office Excel, and another two studies [21, 22] used the randomization allocation method according to sequence of patients' attendance. All of the four studies did not describe the allocation concealment in sufficient detailed ways. Only one study [21] reported the blinding of the participants, and two studies [20, 21] reported the blinding of the outcome assessment, in which one [20] was assessed by an assessor who had no knowledge of acupuncture and another one [21] was assessed by a blinded study nurse. Two trials [21, 22] had low risk of attrition bias, which reported that no participants dropped out or were excluded from the primary analysis, and another two trials [20, 23] also had low risk for reporting the number of dropouts. All of the relevant outcomes were reported in detail in the four trials [20–23], which had low risk of reporting bias. None of the four trials [20–23] reported the source of financial support, declared that no financial interests exist, or mentioned that the research was approved by ethics committee.

3.4. Measures of Effect

3.4.1. Elbow Functional Status

Acupuncture versus Sham Acupuncture. The clinical heterogeneity of two trials [20, 21] comparing acupuncture with sham acupuncture is considerable. Pooled analysis showed no statistical heterogeneity among the studies ($P > 0.1$) and was statistically significant (SMD −0.56, 95% CI −0.98 to −0.15, $P = 0.008$), which suggested that the effectiveness of acupuncture on treating function disability of LE is better than sham acupuncture (see Figure 4).

Acupuncture Plus Moxibustion with Material Insulation versus Blockage Therapy. Only one trial [22] compared the acupuncture plus moxibustion with material insulation with acupuncture alone (MD 12.10, 95% CI 10.65 to 13.55). The result showed that acupuncture plus moxibustion with material

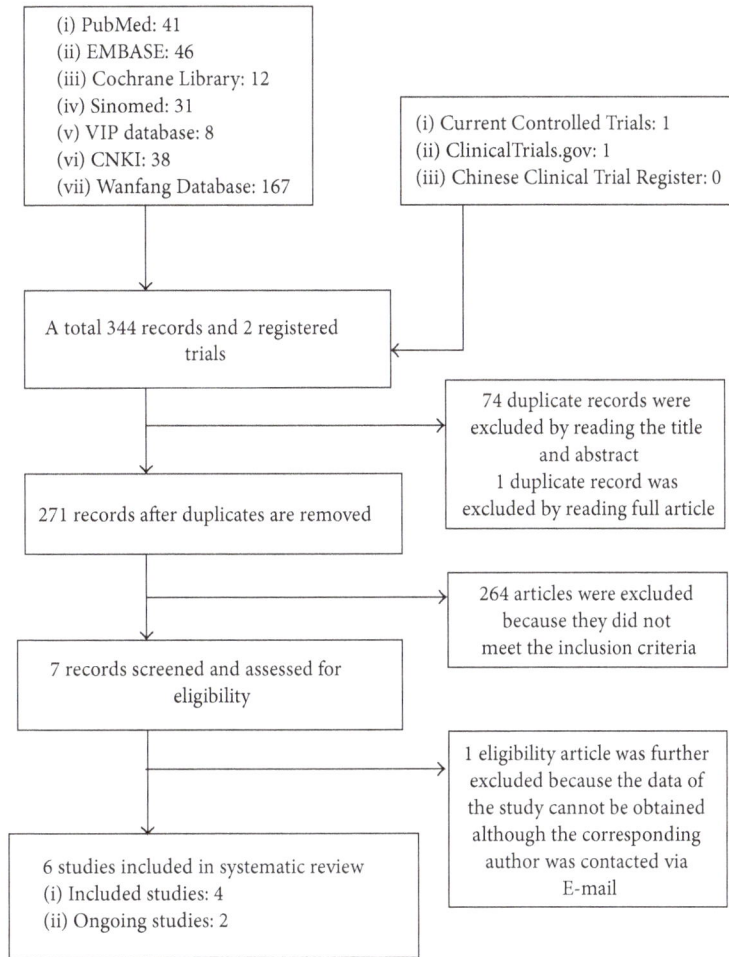

FIGURE 1: Flow diagram for search and selection of the included studies.

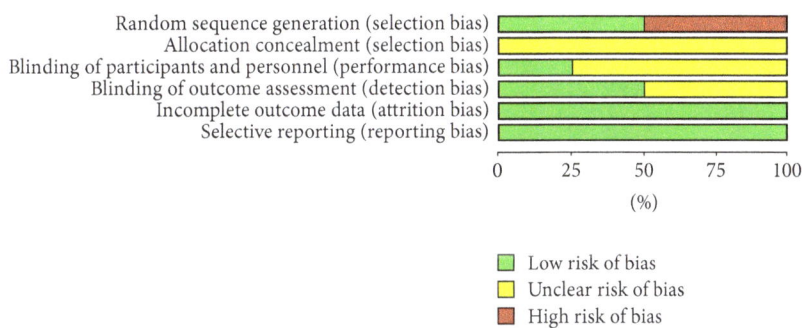

FIGURE 2: Risk of bias graph: review authors' judgements about each risk of bias item presented as percentages across all included studies.

insulation is superior for improving the function disability to acupuncture alone (see Figure 5).

Acupuncture Plus Blockage Therapy versus Blockage Therapy. One trial [23] revealed no statistically significant difference between acupuncture plus blockage therapy and blockage therapy alone (MD 2, 95% CI −0.98 to 4.98), which demonstrated that acupuncture plus blockage therapy was not superior to blockage therapy alone in improving function disability of LE (see Figure 6).

3.4.2. Myodynamia

Acupuncture versus Sham Acupuncture. Two trials [20, 21] were included to pool-analyze the change in myodynamia, which showed that acupuncture group had better effect than

TABLE 1: The characteristics of included studies in this systematic review.

Author, year	Method	Participants total (T/C)	Mean (SD)/range age		Intervention		Acupuncture points	Frequency and duration of acupuncture intervention	Outcomes
			Treatment	Control	Treatment	Control			
Fink et al., 2002 [20]	RCT	45 (23/22)	52.5 ± 8.7	51.6 ± 10.0	Real acupuncture	Sham acupuncture	Ashi, LI10, LI11, LU5, LI4, and SJ5	25 min/treatment; 10 treatments, with 2 treatments per week	(1) Maximal muscle strength (2) VAS (3) DASH
Irnich et al., 2003 [21]	RCT	50 (25/25)	31–70	38–65	Real acupuncture	Sham acupuncture	LI4, LI10, SI3, SJ5, and GB34	25 min/treatment; 3 treatments within 10 days	(1) PPT (2) GS (3) IP
Jiang et al., 2005 [22]	RCT	128 (64/64)	42.14 ± 5.62	41.68 ± 5.76	Electroacupuncture plus moxibustion with material insulation	Blockage therapy	LI4, LR3	20 min/treatment; 10 treatments within 5 treatments per week	Elbow function status
Li et al., 2014 [23]	RCT	86 (43/43)	18–22	18–22	Electroacupuncture plus massage and blockage therapy	Blockage therapy	Ashi, LI11, LI12, LI10, SJ5, and LI4	30 min/treatment; once per day for 10 days	(1) VAS (2) GSI (3) MEPS

VAS: Visual Analog Scale; DASH: disabilities of the arm, shoulder, and hand; PPT: pressure pain threshold; GS: grip strength; IP: impairment caused by pain; GSI: grip strength index; MEPS: Mayo Elbow Performance Score.

TABLE 2: The characteristics of ongoing studies in this systematic review.

Title	Country	Trial registration	Inclusion criteria	Exclusion criteria	Method	Participants total	Intervention Treatment	Intervention Contralateral	Control	Outcomes Primary outcome	Outcomes Second outcome
Acupuncture for Lateral Epicondylitis (Tennis Elbow): Study Protocol for a Randomized Practitioner-Assessor Blinded, Controlled Pilot Clinical Trial	Korea	Clinical Research Information Service (CRIS), Republic of Korea: KCT0000628	(1) Individuals between the ages of 19 and 65 years with lateral epicondylitis on one arm and pain persisting for at least 4 weeks; (2) individuals with tenderness limited to the elbow joint and surrounding area; (3) individuals reporting pain under resisted extension of the middle finger and wrist; (4) individuals with an average pain of 40 or more (0–100) on the Visual Analogue Scale (VAS) in the week prior to the screening visit; (5) individuals who volunteered to participate in the study and who signed a consent form	(1) Individuals whose radiological examinations show abnormalities such as calcification, arthritis, and inflammatory arthropathy of the elbow joint; (2) individuals with a history of trauma, ligament damage, fracture, tumor, or surgery of the elbow joint; (3) individuals who have been diagnosed with or treated for cervical radiculopathy or herniation of intervertebral disc; (4) individuals who have received injections for lateral epicondylitis during the last 6 months; (5) individuals who have received treatments such as nonsteroidal anti-inflammatory drugs (NSAIDs), acupuncture, and physiotherapy for lateral epicondylitis during the last 2 weeks; (6) individuals judged by the person in charge of the clinical trial as unsuitable for participation, such as those with mental disorders, those who are pregnant, or those that have other acute or chronic disorders	RCT	45	Ipsilateral acupuncture group	Contralateral acupuncture group	Control group	The Visual Analog Scale (VAS) at 4 weeks	(1) The Visual Analog Scale (VAS) at 8 and 12 weeks; (2) the patient-rated tennis elbow evaluation (PRTEE); (3) pain-free/maximum grip strength; (4) pressure pain threshold; (5) clinically relevant improvement, patient global assessment, and EuroQol at 4, 8, and 12 weeks
Clinical Comparative Effect of Physiotherapy or Acupuncture Treatment of Lateral Epicondylitis: A Randomized Controlled Pilot Trial	Norway	ClinicalTrials.gov: NCT02321696	(1) Lateral epicondylitis (LE) (duration: >2 weeks); (2) unilateral localization; (3) individuals with average pain of NRS 4 or higher during the last week prior to screening; (4) age between 18 and 67 years; (5) written informed consent	(1) Corticosteroid injections during the last 4 weeks; (2) diseases of the central or peripheral nervous system; (3) inflammatory rheumatic diseases; (4) radioulnar or radiohumeral osteoarthritis; (5) unwillingness to participate	RCT	36	Acupuncture and eccentric exercise	Physiotherapy and eccentric exercise	Watchful waiting and eccentric exercise	Elbow pain on Numeric Rating Scale (0–10)	(1) The disabilities of the arm, shoulder, and hand (quick-DASH); (2) quality of life by EQ-5D; (3) sick listing; (4) patients satisfaction; global perceived effect and satisfaction with treatment; (5) use of analgesics; (6) number of treatment sessions

FIGURE 3: Risk of bias summary: review authors' judgments about each risk of bias item for each included study.

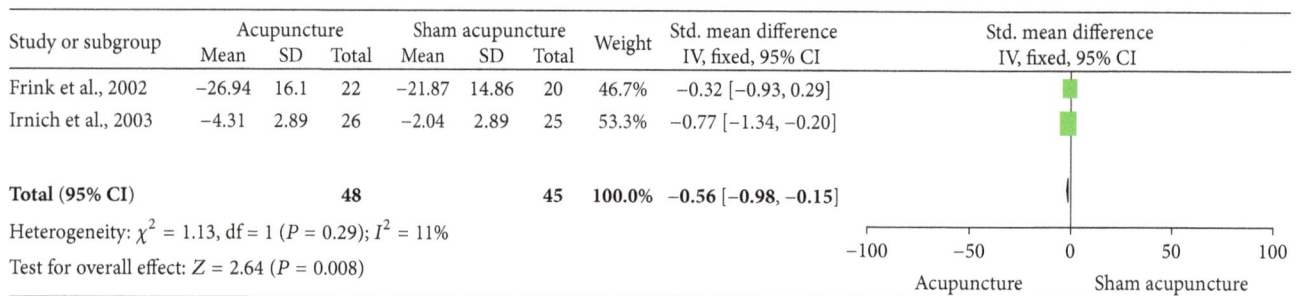

FIGURE 4: The effect of acupuncture versus sham acupuncture on elbow functional status.

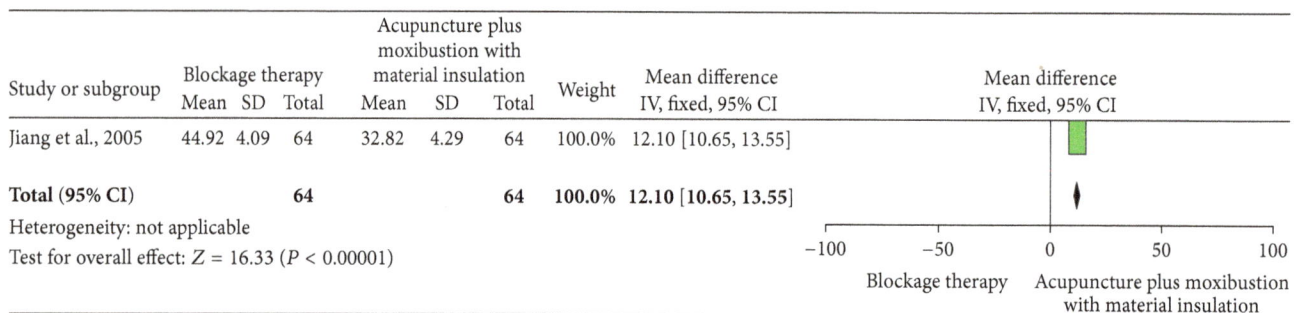

FIGURE 5: The effect of acupuncture plus moxibustion with material insulation versus blockage therapy on elbow functional status.

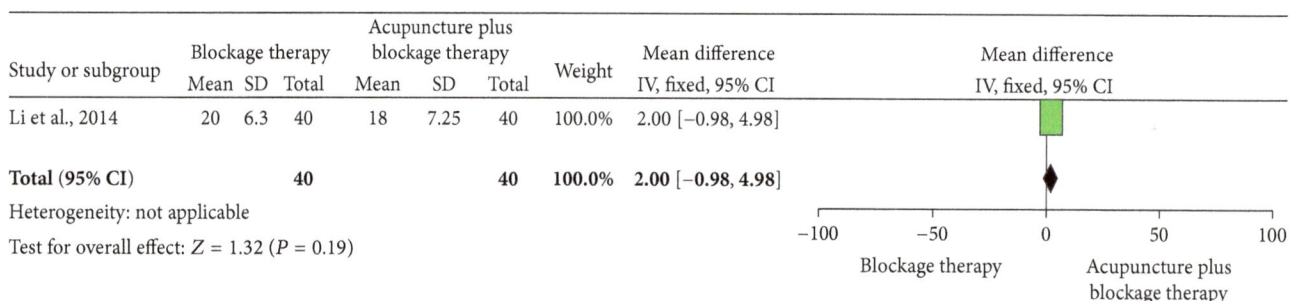

FIGURE 6: The effect of acupuncture plus blockage therapy versus blockage therapy on elbow functional status.

Study or subgroup	Sham acupuncture			Acupuncture			Weight	Std. mean difference	Std. mean difference
	Mean	SD	Total	Mean	SD	Total		IV, fixed, 95% CI	IV, fixed, 95% CI
Frink et al., 2002	52.4	49.3	22	36.5	46.73	20	45.7%	0.33 [−0.29, 0.93]	
Irnich et al., 2003	21.54	28.27	26	8.53	17.9	25	54.3%	0.54 [−0.02, 1.10]	
Total (95% CI)			48			45	100.0%	0.44 [0.03, 0.85]	

Heterogeneity: $\chi^2 = 0.26$, df = 1 ($P = 0.61$); $I^2 = 0\%$
Test for overall effect: $Z = 2.10$ ($P = 0.04$)

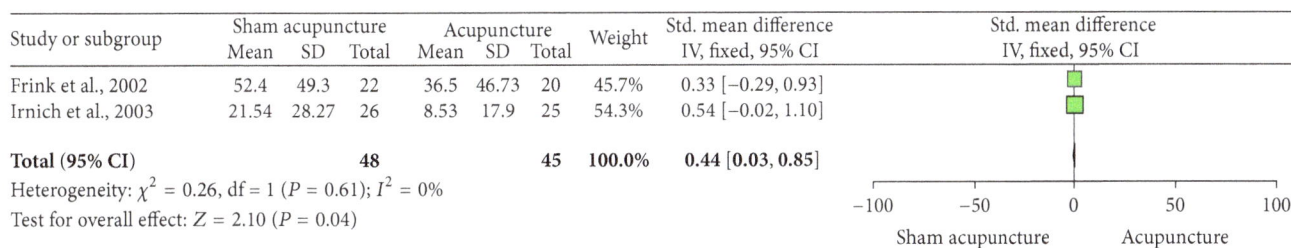

FIGURE 7: The effect of acupuncture versus sham acupuncture on elbow myodynamia.

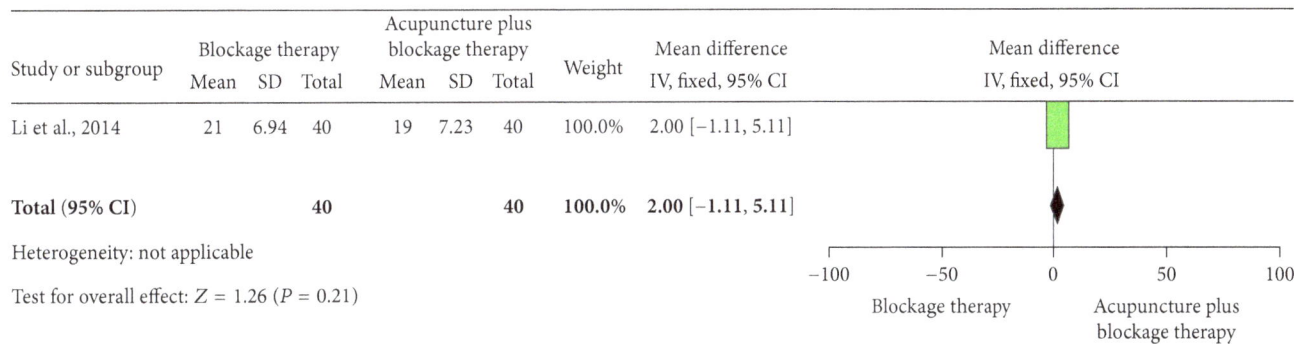

Study or subgroup	Blockage therapy			Acupuncture plus blockage therapy			Weight	Mean difference	Mean difference
	Mean	SD	Total	Mean	SD	Total		IV, fixed, 95% CI	IV, fixed, 95% CI
Li et al., 2014	21	6.94	40	19	7.23	40	100.0%	2.00 [−1.11, 5.11]	
Total (95% CI)			40			40	100.0%	2.00 [−1.11, 5.11]	

Heterogeneity: not applicable

Test for overall effect: $Z = 1.26$ ($P = 0.21$)

FIGURE 8: The effect of acupuncture plus blockage therapy versus blockage therapy on elbow myodynamia.

sham acupuncture (SMD 0.44, 95% CI 0.03 to 0.85, $P = 0.04$), and the statistical heterogeneity was not significant ($P = 0.61$) (see Figure 7).

Acupuncture Plus Blockage Therapy versus Blockage Therapy. One trial [23] showed no statistically significant difference between acupuncture plus blockage therapy and blockage therapy alone (MD 2, 95% CI −1.11 to 5.11, $P = 0.21$) (see Figure 8).

3.5. *Adverse Events.* Of the four studies, three studies [20, 21, 23] reported the adverse events. One study [20] reported that no serious adverse event was observed during the study. The other two studies [20, 22] reported that the pain would be the main reason for the dropout.

3.6. *Quality of Evidence.* The quality of evidence evaluated using the Grading of Recommendations Assessment, Development, and Evaluation (GRADE) system was from very low to low (Table 3). All of the studies reported the randomization method, but two of the studies [21, 22] used the wrong random method, according to the sequence of attendance. Besides, all of the studies did not describe the method of allocation concealment in a detailed way, and only one study [21] reported the blinding of the participants, which downgraded the outcomes. In addition, the small number of participants of all outcomes also downgraded all outcomes.

4. Discussion

Comprehensive search was conducted through 7 electronic databases and WHO International Clinical Trials Registry Platform Search Portal for acupuncture in treating LE. The studies identification, data extraction, and analysis were carried out independently by two review authors. In this systematic review, we included a total of four randomized controlled trials [20–23] with 309 participants suffering from LE. Of all studies, two studies [20, 21] were designed to compare acupuncture with sham acupuncture, one study [22] compared acupuncture combined with moxibustion with material insulation to blockage therapy, and another study [23] was designed to compare acupuncture plus blockage therapy with blockage therapy. In the outcomes, two studies [20, 21] that compared acupuncture with sham acupuncture showed that acupuncture significantly improves elbow functional disabilities and myodynamia. Besides, one trial [22] also showed that electroacupuncture combined with moxibustion with material insulation improved elbow functional disabilities and myodynamia when compared with blockage therapy. However, when combining electroacupuncture with blockage therapy to compare with blockage therapy alone, there is no change in elbow functional status and myodynamia. Up to the present, there were five systematic reviews that have assessed acupuncture for LE. All of the systematic reviews have assessed the effectiveness and safety of acupuncture for LE by evaluating the pain and suggested that acupuncture has some effect on treating elbow pain. Although there are two systematic reviews that have assessed the strength of arm and functional status of arms, they did not draw a definitive conclusion on whether acupuncture is effective for LE or not. Therefore, we conducted this systematic review to assess the effectiveness and safety of acupuncture for LE on elbow functional disability and myodynamia. In the present review, we analyzed four studies accounting for

TABLE 3: The quality of evidence.

(a) Acupuncture versus sham acupuncture

Number of studies	Design	Quality assessment					Number of patients		Effect		Quality	Importance
		Risk of bias	Inconsistency	Indirectness	Imprecision	Other considerations	Acupuncture	Sham acupuncture	Relative (95% CI)	Absolute		
Function (follow-up: 14–60 days, measured with scale, range of scores: 10–20, better indicated by lower values)												
2	Randomized trials	Serious[1]	No serious inconsistency	No serious indirectness	Serious[2]	None	48	45	—	SMD 0.56 lower (0.98 to 0.15 lower)	Low	Critical
Myodynamia (follow-up: 4 to 60 days, measured with scale, range of scores: 10–20, better indicated by higher values)												
2	Randomized trials	Serious[1]	No serious inconsistency	No serious indirectness	Serious[2]	None	48	45	—	SMD 0.44 higher (0.53 to 0.85 higher)	Low	Critical

[1]The trial used the wrong random method, which according to sequence of attendance and the method of allocation concealment is not described.
[2]Total population size is less than 400, and effect size is considered a small effect; the upper or lower confidence limit crosses an effect size of 0.5 in either direction.

(b) Acupuncture plus moxibustion with material insulation versus blockage therapy

Number of studies	Design	Quality assessment					Number of patients		Effect		Quality	Importance
		Risk of bias	Inconsistency	Indirectness	Imprecision	Other considerations	Acupuncture plus moxibustion with material insulation	Blockage therapy	Relative (95% CI)	Absolute		
Function (measured with scales, range of scores: 10–20, better indicated by higher values)												
1	Randomized trials	Very serious[1]	No serious inconsistency	No serious indirectness	Serious[2]	None	64	64	—	MD 12.10 higher (10.65 to 13.55 higher)	Very low	Critical

[1]The method of allocation concealment is not described.
[2]Total population size is less than 400, and effect size is considered a small effect; the upper or lower confidence limit crosses an effect size of 0.5 in either direction.

(c) Acupuncture plus blockage therapy versus blockage therapy

Number of studies	Design	Quality assessment					Number of patients		Effect		Quality	Importance
		Risk of bias	Inconsistency	Indirectness	Imprecision	Other considerations	Acupuncture plus blockage therapy	Blockage therapy	Relative (95% CI)	Absolute		
Function (follow-up mean: 12 months, measured with scales, range of scores: 10–20, better indicated by higher values)												
1	Randomized trials	Serious[1]	No serious inconsistency	No serious indirectness	Serious[2]	None	40	40	—	MD 2 higher (0.96 lower to 4.98 higher)	Low	Critical

(c) Continued.

Number of studies	Quality assessment						Number of patients		Effect		Quality	Importance
	Design	Risk of bias	Inconsistency	Indirectness	Imprecision	Other considerations	Acupuncture plus blockage therapy	Blockage therapy	Relative (95% CI)	Absolute		
Myodynamia (follow-up mean: 12 months, measured with scales, range of scores: 10–20, better indicated by higher values)												
1	Randomized trials	Serious[1]	No serious inconsistency	No serious indirectness	Serious[2]	None	40	40	—	MD 2 higher (1.11 lower to 5.11 higher)	Low	Critical

[1]The method of allocation concealment is not described.
[2]Total population size is less than 400, and effect size is considered a small effect; the upper or lower confidence limit crosses an effect size of 0.5 in either direction.

309 participants on elbow functional status and myodynamia, which showed that acupuncture has some effect on elbow functional disability. While this finding seems promising, it should be interpreted with caution because of the small number of included studies and participants. Besides, there were no trials reporting a formal sample size calculation which is essential to ensure adequate statistical power.

There are still several limitations in this review. The key limitation was the small number of the included studies and participants, which limited the reliability of the pooled results. Another limitation was the quality of the included studies. Mostly included studies were of low quality due to no detailed definition on random sequence generation, allocation concealment, and blinding of participants and personnel. The low quality of the included studies also limited the reliability of conclusion of this review. Besides, all the included studies were from Germany and China, but LE is a worldwide disease. Last, because of ununiformed assessment scale of elbow functional status and upper limb myodynamia, even though SMD method was applied to standardize the results of the studies to a uniform scale before they were combined, we still cannot ignore the report bias caused by the ununiformed assessment scale.

Thus, based on the current systematic review, no firm conclusion can be drawn regarding the effect of acupuncture for LE. Although four randomized controlled trials were identified, the methodological quality of the four studies was low due to high risk in selection bias and blinding of participants and personnel, and the number of the patients recruited in each trial was small, which limited the reliability of the pooled results. Besides, the small number of the included studies also makes the results of this review inconclusive. In the end, in order to confirm the effectiveness of acupuncture for LE, large prospective trials with rigorous design should be conducted more rigorously in the future trials and the assessment scale as well as the evaluation standard needs to be unified from international institute of health as soon as possible.

Appendix

A. Search Strategies

A.1. Search Strategy Used in Cochrane Library

#1 "lateral epicondyle":ti,ab,kw

#2 lateral epicondylitis:ti,ab,kw

#3 "tennis elbow":ti,ab,kw

#4 external humeral epicondylitis:ti,ab,kw

#5 Lateral Humeral Epicondylitis:ti,ab,kw

#6 #1 or #2 or #3 or #4 or #5

#7 "acupuncture":ti,ab,kw

#8 "electroacupuncture":ti,ab,kw

#9 warm acupuncture:ti,ab,kw

#10 neddle acupuncture:ti,ab,kw

#11 mannual acupuncture:ti,ab,kw

#12 #7 or #8 or #9 or #10 or #11

#13 "controlled clinical trial":ti,ab,kw

#14 "randomised clinical trial":ti,ab,kw

#15 "randomised control trial":ti,ab,kw

#16 #13 or #14 or #15

#17 "animal":ti,ab,kw and "human":ti,ab,kw

#18 "animal":ti,ab,kw

#19 #18 not #17

#20 #16 not #19

#21 #6 and #12 and #20

A.2. Search Strategy Used in EMBASE

#1 lateral AND epicondylitis

#2 tennis AND elbow

#3 lateral AND epicondyle

#4 external AND humeral AND epicondylitis

#5 lateral AND humeral AND epicondylitis

#6 #1 OR #2 OR #3 OR #4 OR #5

#7 Acupuncture

#8 electroacupuncture

#9 warm AND acupuncture

#10 neddle AND acupuncture

#11 mannual AND acupuncture

#12 #7 OR #8 OR #9 OR #10 OR #11

#13 controlled AND clinical AND trial

#14 randomised AND clinical AND trial

#15 randomised AND control AND trial

#16 #13 OR #14 OR #15

#17 #6 AND #12 AND #16

A.3. Search Strategy Used in PubMed

#1 acupuncture

#2 acupuncture therapy

#3 manual acupuncture

#4 electroacupuncture

#5 acupoint

#6 acupuncture[MeSH Terms]

#7 acupuncture therapy[MeSH Terms]

#8 acupoint[MeSH Terms]

#9 #1 OR #2 OR #3 OR #4 OR #5 OR #6 OR #7 OR #8

#10 Tennis Elbow

#11 Elbow, Tennis

#12 Elbows, Tennis

#13 Tennis Elbows

#14 Epicondylitis, Lateral Humeral

#15 Epicondylitides, Lateral Humeral

#16 Humeral Epicondylitides, Lateral

#17 Humeral Epicondylitis, Lateral

#18 Lateral Humeral Epicondylitides

#19 Lateral Humeral Epicondylitis

#20 lateral epicondylitis

#21 lateral epicondyle

#22 external humeral epicondylitis

#23 epicondylitis

#24 Tennis Elbow[MeSH Terms]

#25 #10 OR #11 OR #12 OR #13 OR #14 OR #15 OR #16 OR #17 OR #18 OR #19 OR #20 OR #21 OR #22 OR #23 OR #24

#26 randomised controlled trial

#27 controlled clinical trial

#28 randomized controlled trial

#29 randomised

#30 randomly

#31 placebo

#32 trial

#33 randomized controlled trial[MeSH Terms]

#34 #26 OR #27 OR #28 OR #29 OR #30 OR #31 OR #32 OR #33

#35 (animals) AND humans

#36 animals

#37 #36 NOT #35

#38 #34 NOT #37

#39 #9 AND #25 AND #38

A.4. Search Strategy Used in Sinomed

#1 "网球肘"[不加权:扩展]

#2 网球肘

#3 肱骨外上髁炎

#4 (#3) OR (#2) OR (#1)

#5 "针刺疗法"[不加权:扩展]

#6 "针刺穴位"[不加权:扩展]

#7 "电针"[不加权:扩展]

#8 "温针疗法"[不加权:扩展]

#9 "针刺"[不加权:扩展]

#10 针刺疗法

#11 针刺

#12 电针

#13 温针

#14 针刺穴位

#15 (#14) OR (#13) OR (#12) OR (#11) OR (#10) OR (#9) OR (#8) OR (#7) OR (#6) OR (#5)

#16 "随机对照试验"[不加权:扩展]

#17 "随机分配"[不加权:扩展]

#18 随机对照试验

#19 随机分配

#20 (#19) OR (#18) OR (#17) OR (#16)

#21 (#20) AND (#15) AND (#4)

#22 ((#21)) AND (人类[特征词])

Conflict of Interests

All authors declare that there is no conflict of interests regarding the publication of this paper.

Authors' Contribution

H. Tang and H. Fan contributed equally to the conception of the study. The paper was drafted by H. Tang and H. Fan and revised by J. Chen. The search strategy was developed by all authors and run by L. Tang and H. Rong, who also independently screened the potential studies. J. Wu and M. Yang extracted data from the included studies, and J. Chen assessed the risk of bias and finished data synthesis. F. Liang arbitrated any disagreements and ensured that no errors occur during the study. Besides, H. Tang, H. Fan, J. Chen, M. Yang, F. Liang, X. Yi, G. Dai, and J. Chen contributed to the registration of this systematic review. All authors have approved the publication of the systematic review.

Acknowledgment

This work was supported by funds from the Science and Technology Department of Sichuan province, Grants nos. 2011SZ0302 and 2015SZ0096.

References

[1] B. Silverstein, E. Welp, N. Nelson, and J. Kalat, "Claims incidence of work-related disorders of the upper extremities: Washington State, 1987 through 1995," *American Journal of Public Health*, vol. 88, no. 12, pp. 1827–1833, 1998.

[2] E. Allander, "Prevalence, incidence, and remission rates of some common rheumatic diseases or syndromes," *Scandinavian Journal of Rheumatology*, vol. 3, no. 3, pp. 145–153, 1974.

[3] R. Shiri, E. Viikari-Juntura, H. Varonen, and M. Heliövaara, "Prevalence and determinants of lateral and medial epicondylitis: a population study," *American Journal of Epidemiology*, vol. 164, no. 11, pp. 1065–1074, 2006.

[4] V. S. Kumar, A. A. Shetty, K. J. Ravikumar, and M. J. Fordyce, "Tennis elbow—outcome following the garden procedure: a retrospective study," *Journal of Orthopaedic Surgery*, vol. 12, no. 2, pp. 226–229, 2004.

[5] J. A. Martinez-Silvestrini, K. L. Newcomer, R. E. Gay, M. P. Schaefer, P. Kortebein, and K. W. Arendt, "Chronic lateral

epicondylitis: comparative effectiveness of a home exercise program including stretching alone versus stretching supplemented with eccentric or concentric strengthening," *Journal of Hand Therapy*, vol. 18, no. 4, pp. 411–420, 2005.

[6] K. Kurppa, E. Viikari-Juntura, E. Kuomas, M. Huuskonen, and P. Kivi, "Incidence of tenosynovitis or peritendinitis and epicondylitis in a meta-processing factory," *Scandinavian Journal of Work, Environment and Health*, vol. 17, no. 1, pp. 32–37, 1991.

[7] J. A. N. Verhaar, "Tennis elbow. Anatomical, epidemiological and therapeutic aspects," *International Orthopaedics*, vol. 18, no. 5, pp. 263–267, 1994.

[8] R. Buchbinder, R. V. Johnston, L. Barnsley, W. J. Assendelft, S. N. Bell, and N. Smidt, "Surgery for lateral elbow pain," *Cochrane Database of Systematic Reviews*, vol. 3, Article ID CD003525, 2011.

[9] P. Hoogvliet, M. S. Randsdorp, R. Dingemanse, B. W. Koes, and B. M. A. Huisstede, "Does effectiveness of exercise therapy and mobilization techniques offer guidance for the treatment of lateral and medial epicondylitis? A systematic review," *British Journal of Sports Medicine*, vol. 47, no. 17, pp. 1112–1119, 2013.

[10] P. Pattanittum, T. Turner, S. Green, and R. Buchbinder, "Nonsteroidal anti-inflammatory drugs (NSAIDs) for treating lateral elbow pain in adults," *The Cochrane Database of Systematic Reviews*, vol. 5, Article ID CD003686, 2013.

[11] P. A. A. Struijs, N. Smidt, H. Arola, C. N. Van Dijk, R. Buchbinder, and W. J. J. Assendelft, "Orthotic devices for tennis elbow: a systematic review," *British Journal of General Practice*, vol. 51, no. 472, pp. 924–929, 2001.

[12] R. Buchbinder, S. E. Green, J. M. Youd, W. J. J. Assendelft, L. Barnsley, and N. Smidt, "Systematic review of the efficacy and safety of shock wave therapy for lateral elbow pain," *Journal of Rheumatology*, vol. 33, no. 7, pp. 1351–1363, 2006.

[13] B. K. Coombes, L. Bisset, and B. Vicenzino, "Efficacy and safety of corticosteroid injections and other injections for management of tendinopathy: a systematic review of randomised controlled trials," *The Lancet*, vol. 376, no. 9754, pp. 1751–1767, 2010.

[14] NIH, "Acupuncture," *NIH Consensus Statement*, vol. 15, no. 5, pp. 1–34, 1997.

[15] S. Green, R. Buchbinder, L. Barnsley et al., "Acupuncture for lateral elbow pain," *Cochrane Database of Systematic Reviews*, no. 1, Article ID CD003527, 2002.

[16] R. Buchbinder, S. E. Green, and P. Struijs, "Tennis elbow," *BMJ Clinical Evidence*, vol. 2008, article 1117, 2008.

[17] K. V. Trinh, S.-D. Phillips, E. Ho, and K. Damsma, "Acupuncture for the alleviation of lateral epicondyle pain: a systematic review," *Rheumatology*, vol. 43, no. 9, pp. 1085–1090, 2004.

[18] L. Bisset, A. Paungmali, B. Vicenzino, and E. Beller, "A systematic review and meta-analysis of clinical trials on physical interventions for lateral epicondylalgia," *British Journal of Sports Medicine*, vol. 39, no. 7, pp. 411–422, 2005.

[19] M. Gadau, W.-F. Yeung, H. Liu et al., "Acupuncture and moxibustion for lateral elbow pain: a systematic review of randomized controlled trials," *BMC Complementary and Alternative Medicine*, vol. 14, article 136, 2014.

[20] M. Fink, E. Wolkenstein, M. Karst, and A. Gehrke, "Acupuncture in chronic epicondylitis: a randomized controlled trial," *Rheumatology*, vol. 41, no. 2, pp. 205–209, 2002.

[21] D. Irnich, H. Karg, N. Behrens et al., "Controlled trial on point specificity of acupuncture in the treatment of lateral epicondylitis (Tennis elbow)," *Physikalische Medizin, Rehabilitationsmedizin, Kurortmedizin*, vol. 13, no. 4, pp. 215–219, 2003.

[22] Z. Y. Jiang, C. D. Li, J. H. Guo, J. C. Li, and L. Gao, "Controlled observation on electroacupuncture combined with cake-separated moxibustion for treatment of tennis elbow," *Zhongguo Zhen Jiu*, vol. 25, no. 11, pp. 763–764, 2005.

[23] X. Li, K. Zhou, E. Zhang et al., "Therapeutic effect of electroacupuncture, massage, and blocking therapy on external humeral epicondylitis," *Journal of Traditional Chinese Medicine*, vol. 34, no. 3, pp. 261–266, 2014.

[24] G. H. Guyatt, A. D. Oxman, R. Kunz et al., "What is 'quality of evidence' and why is it important to clinicians?" *British Medical Journal*, vol. 336, no. 7651, pp. 995–998, 2008.

[25] G. H. Guyatt, A. D. Oxman, G. E. Vist et al., "GRADE: an emerging consensus on rating quality of evidence and strength of recommendations," *British Medical Journal*, vol. 336, no. 7650, pp. 924–926, 2008.

[26] Clinical Comparative Effect of Physiotherapy or Acupuncture Treatment of Lateral Epicondylitis: a Randomized Controlled Pilot Trial, NCT02321696, https://clinicaltrials.gov/.

[27] K.-M. Shin, J.-H. Kim, S. Lee et al., "Acupuncture for lateral epicondylitis (tennis elbow): study protocol for a randomized, practitioner-assessor blinded, controlled pilot clinical trial," *Trials*, vol. 14, no. 1, article 174, 2013.

Berberine in Combination with Insulin Has Additive Effects on Titanium Implants Osseointegration in Diabetes Mellitus Rats

Li Lu, Huang Zhijian, Li Lei, Chen Wenchuan, and Zhu Zhimin

Department of Prosthodontics, West China Hospital of Stomatology, State Key Laboratory of Oral Diseases, Sichuan University, Chengdu 610041, China

Correspondence should be addressed to Chen Wenchuan; hxkqcwc@scu.edu.cn and Zhu Zhimin; zzhimin@163.com

Academic Editor: Bhushan Patwardhan

This study evaluated the effects of berberine in combination with insulin on early osseointegration of implants in diabetic rats. Fifty male Sprague-Dawley rats were randomly divided into 5 groups: healthy rats were used as control (HC), and streptozotocin-induced diabetic rats were treated with insulin, berberine, berberine + insulin (IB), or no treatment. Each rat received one machined-surface cp-Ti implant into the right tibia and was given insulin injection and/or gavage feeding with berberine daily for 8 weeks until being sacrificed. Serum levels of alkaline phosphatase (ALP) and bone gamma-carboxyglutamic acid-containing protein (BGP) were analyzed in each group. Peri-implant mineral apposition was marked by fluorochrome double-labeling and osseointegration was histomorphologically examined. The ALP and BGP levels decreased in diabetic rats but were successfully corrected by insulin and berberine combined treatment. Moreover, untreated diabetic rats had less labeled mineral apposition and impaired osseointegration. In contrast, Groups I, B, and IB were observed with increased peri-implant bone formation. The combination treatment of insulin and berberine was more effective than each administrated as a monotherapy. These results suggest that berberine combined with insulin could promote osseointegration in diabetic rats, thereby highlighting its potential application to patients, though further studies are needed.

1. Introduction

"Osseointegration" refers to the formation process of a direct interface between an implant and living bone [1]. Thereafter, implant has been extensively studied and widely used in clinics to replace missing teeth and restore oral functions. However, many systemic diseases such as osteoporosis, diabetes, and autoimmune diseases may interfere with the implant osseointegration in clinical practice [2]. Studies have shown that diabetes caused a higher failure rate of implants and poorer bone implant integration [3, 4]. Type 2 diabetes mellitus (T2DM), the most common form of diabetes mellitus, is a metabolic disorder characterized by hyperglycemia resulting from peripheral insulin resistance with defective insulin secretion. T2DM is also associated with systemic chronic progressive disorders in kidneys, nerves, blood vessels, bones, and other tissues, which can lead to diminished immune response and increased inflammatory effect [5, 6]. Also, substances such as advanced glycation end products (AGEs) and cytokines have deleterious effects on osteoblasts and the bone marrow microenvironment [7]. All of the systemic changes above would impair the osseointegration, as well as the long-term function of dental implants.

It is accepted that survival of implant can be improved when plasma glucose level is brought under control [8]. However, others admit that insulin alone is insufficient to reverse all the negative impact of diabetes on bone healing, with impaired bone implant integration in both animal models and patients [9–11]. One explanation may be the impossibility of continuously monitoring glucose and automatically adjusting insulin delivery; another important reason may lie in insulin resistance. Hence, there is a considerable interest in seeking complementary and alternative approaches in improving implant success in diabetes, especially orally available drugs which could mimic insulin action and somehow overcome insulin resistance [12].

Berberine (BBR, $C_{20}H_{18}NO_4$) is an isoquinoline alkaloid purified from herbal plants including *Coptis chinensis*, *Hydrastis canadensis*, and *Berberis aquifolium* [13]. This naturally occurring molecule displays a broad array of pharmacological effects beneficial to a number of diseases. For example, it has been used as a nonprescription drug for treating infectious diseases like diarrhea in Asia for centuries. The hypoglycemic effect of berberine was first discovered in 1988 by accident when diabetic patients were found to have lowered serum glucose level with berberine playing its antidiarrheal role [14]. Thereafter, more studies have shown that berberine could potently augment glucose uptake into adipose and muscle tissues through multiple mechanisms, including insulin-dependent PTP1B, insulin-independent AMPK, increasing the affinity of low-activity glucose transporters (gluT1), and improving insulin sensitivity [15–17]. In STZ-induced diabetic rats, berberine potently lowered rats fasting blood glucose levels and improved oral glucose tolerance. Additionally, berberine also lowered multiple factors related to insulin resistance including blood cholesterol and triacylglycerols levels [18]. In diabetic patients, the hypoglycemic effect of berberine was similar to that of metformin [19]. In another aspect, berberine has been reported to promote osteogenic differentiation of bone marrow-derived mesenchymal stem cells (MSCs) through canonical Wnt/β-catenin signaling [20]. Also, osteogenic genes expression, including *osteopontin*, *osteocalcin*, and *Runx2* (Runt-related transcription factor 2), was upregulated in osteoblasts by berberine [21]. Furthermore, berberine inhibited osteoclasts activity through suppressing the NF-kappaB and Akt pathways [22, 23]. In vivo, osteoporosis in both glucocorticoid-induced rat model and senescence accelerated mice P6 (SAMP6) was prevented by berberine [24, 25]. Since functions of berberine in glucose homeostasis, insulin sensitizing, and bone anabolism are closely related to the promotion of bone formation in diabetic patients, we therefore hypothesize that berberine alone and in combination with insulin therapy may be beneficial to the implant osseointegration in T2DM. The combination therapy seems to be more promising for the different and complementary mechanisms of action of berberin and insulin.

2. Experimental Section

2.1. Experimental Implants.
The implants were provided by Professor Liu Xiaoguang (the National Engineering Research Center of Biomaterials, Sichuan University, Chengdu, China). The cp-Ti implants are 4 mm in length and 1 mm in diameter with machined surface. All implants were washed with deionized water in the ultrasonic bath and sterilized in an autoclave before surgery.

2.2. Experimental Animals.
This experiment protocol was approved by the Animal Research Bioethics Committee of Sichuan University and was conducted following the international animal welfare standards. A total of 50 male Sprague-Dawley (SD) rats, provided by the Experimental Animal Center at Sichuan University, were selected for study. They were 8 weeks of age, weighing around 190 g. Every two rats were housed in each cage in a 12-hour day/night cycle and had free access to water and rat normal pellet diet (NPD, DaShuo Laboratory Animal Co., Ltd., Chengdu, China).

After 1 week of acclimation (start of the study), the rats were randomly assigned into 5 groups ($n = 10$ per group): (1) healthy rats without treatment (Group HC); (2) diabetic rats without treatment (Group D); (3) diabetic rats treated with insulin (Group I); (4) diabetic rats treated with berberine (Group B); (5) diabetic rats treated with both insulin and berberine (Group IB). Type 2 diabetes rat model was built according to the combination of high-fat diet-fed and low-dose streptozotocin-treatment method [26]. Four diabetic groups were fed with high-fat diet (HFD, 58% total kcal of fat, 25% of protein, and 17% of carbohydrate) while Group HC were continually fed with NPD. After 2 weeks of dietary manipulation, the high-fat diet rats (i.e., Groups D, I, B, and IB) were given intraperitoneally 35 mg/kg freshly prepared streptozotocin (STZ, Sigma, St. Louis, MO, USA), while the healthy control rats (Group HC) were injected with 1 mL of vehicle citrate buffer (pH 4.4). The plasma glucose levels (PGLs) were measured 72 hours after the STZ administration and rats with nonfasting PGLs higher than 16.7 mmol/L threshold were considered to be diabetic and chosen for further studies. All the rats were continually fed on their respective diets until being sacrificed.

2.3. Implant Surgery.
After diabetic rat model establishment (0 days), animals were anesthetized intraperitoneally (10% chloral hydrate, 3 mL/kg). The surgical area was shaved and disinfected with 75% ethanol. Then, the implant bed was prepared by standardized drilling procedure with saline irrigation [27], followed by inserting the implant perpendicularly to the long axis of the right tibia in distal tibia metaphysis (2 mm distal to the proximal growth plate) (Figure 1). After surgery, the skins were carefully and separately sutured to ensure the submerged healing of implants with no functional loading. All animals received the intramuscular antibiotic prophylaxis in the first three days after surgery.

2.4. Pharmaceutical Treatment.
Group I rats received a daily subcutaneous injection of 1-2 UI NPH insulin (Humulin N, Lilly, Fegersheim, France) for 8 weeks according to literature review [28]. Based on prior study, Group B received daily 300 mg/kg of berberine (Sigma, St. Louis, MO, USA) dissolved in 0.5% carboxymethyl cellulose via oral gavage [29]. Group IB received insulin and berberine with doses and methods similar to those of Groups I and B. Group HC received a daily gavage of saline solution. A summary of the animal grouping and treatments is presented in Figure 2.

2.5. Fluorochrome Double-Labeling.
Two fluorochromes were injected sequentially: alizarin red (25 mg/kg/im, Sigma, St. Louis, MO, USA) at 1 week after surgery and calcein green (30 mg/kg/im, Sigma, St. Louis, MO, USA) at 7 weeks after surgery. Both fluorochrome labels could bind to the sites of active bone deposition shortly after injection. This enabled

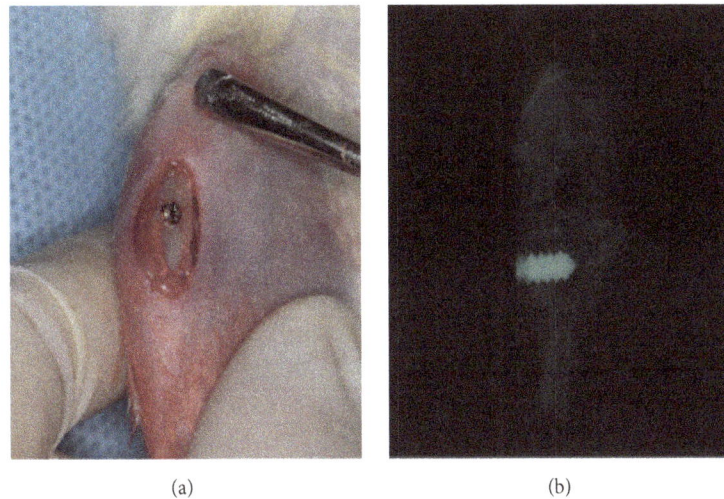

(a)   (b)

FIGURE 1: Implant surgery and postsurgery radiograph. (a) The implant was placed into the hole prepared in the tibia metaphysis. (b) Radiograph of tibia with implant after surgery.

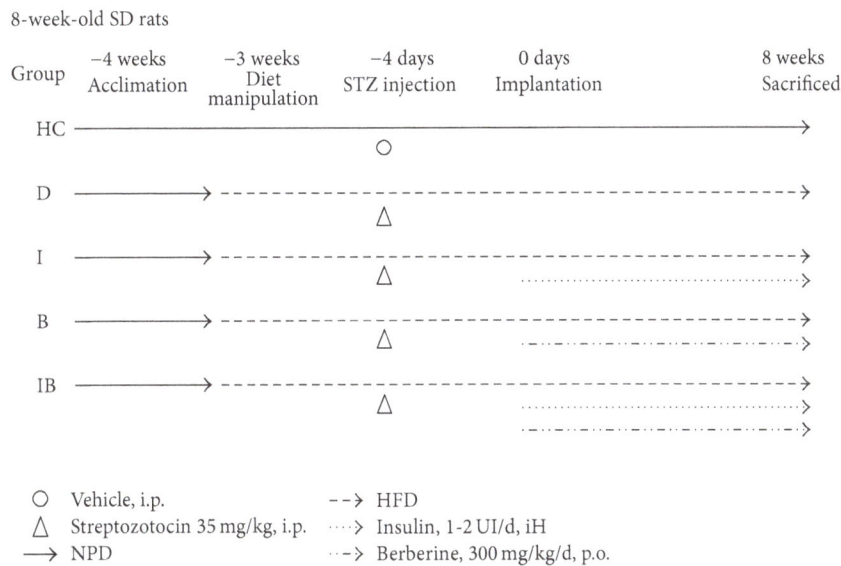

FIGURE 2: Summary of animal grouping and treatments. Animals were randomly allocated into five groups: healthy rats as control (HC) and 4 groups of diabetic rats including (1) no additional treatment, (2) insulin, (3) berberine, and (4) berberine + insulin therapies; the treatments were given to animals for 8 weeks until being sacrificed.

the identification of bone deposition around implants at different time points.

2.6. Measuring of Blood Glucose and Body Weight.
Blood samples were randomly obtained from the animals by tail snipping, with plasma glucose levels (PGLs) measuring by an Accu-Chek glucose meter (Roche Diagnostics, Laval, QC, Canada). PGLs and body weights of the rats ($n = 10$ specimens per group) were measured at −3 weeks, 0 days, 1 week, 4 weeks, and 8 weeks, respectively.

2.7. Serum Biochemical Assays.
All the animals were sacrificed 8 weeks after surgery with a lethal dose of pentobarbital.

Blood samples ($n = 10$ specimens per group) were collected at the time of sacrifice and analyzed for serum alkaline phosphatase (ALP) and bone gamma-carboxyglutamic acid-containing (also known as osteocalcin) protein (BGP). Serum values of BGP were measured by rat osteocalcin Enzyme-Linked Immunosorbent Assay (ELISA) Kit (DRG International Inc., NJ, USA). ALP activity was analyzed using a pNPP Alkaline Phosphatase Assay Kit (AnaSpec Inc., CA, USA).

2.8. Fluorochrome Double-Labeling Analysis.
The tibias with implants ($n = 10$ specimens per group) were harvested after the removal of soft tissue and maintained in a 4% neutral-buffered solution of formalin at 4°C for fixation.

TABLE 1: Plasma glucose levels (mmol/L) of rats during the whole study.

Animal status	−3 weeks	0 days	1 week	4 weeks	8 weeks
Group HC	5.8 ± 0.7^1	6.4 ± 0.8^1	6.3 ± 0.8^1	6.6 ± 0.8^1	6.7 ± 0.7^1
Group D	6.2 ± 0.7^1	27.1 ± 2.2^2	24.0 ± 2.4^5	29.1 ± 1.9^3	25.4 ± 1.2^3
Group I	6.1 ± 0.8^1	26.8 ± 3.0^2	11.2 ± 1.8^3	8.7 ± 1.2^1	7.1 ± 0.6^1
Group B	6.2 ± 0.7^1	26.8 ± 3.7^2	20.1 ± 1.6^4	17.5 ± 2.2^2	11.2 ± 1.3^2
Group IB	6.3 ± 0.6^1	24.4 ± 1.4^2	8.7 ± 1.7^2	6.4 ± 1.2^1	6.7 ± 0.9^1

Means with identical superscripts in a given column are not statistically significant at the 5% alpha level.

TABLE 2: Weights (g) of rats during the whole study.

Animal status	−3 weeks	0 days	1 week	4 weeks	8 weeks
Group HC	207 ± 2.8^1	262 ± 21.9^1	275 ± 20.3^1	344 ± 19.7^2	424 ± 20.0^3
Group D	212 ± 2.9^1	314 ± 15.4^2	291 ± 13.8^1	289 ± 18.4^1	267 ± 18.1^1
Group I	209 ± 3.9^1	323 ± 30.1^2	301 ± 19.5^1	308 ± 23.4^2	374 ± 30.6^2
Group B	212 ± 5.3^1	314 ± 29.4^2	302 ± 25.4^1	284 ± 28.9^1	277 ± 27.7^1
Group IB	210 ± 3.9^1	317 ± 20.7^2	307 ± 26.8^1	313 ± 30.0^2	397 ± 27.9^2

Means with identical superscripts in a given column are not statistically significant at the 5% alpha level.

The specimens were dehydrated in an ascending series of alcohol concentrations and embedded with methyl methacrylate. Afterwards, the samples were sectioned along the longitudinal direction of the implant by a rotary diamond saw (SP1600/2600, Leica, Nussloch, Germany) and each tibia specimen could get 3 to 4 slides, which were ground to a final thickness of approximately 30 μm by a microtome (Leica SP2600 Ultramiller, Nussloch, Germany). The slides were first observed under a Nikon Eclipse 300 fluorescence microscope (Compix Inc., Sewickley, PA, USA) to determine the mineral apposition at different time points.

2.9. Histomorphological Analysis. After the labeling analysis, the slides with section through the central part of screw in each tibia specimen were selected and stained with 1% toluidine blue (n = 10 slides per group). Images were captured through a microscope (DXM 1200, Nikon, Tokyo, Japan) and evaluated using a computerized image analyzer (Image Pro Plus V6.0, Media Cybernetics, Bethesda, MD, USA). Values of bone-to-implant contact ratio (BIC, the percentage of linear surface of the implant directly contacted by mineralized bone) were measured along the whole implant surface and bone area fraction occupancy (BAFO, the percentage of bone filling the spaces between implant threads) was evaluated in the spaces within the whole implant threads [30].

2.10. Statistical Analysis. All of the experiments were repeated three times, and means ± SDs (standard deviations) were calculated for each array of treatments for preliminary numerical comparisons. Intergroup differences were first analyzed using one-way ANOVA followed by Fisher's Least Significant Difference (LSD) post hoc tests at a significance level of α = 0.05. All data was analyzed with SPSS 19.0 software (SPSS, Inc., Chicago, USA).

3. Results

At 8 weeks postoperatively, all the surgery sites showed adequate healing, with no implant loss or infection.

3.1. Plasma Glucose Levels. Plasma glucose levels were presented in Table 1. Before STZ administration, the average of PGLs in each treatment group ranged from 5.8 to 6.3 mmol/L, considered to be normal in this study. After STZ administration, PGLs in the diabetic rats showed a significant increase. After treatment, both insulin and/or berberine effectively lowered the PGLs. At the end of the study, Groups I and IB had PGLs restored to their prestudy levels. Berberine moderately lowered PGLs to 11.2 mmol/L.

3.2. Body Weight. Table 2 shows the fluctuation of animal weights. After diet manipulation, animals fed with HFD weighed significantly greater than those fed with NPD ($P < 0.05$). However, the induction of diabetes caused a rapid loss of weights. At the end of study, DM rats in Groups I and IB gained weight; nevertheless, rats in Groups D and B continued to lose weight.

3.3. Plasma Levels of BGP and ALP. Figure 3 showed that, after 8 weeks, insulin and/or berberine substantially increased the plasma BGP levels compared to that of Group D. Moreover, the plasma BGP levels in Group IB were significantly higher than that in Group HC ($P < 0.05$). As for the plasma ALP levels, the values in Groups B and IB seem to be higher than Group D; the differences were not significant ($P > 0.05$).

3.4. Fluorescence Observations. Figure 4 showed mineral appositions around the implant, which was determined by fluorochrome double-labeling. The areas in green or red

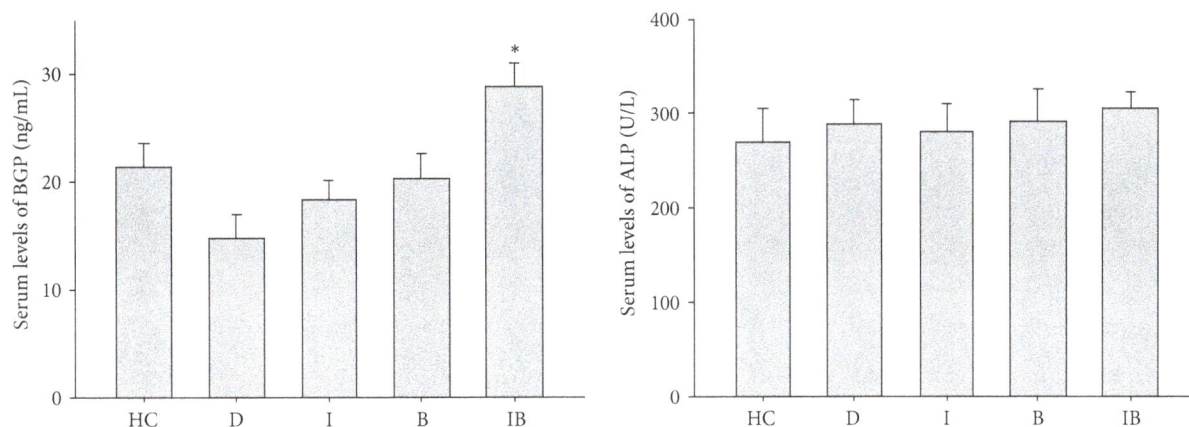

FIGURE 3: Plasma BGP and ALP levels at 8 weeks after implantation. $^{*}P < 0.05$, for Group HC versus Group IB.

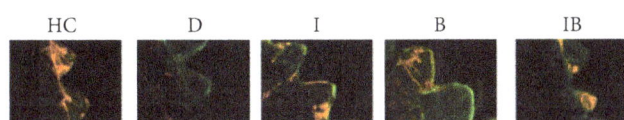

FIGURE 4: Fluorochrome double-labeling images of peri-implant osseointegration under microscopy at 10x (HC: healthy control; D: nontreated diabetic; I: insulin-treated diabetic; B: berberine-treated diabetic; IB: berberine + insulin-treated diabetic). Red was labeled by alizarin red at week 1 after surgery and green was labeled by calcein green at week 7 after surgery.

represented regions of calcium precipitation labeled by fluorochromes during the healing phases: red being at week 1 and green at week 7 after surgery. All groups but the diabetic exhibited obvious red labeling: larger scales of red labeling were observed in Groups HC and IB, whereas only a few red spots were observed in Group D. In addition, only faint green labeling was observed in all groups.

3.5. Histomorphometric Analyses. Figure 5(a) showed bone formation around implants. Comparison of bone filling the spaces between threads: there was the least osseointegration (discontinuance bone, minor direct contact) in Group D and the most osseointegration (mostly lamellar bone, dense and well organized, major contact) in Groups HC and IB. In quantitative analysis (Figures 5(b) and 5(c)), insulin increased BIC 1.7-fold and BAFO 1.3-fold compared with Group D. Berberine increased BIC 1.3-fold and slightly increased BAFO. The BIC and BAFO were successfully restored to normal level after insulin and berberine combined treatment (no significant differences compared with those of Group HC ($P > 0.05$)).

4. Discussion

Diabetes mellitus has been widely studied for its influence on bone healing and remodeling and is shown to be detrimental to dental implants osseointegration. Consistent with previous studies [11], impaired new bone formation (little

fluorochrome labeling) and poor osseointegration (decreased BIC and BAFO values) were observed in the untreated diabetic rats.

Previous studies have mainly discussed application of insulin to control serum glucose and improve implant osseointegration. However, the effects remained controversial due to the heterogeneity of diabetic models and the methodologies of insulin therapy used in their studies. The diabetic rat model in this study was induced by two steps: first, high-fat chow feeding to induce obesity, compensatory hyperinsulinemia, and insulin resistance, and second, the administration of low-dose STZ to destroy a part of pancreatic beta cells, leading to a reduction of insulin in serum and causing hyperglycemia. This STZ model is a widely used model in type 2 diabetic research that replicates metabolic characteristics of the human syndrome [26]. In this study, the changes of plasma glucose levels and weight substantiated onset of diabetic symptoms. The rats in Group D had significantly higher PGLs and increased body weight loss. The diabetic animals treated by insulin had their PGLs gradually restored to the normal range, indicating continuous regulation of plasma glucose levels in this study, which would avoid the major side effect of hypoglycemia usually seen in an intensive insulin therapy [31]. In fact, the fear of hypoglycemia commonly complicated the effective glycemic control both in patients and in physicians [32]. In this study, insulin only moderately increased BIC and BAFO, which were not comparable to the healthy controls. This might contribute to the fact that the body cells could not use insulin effectively due to insulin resistance (defects in insulin-related signaling). Our study showed that insulin could not counterbalance all the negative changes caused by diabetes, which was in agreement with former studies showing that the BIC and removal torque were significantly lower compared to the healthy controls [9, 10].

Berberine has been recently reported for its dual functions in boosting bone remodeling and maintaining glucose homeostasis. Consistent with previous observations, the administration of berberine alone could effectively lower PGL but failed to restore it to the normal level [18]. The explanation might be that although berberine could activate

(a)

(b)

(c)

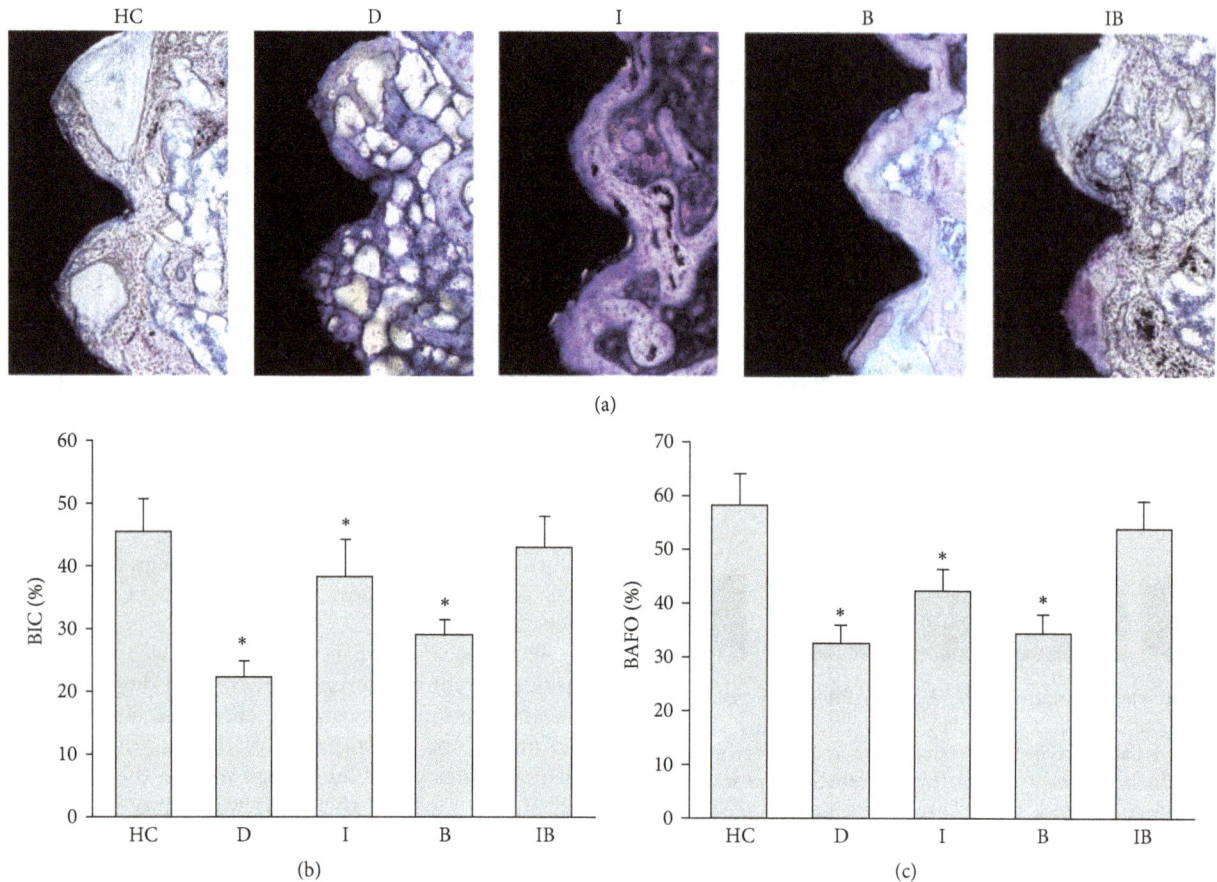

FIGURE 5: Histological images and quantitative analysis of implants 8 weeks after surgery by toluidine blue staining (10x). (a) HC: healthy control; D: nontreated diabetic; I: insulin-treated diabetic; B: berberine-treated diabetic; IB: berberine + insulin-treated diabetic. (b) Bone-to-implant contact ratio. (c) Bone area fraction occupancy ratio. Data are expressed as mean $\pm$ SD, $n = 10$. $^*P < 0.05$, for healthy control rats versus others.

both insulin and AMPK signaling to increase glucose uptake, it could not alter the insulin secretion and synthesis therefore did not reverse total insulin reduction caused by destroyed pancreas beta cells [33]. This incomplete control of hyperglycemia may further explain weaker promotion of berberine on osseointegration compared with insulin. Interestingly, no weight gains were observed in Group B though PGLs were reduced, implying that berberine might have weaker or delayed regulation on body energy homeostasis compared to its effect on glucose modulation.

We further investigated the effect of berberine and insulin combined treatment on implant osseointegration and whether the effect is additive. As is shown in PGLs result, berberine together with insulin treatment successfully corrected PGLs after 4 weeks. Furthermore, values of BIC and BAFO in Group IB increased and were equivalent to those observed in Group HC. As ALP and BGP secreted by osteoblasts are associated with early and subsequent bone formation stages [34, 35], serum measurement of these two biomarkers in correlation with histological assessments of osseointegration can provide important information about the influence of the treatment on bone metabolism. The serum total ALP level in Groups B and IB was higher than

that of Group D, while the difference was not significant ($P > 0.05$). Interestingly, the correlation between serum ALP levels and localized osseointegration was not reflected. This might be due to the fact that alkaline phosphates are secreted by various sources including nonskeletal tissues, such as liver, intestine, and spleen. We also found significantly increased serum BGP levels in Groups I, B, and IB, with the highest value in Group IB. Taken together, the corrected PGLs, improved osseointegration, and highest levels of BGP in Group IB suggest that berberine in combination with insulin may lead to an additive or synergistic effect on glycemic control and bone activity. The improved osseointegration might be attributed to multiple factors mainly including corrected hyperglycemia, enhanced bone formation, and inhibited bone resorption: (1) abnormality in insulin receptor (InsR) is the major cause for the development of insulin resistance and type 2 diabetes mellitus. Berberine mimics insulin action and attenuates insulin resistance by increasing IR phosphorylation [15]. Therefore, when applied together, berberine and insulin may have additive effect in glucose uptake. (2) Berberine has potent antioxidant effects in reducing protein damage, DNA stand breaking, and inflammatory markers level in diabetic rats, which is beneficial for maintaining a suitable environment for bone healing [36, 37]. (3) Berberine decreases the level of bone loss by inhibiting osteoclasts formation and differentiation [22].

With the steady increase of diabetes patients, therapies that promote higher clinical efficiency and shorter rehabilitation duration are of great urgency in dental implant treatment. This study took advantage of the multiple functions of berberine in glucose homeostasis, insulin sensitizing, and bone anabolism, which are closely related to the promotion of bone formation in diabetic patients. We found that a combination of insulin and berberine (two existing drugs) seemed to be more effective than each applied alone, which may be because of their different and complementary mechanisms of action. Admittedly, differences of development and characterization could exist between the tibia and jaw. Further analysis at the cellular and molecular levels is also helpful to elucidate the intrinsic mechanism of action of the combination therapy. Also, modifying the chemistry of berberine to enhance its properties in glucose homeostasis and bone anabolism may also be encouraged.

Conflict of Interests

The authors declare that there is no conflict of interests regarding the publication of this paper.

Acknowledgments

This study was supported by a grant from the National Natural Science Foundation of China 81000455 (Chen Wenchuan) and Sichuan University. Supports provided by Drs. Ga Liao and Ning Ji of the State Key Laboratory of Oral Diseases at Sichuan University are greatly appreciated.

References

[1] P.-I. Brånemark, U. Breine, R. Adell, B. O. Hansson, J. Lindström, and A. Ohlsson, "Intra-osseous anchorage of dental prostheses. I. Experimental studies," *Scandinavian Journal of Plastic and Reconstructive Surgery and Hand Surgery*, vol. 3, no. 2, pp. 81–100, 1969.

[2] A. Mombelli and N. Cionca, "Systemic diseases affecting osseointegration therapy," *Clinical Oral Implants Research*, vol. 17, supplement 2, pp. 97–103, 2006.

[3] F. Marchand, A. Raskin, A. Dionnes-Hornes et al., "Dental implants and diabetes: conditions for success," *Diabetes and Metabolism*, vol. 38, no. 1, pp. 14–19, 2012.

[4] F. Wang, Y.-L. Song, D.-H. Li et al., "Type 2 diabetes mellitus impairs bone healing of dental implants in GK rats," *Diabetes Research and Clinical Practice*, vol. 88, no. 1, pp. e7–e9, 2010.

[5] M. A. Pfeffer, E. A. Burdmann, C.-Y. Chen et al., "A trial of darbepoetin alfa in type 2 diabetes and chronic kidney disease," *New England Journal of Medicine*, vol. 361, no. 21, pp. 2019–2032, 2009.

[6] J. H. DeVries, "Therapies for type 2 diabetes and coronary artery disease," *The New England Journal of Medicine*, vol. 361, no. 14, pp. 1408–1409, 2009.

[7] M. J. Tolosa, S. R. Chuguransky, C. Sedlinsky et al., "Insulin-deficient diabetes-induced bone microarchitecture alterations are associated with a decrease in the osteogenic potential of bone marrow progenitor cells: preventive effects of metformin," *Diabetes Research and Clinical Practice*, vol. 101, no. 2, pp. 177–186, 2013.

[8] F. Javed and G. E. Romanos, "Impact of diabetes mellitus and glycemic control on the osseointegration of dental implants: a systematic literature review," *Journal of Periodontology*, vol. 80, no. 11, pp. 1719–1730, 2009.

[9] R. Margonar, C. E. Sakakura, M. Holzhausen, M. T. Pepato, J. R. C. Alba, and J. E. Marcantonio, "The influence of diabetes mellitus and insulin therapy on biomechanical retention around dental implants: a study in rabbits," *Implant Dentistry*, vol. 12, no. 4, pp. 333–339, 2003.

[10] B. Wang, Y. Song, F. Wang et al., "Effects of local infiltration of insulin around titanium implants in diabetic rats," *British Journal of Oral and Maxillofacial Surgery*, vol. 49, no. 3, pp. 225–229, 2011.

[11] S. Kotsovilis, I. K. Karoussis, and I. Fourmousis, "A comprehensive and critical review of dental implant placement in diabetic animals and patients," *Clinical Oral Implants Research*, vol. 17, no. 5, pp. 587–599, 2006.

[12] M. Eddouks, A. Bidi, B. El Bouhali, L. Hajji, and N. A. Zeggwagh, "Antidiabetic plants improving insulin sensitivity," *Journal of Pharmacy and Pharmacology*, vol. 66, no. 9, pp. 1197–1214, 2014.

[13] Y. Liu, L. Zhang, H. Song, and G. Ji, "Update on berberine in nonalcoholic fatty liver disease," *Evidence-Based Complementary and Alternative Medicine*, vol. 2013, Article ID 308134, 8 pages, 2013.

[14] Y. X. Ni, "Therapeutic effect of berberine on 60 patients with type II diabetes mellitus and experimental research," *Zhong Xi Yi Jie He Za Zhi*, vol. 8, no. 12, Article ID 707, pp. 711–713, 1988.

[15] C. Chen, Y. Zhang, and C. Huang, "Berberine inhibits PTP1B activity and mimics insulin action," *Biochemical and Biophysical Research Communications*, vol. 397, no. 3, pp. 543–547, 2010.

[16] A. Cok, C. Plaisier, M. J. Salie, D. S. Oram, J. Chenge, and L. L. Louters, "Berberine acutely activates the glucose transport activity of GLUT1," *Biochimie*, vol. 93, no. 7, pp. 1187–1192, 2011.

[17] P. Yi, F.-E. Lu, L.-J. Xu, G. Chen, H. Dong, and K.-F. Wang, "Berberine reverses free-fatty-acid-induced insulin resistance in 3T3-L1 adipocytes through targeting IKKβ," *World Journal of Gastroenterology*, vol. 14, no. 6, pp. 876–883, 2008.

[18] Y. Chen, Y. Wang, J. Zhang, C. Sun, and A. Lopez, "Berberine improves glucose homeostasis in streptozotocin-induced diabetic rats in association with multiple factors of insulin resistance," *ISRN Endocrinology*, vol. 2011, Article ID 519371, 8 pages, 2011.

[19] J. Yin, H. Xing, and J. Ye, "Efficacy of berberine in patients with type 2 diabetes mellitus," *Metabolism: Clinical and Experimental*, vol. 57, no. 5, pp. 712–717, 2008.

[20] K. Tao, D. Xiao, J. Weng, A. Xiong, B. Kang, and H. Zeng, "Berberine promotes bone marrow-derived mesenchymal stem cells osteogenic differentiation via canonical Wnt/β-catenin signaling pathway," *Toxicology Letters*, vol. 240, no. 1, pp. 68–80, 2016.

[21] H. W. Lee, J. H. Suh, H. N. Kim et al., "Berberine promotes osteoblast differentiation by Runx2 activation with p38 MAPK," *Journal of Bone and Mineral Research*, vol. 23, no. 8, pp. 1227–1237, 2008.

[22] P. Wei, L. Jiao, L.-P. Qin, F. Yan, T. Han, and Q.-Y. Zhang, "Effects of berberine on differentiation and bone resorption of

osteoclasts derived from rat bone marrow cells," *Zhong Xi Yi Jie He Xue Bao*, vol. 7, no. 4, pp. 342–348, 2009.

[23] J.-P. Hu, K. Nishishita, E. Sakai et al., "Berberine inhibits RANKL-induced osteoclast formation and survival through suppressing the NF-kappaB and Akt pathways," *European Journal of Pharmacology*, vol. 580, no. 1-2, pp. 70–79, 2008.

[24] D. Xu, W. Yang, C. Zhou, Y. Liu, and B. Xu, "Preventive effects of berberine on glucocorticoid-induced osteoporosis in rats," *Planta Medica*, vol. 76, no. 16, pp. 1809–1813, 2010.

[25] H. Li, T. Miyahara, Y. Tezuka, Q. Le Tran, H. Seto, and S. Kadota, "Effect of berberine on bone mineral density in SAMP6 as a senile osteoporosis model," *Biological and Pharmaceutical Bulletin*, vol. 26, no. 1, pp. 110–111, 2003.

[26] K. Srinivasan, B. Viswanad, L. Asrat, C. L. Kaul, and P. Ramarao, "Combination of high-fat diet-fed and low-dose streptozotocin-treated rat: a model for type 2 diabetes and pharmacological screening," *Pharmacological Research*, vol. 52, no. 4, pp. 313–320, 2005.

[27] R. P. Guimarães, P. A. D. de Oliveira, and A. M. S. D. Oliveira, "Effects of induced diabetes and the administration of aminoguanidine in the biomechanical retention of implants: a study in rats," *Journal of Periodontal Research*, vol. 46, no. 6, pp. 691–696, 2011.

[28] J. T. Siqueira, S. C. Cavalher-Machado, V. E. Arana-Chavez, and P. Sannomiya, "Bone formation around titanium implants in the rat tibia: role of insulin," *Implant dentistry*, vol. 12, no. 3, pp. 242–251, 2003.

[29] T. Lu, Y. Liang, J. Song, L. Xie, G. J. Wang, and X. D. Liu, "Simultaneous determination of berberine and palmatine in rat plasma by HPLC-ESI-MS after oral administration of traditional Chinese medicinal preparation Huang-Lian-Jie-Du decoction and the pharmacokinetic application of the method," *Journal of Pharmaceutical and Biomedical Analysis*, vol. 40, no. 5, pp. 1218–1224, 2006.

[30] Y. Gao, E. Luo, J. Hu, J. Xue, S. Zhu, and J. Li, "Effect of combined local treatment with zoledronic acid and basic fibroblast growth factor on implant fixation in ovariectomized rats," *Bone*, vol. 44, no. 2, pp. 225–232, 2009.

[31] E. C. McNay, J. A. Teske, C. M. Kotz et al., "Long-term, intermittent, insulin-induced hypoglycemia produces marked obesity without hyperphagia or insulin resistance: a model for weight gain with intensive insulin therapy," *American Journal of Physiology—Endocrinology and Metabolism*, vol. 304, no. 2, pp. E131–E138, 2013.

[32] S. A. Ross, H. D. Tildesley, and J. Ashkenas, "Barriers to effective insulin treatment: the persistence of poor glycemic control in type 2 diabetes," *Current Medical Research and Opinion*, vol. 27, supplement 3, pp. 13–20, 2011.

[33] J. Zhou, S. Zhou, J. Tang et al., "Protective effect of berberine on beta cells in streptozotocin- and high-carbohydrate/high-fat diet-induced diabetic rats," *European Journal of Pharmacology*, vol. 606, no. 1-3, pp. 262–268, 2009.

[34] Z. Du, J. Chen, F. Yan, N. Doan, S. Ivanovski, and Y. Xiao, "Serum bone formation marker correlation with improved osseointegration in osteoporotic rats treated with simvastatin," *Clinical Oral Implants Research*, vol. 24, no. 4, pp. 422–427, 2013.

[35] F. J. de Paula and C. J. Rosen, "Bone remodeling and energy metabolism: new perspectives," *Bone Research*, vol. 1, no. 1, pp. 72–84, 2013.

[36] W. Liu, P. Liu, S. Tao et al., "Berberine inhibits aldose reductase and oxidative stress in rat mesangial cells cultured under high glucose," *Archives of Biochemistry and Biophysics*, vol. 475, no. 2, pp. 128–134, 2008.

[37] J.-Y. Zhou and S.-W. Zhou, "Protective effect of berberine on antioxidant enzymes and positive transcription elongation factor b expression in diabetic rat liver," *Fitoterapia*, vol. 82, no. 2, pp. 184–189, 2011.

14

Diuretic Properties and Chemical Constituent Studies on *Stauntonia brachyanthera*

Xuan Li Liu, Dan Dan Wang, Zi Hao Wang, and Da Li Meng

School of Traditional Chinese Materia Medica, Key Laboratory of Structure-Based Drug Design and Discovery (Shenyang Pharmaceutical University), Ministry of Education, Wenhua Road 103, Shenyang 110016, China

Correspondence should be addressed to Da Li Meng; mengdl@163.com

Academic Editor: Nunziatina De Tommasi

The pharmacological evaluation demonstrated that the extracts from the stem of *S. brachyanthera* could significantly increase the outputs of urine of rats compared to those of furosemide treated group, and the effect could last for a longer period of time. The best effect appeared in the first two hours, which scientifically confirmed the diuretic effect of the plant. The comparative pharmacognosy study showed that the characters of the crude drugs of the stem of *S. brachyanthera* were similar to those of *Akebia caulis*. Further systemic work on its chemical constituents by chromatographic methods and NMR elucidations led to the isolation of 10 triterpenoids, 6 flavonoids, 4 lignanoids, and 3 phenylethanoid glycosides, whose structural types were much similar to those of *A. quinata*. Among them, 7 compounds were firstly reported in the genus of *Stauntonia* and calceolarioside B was the common characteristic constituent in both plants. From the similar pharmacognosy characters, pharmacological effects, and chemical constituents, it could be concluded that *S. brachyanthera* have a great possibility to be a succedaneum of *Akebia caulis*, whose supply is extremely short in recent years.

1. Introduction

Recent studies demonstrated that the impaired renal function, hypertension, hyperkalemia, and the side-effect of immunosuppressant might lead to severe disruption of the water homeostasis, and the retention of urine flow is crucial compensatory mechanisms of water retention [1–4]. The treatments of some diseases such as ascites of liver, heart failure, edema, and glaucoma also need intakes of diuretics [5, 6]. With an aim to resist the retention of urine caused by the above factors and to find effective medicines to treat diseases mentioned above, an effective and safe diuretic agent is very necessary.

Although so many synthetic medicines were used for this purpose, natural resources medicines are still an important choice because of their higher efficiency and better safety. As we all know that China is famous for its extensive utilization of herbal medicines, among which *Akebia caulis*, a traditional Chinese medicine called Mutong by Chinese people, has been proved for its distinguished effects of diuresis, tranquilization, and promoting menstruation [7, 8] and used for thousands of years as analgesics, antiphlogistics, and diuretics to treat the diseases such as edema, stranguria, and amenorrhea [9–11]. In Chinese Pharmacopeia [12], *Akebia caulis* used to have two main resources, *Akebia quinata* (Thunb.) Decne and *Aristolochia manshuriensis* Kom. However, with the discovery of the harm of aristolochic acid, which could induce the injury of kidney, *A. manshuriensis* has been banned in China. Thus, although some alternatives including *Akebia trifoliata* (Thunb.) Koidz and *Akebia trifoliata* (Thunb.) Koidz. var. *australis* (Diels) Rehd have been applied, the supply of *Akebia caulis* is still scarce. In the current market of Chinese Materia Medica, the price of *Akebia caulis* is about 30–50 RMB/kg, which is obviously higher than a decade ago and still rising. In this situation, the discovery of a new source becomes particularly urgent.

Stauntonia brachyanthera Hand-Mazz., an evergreen shrub, is naturally growing in the southwest of China including Hunan, Guizhou, and Guangxi provinces. Just as *A. trifoliata* or *A. trifoliate*, *S. brachyanthera* also belongs to the family of Lardizabalaceae. In local areas, this plant is a main economic crop, whose fruits are not only consumed for its delicious taste, but also used as raw materials to produce beverages and vinegar [13]. Meanwhile, its seeds are utilized to extracting oil for edible purposes. In addition, *S. brachyanthera* also has its medicinal values. In Dong and Yao minorities of China, it has been used as the alternative of *Akebia caulis* for the purpose of diuresis and the treatments of inflammation, pain, and edema [14]. Besides, the constituents from *S. brachyanthera* are also proved to have antioxidant, cytotoxic [15], and hepatic protectant activities [16].

From the aspect of medicines, *S. brachyanthera* has not only the same origin as other plants of *Akebia caulis*, but also similar pharmacological effect, which has been applied in some regions. So, *S. brachyanthera* is probably the succedaneum and new resource of *Akebia caulis*. It is interesting to note that in local countryside of the southwest of China, farmers usually use the stem of *S. brachyanthera* as pipe to blow toward the fire to make the flame more exuberant when cooking. This utilization is just the folk usage of *Akebia caulis* and the origin of the name of *Akebia caulis* (Mutong, in China). So, it could be presumed that the physiologic structures of *S. brachyanthera* and *Akebia caulis* might be much alike. Therefore, in order to scientifically verify this thesis and find more effective diuretics, a serious of researches including the microscopic features, the diuretic effect and the analysis and identification of main constituents of *S. brachyanthera* were carried out. Herein, the details of these works will be discussed comprehensively.

2. Materials and Methods

2.1. Plant Material. Samples of *S. brachyanthera* were collected in Hunan by Shumo Mei, Huaihua Medical College in October 2009, and were identified by Professor Jincai Lu, School of Traditional Chinese Materia Medica, Shenyang Pharmaceutical University. A voucher specimen (number HLG-0910) was deposited in the School of Traditional Chinese Material Medica, Shenyang Pharmaceutical University.

2.2. The Preparation of Microtome Section. Dried stems of plants were boiled for 3 hours in water and then cut into 20 μm of slices. After dyeing with sarranine and red orange, the samples were mounted for further observation.

2.3. Animals and Drugs. Male albino rats of the Wistar strain, weighing approximately 220–280 g, obtained from the Experimental Animal Center of Shenyang Pharmaceutical University, Shenyang, China, were acclimatized under laboratory conditions with free access to commercial chow and water for 2 weeks. Wistar rats under *ad libitum* water conditions and fasted for 18 h prior to the start of the selection were administered with deionized water (2.5% body wt, i.g.) and their urine volume were measured after 2 h following the method of Aston [17]. Only those whose urinary outputs were more than 1% body wt can be used for the experiment.

Animals and all experiments were performed according to the approved protocols of Animal Ethics Committee, Shenyang Pharmaceutical University, China (SCXK (Liao) 2010-0001).

Furosemide was purchased from Tasly Company (Tianjin, China). 0.9% normal saline was purchased from Dubang

Company (Jilin, China). Furosemide and the extracts of *S. brachyanthera* were dissolved in normal saline.

2.4. Diuresis Study. In the diuretic experiments, animals were randomly divided into 5 groups of eight animals. The normal control group received vehicle only and the furosemide-treated groups were given furosemide (10 mg/kg body wt, i.g.). The treatment groups were intragastrically administered ESB at doses of 150, 300, and 600 mg/kg, respectively.

Wistar rats under *ad libitum* water conditions and fasted for 12 h prior to the start of the experiment were volume-expanded with 0.9% NaCl (4% body wt, i.g.) vehicle, and furosemide and different doses of ESB were administered to each group of rats, respectively, as indicated in the text. Rats were individually housed in metabolic cages, and urine volume was measured every 60 min throughout the experiment (6 h).

2.5. Extraction and Isolation of S. brachyanthera. The stems of *S. brachyanthera* were chopped into small pieces (200 mesh) and then extracted with 70% aqueous EtOH under reflux for 2 h. After evaporation of the combined EtOH extracts *in vacuo*, the resultant aqueous residues were heated into dryness to get the extracts (ESB). The 2.0 kg of ESB was suspended in water and passed through macroporous adsorptive resin (HPD-100, Cangzhou Bon Adsorber Technology Co., Ltd., Cangzhou, China) and eluted sequentially with H_2O, 40% EtOH, and 95% EtOH to afford 40% EtOH eluates (MR40) and 95% EtOH eluates (MR95), respectively.

MR40 (180 g) was chromatographed on silica gel (200–300 mesh, Qingdao Haiyang Chemical Group Corporation, Qingdao, China) column with a gradient CH_2Cl_2-MeOH system (100 : 1–0 : 100) to give nine fractions (Fr. 40A–40I). Those fractions were further purified by repeated silica gel column chromatography (CC) with PE/EtOAc and $CHCl_3$/MeOH as eluants, Sephadex LH-20 (GE Healthcare, Uppsala, Sweden) CC with MeOH as mobile phase, ODS CC (YMC-Pack-ODS, 50 μm, YMC Co. Ltd., Kyoto, Japan) eluted by MeOH/H_2O (10 : 100–100 : 80), and preparative reverse phase high pressure liquid chromatography (RP-HPLC, YMC-Pack ODS-A, 250 × 20 mm, 5 μm) to give **4** (24.7 mg) from fraction **C**, **12** (380 mg) and **18** (12.0 mg) from fraction **D**, **2** (25.0 mg), **3** (16.4 mg), **19** (14.9 mg), and **20** (21.2 mg) from fraction **E**, **8** (12.0 mg) and **7** (36.6 mg) from fraction **G**, **16** (962.5 mg) and **21** (2.1 g) from fraction **H**, and **1** (586.8 mg), **9** (23.0 mg), and **10** (1.2 g) from fraction **I**, respectively. MR95 (65 g) was also chromatographed on silica gel column with a gradient CH_2Cl_2-MeOH system (100 : 1–0 : 100) to give 6 fractions (Fr. 95A–95F). Those fractions were further purified by repeated silica gel CC with PE/EtOAc and $CHCl_3$/MeOH as eluants, Sephadex LH-20 CC with MeOH as mobile phase, and recrystallization method to give compounds **5** (15.3 mg) and **6** (61.2 mg) from fraction **B**, **13** (24.7 mg) and **17** (36.6 mg) from fraction **C**, **11** (20.1 mg) from fraction **E**, **15** (12.0 mg) from fraction **H**, and **22** (23.0 mg), **14** (16.8 mg), and **23** (32.4 mg) from fraction **I**, respectively. All chemicals and solvents used in this study were of analytical grade.

The structures of all isolated compounds were determined by NMR spectra, which were acquired using a Bruker

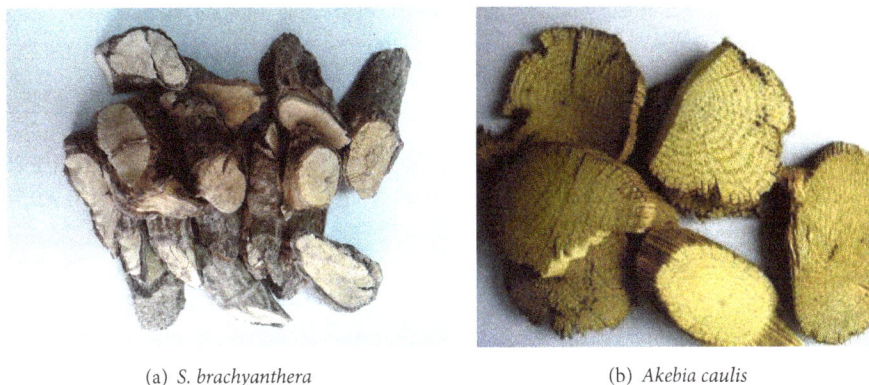

(a) *S. brachyanthera*

(b) *Akebia caulis*

FIGURE 1: The crude drugs of the stems of *S. brachyanthera* and *Akebia caulis*.

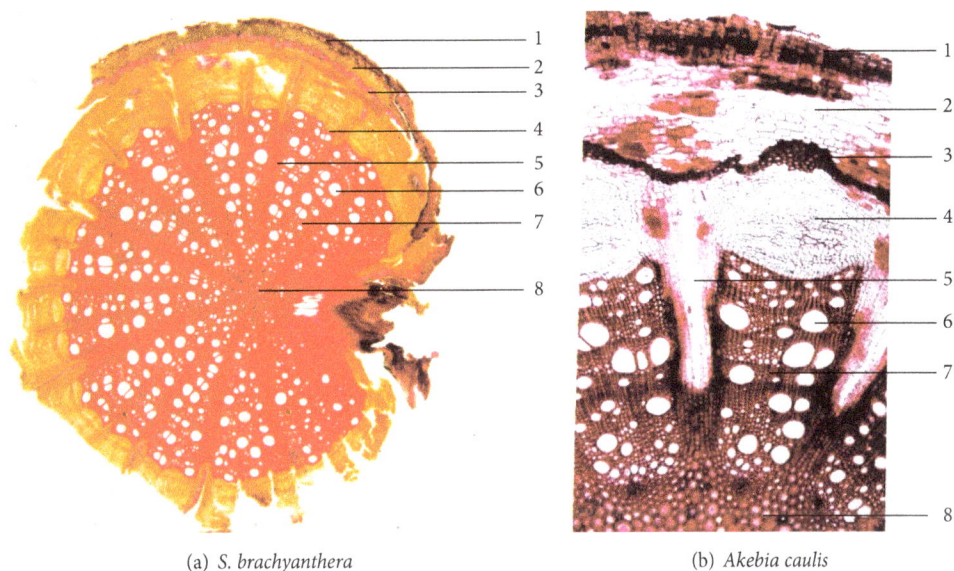

(a) *S. brachyanthera*

(b) *Akebia caulis*

FIGURE 2: Microscopic features of transverse section of stems of *S. brachyanthera* and *Akebia caulis*. 1: cork, 2: cortex, 3: stone cells, 4: phloem, 5: ray, 6: vessel, 7: xylem, and 8: cord.

ARX-300 and ARX-600. Chemical shifts (δ ppm) were relative to TMS as an internal standard.

2.6. Statistical Analysis. Values were expressed as means ± SEM. The significance of differences between means was analyzed by repeated-measure analysis of variance (ANOVA). A p value less than 0.05 was considered significant.

3. Results

3.1. Pharmacognosy Characteristics. The stem of *S. brachyanthera* (Figure 1(a)) was cylindrical with the diameter of 1~3 cm or more thick. Its surface is rough and wrinkled with many irregular furrows and lenticel-like protrusions on it. The plant is light, while the texture is compact and tough. The cortex of the stem was thick and in the color of yellowish-brown or greyish-yellow. The inner wood was also yellowish-white with small port-holes, which ensured the traverse of the air. The

yellowish-brown rays were arranged radially and the pith was also yellowish-brown and small. All of these characteristics of the appearance of the stem of *S. brachyanthera* were much alike to that of *Akebia caulis* according to our observation (Figure 1(b)) and the description in Chinese Pharmacopeia [12].

Observed from the microscope, it could be found that microscopic features of the two kinds of medicinal materials were almost the same. In the transverse section of the stem of *S. brachyanthera* (Figure 2(a)), the thick cork consisted of several layers of cells which filled with yellowish-brown contents. The phellogen consisted of 2~3 rows of tangentially elongated cells. The phelloderm was comprised of several layers of flat cells with intermittent circular belt of rounded stone cells inside. The cortex was composed of rounded parenchyma cells which were filled with yellowish-brown contents. The vascular cylinder was broad, scattered with ectophloic vascular bundle and with wavy pericyclic fiber outside. In the transverse section, it could also be found that the phloem

TABLE 1: The accumulated urine volumes of rats by treating different doses of ESB.

Substance (mg/kg)	Accumulated urine volume (mL)					
	+1 h	+2 h	+3 h	+4 h	+5 h	+6 h
None	0.55 ± 0.38	1.01 ± 0.51	1.36 ± 0.59	1.35 ± 0.58	1.49 ± 0.65	1.56 ± 0.66
ESB 150	$2.98 \pm 0.49^*$	$5.87 \pm 0.48^*$	$7.22 \pm 0.69^*$	$7.66 \pm 0.80^*$	$8.17 \pm 0.88^*$	$8.70 \pm 0.90^*$
ESB 300	$2.59 \pm 0.04^\#$	$6.36 \pm 0.37^*$	$7.38 \pm 0.41^*$	$8.18 \pm 0.51^*$	$8.61 \pm 0.54^*$	$8.99 \pm 0.54^*$
ESB 600	$2.49 \pm 0.30^\#$	$6.23 \pm 0.70^*$	$7.76 \pm 0.75^*$	$8.41 \pm 0.75^*$	$8.82 \pm 0.74^*$	$9.62 \pm 0.74^*$
Furosemide	$2.64 \pm 0.71^\#$	$5.37 \pm 0.77^*$	$6.66 \pm 0.98^*$	$7.39 \pm 1.00^*$	$7.73 \pm 1.00^*$	$8.36 \pm 1.09^*$

Data are represented as means $\pm$ SEM; number in parenthesis is the number of rats used; nd: not determined; $^\#p < 0.01$ and $^*p < 0.001$ versus control (none).

of the stem of *S. brachyanthera* was narrow, while the xylem was broad. The interfascicular cambium was indistinct and irregular shape stone cells could be observed in the outer of interfascicular cambium. The cells in the pith were thick-walled and lignified.

The similar microscopic features could also be found in the transverse section of *Akebia caulis* (Figure 2(b)), in which there were several rows of cork cells containing brown contents. The phelloderm was filled with plenty of calcium oxalate prisms. The cortex of *Akebia caulis* was composed of 6~10 rows of parenchyma cells which were filled with small prisms too. The stone cells observed from microscope were also arranged in a circular belt. The phloem was narrow. The xylem was composed of vessel, wood fiber, and parenchyma cells, whose cell walls were all lignified. And the rays of *Akebia caulis* were all primary rays [18].

3.2. Diuretic Effect of ESB on Rats.

In order to evaluate acute alterations in diuresis, a 4% body weight volume expansion was produced in all experiments. This magnitude of expansion allowed studies to be performed on the acute effect of substances that either stimulate or inhibit diuresis [19].

From the results of diuretic effects as shown in Table 1 and Figure 3, it could be found that, in the experimental conditions, furosemide (10 mg/kg) could increase the urine volume significantly compared with normal control. For example, furosemide increased urine volume from 0.55 ± 0.38 mL (normal control) to 2.64 ± 0.71 mL ($p < 0.01$) at the first hour and reached to 7.73 ± 1.00 mL ($p < 0.001$) at 5th hour compared with 1.49 ± 0.65 mL of normal control. ESB also showed similar effect as furosemide at a low dose (150 mg/kg), whose accumulated urine volume was 2.98 ± 0.49 mL ($p < 0.001$) at first hour and 8.17 ± 0.88 mL ($p < 0.001$) at 5th hour. Compared with furosemide, the diuretic effects of ESB at middle and higher doses exhibited relative stronger effects. From 2nd hour to 6th hour, for example, the accumulated urine volumes of ESB 300 mg/kg treatment group were all higher than those of furosemide treatment group, and ESB 600 mg/kg could stimulate rats' urine production at the highest level, which could be observed directly from Figure 3.

From Figure 3, it also could be found that both ESB and the furosemide could cause the increase of urine volume at the same manner. They stimulated the urine volume of rats very obviously during the first four hours, especially the first two hours. For example, the accumulated urine volume of ESB at 300 mg/kg dose was 6.36 ± 0.37 mL ($p < 0.001$)

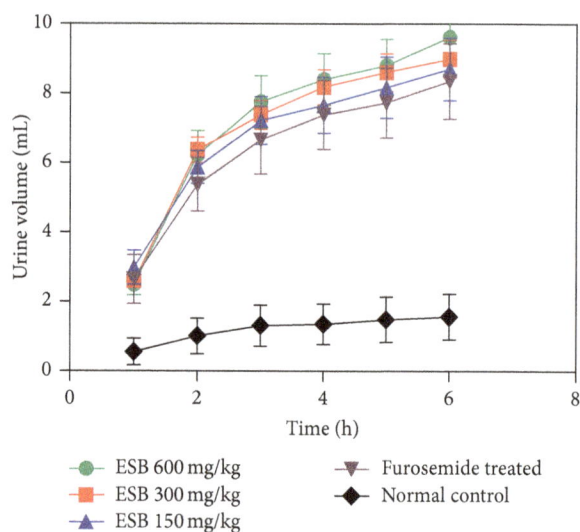

FIGURE 3: The diuretic effects of ESB on rats.

at the first hour and then reached to 8.18 ± 0.51 mL ($p < 0.001$) at the 4th hour. But from 4th hour to 5th hour, it only increased the urine volumes from and 8.18 ± 0.51 mL ($p < 0.001$) to 8.61 ± 0.54 mL ($p < 0.001$). After four hours later, the degree of the increase of urine volumes was lowered. From this result, it can be drawn that the optimal time for ESB to take effect should be the first four hours, especially the first two hours.

Although ESB could stimulate the increase of rat's urine volume at both 300 and 600 mg/kg doses, there were no obvious differences between two doses. So, from the aspect of convenience of drug administration, the optimum dose of ESB for its diuretic action should be at the 300 mg/kg body wt. In addition, it must be pointed out that ESB could continuously play pharmacological effects at all three doses after six hours later, which indicated its longer period of effecting time for the diuretic properties.

3.3. Structural Elucidation of the Chemical Constituents from *S. brachyanthera*.

The detail studies on ESB by various chromatographic methods finally lead to the isolation of 23 compounds. By comparing their ^{1}H and ^{13}C NMR data with reported values, the structures of these compounds were identified as brachyantheraoside A_4 (**1**), brachyantheraoside

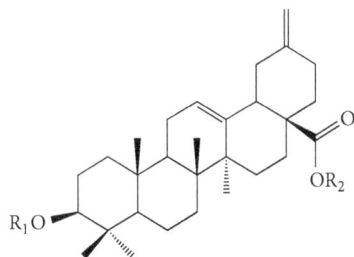

Comp. **1** $R_1 = \alpha\text{-L-ara-}(1 \to 4)\text{-}\alpha\text{-L-ara-}(1 \to 3)\text{-}\alpha\text{-L-ara-}$
        $R_2 = \alpha\text{-L-rha-}(1 \to 4)\text{-}\beta\text{-D-glc-}(1 \to 6)\text{-}\beta\text{-D-glc-}$

Comp. **2** $R_1 = \alpha\text{-L-ara-}(1 \to 3)\text{-}\alpha\text{-L-ara-}(1 \to 3)\text{-}[\beta\text{-D-xyl-}(1 \to 2)]\text{-}\alpha\text{-L-ara-}$
        $R_2 = \alpha\text{-L-rha-}(1 \to 4)\text{-}\beta\text{-D-glc-}(1 \to 6)\text{-}\beta\text{-D-glc-}$

Comp. **6** $R_1 = H$ $R_2 = H$

Comp. **7** $R_1 = \alpha\text{-L-ara-}(1 \to 3)\text{-}\alpha\text{-L-rha-}(1 \to 2)\text{-}\alpha\text{-L-ara-}$ $R_2 = \beta\text{-D-glc-}(1 \to 6)\text{-}\beta\text{-D-glc-}$

Comp. **8** $R_1 = \alpha\text{-L-ara-}(1 \to 3)\text{-}\alpha\text{-L-ara-}$ $R_2 = \alpha\text{-L-rha-}(1 \to 4)\text{-}\beta\text{-D-glc-}(1 \to 6)\text{-}\beta\text{-D-glc-}$

Comp. **9** $R_1 = \alpha\text{-L-rha-}(1 \to 2)\text{-}\alpha\text{-L-ara-}$ $R_2 = \alpha\text{-L-rha-}(1 \to 4)\text{-}\beta\text{-D-glc-}(1 \to 6)\text{-}\beta\text{-D-glc-}$

Comp. **10** $R_1 = \alpha\text{-L-ara-}$ $R_2 = \beta\text{-D-glc-}(1 \to 6)\text{-}\beta\text{-D-glc-}$

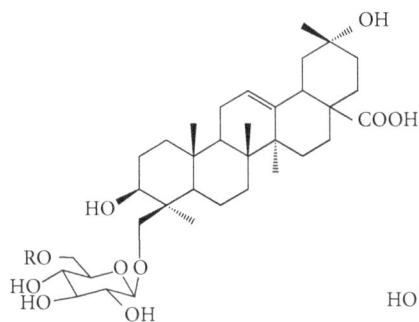

Comp. **3**   R = acetyl
Comp. **4**   R = H

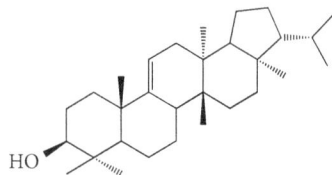

Comp. **5**

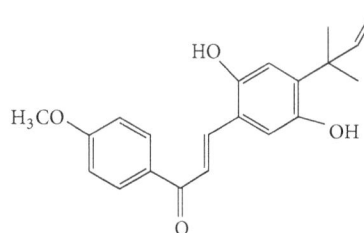

Comp. **11**

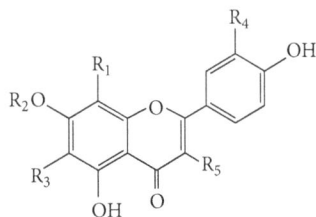

Comp. **12** $R_1 = H$ $R_2 = H$ $R_3 = H$ $R_4 = OH$ $R_5 = \text{Rha}(1 \to 6)\text{-}\beta\text{-D-glc-O-}$
Comp. **13** $R_1 = H$ $R_2 = \text{Glc}$ $R_3 = H$ $R_4 = OH$ $R_5 = H$
Comp. **14** $R_1 = H$ $R_2 = \text{Glc}$ $R_3 = \text{Glc}$ $R_4 = H$ $R_5 = H$
Comp. **15** $R_1 = \text{Glc}$ $R_2 = H$ $R_3 = H$ $R_4 = H$ $R_5 = H$
Comp. **16** $R_1 = H$ $R_2 = H$ $R_3 = H$ $R_4 = H$ $R_5 = \text{Rha}(1 \to 6)\text{-}\beta\text{-D-glc-O-}$

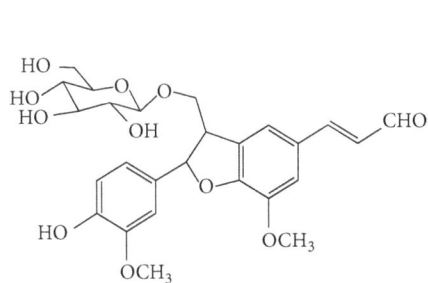

Comp. **17**

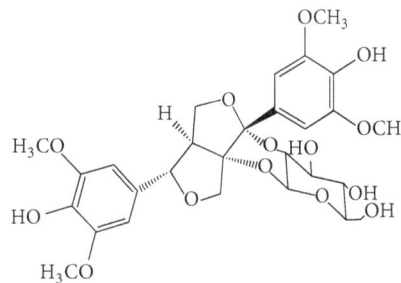

Comp. **18**

Figure 4: Continued.

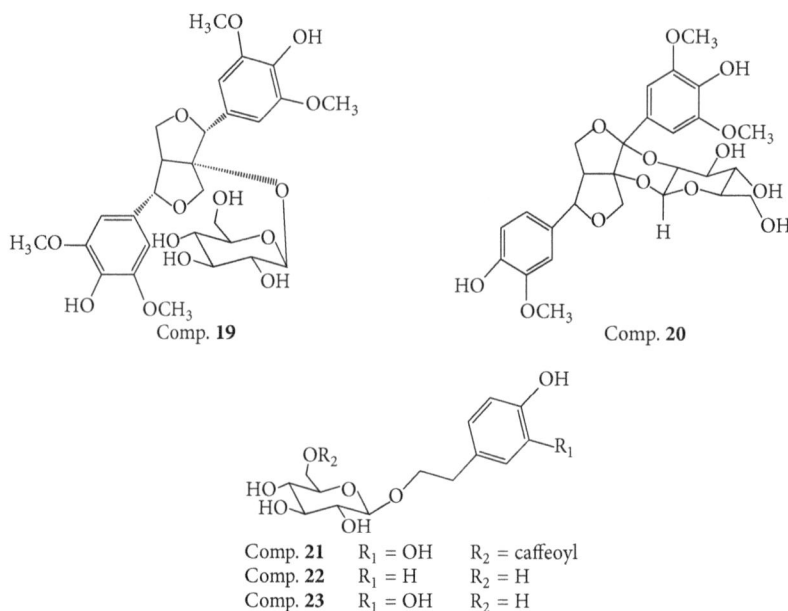

Comp. **19**

Comp. **20**

Comp. **21**   R₁ = OH   R₂ = caffeoyl
Comp. **22**   R₁ = H   R₂ = H
Comp. **23**   R₁ = OH   R₂ = H

FIGURE 4: The structures of isolated compounds from 70% EtOH extracts of S. brachyanthera.

A₅ (**2**), brachyantheraoside B₆ (**3**) [19], 3β, 20α, 24-trihydroxy-29-norolean-12-en-28-oicacid 24-O-β-D-glucopyranoside (**4**) [20], fernenol (**5**) [21], 3β-3-hydroxy-30-norolean-12, 20(29)-dien-28-oic acid (**6**) [22], yemuoside I (**7**) [23], yemuoside YM₇ (**8**), yemuoside YM₁₀ (**9**), yemuoside YM₁₁ (**10**), licochalcone A (**11**) [24], rutin (**12**) [25], luteolin-7-O-glucoside (**13**) [26], saponarin (**14**) [27], vitexin (**15**) [28], kaempferol-3-O-rutinose (**16**) [29], tortoside F (**17**) [30], brachyanin E (**18**) [15], staunoside C (**19**) [31], 7-(4-hydroxy-3-methoxyphenyl)-7′-(4′-hydroxy-3′,5′-dimethoxyphenyl)-7, 9′:7′,9-diepoxylignan-8H,8′-O-β-D-(2″,7′-epoxy)-glucopyranoside (**20**) [32], calceolarioside B (**21**) [33], 2-(4′-hydroxyphenyl)ethyl-β-D-glucopyranoside (**22**) [34], and 2-(3′,4′-dihydroxyphenyl)ethyl-β-D-glucopyranoside (**23**) [35]. Among them, compounds **5**, **6**, **7**, **11**, **12**, **16**, and **17** were firstly reported in the genus of *Stauntonia*, which not only was a breakthrough on the study of *S. brachyanthera*, but enriched the structural types of the genus. Their structures were listed in Figure 4.

4. Discussion and Conclusion

In this paper, by the comparative observation of pharmacognosy characteristics of the fork medicine, *S. brachyanthera* (Figures 1(a) and 2(a)), and the traditional Chinese medicine, *Akebia caulis* (Figures 1(b) and 2(b)), it could be found that the characters of crude drugs of the stem of *S. brachyanthera* are similar to the properties of *Akebia caulis*. The transverse sections of two plants were all presented in the form of spider's web, which marks Mutong off from other medicinal materials. As observed from microscope, it could be found that the ratios of xylem in both medicinal materials were significantly higher than the other parts, while those of core were little. Meanwhile in the xylem, there were abundant of vessels,

whose diameters were obviously big. Another important feature in common between two medicinal materials was that there were all a distinct layer of stone cells filled with prisms of calcium oxalate in phelloderm, which was usually the main evidence for the identification of medicinal materials. Therefore, as concluded, all those common characteristics, including the spider's web transverse section, plentiful vessels in xylem, and stone cells circular band, indicated that *S. brachyanthera* were almost similar to *Akebia caulis* and might be used as the substitution of *Akebia caulis* from the point of pharmacognosy.

Just as discussed above, *Akebia caulis* has been used in China as diuretics for a long time and its effect diuresis has also been proved [36–38]. In our present studies, the diuretic studies also showed that the ethanol extracts of the stems of *S. brachyanthera* have significant effects on diuresis in normal rats. At low dosage (150 mg/kg body wt), the effects of ESB are consistent with the furosemide treatment group. While the outputs of urine of ESB at middle and high dosages (300 mg/kg, 600 mg/kg body wt) were obviously increased compared to that of furosemide treatment group, the trends of later four hours were similar to the furosemide treatment group. Therefore the results of pharmacological study *in vivo* demonstrated that ESB have strong diuretic effect, and the optimum time for ESB to take effects is the first four hours, especially the first two hours, which could reveal that *S. brachyanthera* might be a succedaneum of the *Akebia caulis* from the level of pharmacology.

The chemical studies on ESB led to the isolation of a variety of compounds including triterpenoids (Comp. **1–10**), flavonoids (Comp. **10–16**), lignanoids (Comp. **17–20**), and phenylethanoid glycosides (Comp. **21–23**). The types of these compounds were much similar to those of *A. quinata* and consistent with those of the plants in Lardizabalaceae family

[14]. Among them, the amounts of brachyantheraoside A_4 **1** (586.8 mg), yemuoside YM_{11} **10** (1.2 g), rutin **12** (380 mg), kaempferol-3-O-rutinose **16** (962.5 mg), and calceolarioside B **21** (2.1 g) were significantly higher than the other compounds, which could be designated as characteristic components for the qualitative identification of the plant. Calceolarioside B, the characteristic component of *Akebia caulis* in Chinese Pharmacopeia [12], could also be served as indicator because of its absolutely higher amount for the quality control of the *S. brachyanthera*. Thus, from the chemical aspect including the structural types and the amount of calceolarioside B, it could be deduced that *S. brachyanthera* has the similar chemical composition and might be applied as the succedaneum of *Akebia caulis*.

Akebia caulis and *S. brachyanthera* come from different genus of the same family. Their consistent pharmacognosy characteristics and similar chemical constituents further confirmed the close genetic relationship between them and revealed the similar pharmacodynamic materials and the same pharmacological effect. Our study presented sufficient evidences for the substitution of *S. brachyanthera* for *Akebia caulis*, which will probably expand the resources of *Akebia caulis*, solve the supply shortage, and promote the full utilization of this economic crop.

As for the diuretic effect, *S. brachyanthera* can be considered as a promising plant for further studies and applications in the production of bioactive ingredients, not only in food or functional food industry, but also in pharmaceutical industry. Thus, more comprehensive studies should be focused on the diuretic effects of the main composition such as yemuoside YM_{11}, kaempferol-3-O-rutinose, or calceolarioside B by *in vivo* and *in vitro* experiments, which are undergoing in our group and will be reported later.

Conflict of Interests

The authors declare that there is no conflict of interests regarding the publication of this paper.

Acknowledgment

This work was supported by the National Natural Science Foundation of China (Grant nos. 81073154, 81374061, and 81573694), the Program for Innovative Research Team of the Ministry of Education, Program for Liaoning Innovative Research Team in University, and Program for Innovation team of Liaoning province (LT2015027). The authors appreciate the help of Association Professor Shumo Mei at Huaihua Medical College and Professor Jincai Lu at Shenyang Pharmaceutical University for providing and identifying the plant material.

References

[1] S. U. Nigwekar and S. S. Waikar, "Diuretics in acute kidney injury," *Seminars in Nephrology*, vol. 31, no. 6, pp. 523–534, 2011.

[2] Y. Joko, N. Ikemura, K. Miyata et al., "Efficacy of tolvaptan in a patient with right-sided heart failure and renal dysfunction refractory to diuretic therapy," *Journal of Cardiology Cases*, vol. 9, no. 6, pp. 226–229, 2014.

[3] Y.-Y. Chang, H.-H. Lee, C.-S. Hung et al., "Association between urine aldosterone and diastolic function in patients with primary aldosteronism and essential hypertension," *Clinical Biochemistry*, vol. 47, pp. 1329–1332, 2014.

[4] C. S. Oxlund, K. B. Buhl, I. A. Jacobsen et al., "Amiloride lowers blood pressure and attenuates urine plasminogen activation in patients with treatment-resistant hypertension," *Journal of the American Society of Hypertension*, vol. 8, no. 12, pp. 872–881, 2014.

[5] M. H. Rosner, R. Gupta, D. Ellison, and M. D. Okusa, "Management of cirrhotic ascites: physiological basis of diuretic action," *European Journal of Internal Medicine*, vol. 17, no. 1, pp. 8–19, 2006.

[6] R. J. Cody, "Diuretics and newer therapies for sodium and edema management in cute decompensated heart failure," *Cardiac Intensive Care*, vol. 39, pp. 479–487, 2010.

[7] National Pharmacopoeia Committee, *Pharmacopoeia of the People's Republic of China*, part 1, China Medical Science Press, 2010.

[8] C. Chen and D. L. Meng, "Chemical constituents from *Stauntonia brachyanthera* Hand-Mazz," *Biochemical Systematics and Ecology*, vol. 48, pp. 182–185, 2013.

[9] D. Jiang, S.-P. Shi, J.-J. Cao, Q.-P. Gao, and P.-F. Tu, "Triterpene saponins from the fruits of *Akebia quinata*," *Biochemical Systematics and Ecology*, vol. 36, no. 2, pp. 138–141, 2008.

[10] Y. Y. Sung, D. S. Kim, and H. K. Kim, "*Akebia quinata* extract exerts anti-obesity and hypolipidemic effects in high-fat diet-fed mice and 3T3-L1 adipocytes," *Journal of Ethnopharmacology*, vol. 168, pp. 17–24, 2015.

[11] X. Xue, Y. Xiao, L. K. Gong et al., "Comparative 28-day repeated oral toxicity of Longdan Xieganwan, *Akebia trifoliate* (Thunb.) koidz., *Akebia quinata* (Thunb.) Decne. and *Caulis aristolochiae manshuriensis* in mice," *Journal of Ethnopharmacology*, vol. 119, no. 1, pp. 87–93, 2008.

[12] Chinese Pharmacopoeia Commission, "Mutong (AKEBIAE CAULIS)," *Chinese Pharmacopoeia*, vol. 1, pp. 63–64, 2015.

[13] Z. Wang, S. M. Mei, L. Zhen, and C. Y. Xiao, "The preparation method of *Stauntoniabrachyanthera* Hand-Mazz vinegar juice," Tech. Rep. CN101376872A, 2009 (Chinese).

[14] Y. Liu, W. X. Liu, and C. S. Fan, "Medicinal plant resource and development value of *Stauntonia*," *Journal of Jiangxi University of TCM*, vol. 18, pp. 41–44, 2006 (Chinese).

[15] J. Zhao, J. Guo, Y. Zhang, D. Meng, and Z. Sha, "Chemical constituents from the roots and stems of *Stauntonia brachyanthera* Hand-Mazz and their bioactivities," *Journal of Functional Foods*, vol. 14, pp. 374–383, 2015.

[16] D.-L. Meng, L.-H. Xu, C. Chen, D. Yan, Z.-Z. Fang, and Y.-F. Cao, "A new resource of hepatic protectant, nor-oleanane triterpenoid saponins from the fruit of *Stauntonia brachyanthera*," *Journal of Functional Foods*, vol. 16, pp. 28–39, 2015.

[17] R. Aston, "A rat diuretic screening procedure," *Toxicology and Applied Pharmacology*, vol. 1, no. 3, pp. 277–282, 1959.

[18] P. Li, "Akebia caulis," in *Pharmacognosy*, pp. 216–219, China Medical Science Press, 2nd edition, 2012.

[19] L. R. L. Diniz, P. C. Santana, A. P. A. F. Ribeiro et al., "Effect of triterpene saponins from roots of *Ampelozizyphus amazonicus* Ducke on diuresis in rats," *Journal of Ethnopharmacology*, vol. 123, no. 2, pp. 275–279, 2009.

[20] H. Fu, K. Koike, Q. Zheng et al., "Fargosides A-E, triterpenoid saponins from *Holboellia fargesii*," *Chemical & Pharmaceutical Bulletin*, vol. 49, no. 8, pp. 999–1002, 2001.

[21] X. X. Wu, M. Li, Q. Zhang, and L. Cheng, "Chemical constituents from Arenaria polytrichoides (II)," *Chemical Research Application*, vol. 25, no. 3, pp. 333–335, 2013.

[22] S. H. Wu, S. M. Yang, D. G. Wu et al., "Three novel 24,30-dinortriterpenoids, paeonenoides A-C, from *Paeonia veitchii*," *Helvetica Chimica Acta*, vol. 88, no. 2, pp. 259–265, 2005.

[23] H.-B. Wang, D.-Q. Yu, and X.-T. Liang, "Yemuoside I, a new nortriterpenoid glycoside from Stauntonia Chinensis," *Journal of Natural Products*, vol. 54, no. 4, pp. 1097–1101, 1991.

[24] L. Yang, Q. M. Che, C. Bi, and Q. S. Sun, "Flavonoids from waste residue of Radix glycytthizae," *Chinese Traditional and Herbal Drugs*, vol. 38, no. 5, pp. 671–673, 2007.

[25] Z.-L. Zhang, Y.-M. Zuo, L. Xu, X.-S. Qu, and Y.-M. Luo, "Studies on chemical components of flavonoids in aerial part of *Saururus chinensis*," *Chinese Traditional and Herbal Drugs*, vol. 42, no. 8, pp. 1490–1493, 2011.

[26] X.-M. Ma, Y. Liu, and Y.-P. Shi, "Phenolic derivatives with free-radical-scavenging activities from *Ixeridium gracile* (DC.) SHIH," *Chemistry & Biodiversity*, vol. 4, no. 9, pp. 2172–2181, 2007.

[27] C.-R. Yang, Y.-X. Jin, J.-Z. Zhang, L. Zhang, H.-W. Fu, and J.-K. Tian, "Studies on chemical constituents from leaves of *Dipsacus sativus*," *Chinese Pharmaceutical Journal*, vol. 45, no. 8, pp. 578–580, 2010.

[28] M. Y. Shang, S. Q. Cai, J. Han, J. Li, Y. Y. Zhao, and J. H. Zheng, "Studies on flavonoids from Fenugreek (*Trigonella foenumgraecum* L.)," *Journal of Chinese Materia Medica*, vol. 23, no. 10, pp. 614–616, 1998.

[29] Y.-Y. Wang, X. Liang, and H.-M. Zhong, "Chemical constituents of *Lysimachia stenosepala* var. flavescens," *Chinese Traditional and Herbal Drugs*, vol. 43, no. 7, pp. 1280–1284, 2012.

[30] C. Z. Wang and Z. J. Jia, "Lignan, phenylpropanoid and iridoid glycosides from *Pedicularis torta*," *Phytochemistry*, vol. 45, no. 1, pp. 159–166, 1997.

[31] W. Huai-Bin, R. Mayer, G. Rücker, and M. Neugebauer, "Bisepoxylignan glycosides from *Stauntonia hexaphylla*," *Phytochemistry*, vol. 34, no. 6, pp. 1621–1624, 1993.

[32] B. Liu, A.-J. Deng, J.-Q. Yu, A.-L. Liu, G.-H. Du, and H.-L. Qin, "Chemical constituents of the whole plant of *Elsholtzia rugulosa*," *Journal of Asian Natural Products Research*, vol. 14, no. 2, pp. 89–96, 2012.

[33] X. K. Zheng, J. Li, and W. S. Feng, "Studies on phenylethanoid glycosides from Corallodiscus flabellate," *Chinese Traditional and Herbal Drugs*, vol. 33, no. 10, pp. 881–883, 2002.

[34] X. K. Zheng, Y. B. Liu, J. Li, and W. S. Feng, "One new phenylethanoid glycoside from *Corallodiscus flabellata*," *Acta Pharmacologica Sinica*, vol. 39, no. 9, pp. 716–718, 2004.

[35] S. Lin, M. Liu, S. Wang, S. Li, Y. Yang, and J. Shi, "Phenolic and phenylethanoidal glycosides from branch of *Fraxinus sieboldiana*," *Journal of Chinese Materia Medica*, vol. 35, no. 8, pp. 992–996, 2010.

[36] M. R. Bai, B. Zhang, X. Q. Liu, X. Y. Gao, and L. Ni, "A comparative study on pharmacodynamic action of *Akebia trifoliata* (Thunb.) Koidz and *Akebia quinata* (Thunb) decne and effect on drug metabolIzing-enzymes," *Chinese Archives of Traditional Chinese Medicine*, vol. 26, no. 4, 2008.

[37] H. Feng, "On current research of chemical compositions and pharmacological action of *Akebia trifoliata*," *Journal of Xi'an University of Arts And Science (Natural Science Edition)*, vol. 13, no. 4, 2010.

[38] H. M. Gao and Z. M. Wang, "Advances in the study on medicinal plants of Akebia," *China Journal of Chinese Materia Medica*, vol. 31, no. 1, pp. 10–14, 2006.

15

AHCC Activation and Selection of Human Lymphocytes via Genotypic and Phenotypic Changes to an Adherent Cell Type: A Possible Novel Mechanism of T Cell Activation

Loretta Olamigoke,[1] **Elvedina Mansoor,**[1] **Vivek Mann,**[1]
Ivory Ellis,[1] **Elvis Okoro,**[1] **Koji Wakame,**[2,3] **Hajime Fuji,**[3] **Anil Kulkarni,**[4]
Marie Francoise Doursout,[4] **and Alamelu Sundaresan**[1,4]

[1]*Texas Southern University, Houston, TX 77004, USA*
[2]*Hokkaido School of Pharmacy, Sapporo 004-0839, Japan*
[3]*Amino Up, Sapporo 004-0839, Japan*
[4]*University of Texas Medical School, Houston, TX 77004, USA*

Correspondence should be addressed to Alamelu Sundaresan; lalita1@comcast.net

Academic Editor: José L. Ríos

Active Hexose Correlated Compound (AHCC) is a fermented mushroom extract and immune supplement that has been used to treat a wide range of health conditions. It helps in augmentation of the natural immune response and affects immune cell activation and outcomes. The goal of this project was to study and understand the role and mechanisms of AHCC supplementation in the prevention of immunosuppression through T cell activation. The method described here involves "*in vitro*" culturing of lymphocytes, exposing them to different concentrations of AHCC (0 μg/mL, 50 μg/mL, 100 μg/mL, 250 μg/mL, and 500 μg/mL) at 0 hours. Interestingly, clumping and aggregation of the cells were seen between 24 and 72 hours of incubation. The cells lay down extracellular matrix, which become adherent, and phenotypical changes from small rounded lymphocytes to large macrophage-like, spindle shaped, elongated, fibroblast-like cells even beyond 360 hours were observed. These are probably translated from genotypic changes in the cells since the cells propagate for at least 3 to 6 generations (present observations). RNA isolated was subjected to gene array analysis. We hypothesize that cell adhesion is an activation and survival pathway in lymphocytes and this could be the mechanism of AHCC activation in human lymphocytes.

1. Introduction

The immune system is a dynamic network of cells tissues and organs which protects the body from infection. The immune system has beneficial and nonbeneficial aspects and fights against invading foreign materials. This can be linked to genetic makeup and thus paves a way for novel prevention and treatment measures to be generated against infectious and immune mediated diseases [1]. Being an intricate system, it comprises two major divisions that encompass various cell types which have unique roles: the innate immune system which involves a nonspecific defense mechanism and adaptive immune system which involves antigen specific

immune response. A proper understanding of the different cell types that make up these systems and their mode of communication and action would give researchers an in-depth knowledge of the immune system as a whole [2]. Further in-depth knowledge on how they behave under physiological stress will also help in the study of immune augmenting agents.

We used lymphocytes as our model choice since they are responsible for the astounding specificity of the adaptive immune response. They are well populated in the human body about 2×10^{12} lymphocytes especially in the blood, lymph, and also the lymphoid organs such as thymus, lymph nodes, spleen, and appendix [3, 4]. Despite their abundance, their central role in adaptive immunity was not demonstrated until the late 1950s. The crucial experiments were performed in mice and rats that were heavily irradiated to kill most of their white blood cells, including lymphocytes. This treatment makes the animals unable to mount adaptive immune responses. Then, by transferring various types of cells into the animals, it was possible to determine which cells reversed the deficiency. Only lymphocytes restored the adaptive immune responses of irradiated animals, indicating that lymphocytes are required for these responses [3].

It is seen that both immune systems, innate and adaptive, work hand in hand to eliminate harmful foreign pathogens, such that an activation of the innate immune system usually at the site of infection could trigger a lymphocytic response. Unlike innate immune responses, adaptive responses are activated in peripheral lymphoid organs and provide specific and long-lasting protection against the particular pathogen that induced them.

Different strategies have been looked into to try and develop a favorable approach that aids in boosting of our immune cells and so for this reason a number of substances are being synthesized, produced, extracted, and thus used for augmentation of the immune system [5]. Most of these substances are desirable since they have proven to be nontoxic to humans. AHCC is a dietary nutritional supplement/extract prepared from mycelia of the basidiomycetemushroom *Lentinula edodes* [5, 6]. It is a complex compound that contains a mixture of polysaccharides, amino acids, lipids, and minerals [7]. It is readily bioavailable and has been seen to have no adverse toxic health effect [8]. The main component of AHCC is acetylated α-glucan, which is relatively much easier to absorb than β-glucan (the main component of mushroom products) [8]. α-1,4-Glucan has a much lower molecular weight (5,000 Daltons) than β-glucan (10,000–500,000 Daltons) [7, 8]. From various experiments, which have been performed, AHCC is seen to have anticancer action, immunostimulative action, and reduction of side effects due to chemotherapy as well as defence against infection [8]. Partially acetylated alpha-glucans are known active components of AHCC as per Amino Up (see Scheme 1).

2. Materials and Methods

2.1. Materials. They include RPMI 1640 medium is purchased from Sigma-Aldrich Co. (St. Louis, MO, USA), 10% Fetal Bovine Serum (FBS), 5% Pen/Strep, and buffy coats are purchased from the Gulf Coast Regional Blood Center in Houston Texas (units accepted are those that test normal nonreactive or negative for alt, hbc, hbs, hcv, h17, hti, and sts), Hanks Balanced Salt Solution (HBBS), ficoll, and Active Hexose Correlated Compound (AHCC) are obtained from Amino Up Chemical, Japan, and Phosphate Buffer Saline (PBS), acetic acid 0.3%, trypan blue, and RNeasy mini kit are purchased from Qiagen, USA (Cat. number 74104, Inverted Microscope: Eclipse TS100 (Nikon)).

2.2. Complete Media Preparation. For culturing of lymphocytes isolated from normal human buffy coat, complete RPMI

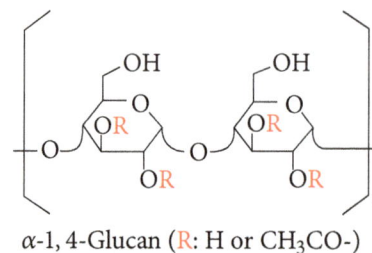

α-1, 4-Glucan (R: H or CH$_3$CO-)

SCHEME 1: Structure of AHCC [8].

media has to be used. Each bottle contains 500 mL of RPMI media. This was supplemented with 10% Fetal Bovine Serum (FBS) and 5% Penicillin-Streptomycin (Pen-Strep). Complete media was prepared by taking out 50 mL of RPMI from the 500 mL bottle and adding 50 mL of FBS and 5 mL of Pen-Strep.

2.3. Lymphocyte Isolation. The buffy coat unit (60 mL) was diluted in 100 mL of Hanks Balanced Salt Solution (HBBS) in a T-flask for a total volume of 160 mL diluted buffy coat and thoroughly mixed. 10 mL of ficoll was added to 4 polypropylene 50 mL centrifuge tubes each and was layered with 40 mL of buffy coat at a slow steady pace preventing penetration of the ficoll layer. The tubes were then centrifuged at 2100 rpm (700 to 800 g) for 20 minutes at room temperature. (Two 50 mL tubes with 10 mL of HBBS were prepared.) Using 1 mL pipette, lymphocytes layer, formed above the ficoll, was aspirated and placed into prepared tubes. HBBS was added to top it off and centrifuged at 2100 (700–800 g) for 12 minutes at room temperature. One tube was prepared containing 10 mL of HBBS to which pelleted lymphocytes from the 2 tubes were added and centrifuged at 2100 rpm (700–800 g) for 12 minutes at room temperature. The supernatant was discarded and the resulting pellet was resuspended in 20 mL of complete RPMI. Cell counts were performed after which the AHCC experiment was set up.

2.4. Cell Counts. We combined 50 μL of the lymphocyte cell suspension with 500 μL trypan blue and 950 μL of 0.3% acetic acid in an eppendorf tube and mixed well to obtain an appropriate dilution. Then, we covered a clean haemocytometer with a cover slip and using a pipettor we added, from an angle, a small amount of the stained, diluted cell suspension onto the covered haemocytometer without moving the cover slip. We allowed the cells to settle before counting.

Once we obtained the cell counts, the cell concentration was calculated using the following formula:

$$\text{Cell concentration} = \frac{\text{Total number of cells}}{4} \tag{1}$$
$$\times \text{ dilution factor } (30) \times 10^4.$$

2.5. AHCC Preparation and Experimental Setup. In the manufacturing process of AHCC, it was sterilized at 121 degrees C for 45 minutes after separation of insoluble fungal parts. Then, this AHCC sample obtained from Amino Up Chemical, Japan, is freshly prepared in sterile complete media (RPMI1640) at a 5 mg/mL stock concentration. Total volume of this sample prepared varies as per experimental need. Cells were resuspended at $1 * 10^6$ cells/mL in 10 mL tissue culture flasks in triplicate. Each flask corresponds to the different experimental concentrations and the corresponding volumes of AHCC were added to achieve the desired concentrations: $0 \mu g/mL$ (control), $50 \mu g/mL$, $100 \mu g/mL$, $250 \mu g/mL$, and $500 \mu g/mL$. The flasks containing the cell cultures were incubated at optimal conditions $37°C$ and 5% CO_2. Daily observations were recorded and microscopic images taken over several days.

2.6. MTT Assay. The cells were isolated, counted, and plated to 96-well plates on the same day as blood collection. $97 \mu L$ of RPMI1640 culture medium was added to 21 wells of a 96-well plate. A final volume of $100 \mu L/well$ was achieved by adding $3 \mu L$ of cell suspension (containing 1×10^5 cells) into each well. To the wells designated for the different AHCC, $0 \mu g/mL$ (control), $50 \mu g/mL$, $100 \mu g/mL$, $250 \mu g/mL$, and $500 \mu g/mL$ concentrations corresponding volumes of AHCC were added to achieve the desired concentrations. The cells were incubated at $37°C$ for 48 hours and then dye solution was added to each well ($15 \mu L/well$) and incubated for 4 hours in a humidified, 5% CO_2 atmosphere. After 4 hours of incubation, the solubilization solution/stop mix was added ($100 \mu L/well$) to stop the cellular conversion of the MTT dye and was again incubated for 1 hour. Finally, cell proliferation was measured using Tecan 96-well plate reader and absorbance at 570 nm wavelength was recorded *(CellTiter 96 Non-Radioactive Cell Proliferation Assay, Promega Corporation, Madison, WI, USA)*.

2.7. RNA Isolation. RNA was isolated according to the protocol obtained from the RNeasy mini kit purchased from Qiagen.

2.8. RNA Analysis by Illumina. Three hundred nanograms of total RNA was amplified and purified using Illumina TotalPrep RNA Amplification Kit (Ambion, Cat.# IL1791) following kit instructions. Briefly, first strand cDNA was synthesized by incubating RNA with T7 oligo (dT) primer and reverse transcriptase mix at $42°C$ for 2 hours. RNase H and DNA polymerase master mix were immediately added to the reaction mix following reverse transcription and were incubated for 2 hours at $16°C$ to synthesize second strand cDNA. RNA, primers, enzymes, and salts that would inhibit *in vitro* transcription were removed through cDNA filter cartridges (part of the amplification kit). *In vitro* transcription was performed and biotinylated cRNA was synthesized by 14-hour amplification with dNTP mix containing biotin-dUTP and T7 RNA polymerase. Amplified cRNA was subsequently purified and concentration was measured by NanoDrop ND-1000 Spectrophotometer (NanoDrop Technologies, DE). An aliquot of 750 nanograms of amplified products was loaded onto Illumina Sentrix Beadchip Array HumanHT12_V4 arrays, hybridized at $58°C$

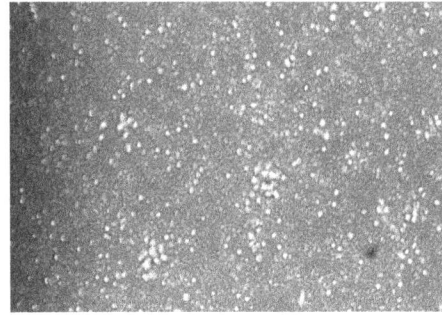

FIGURE 1: Control-$0 \mu g/mL$ treated lymphocytes, 96 hours.

in an Illumina Hybridization Oven (Illumina, Cat.# 198361) for 17 hours, washed, and incubated with streptavidin-Cy3 to detect biotin-labeled cRNA on the arrays. Arrays were dried and scanned with BeadArray Reader (Illumina, CA). Data were analyzed using GenomeStudio software (Illumina, CA). Clustering and pathway analysis were performed with GenomeStudio and Ingenuity Pathway Analysis (Ingenuity Systems, Inc.) software, respectively.

2.9. Statistical Analysis. Standard error was calculated based on the mean and the standard deviation and the standard error bars were included in the data. A "P" value less than 0.05 was considered statistically significant.

3. Results and Discussion

3.1. Phenotypic Observations of the Cells. Control-$0 \mu g/mL$ treated lymphocytes, as shown in Figure 1, live only until 96 hours and die thereafter. Interestingly in AHCC treated cells, after a time lag, clumping and aggregation of the cells were seen between 24 and about 72 hours of incubation. The cells then become *adherent* and *phenotypical changes* were observed even at low doses such as $50 \mu g/mL$ (Figure 2(a)), that is, macrophage-like, spindle shaped, elongated, and fibroblast-like up until 360 hours and beyond. Similar changes were observed in the other doses: $100 \mu g/mL$ to $500 \mu g/mL$ (Figures 2(b), 2(c), and 2(d)). Cell proliferation also increased (cell count assays). The cells were not subjected to stress as the media was changed at various intervals, so stress due to nutrient depletion was eliminated. These are probably translated from genotypic changes in the cells since the cells propagate for at least three to six generations (present observations). Cell count data is shown for up to 72 hours since after that cells become adherent and cannot be counted. Cell viability was high throughout, indicating that AHCC is able to boost cell health (Figure 3). Cell proliferation was further demonstrated via the cell metabolism and proliferation MTT assay (Figure 4). This further elaborated that there was a dose response dependent increase of resting lymphocyte proliferation in response to AHCC treatment. The AHCC treated adherent phenotypic cells can be trypsinized for two generations after which they visibly lay down a lot of extracellular matrixes (ECM). These genotypic changes possibly involve signal transduction of cell adhesion molecules and adhesive cytokines and growth

96-hours incubation   360-hours incubation

(a) 50 μg/mL AHCC, 20x

96-hours incubation   360-hours incubation

(b) 100 μg/mL AHCC, 20x

96-hours incubation   360-hours incubation

(c) 250 μg/mL AHCC, 20x

96-hours incubation   360-hours incubation

(d) 500 μg/mL AHCC, 20x

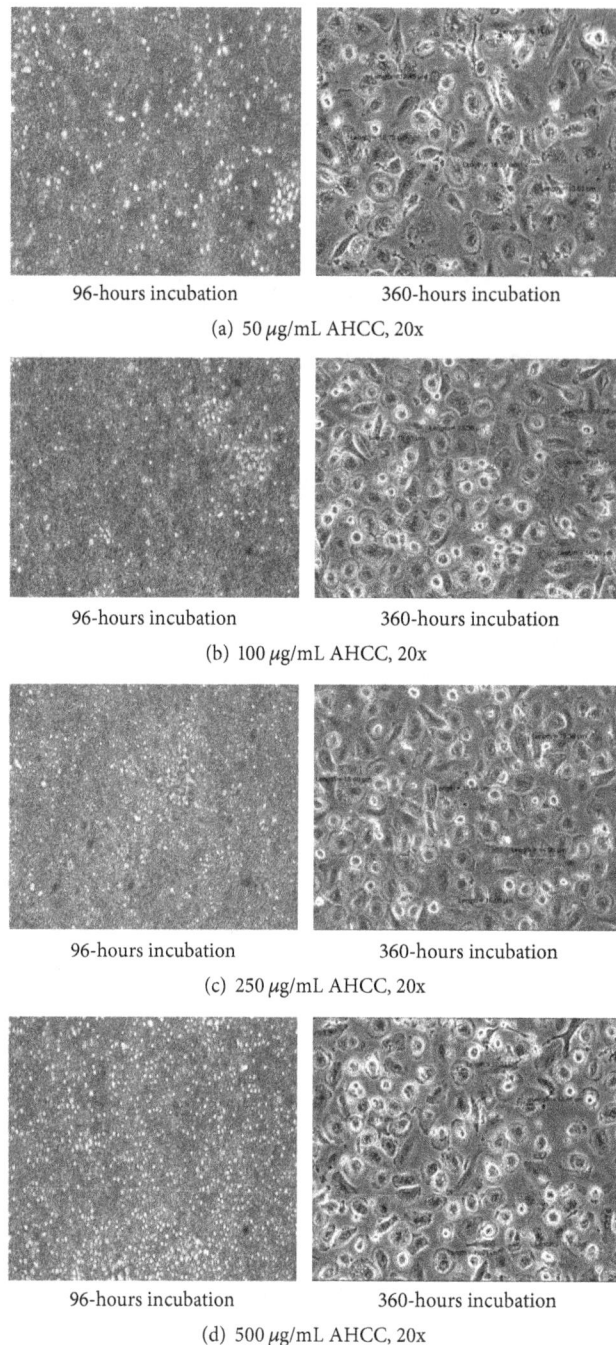

FIGURE 2: Representative image of different concentrations of AHCC treated lymphocytes: (a) 50 μg/mL AHCC 20x, (b) 100 μg/mL AHCC 20x, (c) 250 μg/mL AHCC, and (d) 500 μg/mL AHCC. Note: the morphological changes of lymphocytes from 96 hours to 360 hours posttreatment with AHCC. Cells become adherent and phenotypical changes were observed even at low doses such as 50 μg/mL (a) that is macrophage-like, spindle shaped, elongated, and fibroblast-like up until 360 hours and beyond. Similar changes were observed in the other doses: 100 μg/mL to 500 μg/mL (b, c, d).

factors. Cell adhesion is an activation and survival pathway in lymphocytes and we hypothesize that this could be the mechanism of AHCC activation in human lymphocytes. From the gene array analysis it was seen that certain genes responsible for T cell proliferation and differentiation as well as cell adhesion were significantly upregulated (Figure 5). Of great importance is the LAT gene (linker for activation of T cells) which is required for TCR (T cell antigen receptor) and pre-TCR-mediated signaling in both developing and mature T cells. The possible mode of LAT action in lymphocyte activation in response to AHCC in our experiments is illustrated in Figure 6. In our experiments, AHCC possibly induces upregulation of LAT and promotes cell adhesion to activate resting lymphocytes.

Cell counts

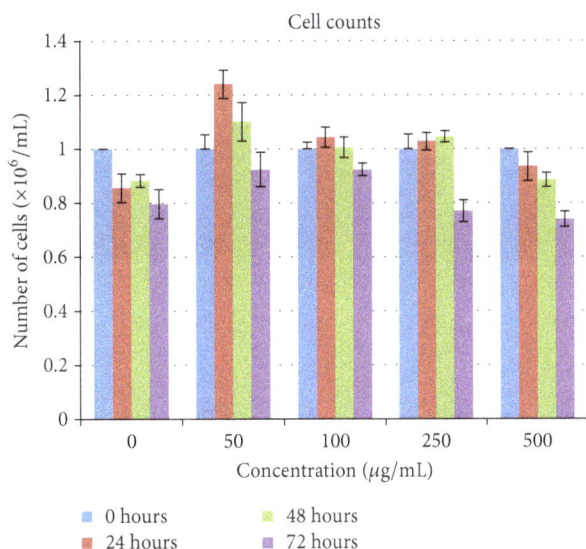

FIGURE 3: Cell counts until 72 hours: overall increase in the cell count is observed 24 hours after culture (except for the control flask) which later decreases over 48 and 72 hours as the cells begin to aggregate, clump, and adhere to the bottom of the flask. The most significant increase was seen in 50 μg/mL from "0" hours to "24" hours compared to the other treated flasks. (Note that lymphocytes are resting cells which have been induced to multiply.)

MTT assay-AHCC

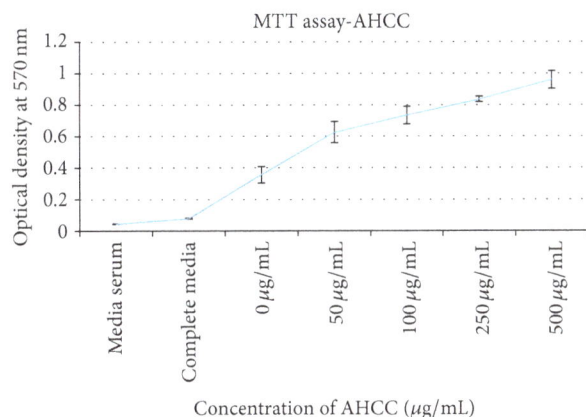

FIGURE 4: Cell proliferation data for AHCC treated lymphocytes. 1×10^5 cells were seeded into the desired well of the 96-well plate. These cells were then treated with different concentrations of the nutritional supplement AHCC at "0" hours. At 48 hours after culture, the cells were treated with MTT reagent according to the protocol. Absorbance was measured at 570 nm.

Results are described as representative of five experiments with the following concentrations: 0 μg/mL, 50 μg/mL, 100 μg/mL, 250 μg/mL, and 500 μg/mL.

The control flask, after a period of about 96 hours, dies off as the cells are not treated with AHCC and so there is no further stimulation of growth/proliferation. From 50 μg/mL to 500 μg/mL, a pictorial representation is given showing 96 hours and 360 hours of incubation (Figures 2(a)–2(d)). The differences in the phenotypic appearance of the cells are distinct; these cells being activated by AHCC adhere,

differentiate, and also vary in sizes ranging from about 11 μm to about 26 μm in diameter. It was also observed that these cells once in contact with each other do not exhibit a contact inhibition, but they begin to merge resulting in a single cell and also continue to grow within the plate. After reaching a confluent stage, the cells were trypsinized and passaged and, after a time lag, the exact same phenomenon was observed. It should be noted that AHCC was only added once, at the start of the experiment, and supplemented with complete media when needed even after cell adhesion had occurred, to avoid nutrient deprivation. The exact mechanism of how AHCC acts on and activates these cells causing them to proliferate, adhere, and differentiate is unknown.

3.2. Cell Counts. After isolation of these lymphocytes, they were resuspended at a concentration of 1×10^6 cells/mL for a total of 10 mL. This was done for all concentrations. A cell count gives an idea of cell proliferation, that is, live versus dead cells. In order to assess if AHCC induced cell proliferation after treatment, cells were counted and we found that after 24 hours an increase was observed in the treated flasks as opposed to the control flask. From 48 to 72 hours there was an observable decrease in the cell count (Figure 3); the reason for this is that, at this period of time, the cells began to aggregate and so a true cell count could not be achieved. For this reason, cell counts were only carried out for 3 days from experimental setup.

3.3. MTT Assay. The CellTiter 96 Non-Radioactive Cell Proliferation Assay is a collection of qualified reagents that provide a rapid and convenient method of determining viable cell number in proliferation, cytotoxicity [9, 10], cell attachment [11, 12], chemotaxis [13], and apoptosis [14] assays. The MTT assay is a colorimetric assay for assessing cell metabolic activity. NAD(P)H-dependent cellular oxidoreductase enzymes may, under defined conditions, reflect the number of viable cells present. These enzymes are capable of reducing the tetrazolium dye MTT 3-(4,5-dimethylthiazol-2-yl)-2,5-diphenyltetrazolium bromide to its insoluble formazan product, which has a purple color; a solubilization solution is added to dissolve the insoluble purple formazan product into a colored solution that is easily detected using a 96-well plate reader. The absorbance of this colored solution can be quantified by measuring at a certain wavelength (usually between 500 and 600 nm) by a spectrophotometer [15].

The CellTiter 96 Assay has several advantages over conventional cell number or 3[H]thymidine incorporation assays. There is a minimum amount of labor involved in doing the CellTiter 96 Assay. The assay is done entirely in a 96-well plate with no steps that require washing the cells or the removal of solution from the wells. The assay can be used for both anchorage-dependent or suspension cells with no change in the protocol. The assay plates are read using a 96-well plate reader, making it easy to computerize data collection, calculations, and report generation [16].

MTT assay gives an idea of cell metabolism and is widely used to measure metabolic activity; thus, it is considered

Gene array data

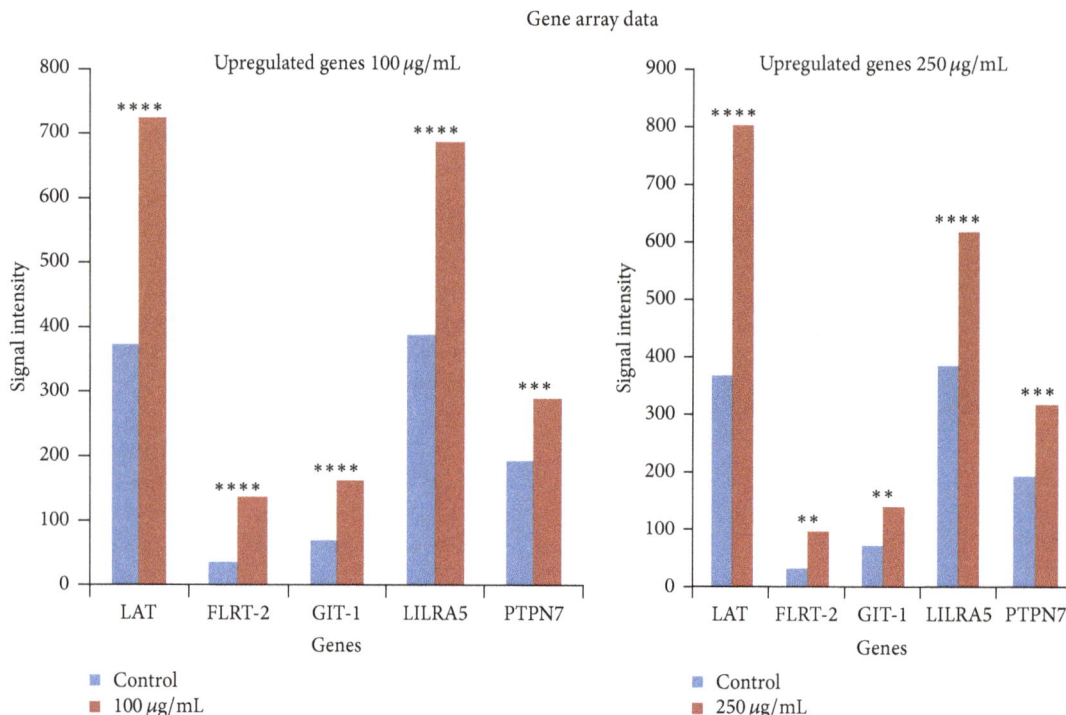

FIGURE 5: Graphical representation of genes responsible for cell proliferation, adhesion, differentiation, receptor signaling, and signal transduction leading to activation of the immune system thus evoking an immune response. It shows upregulated genes (100 μg/mL and 250 μg/mL concentrations); their corresponding signal intensity after a gene array analysis was performed. $P < 0.05$ was considered statistically significant. "$**$" means $P < 0.01$, "$***$" means $P < 0.001$, and "$****$" means $P < 0.0001$.

a real proliferation assay. Our results show a significant increase from control (0 μg/mL) to 500 μg/mL.

3.4. Gene Array Data.

This phenomenon of adhesion has previously not been seen in previous experiments conducted with lymphocytes treated with other agents. In order to delineate the cause of these genotypic and phenotypic effects, RNA isolated from harvested cells is subjected to a gene array analysis to get a bigger picture. This is then narrowed down to pathways that get turned on as a result of AHCC treatment, as the phenotypic effects are seen after a genotypic change has occurred.

In order to specifically characterize the unique phenotypic and proliferation phenomena seen with AHCC treatment in resting lymphocytes compared to control, we analyzed cells harvested and subjected them to the Illumina platform.

From the gene array data that was obtained (Figure 5), a group of significant genes LAT, FLRT-2, GIT-1, LILRA5, and PTPN7 responsible for cell proliferation, cell adhesion and/or receptor signaling, triggering of innate immune responses, differentiation, and regulation of T-lymphocytes as well as signal transduction were identified. Of primary importance is the LAT gene. The gene array data revealed possible direct activation of the lymphocytes via direct engagement of the T cell receptor complex. The linker for activated T cells (LAT), which is the primary activator after TCR engagement in AHCC treated lymphocytes, increased by 2.7-fold compared

to control even at 360 hours posttreatment. This is high for resting cells. As an adaptor protein, the function of LAT in TCR signaling centers upon its tyrosine phosphorylation and subsequent recruitment of other signaling proteins. Upon TCR engagement, phosphorylation of LAT allows it to interact with several SH2 domain-containing proteins, such as Grb2, Gads, and PLC-γ1. We have already seen inhibition of LAT and PLC-γ1 in lymphocytes in microgravity (an immune suppressive scenario) related to reduced T cell activation. Hence, AHCC might be able to directly activate LAT and thus might be a possible future countermeasure candidate to restore T cell activation in immunosuppressive scenarios. It is already in human use as an immune augmentation supplement in conjunction with cancer chemotherapy. AHCC thus might be a possible future countermeasure candidate to restore T cell activation in immunosuppressive scenarios on earth and in space.

Phosphorylation of the ITAMs enables the recruitment of ZAP70 (ζ-chain associated protein kinase of 70 kDa), its phosphorylation by LCK, and its activation. Activated ZAP70 phosphorylates four key tyrosine residues on linker for activation of T cells (LAT), which recruits numerous signaling molecules to form a multiprotein complex, termed the LAT signalosome. Important molecules that constitute this complex include phospholipase Cγ1 (PLCγ1), growth factor receptor-bound protein 2 (GRB2), GRB2-related adaptor protein GADS, SLP76 (SH2 domain-containing leukocyte protein of 76 kDa), adhesion- and degranulation-promoting

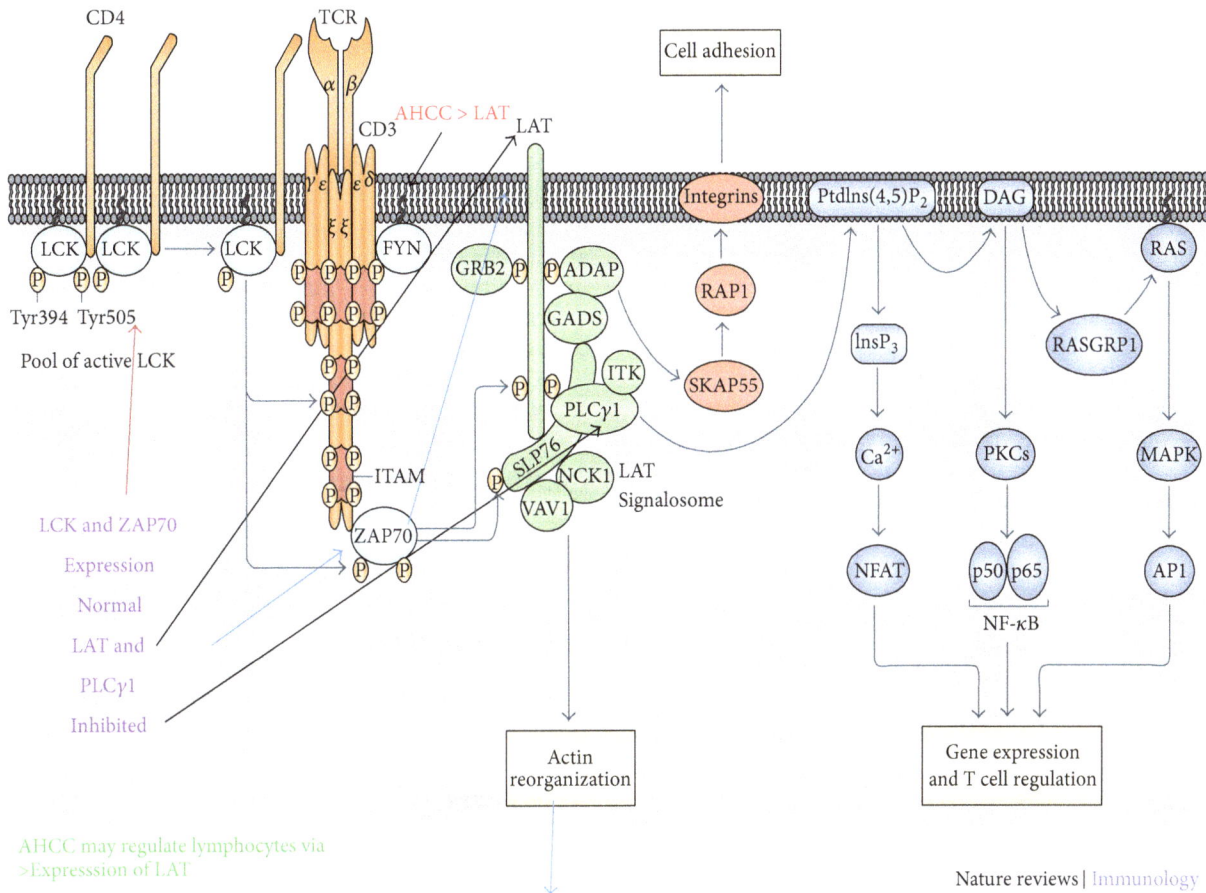

FIGURE 6: T cell receptor (TCR) signal transduction is initiated by the recognition of cognate peptide-MHC molecules. The first molecule to be recruited to the TCR-CD3 complex is the SRC family kinase (SFK) member LCK, which phosphorylates immunoreceptor tyrosine-based activation motifs (ITAMs) of the CD3γ chain, CD3δ chain, CD3ε chains, and the ζ-chains.

adaptor protein (ADAP), interleukin-2-inducible T cell kinase (ITK), NCK1, and VAV1. The LAT signalosome propagates signal branching to three major signaling pathways, the Ca^{2+}, the mitogen-activated protein kinase (MAPK) kinase, and the nuclear factor-κB (NF-κB) signaling pathways, leading to the mobilization of transcription factors that are critical for gene expression and essential for T cell growth and differentiation. Signals initiated from the TCR also result in actin reorganization and the activation of integrins by inside-out signaling. Note the following abbreviations: AP1, activator protein 1; DAG, diacylglycerol; InsP$_3$, inositol-1,4,5-trisphosphate; NFAT, nuclear factor of activated T cells; PKC, protein kinase C; PtdIns(4,5)P$_2$, phosphatidylinositol-4,5-bisphosphate; RASGRP1, RAS guanyl-releasing protein 1; SKAP55, SRC kinase-associated phosphoprotein of 55 kDa [17]. Our key culprits implicated thus far from our experiments are LAT, PLC-γ1, and ZAP 70. AHCC thus might modulate LAT and promote cell adhesion.

FLRT-2 is a gene that encodes a member of the fibronectin leucine-rich transmembrane protein (FLRT) family. FLRT family members may function in cell adhesion and/or receptor signaling. Their protein structures resemble small leucine-rich proteoglycans found in the extracellular matrix (provided by Ref. Seq., Jul. 2008).

GIT-1 (G Protein-Coupled Receptor Kinase Interacting ArfGAP 1) is a protein coding gene. GTPase-activating protein for the ADP ribosylation factor family, which may serve as a scaffold to bring together molecules to form signaling modules controlling vesicle trafficking, adhesion, and cytoskeletal organization, increases the speed of cell migration, as well as the size and rate of formation of protrusions. Among its related pathways are regulations of actin cytoskeleton. It localizes synaptically especially in dendritic cells [18]. If synaptic localization is disturbed, dendritic cells lose their morphology. It is responsible for differentiation and preservation of dendritic cell morphology and it interacts with PLCγ1.

LILRA5 leukocyte immunoglobulin-like receptor, subfamily A, member 5: the protein encoded by this gene is a member of the leukocyte immunoglobulin-like receptor (LIR) family. LIR family members are known to have activating and inhibitory functions in leukocytes. Crosslink of this receptor protein on the surface of monocytes has been shown to induce calcium flux and secretion of several proinflammatory cytokines, which suggests the roles of this protein in triggering innate immune responses (provided by Ref. Seq., Jul. 2008).

PTPN7 protein tyrosine phosphatase, nonreceptor type 7: the protein encoded by this gene is a member of the protein tyrosine phosphatase (PTP) family. PTPs are known to be signaling molecules that regulate a variety of cellular processes including cell growth, differentiation, mitotic cycle, and oncogenic transformation. This gene is preferentially expressed in a variety of hematopoietic cells and is an early response gene in lymphokine stimulated cells. The noncatalytic N-terminus of this PTP can interact with MAP kinases and suppress the MAP kinase activities. This PTP was shown to be involved in the regulation of T cell antigen receptor (TCR) signaling, which was thought to function through dephosphorylating the molecules related to MAP kinase pathway. Multiple alternatively spliced transcript variants have been found for this gene (provided by Ref. Seq., Dec. 2010).

4. Conclusion

From the above concrete observations, it can be hypothesized that AHCC is promoting proliferation and differentiation of leukocytes (multipotent stem cells), as it is seen that the genes responsible for these such as LAT, FLRT2, GIT-1, and so forth, as seen in Figure 5, are upregulated and highly significant ($P < 0.0005$). Gene array and adhesion molecule experiments are ongoing. Cell adhesion is an activation and survival pathway in lymphocytes and we hypothesize that this could be the mechanism of AHCC activation in human lymphocytes. This is a unique phenomenon and has previously not been observed before in our laboratory when we used other agents such as mitogens, transferrin, and nucleotides for rescue of lymphocyte activation and locomotion. We have conducted these studies up to date in 8 normal donors and have found this phenomenon to be donor independent. The study of the adhesion molecules and the ECM could provide valuable insight into the mode of action of AHCC in augmenting the immune system, which has been observed in human subjects. AHCC has immunomodulatory effects via T cell activation, which could be useful for further studies in immunosuppression in microgravity and stressed physiological environments. Physical stressors include microgravity, radiation, malnutrition, and microbial contamination and atmospheric pollutants due to recycled air and water [19, 20]. Microgravity is one of the most detrimental stressors for space travelers and aggravates bone structure and composition, immune function, and the psychoneuroendocrine system and induces muscle atrophy. Immune suppression in microgravity has been documented for many years. With human exploration and long-term space travel, the immune system of the astronaut has to be optimally maintained. Individual risks to organs, such as the heart, bone, muscle, and the immune system, occur in microgravity.

Spaceflight causes various changes in the immune system, including decreases in T cell proliferation, cell-mediated activity, natural killer (NK) cell activity, macrophage function, and responses of bone marrow cells to colony stimulating factors and alteration in cytokine production [19, 20].

However, because of the limited sample number, different mission durations, and different experimental conditions, spaceflight-induced immune changes have not been fully elucidated and ground-based studies have also been required. AHCC (Active Hexose Correlated Compound, Amino Up, Japan) might potentially play a core nutritional metabolic role in regulating physiological stress. Since our lab studies lymphocyte activation in immunosuppressive scenarios such as microgravity, the next step is to expose lymphocytes to modeled microgravity (mmg) using the NASA rotating wall vessel, and unit earth gravity or 1 g, in the presence and absence of the same concentrations of AHCC to evidence if LAT is upregulated in mmg AHCC treated lymphocytes compared to controls grown in mmg alone.

Conflict of Interests

The authors declare that there is no conflict of interests regarding the publication of this paper.

Acknowledgment

This work was supported by Amino Up Chemical, Sapporo, Japan.

References

[1] http://www.niaid.nih.gov/topics/immunesystem/Pages/default.aspx.

[2] http://www.niaid.nih.gov/topics/immuneSystem/Pages/overview.aspx.

[3] B. Alberts, A. Johnson, J. Lewis et al., "Lymphocytes and the cellular basis of adaptive immunity," in *Molecular Biology of the Cell*, Garland Science, New York, NY, USA, 4th edition, 2002.

[4] http://bionumbers.hms.harvard.edu/bionumber.aspx?&id=103587&ver=0.

[5] Z. Yin, H. Fujii, and T. Walshe, "Effects of active hexose correlated compound on frequency of $CD4^+$ and $CD8^+$ T cells producing interferon-γ and/or tumor necrosis factor—α in healthy adults," *Human Immunology*, vol. 71, no. 12, pp. 1187–1190, 2010.

[6] B. E. Roman, E. Beli, D. M. Duriancik, and E. M. Gardner, "Short-term supplementation with active hexose correlated compound improves the antibody response to influenza B vaccine," *Nutrition Research*, vol. 33, no. 1, pp. 12–17, 2013.

[7] S. Nogusa, J. Gerbino, and B. W. Ritz, "Low-dose supplementation with active hexose correlated compound improves the immune response to acute influenza infection in C57BL/6 mice," *Nutrition Research*, vol. 29, no. 2, pp. 139–143, 2009.

[8] http://www.aminoup.co.jp/e/products/AHCC/.

[9] B. G. Campling, J. Pym, P. R. Galbraith, and S. P. C. Cole, "Use of the mtt assay for rapid determination of chemosensitivity of human leukemic blast cells," *Leukemia Research*, vol. 12, no. 10, pp. 823–831, 1988.

[10] R. Jover, X. Ponsoda, J. V. Castell, and M. J. Gómez-Lechón, "Acute cytotoxicity of ten chemicals in human and rat cultured hepatocytes and in cell lines: correlation between in vitro data and human lethal concentrations," *Toxicology In Vitro*, vol. 8, no. 1, pp. 47–54, 1994.

[11] R. L. Klemke, M. Yebra, E. M. Bayna, and D. A. Cheresh, "Receptor tyrosine kinase signaling required for integrin alpha v beta 5-directed cell motility but not adhesion on vitronectin," *The Journal of Cell Biology*, vol. 127, no. 3, pp. 859–866, 1994.

[12] A. L. Prieto, G. M. Edelman, and K. L. Crossin, "Multiple integrins mediate cell attachment to cytotactin/tenascin," *Proceedings of the National Academy of Sciences of the United States of America*, vol. 90, no. 21, pp. 10154–10158, 1993.

[13] Y. Shi, B. S. Kornovski, R. Savani, and E. A. Turley, "A rapid, multiwell colorimetric assay for chemotaxis," *Journal of Immunological Methods*, vol. 164, no. 2, pp. 149–154, 1993.

[14] G. H. W. Wong and D. V. Goeddel, "Fas antigen and p55 TNF receptor signal apoptosis through distinct pathways," *The Journal of Immunology*, vol. 152, no. 4, pp. 1751–1755, 1994.

[15] https://en.wikipedia.org/wiki/MTT_assay.

[16] http://www.promega.com/~/media/files/resources/protocols/technical%20bulletins/0/celltiter%2096%20non-radioactive%20cell%20proliferation%20assay%20protocol.pdf.

[17] R. J. Brownlie and R. Zamoyska, "T cell receptor signalling networks: branched, diversified and bounded," *Nature Reviews Immunology*, vol. 13, no. 4, pp. 257–269, 2013.

[18] http://www.genecards.org/cgi-bin/carddisp.pl?gene=GIT1&keywords=GIT1.

[19] V. M. Aponte, D. S. Finch, and D. M. Klaus, "Considerations for non-invasive in-flight monitoring of astronaut immune status with potential use of MEMS and NEMS devices," *Life Sciences*, vol. 79, no. 14, pp. 1317–1333, 2006.

[20] A. T. Borchers, C. L. Keen, and M. E. Gershwin, "Microgravity and immune responsiveness: implications for space travel," *Nutrition*, vol. 18, no. 10, pp. 889–898, 2002.

The Preventive Effect on Ethanol-Induced Gastric Lesions of the Medicinal Plant *Plumeria rubra*: Involvement of the Latex Proteins in the NO/cGMP/K$_{ATP}$ Signaling Pathway

Nylane Maria Nunes de Alencar,[1] Rachel Sindeaux Paiva Pinheiro,[1] Ingrid Samantha Tavares de Figueiredo,[2] Patrícia Bastos Luz,[1] Lyara Barbosa Nogueira Freitas,[1] Tamiris de Fátima Goebel de Souza,[1] Luana David do Carmo,[1] Larisse Mota Marques,[1] and Marcio Viana Ramos[3]

[1]*Departamento de Fisiologia e Farmacologia, UFC, Coronel Nunes de Melo 1127, Rodolfo Teófilo, 60430-270 Fortaleza, CE, Brazil*
[2]*Centro Universitário Estácio do Ceará, Via Corpvs, Rua Eliseu Uchoa Becco, No. 600, Bairro Água Fria, 60810-270 Fortaleza, CE, Brazil*
[3]*Departamento de Bioquímica e Biologia Molecular, UFC, Campus do Pici, Caixa Postal 6033, 60451-970 Fortaleza, CE, Brazil*

Correspondence should be addressed to Nylane Maria Nunes de Alencar; nylane@gmail.com

Academic Editor: Guillermo Schmeda-Hirschmann

Plumeria rubra (Apocynaceae) is frequently used in folk medicine for the treatment of gastrointestinal disorders, hepatitis, and tracheitis, among other infirmities. The aim of this study was to investigate the gastroprotective potential of a protein fraction isolated from the latex of *Plumeria rubra* (PrLP) against ethanol-induced gastric lesions and describe the underlying mechanisms. In a dose-dependent manner, the pretreatment with PrLP prevented ethanol-induced gastric lesions in mice after single intravenous administration. The gastroprotective mechanism of PrLP was associated with the involvement of prostaglandins and balance of oxidant/antioxidant factors. Secondarily, the NO/cGMP/K$_{ATP}$ pathway and activation of capsaicin-sensitive primary afferents were also demonstrated as part of the mechanism. This study shows that proteins extracted from the latex of *P. rubra* prevent gastric lesions induced in experimental animals. Also, the results support the use of the plant in folk medicine.

1. Introduction

Peptic ulcer is a multifactorial disease that affects an increasing number of people worldwide. Etiological factors include emotional stress, improper diet, excessive ethanol ingestion, genetic factors, continuous or indiscriminate use of NSAIDs, and infection by *Helicobacter pylori* [1, 2]. Antagonists of histamine H2–6 receptors and inhibitors of the proton pump are currently the main classes of drugs used in the clinic for the treatment of peptic ulcer [3]. However, some adverse effects are associated with their long-term use, such as hypergastrinemia and an increased risk of *Helicobacter pylori* and *Clostridium difficile* infections [4, 5]. Furthermore, the high costs of these drugs are still concerns to be addressed.

These inconsistencies stimulate the search for alternative or complementary strategies to improve the prevention and healing of ulcers.

Latex fluids have been reported to display numerous pharmacological properties. This is in good agreement with the traditional and folk medicinal use of latex-bearing plants worldwide [6, 7]. *Plumeria rubra* is a laticifer plant, commonly known as the frangipani or temple tree and distributed mainly in tropical and subtropical regions [8]. It is used in folk medicinal purposes to treat or relieve fever, cold, cutaneous infections, tracheitis, gastrointestinal disorders, ureterolithiasis, and hepatitis and to induce coughing up. The traditional uses have been further certified by scientific documentation [9, 10]. Active phytoconstituents (plumericin and isoplumericin) isolated from *P. rubra* showed antialgal, antifungal, antibacterial, and molluscicidal effects and cytotoxic properties [11–13]. The n-hexane fraction of crude methanolic extract stem bark showed *in vitro* antimicrobial activity [14]. The flavone glycoside isolated from the flowers exhibited a significant reduction in serum triglycerides of animals [15]. More recently, the involvement of proteins in pharmacological activities of *P. rubra* was reported. A protease Plumerin-R was isolated from the latex by acetone precipitation and displayed anti-inflammatory activity [16]. In our previous findings, the soluble proteins extracted from the latex (PrLP) showed antioxidant and proteolytic activity [17] and endothelial relaxation of rat thoracic aortic rings [18]. Furthermore, studies with the proteins extracted from latex of other plants have suggested that the proteins are strongly associated with the pharmacological properties claimed by the popular medicine [6, 7]. In the present study, the aqueous protein fraction extracted from the latex of *P. rubra* was examined *in vivo* to determine its gastroprotective potential.

2. Materials and Methods

2.1. Latex Extraction and Protein Recovered. The fresh latex from *Plumeria rubra* L. (Jasmine) was collected in specimens growing in the Garden of Medicinal Plants, Universidade Federal do Ceará (UFC), Brazil. The plant material was identified by a taxonomist and a voucher specimen (number 15018) was deposited at Prisco Bezerra Herbarium of the UFC. Briefly, terminal branches were used to extract fresh latex. The fluid was taken into plastic tubes containing distilled water to yield a dilution ratio of 1 : 2 (v/v). The samples were centrifuged at 5,000 ×g at 10°C for 10 minutes. The precipitated rubber-like material was discarded and the supernatant was submitted to dialysis against distilled water using a membrane with a cutoff of 8000 Da. After 48 h, the nondialyzable material (PrLP) was obtained after centrifugation under the same conditions described above. The supernatant lyophilized was stored at 25°C until use. Soluble proteins from the latex of *Plumeria rubra* (PrLP) used in this study were previously characterized [17]. The summary of their properties will be presented later in this paper.

2.2. Animals. Adult male Swiss mice weighing 25 ± 3.0 g were obtained from the Central Animal House of the Universidade Federal do Ceará, Brazil. The animals were kept in plastic cages under controlled environmental conditions (12/12 h light/dark cycles, temperature 25°C, and humidity $55 \pm 10\%$) with free access to water and fed with a commercial feed (Purina, Paulínia, SP, Brazil) until 16 hours before the experiments. All experimental procedures were handled according to the current *Guide for the Care and Use of Laboratory Animals* of the National Research Council after approval by the "Ethical Committee for Animal Use" of the Universidade Federal do Ceará (protocol number 57/2010).

2.3. Chemicals. Capsaicin, capsazepine, indomethacin, glibenclamide, diazoxide, L-arginine, Nω-nitro-L-arginine

methyl ester (L-NAME), 1H-[1,2,4]oxadiazolo[4,3-a]quinoxalin-1-one (ODQ), and absolute ethanol were purchased from Sigma-Aldrich (St. Louis, MO, USA). Prostaglandin analog 16,16-dimethyl PGE2 (misoprostol) was purchased from Continental Pharma (Cytotec, Italy). N-Acetylcysteine was purchased from União Química (São Paulo, Brazil). All other chemicals were of analytical grade unless otherwise specified.

2.4. Ethanol-Induced Gastric Lesions. The animals were randomly distributed into six groups ($n = 8$ per group) and pretreated intravenously (i.v.) with vehicle (0.9% NaCl, 10 mL/kg; positive control group) or PrLP (0.05, 0.5, 5, or 50 mg/kg) or orally (p.o.) with N-acetylcysteine, the standard antioxidant drug (NAC, 750 mg/kg). After 30 minutes, a single intragastric dose of absolute ethanol (0.2 mL) was administered to positive control (vehicle) or PrLP groups and after 60 minutes to NAC group. One hour after ethanol treatments, the animals were sacrificed with anesthetic overdose. The stomachs were excised, opened along the greater curvature, and rinsed with saline (0.9%), according to the method described by Robert et al. [19]. The stomachs were scanned and the extension of the ulcerated area (%) was estimated using a computer planimetry program (ImageJ; National Institutes of Health, USA) [20]. After the statistical analysis of the data, the lower effective dose of the 4 doses tested was used for all other assays. Subsequently, gastric corpus samples were then weighed, frozen, and stored at −70°C until being assayed to determine glutathione (GSH) levels [21].

2.5. Microscopic Analyses. Samples of the gastric mucosa were fixed in formaldehyde (10%, v/v) and prepared in 0.01 M PBS, pH 7.2, over 24 h for histopathology procedures. Sections (5 μm) were stained with hematoxylin-eosin to evaluate gastric mucosal injury according to the criteria of Laine and Weinstein [22], as follows: edema in the upper mucosa (0–4), hemorrhagic damage (0–4), epithelial cell loss (0–3), and the presence of inflammatory cells (0–3). Photomicrographs of sections were obtained with a Leica DM microscope equipped with a Leica DFC 280 camera (200x magnification).

2.6. Role of Prostaglandins in Gastroprotective Effect of the PrLP. The influence of endogenous prostaglandins was investigated as previously described by Morais et al. [23]. The animals ($n = 8$ per group) were pretreated with the cyclooxygenase inhibitor (indomethacin 10 mg/kg, p.o.), 60 min before the PrLP (0.5 mg/kg, i.v.) or a synthetic prostaglandin E1 analog (misoprostol 50 μg/kg, p.o.). Other groups of animals were treated only with vehicle (0.9% NaCl, 10 mL/kg, i.v.), PrLP (0.5 mg/kg, i.v.), or misoprostol (50 μg/kg, p.o.). After 30 minutes, a single intragastric dose of absolute ethanol (0.2 mL) was administered to positive control (vehicle) or PrLP groups and after 60 minutes to misoprostol groups. One hour after ethanol treatments, the animals were sacrificed with anesthetic overdose. The stomachs were excised and opened along the greater curvature [19]. The extension of the ulcerated area (%) was estimated using ImageJ software [20].

2.7. Role of Nitric Oxide in Gastroprotective Effect of the PrLP. The involvement of nitric oxide was investigated, as previously described [23]. The animals (n = 8 per group) were pretreated with inhibitor of the nitric oxide synthase (L-NAME 20 mg/kg) by intraperitoneal (i.p.) administration, 30 min prior to the treatment with PrLP (0.5 mg/kg, i.v.) or a substrate for nitric oxide synthase (L-arginine 600 mg/kg, i.p.). Other groups of animals were treated only with vehicle (0.9% NaCl, 10 mL/kg, i.v.), PrLP (0.5 mg/kg, i.v.), or L-arginine (600 mg/kg, i.p.). After 30 minutes, all animals received a single intragastric dose of absolute ethanol (0.2 mL). One hour later, the animals were sacrificed with anesthetic overdose. The stomachs were excised and opened along the greater curvature [19]. The extension of the ulcerated area (%) was estimated using ImageJ software [20]. Subsequently, samples from gastric mucosa were then weighed, frozen, and stored at −70°C until being assayed for NO_3/NO_2 production [24].

2.8. Evaluation of Transient Receptor Potential Vanilloid Type 1 (TRPV1) Triggers. The activation of capsaicin-sensitive primary afferents was investigated using a TRPV1 antagonist, capsazepine [25]. The animals (n = 8 per group) were pretreated with capsazepine (5 mg/kg, i.p.), 30 min prior to the treatment with PrLP (0.5 mg/kg, i.v.) or a vanilloid agonist (capsaicin 0.3 mg/kg, p.o.). Other groups of animals were treated only with vehicle (0.9% NaCl, 10 mL/kg, i.v.), PrLP (0.5 mg/kg, i.v.), or capsaicin (0.3 mg/kg, p.o.). After 30 minutes, a single intragastric dose of absolute ethanol (0.2 mL) was administered to positive control (vehicle) or PrLP groups and after 60 minutes to capsaicin groups. One hour after ethanol treatments, the animals were sacrificed with anesthetic overdose. The stomachs were excised and opened along the greater curvature [19]. The extension of the ulcerated area (%) was estimated using ImageJ software [20].

2.9. Evaluation of Soluble Guanylate Cyclase Activation. A soluble guanylate cyclase inhibitor (ODQ) was used to investigate the involvement of cGMP [26]. The animals (n = 8 per group) were pretreated with ODQ (10 mg/kg, i.p.), 30 min prior to the treatment with PrLP (0.5 mg/kg, i.v.). Other groups of animals were treated only with vehicle (0.9% NaCl, 10 mL/kg, i.v.) or PrLP (0.5 mg/kg, i.v.). After 30 minutes, all animals received a single intragastric dose of absolute ethanol (0.2 mL). One hour later, the animals were sacrificed with anesthetic overdose. The stomachs were excised and opened along the greater curvature [19]. The extension of the ulcerated area (%) was estimated using ImageJ software [20].

2.10. Role of ATP-Sensitive Potassium Channels (K_{ATP}) in Gastroprotective Effect of PrLP. Pharmacological modulation of K_{ATP} with diazoxide (agonist) or glibenclamide (antagonist) was used to investigate the involvement of these channels in the gastroprotective effect of PrLP [22]. The animals (n = 8 per group) were pretreated with glibenclamide (5 mg/kg, i.p.), 30 min prior to the treatment with PrLP (0.5 mg/kg, i.v.) or diazoxide (3 mg/kg, i.p.). Other groups of animals were treated only with vehicle (0.9% NaCl, 10 mL/kg, i.v.),

PrLP (0.5 mg/kg, i.v.), or diazoxide (3 mg/kg, i.p.). After 30 minutes, all animals received a single intragastric dose of absolute ethanol (0.2 mL). One hour later, the animals were sacrificed with anesthetic overdose. The stomachs were excised and opened along the greater curvature [19]. The extension of the ulcerated area (%) was estimated using ImageJ software [20].

2.11. Measurement of Nitrate/Nitrite Levels in the Gastric Mucosa. Nitrite levels in biopsy lysates from the gastric mucosa were determined indirectly as the total content of nitrite and nitrate (NO_3^-/NO_2^-) by a spectrophotometric method based on the Griess reaction [24]. Samples of the gastric mucosa were homogenized in 50 mM potassium phosphate buffer (pH 7.8) and centrifuged at 11,000 ×g for 15 minutes at 4°C. An aliquot of each sample (80 μL) was incubated in a microplate with nitrate reductase for 12 h to convert NO_3 into NO_2. At room temperature (25°C), 100 μL of Griess reagent (1% sulphanilamide in 1% phosphoric acid and 0.1% naphthalene diamine dihydrochloride in water) was added and incubated for 10 minutes. The optical densities were measured at 540 nm in a microplate reader. Nitrite concentrations in the samples were determined from a standard curve generated by different concentrations of sodium nitrite (0.1–100 mM). The data are expressed as micromoles of nitrite. All analyses were performed in triplicate and were reproduced without significant differences.

2.12. Glutathione (GSH) Levels in the Gastric Mucosa. Samples of the gastric mucosa were homogenized in a solution that contained 1 mL of a 0.02 M EDTA cooled solution, 320 μL of distilled water, and 400 μL of trichloroacetic acid (TCA) 50% (w/v). The homogenates were centrifuged at 3000 ×g for 15 minutes. The supernatants (400 μL) were mixed with 800 μL of Tris buffer (40 mM, pH 8.9) and 5,5′-dithiobis(2-nitrobenzoic acid) (DTNB, 10 mM) was added. The absorbance was measured within 3 minutes after addition of DTNB at 412 nm against a blank reagent without homogenate [21]. The absorbance values were extrapolated from a reduced glutathione standard curve and expressed as NP-SH/g of stomach tissue.

2.13. Statistical Analysis. Values are expressed as the mean ± standard errors mean (SEM) or median. Analysis of Variance (ANOVA) followed by Student-Newman-Keuls test was used to compare means and Kruskal-Wallis nonparametric test, followed by Dunn's test, to compare medians; $P < 0.05$ was defined as statistically significant.

3. Results and Discussion

PrLP comprises the water soluble protein fraction extracted from the whole latex of *Plumeria rubra*. The antioxidative enzymes ascorbate peroxidase and superoxide dismutase were detected in PrLP while catalase was absent. Chitinases were also found. Proteolytic enzymes that were best inhibited by E-64 were reported [17]. These authors reported that PrLP represents nearly 0.33 mg of protein in 1 mL of crude latex.

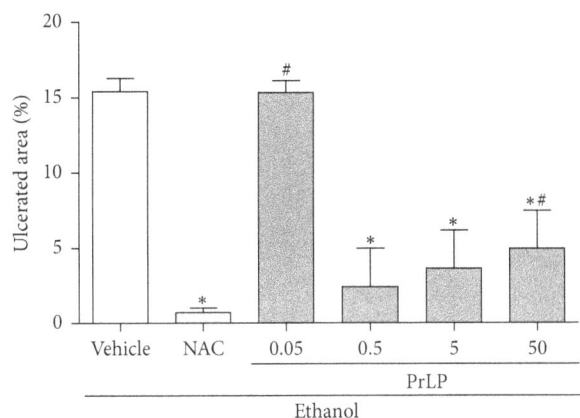

FIGURE 1: Ethanol-induced gastric lesions. Animals were sacrificed, and their stomachs were immediately excised to evaluate the extension of the ulcerated area. Data are expressed as the mean ± standard error mean (SEM) of the number of lesions (8 animals per group), expressed in percent. $^*P < 0.05$ indicates a significant difference compared with the positive control group (vehicle); $^\#P < 0.05$ indicates a significant difference compared with animals treated with NAC (ANOVA, Newman-Keuls test).

TABLE 1: Semi-quantitative evaluation of gastric lesions.

Groups	Microscopic scores		
	Hemorrhage	Loss epithelial cell	Inflammatory infiltrate
Negative control group	0 (0-0)	0 (0-0)	0 (0-0)
Positive control group	4 (4-4)*	3 (2-3)*	1 (0-1)
PrLP	0.5 (0-1)$^\#$	1 (1-1)$^\#$	0 (0-1)
NAC	0 (0-0)$^\#$	1 (1-1)$^\#$	0 (0-1)

Data represent the median and range of scores from two separate experiments: (0) absent, (1) mild, (2) moderate, (3) intense, (4) edema in the upper mucosa, hemorrhagic damage, epithelial cell loss and the presence of inflammatory cells. $^*P < 0.05$ indicates a significant difference compared with the negative control group. $^\#P < 0.05$ indicates a significant difference compared with the positive control group (vehicle). ($n = 8$ animals/group, Kruskal-Wallis test followed by Dunn's test).

PrLP is free of other metabolites, mainly those produced by the secondary metabolism. Water insoluble compounds are lost by precipitation along dialyses in water and the water soluble ones are lost through the dialyses membrane. Chemical assays for measurement of saponins, flavonoids, phenols, tannins, triterpenes, and alkaloids on PrLP have failed (data not shown). At least the overall profile of proteins present in PrLP can be found in the studies of de Freitas et al. [17] cited above.

Experimental studies to highlight gastroprotective substances have been performed using a model of ethanol-induced gastric lesions [27–29]. Here, we investigated the gastroprotective potential of PrLP, since the properties of latex proteins in different pharmacological models have been successfully confirmed. The venous route for sample administration was selected as the first approach in order to avoid the physiochemical instability and enzymatic barrier of proteins. Moreover, the influence of enterohepatic recirculation could reduce the bioavailability of the soluble proteins. We have initiated approaches to determine the potential subchronic toxicity of PrLP in animals. Serum level of urea and the enzymatic activities of alanine aminotransferase (ALT or TGP) and aspartate aminotransferase (AST or TGO) determined with standardized diagnostic kits were normal in animals given PrLP at tested doses (unpublished data).

In a dose-dependent manner, the pretreatment with PrLP prevented the appearance of gastric mucosal ulceration when compared with positive control group (vehicle) ($P < 0.05$). The effect was similar to that observed in the N-acetylcysteine (NAC) group. The highest gastroprotective effect of PrLP occurred at a dose of 0.5 mg/kg (Figure 1).

Macro- and microscopic aspects of the gastric mucosa are shown in Figures 2(a)–2(d) and Table 1. No type of lesion was observed in the samples of stomach from the negative control group (saline), as seen by the gastric epithelia integrity

(Figures 2(a1) and 2(a2)). Animals pretreated with vehicle (positive control group) and subjected to intragastric absolute ethanol presented a significant number of lesions on the gastric mucosa, with intense signs of hemorrhage and loss of epithelial cells when compared with negative control group (Figures 2(b1) and 2(b2)). The groups of animals pretreated with PrLP or NAC were protected from alterations induced by ethanol (Figures 2(c1), 2(c2), 2(d1), and 2(d2)).

The genesis of ethanol-induced gastric lesions is multifactorial and is associated with a decrease in the intrinsic gastric mucosal defense mechanisms or an increase in aggressive factors, mainly related to changes in the microcirculation and oxidative stress [26]. The existence of cytoprotective effect associated with a significant reduction of the ulcer index, besides free radical scavenging activity, was previously pointed to ethanol and chloroform extract of Plumeria rubra [30]. However, our data shown in this work suggest that the gastroprotective effect observed on animals submitted to induced gastric ulcer was mediated by the latex protein fraction instead of other metabolites.

It is well known that prostaglandin E2 (PGE2), an eicosanoid, has gastroprotective effects through stimulating bicarbonate and mucus release, also provoking vasodilation and increased blood flow [31–33]. The effects of PGE2 on ethanol-induced gastric lesions are due to an increase in intracellular cGMP, mediated by an increase in intracellular calcium concentration and nitric oxide production [34, 35]. The involvement of prostaglandins in the gastroprotective mechanism of PrLP was investigated through pharmacological modulation with indomethacin (an inhibitor of prostaglandin synthesis). A significant extension of the gastric mucosal ulceration was observed in animals pretreated with vehicle (positive control group) and subjected to intragastric absolute ethanol (Figure 3). The appearance of injuries was significantly prevented by the pretreatment with PrLP or misoprostol, when compared with the positive control group (vehicle) ($P < 0.05$). However, the pretreatment of animals with indomethacin reversed the gastroprotective effects promoted by PrLP or misoprostol, significantly increasing the ethanol-induced gastric mucosal lesions ($P < 0.05$).

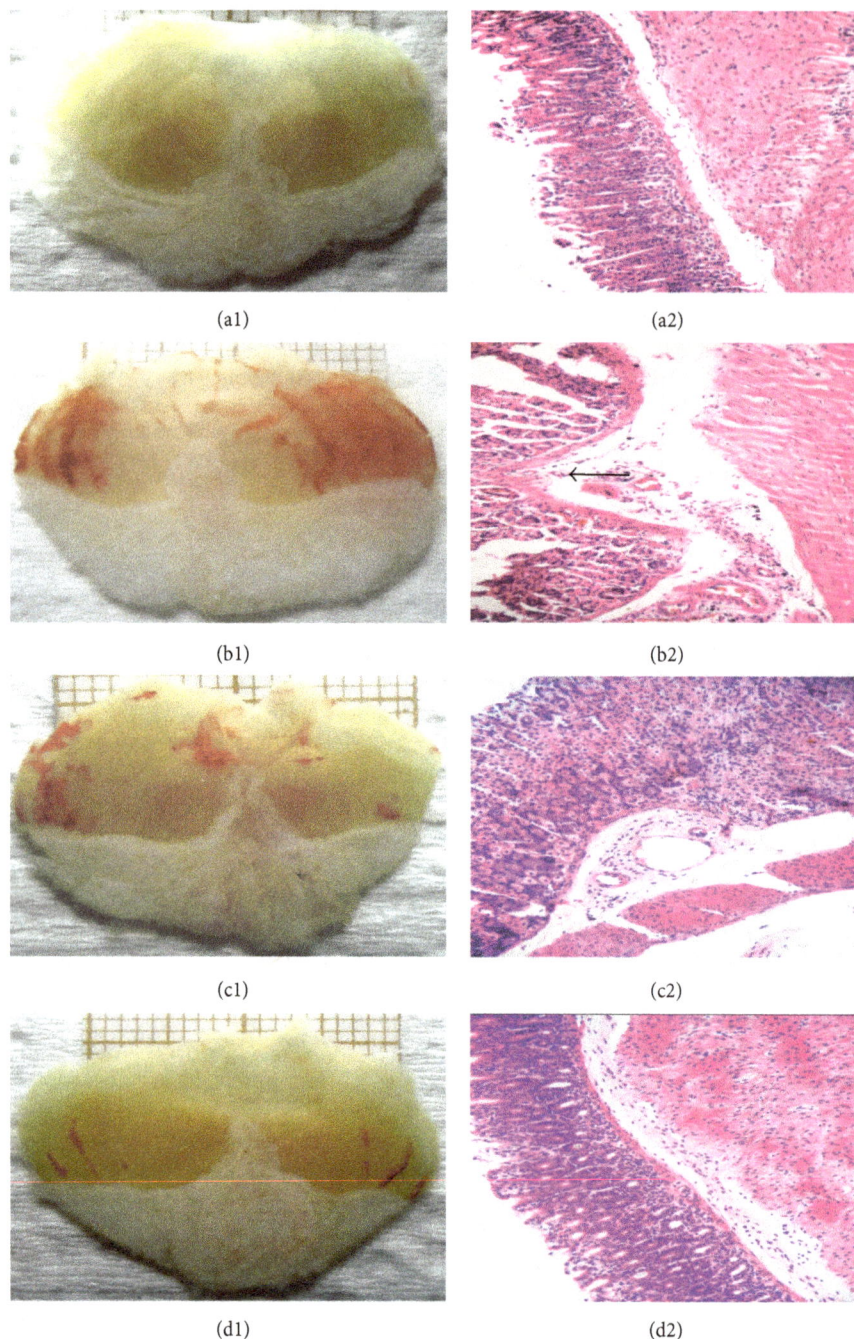

FIGURE 2: Gastric mucosal lesions: macro- and microscopic aspects. Animals were sacrificed, and their stomachs were opened along the greater curvature. For macroscopic evaluation, images were selected from animals belonging to the corresponding experimental groups (a1–d1). Samples of the gastric mucosa were removed to perform histological analyses (a2–d2). Hematoxylin-eosin stained sections were employed to obtain photomicrographs and to estimate hemorrhage, loss of epithelial cells, and inflammatory infiltrates (arrow) among the different experimental groups: (a1, a2) negative control group, (b1, b2) positive control group, (c1, c2) PrLP 0.5 mg/kg, i.v., and (d1, d2) NAC (200x magnification).

These results strongly indicate that PrLP acts through the involvement of prostaglandins, possibly stimulating the production of this mediator. Similarly, the protective response of chloroform and ethanolic extract of leaves from *P. rubra* against ethanol-induced gastric lesions was also a suggestion of its effect on prostaglandin synthesis [22].

Gastric mucosal defense is also mediated physiologically by nitric oxide (NO) through blood flow regulation, mucus release, and inhibition of inflammatory infiltrates [36–38]. Thus, drugs that block the synthesis of NO exacerbate the lesions associated with ethanol. Therefore, an inhibitor of NO synthesis (L-NAME) was used in order to observe the

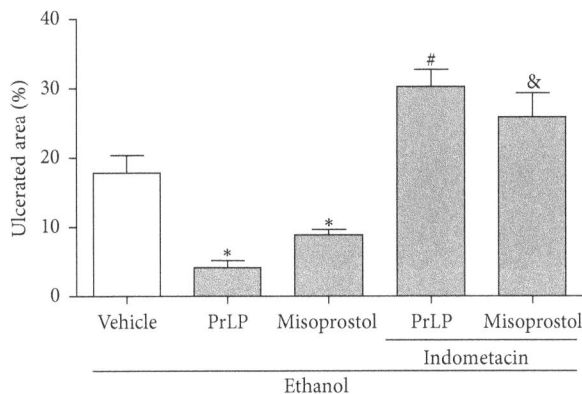

FIGURE 3: Involvement of prostaglandins in ethanol-induced gastric lesions. Animals were sacrificed, and their stomachs were immediately excised to evaluate the extension of the ulcerated area. Data are expressed as the mean ± standard error mean (SEM) of the number of lesions (8 animals per group), expressed in percent. $^*P <$ 0.05 indicates a significant difference compared with the positive control group (vehicle); $^{\#}P < 0.05$ indicates a significant difference compared with animals treated only with PrLP; $^{\&}P < 0.05$ indicates a significant difference compared with animals treated only with misoprostol (ANOVA, Newman-Keuls test).

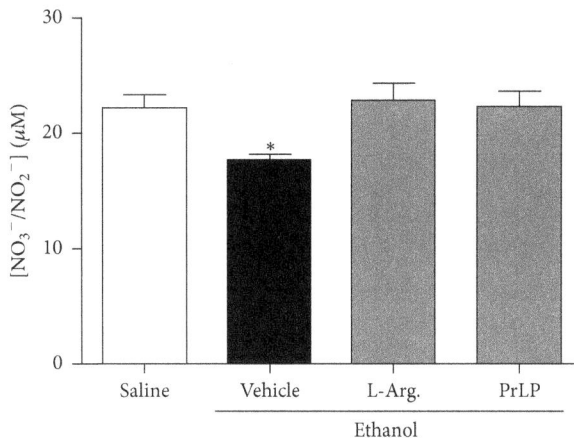

FIGURE 5: Nitrite levels in gastric mucosa. Animals were sacrificed, and their stomachs were immediately excised. Samples of the gastric mucosa were removed to determine nitrite levels by the Griess reaction. Data are the mean of three independent experiments and are expressed as the mean ± standard error mean (SEM) of nitric oxide (NO_3/NO_2) levels (μM). $^*P < 0.05$ indicates a significant difference compared with the negative control group (saline) (ANOVA, Newman-Keuls test).

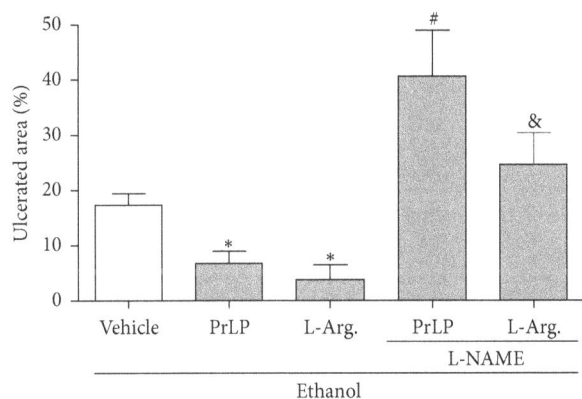

FIGURE 4: Involvement of nitric oxide in ethanol-induced gastric mucosal lesions. Animals were sacrificed, and their stomachs were immediately excised to evaluate the extension of the ulcerated area. Data are expressed as the mean ± standard error mean (SEM) of the number of lesions (8 animals per group), expressed in percent. $^*P < 0.05$ indicates a significant difference compared with the positive control group (vehicle); $^{\#}P < 0.05$ indicates a significant difference compared with animals treated only with PrLP; $^{\&}P < 0.05$ indicates a significant difference compared with animals treated only with L-arginine (ANOVA, Newman-Keuls test).

significantly increased ethanol-induced gastric lesions ($P <$ 0.05). As demonstrated, nitric oxide was involved in the gastroprotective effects of PrLP. To confirm this hypothesis, stomach samples were used to measure nitrite/nitrate levels. Animals pretreated with vehicle (positive control group) and submitted to intragastric absolute ethanol exhibited reduced levels of nitrite in the gastric mucosa, when compared with the negative control group ($P < 0.05$) (Figure 5). The reduction in nitrite levels induced by ethanol was significantly prevented in the group of animals pretreated with PrLP or L-arginine ($P < 0.05$).

These results confirm the involvement of nitric oxide in the gastroprotective effect of PrLP, probably by constitutive overexpression of nitric oxide synthases (NOS) and their efficiency on catalytic actions. According to the published literature, nitric oxide increases vascular permeability and prostaglandin production in the gastric mucosa. Moreover, its effects on gastric microcirculation and the synthesis of mucus also result from cooperative activity with prostaglandins [39, 40].

It is well known that the vasodilator effect of NO is mediated by the stimulation of the enzyme soluble guanylyl cyclase (sGS) and the consequent release of cGMP [41]. In experimental models, a highly selective irreversible heme-site inhibitor of soluble guanylyl cyclase, known as ODQ (1H-[1,2,4]oxadiazolo[4,3-a]quinoxalin-1-one), has been used to identify the correlation of gastroprotective substances with the NO-sGS-cGMP signaling system [42, 43]. According to this approach, animals pretreated with vehicle (positive control group) and subjected to intragastric absolute ethanol exhibited a significant extension of the gastric mucosal ulceration (Figure 6). The appearance of lesions was significantly prevented in the group of animals pretreated with PrLP (i.v.). Another group of animals was pretreated with ODQ, in

involvement of NO in the gastroprotective effect of PrLP. A significant extension of the gastric mucosal ulceration was observed in animals pretreated with vehicle (positive control group) and subjected to intragastric absolute ethanol (Figure 4). The pretreatment with PrLP (i.v.) or L-arginine (i.p.) significantly prevented the appearance of lesions compared with the positive control group ($P < 0.05$). The gastroprotective effects promoted by PrLP or L-arginine were reversed in the group of animals pretreated with L-NAME (i.p.), which

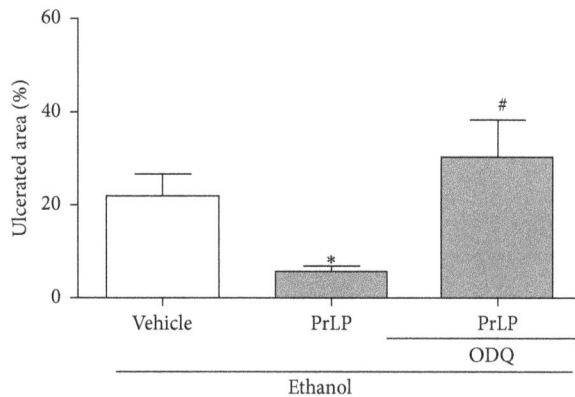

FIGURE 6: Involvement of the NO-sGS-cGMP signaling system in ethanol-induced gastric lesions. Animals were sacrificed, and their stomachs were immediately excised to evaluate the extension of the ulcerated area. Data are expressed as the mean ± standard error mean (SEM) of the number of lesions (8 animals per group), expressed in percent. $^*P < 0.05$ indicates a significant difference compared with the positive control group (vehicle); $^\#P < 0.05$ indicates a significant difference compared with animals treated only with PrLP (ANOVA, Newman-Keuls test).

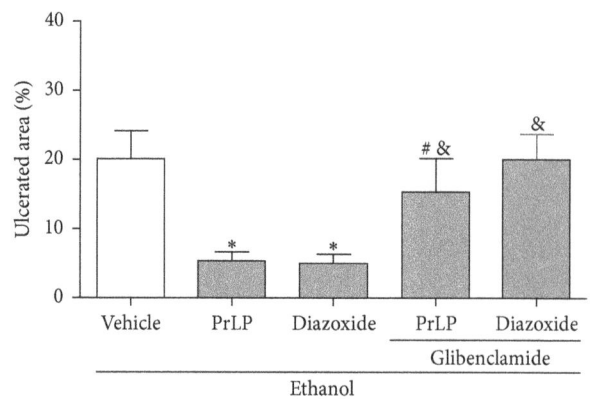

FIGURE 7: Involvement of ATP-dependent potassium channel (K_{ATP}) in ethanol-induced gastric mucosal lesions. Animals were sacrificed, and their stomachs were immediately excised to evaluate the extension of the ulcerated area. Data are expressed as the mean ± standard error mean (SEM) of the number of lesions (8 animals per group), expressed in percent. $^*P < 0.05$ indicates a significant difference compared with the positive control group (vehicle); $^\#P < 0.05$ indicates a significant difference compared with animals treated only with PrLP; $^\&P < 0.05$ indicates a significant difference compared with animals treated only with diazoxide (ANOVA, Newman-Keuls test).

which the protective effects of PrLP against ethanol-induced gastric mucosal injury were reversed ($P < 0.05$). The same involvement of the NO-sGS-cGMP signaling system was also used to explain the gastroprotective mechanism of sildenafil (a drug commercially used to treat erectile dysfunction) by Medeiros et al. [42].

An ATP-dependent potassium channel (K_{ATP}) is associated with the regulation of blood flow, acid secretion, and muscle contractility of the gastric mucosa [44]. Some compounds, such as diazoxide, inhibit ethanol-induced gastric mucosal damage through the opening of K_{ATP} channels, while glibenclamide, a blocker of these channels, attenuates gastric injuries [25, 45, 46]. Thus, to assess the contribution of K_{ATP} channels to the gastroprotective effects of PrLP, pharmacological approaches were employed. A significant extension of the gastric mucosal ulceration was observed in the group of animals pretreated with vehicle (positive control group) and subjected to intragastric absolute ethanol. The damage in the gastric mucosa was significantly prevented by the pretreatment with PrLP (i.v.) or diazoxide (i.p.) ($P < 0.05$). In another group of animals, the prior administration of glibenclamide (i.p.) reversed the gastroprotective effects promoted by PrLP or diazoxide against ethanol-induced gastric mucosal injury ($P < 0.05$) (Figure 7).

The gastroprotective mechanisms involving prostaglandins and nitric oxide are related to the activation of the guanylyl cyclase enzyme and release of the intracellular second messenger cyclic GMP (cGMP). Moreover, the activation of ATP-dependent potassium channels may occur in response to nitric oxide and cyclic GMP [26, 47, 48]. Therefore, this set of results suggests that the NO/cGMP/K_{ATP} pathway is of primary importance in the gastroprotective effect of PrLP.

Capsaicin-sensitive sensory nerves are involved as a defense system to protect against gastric damage. The mechanism involves receptor stimulation at the plasma membrane,

primarily of the transient receptor potential vanilloid type 1 (TRPV1) [49, 50]. A vanilloid antagonist capsazepine has been used to determine the involvement of these receptors as part of the gastroprotective mechanism for different substances [51, 52]. A significant extension of the gastric mucosal ulceration was observed in the group of animals pretreated with vehicle (positive control group) and subjected to intragastric absolute ethanol. As expected, PrLP (i.v.) and capsaicin (p.o.) significantly prevented the appearance of injuries when compared with the positive control group ($P < 0.05$). In the group of animals pretreated with vanilloid antagonist capsazepine, the gastroprotective effect of PrLP (i.v.) and capsaicin (p.o.) was significantly reduced ($P < 0.05$) (Figure 8). Our results indicate that the gastroprotective effect of PrLP is also mediated by the activation of capsaicin-sensitive primary afferents. A similar profile was observed in the gastroprotective effect of barbatusin and 3-beta-hydroxy-3-deoxibarbatusin, diterpenes able to stimulate receptor potential vanilloid type 1 (TRPV1) and promote an increase in nitric oxide, displaying mucosal defense through both of these mechanisms [22].

Ethanol-induced gastric mucosal injury is related to the generation of free radicals and imbalance of oxidant/antioxidant factors [53, 54]. Clinical and experimental evidence suggest that antioxidant substances may promote gastroprotective effects [31, 52]. Therefore, grounded by studies that showed the antioxidative and proteolytic activities of laticifer cells of P. rubra [17], the involvement of PrLP in the antioxidant defense mechanisms was investigated through determination of glutathione (GSH) levels in the gastric mucosa. Animals from the negative control group (saline) displayed glutathione (GSH) levels within normal range, according to the published literature [55]. Animals

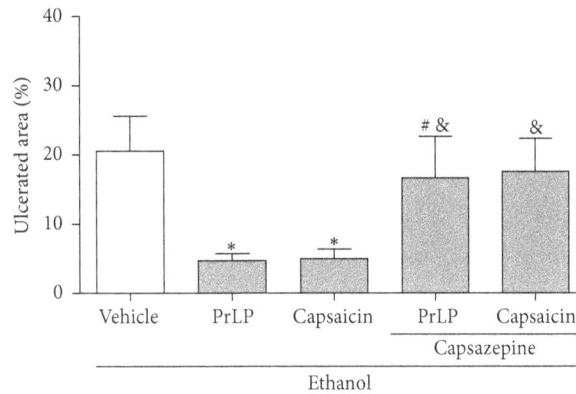

FIGURE 8: Involvement of transient receptor potential vanilloid 1 (TRPV1) in ethanol-induced gastric lesions. Animals were sacrificed, and their stomachs were immediately excised to evaluate the extension of the ulcerated area. Data are expressed as the mean ± standard error mean (SEM) of the number of lesions (8 animals per group), expressed in percent. $^*P < 0.05$ indicates a significant difference compared with the positive control group (vehicle); $^\#P < 0.05$ indicates a significant difference compared with animals treated only with PrLP; $^\&P < 0.05$ indicates a significant difference compared with animals treated only with capsaicin (ANOVA, Newman-Keuls test).

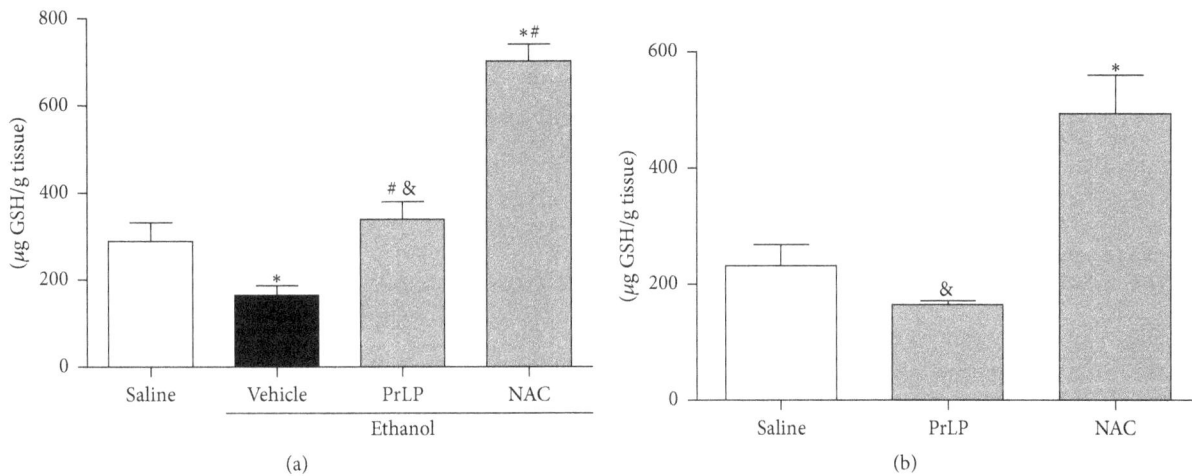

(a)

(b)

FIGURE 9: Glutathione (GSH) levels in ethanol-induced gastric lesions. Animals were sacrificed, and their stomachs were immediately excised. Samples of the gastric mucosa from animals subjected to ethanol (a) or not (b) were removed to determine glutathione levels. Data are the mean of three independent experiments and are expressed as the mean ± standard error mean (SEM) of μg GSH/g of tissue. $^*P < 0.05$ indicates a significant difference compared with the negative control group (saline); $^\#P < 0.05$ indicates a significant difference compared with the positive control group (vehicle); $^\&P < 0.05$ indicates a significant difference compared with the NAC group (ANOVA, Newman-Keuls test).

pretreated with vehicle (positive control group) and subjected to intragastric absolute ethanol displayed significant mucosal GSH depletion when compared with the negative control group ($P < 0.05$). GSH levels were significantly ($P < 0.05$) restored in animals pretreated with NAC (p.o.) or PrLP (i.v.) before administration of intragastric absolute ethanol (Figure 9(a)). A second approach was taken to verify whether PrLP acts by increasing the levels of GSH without influencing ethanol-induced gastric mucosal injury. GSH levels were not altered in animals pretreated with PrLP when compared with the negative control group, while NAC promoted an increase, regardless of the deleterious effects promoted by ethanol (Figure 9(b)).

4. Conclusions

Soluble proteins from the latex of *Plumeria rubra* (PrLP) prevented ethanol-induced gastric lesions through the involvement of prostaglandins and balance of oxidant/antioxidant factors. Secondarily, the NO/cGMP/K$_{ATP}$ pathway and activation of capsaicin-sensitive primary afferents were also demonstrated as part of the mechanism. This study also suggests that the use of the latex of *P. rubra* in folk medicine is pertinent. The diversity of manners in which people use latex as alternative medicine (as topical application or oral ingestion) encourages the scientific studies. However, it still represents a challenge to understand the true potentialities of latex compounds and determine the toxic potential and thus establish the best practices for their use.

Conflict of Interests

The authors declare that there is no conflict of interests regarding the publication of this paper.

Acknowledgments

The study has been supported by grants from the following Brazilian agencies: Concelho Nacional de Desenvolvimento Científico e Tecnológico (CNPq) and Fundação Cearense de Apoio ao Desenvolvimento Científico e Tecnológico (FUNCAP). This study is part of the consortium Molecular Biotechnology of Plant Latex.

References

[1] K. S. Jain, A. K. Shah, J. Bariwal et al., "Recent advances in proton pump inhibitors and management of acid-peptic disorders," *Bioorganic & Medicinal Chemistry*, vol. 15, no. 3, pp. 1181–1205, 2007.

[2] C. Musumba, D. M. Pritchard, and M. Pirmohamed, "Review article: cellular and molecular mechanisms of NSAID-induced peptic ulcers," *Alimentary Pharmacology & Therapeutics*, vol. 30, no. 6, pp. 517–531, 2009.

[3] J. L. Wallace and J. G. P. Ferraz, "New pharmacologic therapies in gastrointestinal disease," *Gastroenterology Clinics of North America*, vol. 39, no. 3, pp. 709–720, 2010.

[4] M. Valko, C. J. Rhodes, J. Moncol, M. Izakovic, and M. Mazur, "Free radicals, metals and antioxidants in oxidative stress-induced cancer," *Chemico-Biological Interactions*, vol. 160, no. 1, pp. 1–40, 2006.

[5] E. Palencia-Herrejón, B. Sánchez, I. Escobar, and M. L. Gómez-Lus, "Proton pump inhibitors and infection risk," *Revista Española de Quimioterapia*, vol. 24, no. 1, pp. 4–12, 2011.

[6] K. C. Mousinho, C. D. C. Oliveira, J. R. D. O. Ferreira et al., "Antitumor effect of laticifer proteins of *Himatanthus drasticus* (Mart.) Plumel—Apocynaceae," *Journal of Ethnopharmacology*, vol. 137, no. 1, pp. 421–426, 2011.

[7] P. Chaudhary, C. D. A. Viana, M. V. Ramos, and V. Kumar, "Antiedematogenic and antioxidant properties of high molecular weight protein sub-fraction of *Calotropis procera* latex in rat," *Journal of Basic and Clinical Pharmacy*, vol. 6, no. 2, pp. 69–73, 2015.

[8] M. E. Endress and P. V. Bruyns, "A revised classification of the Apocynaceae s.l.," *The Botanical Review*, vol. 66, no. 1, pp. 1–56, 2000.

[9] L. M. Perry, *Medicinal Plants of East and Southeast Asia: Attributed Properties and Uses*, MIT Press, Cambridge, UK, 1980.

[10] G. Ye, Z.-X. Li, G.-X. Xia et al., "A new iridoid alkaloid from the flowers of *Plumeria rubra* L. *cv. Acutifolia*," *Magnetic Resonance in Chemistry*, vol. 46, pp. 1195–1197, 2009.

[11] M. O. Hamburger, G. A. Cordell, and N. Ruangrungsi, "Traditional medicinal plants of Thailand XVII Biologically active constituents of *Plumeria rubra*," *Journal of Ethnopharmacology*, vol. 33, no. 3, pp. 289–292, 1991.

[12] M. Grignon-Dubois, B. Rezzonico, A. Usubillaga, and L. B. Vojas, "Isolation of plumieride from *Plumeria inodora*," *Chemistry of Natural Compounds*, vol. 41, no. 6, pp. 730–731, 2005.

[13] G. M. Kuigoua, S. F. Kouam, B. T. Ngadjui et al., "Minor secondary metabolic products from the stem bark of *Plumeria rubra* Linn. displaying antimicrobial activities," *Planta Medica*, vol. 76, no. 6, pp. 620–625, 2010.

[14] A. Dey, T. Das, and S. Mukherjee, "In vitro antibacterial activity of n-Hexane fraction of methanolic extract of *Plumeria rubra* L. (Apocynaceae) stem bark," *Journal of Plant Sciences*, vol. 6, no. 3, pp. 135–142, 2011.

[15] A. J. Merina, D. Sivanesan, V. H. Begum, and N. Sulochana, "Antioxidant and hypolipidemic effect of *Plumeria rubra* L. in alloxan induced hyperglycemic rats," *E-Journal of Chemistry*, vol. 7, no. 1, pp. 1–5, 2010.

[16] I. Chanda, U. Sarma, S. K. Basu, M. Lahkar, and S. K. Dutta, "A protease isolated from the latex of *Plumeria rubra* linn (apocynaceae) 2: Anti-inflammatory and wound-healing activities," *Tropical Journal of Pharmaceutical Research*, vol. 10, no. 6, pp. 755–760, 2011.

[17] C. D. T. de Freitas, D. P. de Souza, E. S. Araújo, M. G. Cavalheiro, L. S. Oliveira, and M. V. Ramos, "Anti-oxidative and proteolytic activities and protein profile of laticifer cells of *Cryptostegia grandiflora*, *Plumeria rubra* and *Euphorbia tirucalli*," *Brazilian Journal of Plant Physiology*, vol. 22, no. 1, pp. 11–22, 2010.

[18] S. V. F. Gaban, W. S. Costa, C. N. Assis et al., "Latex extract of *Plumeria rubra* induces antihypertensive and vasodilator effects on rat aorta," *International Journal of Indigenous Medicinal Plants*, vol. 46, pp. 2051–4263, 2013.

[19] A. Robert, J. E. Nezamis, C. Lancaster, and A. J. Hanchar, "Cytoprotection by prostaglandins in rats. Prevention of gastric necrosis produced by alcohol, HCl, NaOH, hypertonic NaCl, and thermal injury," *Gastroenterology*, vol. 77, no. 3, pp. 433–443, 1979.

[20] N. R. D. Costa, R. O. Silva, L. A. D. Nicolau et al., "Role of soluble guanylate cyclase activation in the gastroprotective effect of the HO-1/CO pathway against alendronate-induced gastric damage in rats," *European Journal of Pharmacology*, vol. 700, no. 1–3, pp. 51–59, 2013.

[21] J. Sedlak and R. H. Lindsay, "Estimation of total, protein-bound, and nonprotein sulfhydryl groups in tissue with Ellman's reagent," *Analytical Biochemistry*, vol. 25, pp. 192–205, 1968.

[22] P. D. A. Rodrigues, S. M. de Morais, C. M. de Souza et al., "Gastroprotective effect of barbatusin and 3-beta-hydroxy-3-deoxibarbatusin, quinonoid diterpenes isolated from *Plectranthus grandis*, in ethanol-induced gastric lesions in mice," *Journal of Ethnopharmacology*, vol. 127, no. 3, pp. 725–730, 2010.

[23] T. C. Morais, N. B. Pinto, K. M. M. B. Carvalho et al., "Protective effect of anacardic acids from cashew (*Anacardium occidentale*) on ethanol-induced gastric damage in mice," *Chemico-Biological Interactions*, vol. 183, no. 1, pp. 264–269, 2010.

[24] J.-C. Chen, H.-M. Chen, M.-H. Shyr et al., "Selective inhibition of inducible nitric oxide in ischemia-reperfusion of rat small intestine," *Journal of the Formosan Medical Association*, vol. 99, no. 3, pp. 213–218, 2000.

[25] A. P. De Vasconcellos Abdon, G. C. De Souza, L. N. C. De Souza et al., "Gastroprotective potential of frutalin, a d-galactose binding lectin, against ethanol-induced gastric lesions," *Fitoterapia*, vol. 83, no. 3, pp. 604–608, 2012.

[26] H. W. Davenport, "Gastric mucosal hemorrhage in dogs. Effects of acid, aspirin, and alcohol," *Gastroenterology*, vol. 56, no. 3, pp. 439–449, 1969.

[27] D. Wong and C. W. Ogle, "Chronic parenterally administered nicotine and stress- or ethanol-induced gastric mucosal damage in rats," *European Journal of Pharmacology: Environmental Toxicology and*, vol. 292, no. 2, pp. 157–162, 1995.

[28] K. Sairam, C. V. Rao, M. D. Babu, and R. K. Goel, "Prophylactic and curative effects of *Bacopa monniera* in gastric ulcer models," *Phytomedicine*, vol. 8, no. 6, pp. 423–430, 2001.

[29] F. M. De-Faria, A. C. A. Almeida, A. Luiz-Ferreira et al., "Antioxidant action of mangrove polyphenols against gastric damage induced by absolute ethanol and ischemia-reperfusion in the rat," *The Scientific World Journal*, vol. 2012, Article ID 327071, 9 pages, 2012.

[30] M. Vimlesh, Y. Garima, U. S. Mubeen, and S. Vivek, "Determination of antiulcer activity of *Plumeria rubra* leaves extracts," *International Research Journal of Pharmacy*, vol. 3, no. 9, pp. 194–197, 2012.

[31] T. Brzozowski, P. C. Konturek, D. Drozdowicz et al., "Grapefruit-seed extract attenuates ethanol and stress-induced gastric lesions via activation of prostaglandin, nitric oxide and sensory nerve pathways," *World Journal of Gastroenterology*, vol. 11, no. 41, pp. 6450–6458, 2005.

[32] L. Laine, K. Takeuchi, and A. Tarnawski, "Gastric mucosal defense and cytoprotection: bench to bedside," *Gastroenterology*, vol. 135, no. 1, pp. 41–60, 2008.

[33] K. Higuchi, E. Umegaki, Y. Yoda, T. Takeuchi, M. Murano, and S. Tokioka, "The role of prostaglandin derivatives in a treatment and prevention for gastric ulcers in the aged patients," *Nippon Rinsho*, vol. 68, no. 11, pp. 2071–2075, 2010.

[34] G. B. Glavin, S. Szabo, B. R. Johnson et al., "Isolated rat gastric mucosal cells: optimal conditions for cell harvesting, measures of viability and direct cutoprotection," *Journal of Pharmacology and Experimental Therapy*, vol. 276, pp. 1174–1179, 1986.

[35] H. Sakai, E. Kumano, A. Ikari, and N. Takeguchi, "A gastric housekeeping Cl⁻ channel activated via prostaglandin EP3 receptor-mediated Ca^{2+}/nitric oxide/cGMP pathway," *The Journal of Biological Chemistry*, vol. 270, no. 32, pp. 18781–18785, 1995.

[36] J. F. Brown, A. C. Keates, P. J. Hanson, and B. J. R. Whittle, "Nitric oxide generators and cGMP stimulate mucus secretion by rat gastric mucosal cells," *The American Journal of Physiology—Gastrointestinal and Liver Physiology*, vol. 265, no. 3, pp. G418–G422, 1993.

[37] J. L. Wallace, W. McKnight, T. L. Wilson, P. D. Del Soldato, and G. Cirino, "Reduction of shock-induced gastric damage by a nitric oxide-releasing aspirin derivative: role of neutrophils," *American Journal of Physiology—Gastrointestinal and Liver Physiology*, vol. 273, no. 6, pp. G1246–G1251, 1997.

[38] J. L. Wallace, "Nitric oxide, aspirin-triggered lipoxins and NO-aspirin in gastric protection," *Inflammation & Allergy—Drug Targets*, vol. 5, no. 2, pp. 133–137, 2006.

[39] M. Ding, Y. Kinoshita, K. Kishi et al., "Distribution of prostaglandin E receptors in the rat gastrointestinal tract," *Prostaglandins*, vol. 53, no. 3, pp. 199–216, 1997.

[40] M. N. Muscara and J. L. Wallace, "Nitric oxide: therapeutic potential of nitric oxide donors and inhibitors," *American Journal of Physiology*, vol. 276, pp. 1313–1316, 1999.

[41] J. W. Denninger, J. P. M. Schelvis, P. E. Brandish, Y. Zhao, G. T. Babcock, and M. A. Marletta, "Interaction of soluble guanylate cyclase with YC-1: kinetic and resonance Raman studies," *Biochemistry*, vol. 39, no. 14, pp. 4191–4198, 2000.

[42] J. V. R. Medeiros, G. G. Gadelha, S. J. Lima et al., "Role of the NO/cGMP/K ATP pathway in the protective effects of sildenafil against ethanol-induced gastric damage in rats," *British Journal of Pharmacology*, vol. 153, no. 4, pp. 721–727, 2008.

[43] A. E. Chávez-Piña, G. R. Tapia-Álvarez, A. Reyes-Ramínrez, and A. Navarrete, "Carbenoxolone gastroprotective mechanism: participation of nitric oxide/cGMP/KATP pathway in ethanol-induced gastric injury in the rat," *Fundamental & Clinical Pharmacology*, vol. 25, no. 6, pp. 717–722, 2011.

[44] H. P. Toroudi, M. Rahgozar, A. Bakhtiarian, and B. Djahanguiri, "Potassium channel modulators and indomethacin-induced gastric ulceration in rats," *Scandinavian Journal of Gastroenterology*, vol. 34, no. 10, pp. 962–966, 1999.

[45] F. F. B. P. Freitas, H. B. Fernandes, C. A. Piauilino et al., "Gastroprotective activity of *Zanthoxylum rhoifolium* Lam. in animal models," *Journal of Ethnopharmacology*, vol. 137, no. 1, pp. 700–708, 2011.

[46] B. Saxena and S. Singh, "Investigations on gastroprotective effect of citalopram, an antidepressant drug against stress and pyloric ligation induced ulcers," *Pharmacological Reports*, vol. 63, no. 6, pp. 1413–1426, 2011.

[47] B. M. Peskar, K. Ehrlich, and B. A. Peskar, "Role of ATP-sensitive potassium channels in prostaglandin-mediated gastroprotection in the rat," *Journal of Pharmacology and Experimental Therapeutics*, vol. 301, no. 3, pp. 969–974, 2002.

[48] M. I. G. Silva, B. A. Moura, M. R. D. Q. Neto et al., "Gastroprotective activity of isopulegol on experimentally induced gastric lesions in mice: investigation of possible mechanisms of action," *Naunyn-Schmiedeberg's Archives of Pharmacology*, vol. 380, no. 3, pp. 233–245, 2009.

[49] G. Mózsik, J. Szolcsányi, and A. Dömötör, "Capsaicin research as a new tool to approach of the human gastrointestinal physiology, pathology and pharmacology," *Inflammopharmacology*, vol. 15, no. 6, pp. 232–245, 2007.

[50] A. P. C. Castelo, B. N. Arruda, R. G. Coelho et al., "Gastroprotective effect of *Serjania erecta* Radlk (Sapindaceae): involvement of sensory neurons, endogenous nonprotein sulfhydryls, and nitric oxide," *Journal of Medicinal Food*, vol. 12, no. 6, pp. 1411–1415, 2009.

[51] J. V. R. Medeiros, V. H. Bezerra, A. S. Gomes et al., "Hydrogen sulfide prevents ethanol-induced gastric damage in mice: role of ATP-sensitive potassium channels and capsaicin-sensitive primary afferent neurons," *Journal of Pharmacology and Experimental Therapeutics*, vol. 330, no. 3, pp. 764–770, 2009.

[52] G. S. Cerqueira, G. S. Silva, E. R. Vasconcelos et al., "Effects of hecogenin and its possible mechanism of action on experimental models of gastric ulcer in mice," *European Journal of Pharmacology*, vol. 683, no. 1–3, pp. 260–269, 2012.

[53] M. G. Repetto and S. F. Llesuy, "Antioxidant properties of natural compounds used in popular medicine for gastric ulcers," *Brazilian Journal of Medical and Biological Research*, vol. 35, no. 5, pp. 523–534, 2002.

[54] R. Nassini, E. Andrè, D. Gazzieri et al., "A bicarbonate-alkaline mineral water protects from ethanol-induced hemorrhagic gastric lesions in mice," *Biological and Pharmaceutical Bulletin*, vol. 33, no. 8, pp. 1319–1323, 2010.

[55] S. R. B. Damasceno, J. C. Rodrigues, R. O. Silva et al., "Role of the No/KATP pathway in the protective effect of a sulfated-polysaccharide fraction from the algae *Hypnea musciformis* against ethanol-induced gastric damage in mice," *Brazilian Journal of Pharmacognosy*, vol. 23, no. 2, pp. 320–328, 2013.

Effects of "Danzhi Decoction" on Chronic Pelvic Pain, Hemodynamics, and Proinflammatory Factors in the Murine Model of Sequelae of Pelvic Inflammatory Disease

Xiaoling Bu,[1] Yanxia Liu,[2] Qiudan Lu,[2] and Zhe Jin[2]

[1]*Beijing University of Traditional Chinese Medicine, North 3rd Ring Road No. 11 School Range, Chaoyang District, Beijing 100029, China*

[2]*Department of Gynecology, Dongfang Hospital of Beijing University of Traditional Chinese Medicine, No. 6 Fangxingyuan 1 Qu, Fengtai District, Beijing 100078, China*

Correspondence should be addressed to Zhe Jin; jinzhe0231@163.com

Academic Editor: Chang-Gue Son

Objective. To evaluate the effect of Danzhi decoction (DZD) on chronic pelvic pain (CPP), hemodynamics, and proinflammatory factors of sequelae of pelvic inflammatory diseases (SPID) in murine model. *Methods.* SPID mice were randomly treated with high-dose DZD, mid-dose DZD, low-dose DZD, aspirin, and vehicle for 3 estrous circles. The Mouse Grimace Scale (MGS) was performed to evaluate CPP; blood flows of the upper genital tract, pelvic wall, and mesentery were used to assess hemodynamics in SPID mice; expressions of vascular endothelial growth factor (VEGF), angiopoietin-2 (Ang-2), and osteopontin (OPN) were measured by Western blot and immunochemistry. *Results.* Treatment with dose-dependent DZD significantly decreased the MGS scores, accelerated blood flows of the pelvis, and reduced expressions of VEGF, Ang-2, and OPN in the upper genital tract. *Conclusions and Discussions.* DZD was effective in relieving CPP and improving hemodynamics of the pelvic blood-stasis microenvironment in SPID mice. There was a relationship between CPP and the pelvic blood-stasis microenvironment. Furthermore, DZD might play a positive role in the anti-inflammatory process.

1. Introduction

PID is most commonly a complication of sexually transmitted infections (STIs), involving any or all of the uterus, oviducts, and/or ovaries [1]. PID may cause sequelae (i.e., chronic pelvic pain, ectopic pregnancy, and infertility) from tubal scarring and adhesions [2], which is called SPID and was once called chronic pelvic inflammatory disease (CPID).

In theory of traditional Chinese medicine (TCM), the main pathogenesis of SPID is blood stasis in collaterals of the pelvis. It refers to abnormal hemodynamics, such as the circulation of blood that is not smooth, blood flow that is stagnant or forms stasis [3], or the decrease of blood flow velocity. Pathogenic factors, like cold and dampness, damage the uterus and uterine collaterals and then lead to qi obstruction that further results in blood stasis in collaterals in the pelvis

[4]. Blood stasis increases microvascular distortion and/or microvascular obstruction, which will aggravate stagnation of blood as well [5]. As a pathogenic factor, it directly affects the delivery of beneficial nutrients and clear of detrimental molecules or waste products. Therefore, blood stasis usually causes organ dysfunction and induces a series of symptoms, mostly in connection with slow-progressing diseases or chronic diseases [6]. In SPID, blood stasis affects the peristalsis of fallopian tubes so that it leads to abnormal pregnancy or infertility; because of microvascular obstruction and abnormal hemodynamics, it causes fixed pain in the pelvis. Thus, an optional therapy of SPID is to normalize the blood-stasis microcirculation in the inflammatory focus.

DZD, as a Chinese medicinal formula, is composed of *Salvia miltiorrhiza Bge., Morus alba L., Liguisticum chuanxiong Hort., Dipsacus asper Wall, Forsythia suspensa Vahl,*

TABLE 1: The composition of Danzhi decoction (DZD).

Scientific name	Chinese name	Medicinal parts	Grams	%
Salvia miltiorrhiza Bge.	Danshen	Root	10	13.0
Morus alba L.	Sangzhi	Twig	10	13.0
Liguisticum chuanxiong Hort.	Chuanxiong	Tuber	6	7.8
Dipsacus asper Wall	Chuanduan	Root	15	19.5
Forsythia suspensa Vahl	Lianqiao	Fruit	10	13.0
Litchi chinensis Sonn.	Lizhihe	Seed	10	13.0
Corydalis turtschaninovii Bess. y. yanhusuo Y. H. Chou et C. C. Hsu	yuanhu	Root	10	13.0
Cyperus rotundus L.	Xiangfu	Tuber	6	7.8
Total amount			77	100

Litchi chinensis Sonn., Corydalis turtschaninovii Bess. y. yanhusuo Y. H. Chou et C. C. Hsu, and *Cyperus rotundus L.* as shown in Table 1. It is effective in dispersing blood stasis and dredging collaterals. In the previous study, we confirmed that DZD could decrease the level of VEGF-A/C/D expressions in endometrial cells in a 3D endometrial cell model. In this way, DZD could regulate endothelium function and improve the blood-stasis microenvironment in SPID [4].

In this study, we would observe MGS and blood flow of the pelvis (including ovarian artery, internal iliac artery, and mesenteric and pelvic wall microvessels) in the SPID murine model, to investigate whether DZD could relieve CPP and hemodynamics of the pelvis. Expressions of VEGF, Ang-2, and OPN were measured to evaluate DZD's influence in the anti-inflammatory process.

2. Materials and Methods

Ethics Statement. All animal experiments were carried out in strict accordance with the guidelines of the Institute of Chinese Materia Medica China Academy of Chinese Medical Sciences Animal Care and Use Committee (license number: SYXK (Jing) 2013-0035).

2.1. Animals. 6–8-week-old female BALB/c mice were purchased from Vital River Laboratories and housed at the Institute of Chinese Materia Medica China Academy of Chinese Medical Sciences China institute of traditional Chinese medicine academy of sciences. The mice were kept under controlled temperature ($23 \pm 3°C$) with 45%–65% humidity.

2.2. Preparation of DZD. The crude drugs of DZD were purchased from the pharmacy of Dongfang Hospital of Beijing University of Traditional Chinese Medicine. Soaked in 8 volumes of double-distilled water for 20 min, all the herbs in proportion were boiled and then decocted over a low heat for 20 min. Repeat twice; the decoction was homogenized and concentrated by heating until the concentration of the crude drug was 1.8 g/mL (high dose), 0.9 g/mL (mid dose), and 0.45 g/mL (low dose), respectively.

2.3. HPLC and Fingerprint Analysis. DZD of 0.9 g/mL was concentrated at $60°C$ in a rotary evaporator under reduced pressure. The yield of final extract was 25.07%. 0.2261 g of the sample was dissolved in 80% methanol, ultrasonicated, and then filtered on a 0.45 μm filter for HPLC analysis. The extract of DZD was analyzed by Waters 2695 HPLC instrument (2998PDA detector). The sample was separated on a Waters Symmetry C18 column (4.6×250 mm, 5 μm) and the linear gradient was 5–95% B (A = 0.1% formic acid water, B = acetonitrile) for 70 min. The flow rate was 1.0 mL/min and the column temperature was maintained at $30°C$. Sample of 10 μL was detected at 280 nm.

Reference compounds consisted of mulberroside A, phillyrin (purchased from Chengdu Pulse Biological Technology Co., Ltd.), tetrahydropalmatine, ferulic acid, and tanshinone IIA (purchased from National Institute for the Control of Pharmaceutical and Biological Products, Beijing, China). The method of HPLC was the same as above.

2.4. The Murine Model of SPID and Animal Treatment. Oestrus was identified by vaginal smear for continuous 3 cycles. Only those with regular cycles were allowed to continue the next experiments. Suitable mice were randomly allocated into 2 groups: a group of 30 mice served as the control group, and the others were used for the model of SPID.

Briefly, except the mice in the control group, the others were anesthetized with an intraperitoneal administration of 5% chloral hydrate at 3.5 mL/kg body weight and intrauterinely injected with *C. muridarum* Everette et al. (Nigg, ATCC VR-123) [7–9] of 10^5 IFUs in 20 μL SPG (sucrose-phosphate-glutamate buffer) to each uterine horn. *C. muridarum* was propagated, purified, and titrated as described elsewhere [10]. Aliquots of the organisms were stored at $-80°C$ till use.

After 7 days, vaginal swabs were taken from 30 mice at random to carry on *C. muridarum* detection. Each swab was suspended in 500 mL of ice-cold SPG followed by vortexing with glass beads, and the released organisms were titrated on HeLa cell monolayers in duplicate until the titer showed negative. The number of IFUs/swab was converted into $\log_{10}$ and the $\log_{10}$ IFUs was used to calculate mean $\pm$ SEM [10].

Six weeks after infection, successfully infected 150 mice were randomly divided into 5 groups as follows: the model group, aspirin group, and high-dose, mid-dose, and low-dose DZD groups (DZD-H, DZD-M, and DZD-L, resp.). Each consisted of 30 mice.

All mice received drugs intragastrically at a dosage of 0.1 mL/10 g/day for 3 estrous cycles. The mice in the model group and the control group received 5‰ carboxymethylcellulose (CMC); in the aspirin group, aspirin 10 mg/(kg·d) was dissolved in 5‰ CMC; in the DZD-H, DZD-M, and DZD-L groups, DZD was dissolved at 18 g/(kg·d), 9 g/(kg·d), and 4.5 g/(kg·d), respectively.

2.5. Evaluation of CPP with MGS. Mice were captured and fixed with the routine method, and a Q-tip was used to press the bilateral lower quadrants of the abdomen in an appropriate intensity for 10 seconds. One researcher, who was blind to the grouping, operated the abdominal stimulation and scored mice's responses according to the MSG standard. The facial expressions included orbital tightening, nose bulge, cheek bulge, and whisker change. Based on different intensities, each feature was coded on a three-point scale that was 0 (not present), 1 (moderately visible), and 2 (severe) [11]. Another took charge of recording the grouping and the MGS score.

2.6. Assessment of Hemodynamics. By observation of vaginal smears, only mice in estuation were selected to assess the following tests in order to avoid the influence of hormone. All mice underwent the following tests in 5 days.

2.6.1. Blood Flow of Ovarian and Internal Iliac Arteries. The blood flows of the ovarian and the internal iliac arteries were measured by the Visual Sonics Vevo 2100 high-resolution ultrasound microimaging system (Visual Sonics, Toronto, Canada) with a 40 MHz probe.

The mice were anesthetized with isoflurane vapor to minimize breathing movement during scans [12]. All hair was removed from the abdomen and lower back with a chemical hair remover [13]. Before imaging, coupling gel was applied between the skin and the probe.

In B-mode, the ovary was identified by locating the kidney firstly when the mouse was in the prone position; each ovary was behind its ipsilateral kidney [12]. The ovarian artery was selected to test blood flow in color mode, and peak systolic velocity (PSV) was measured to be compared between groups.

The internal iliac artery was found when the mouse was in the supine position, which was below the bladder and traced by locating the abdominal aorta and unilateral common iliac artery firstly. In the same way, blood flow and PSV of the internal iliac artery were assessed.

2.6.2. Microvascular Perfusion of Pelvic Wall. Blood flow of pelvic wall was invasively assessed with the flowmeter PeriFlux 5000 (PeriCam PSI, Sweden), utilizing the Doppler shift, that is, the frequency change that laser light undergoes when interacting with objects in motion [14]. Three points

of microvessels of the pelvis were selected randomly to test blood perfusion; the average was taken to evaluate the local microcirculation.

2.6.3. Mesenteric Blood Flow Perfusion. This study was carried on with the PeriCam PSI system. It is a blood perfusion imager based on the Laser Speckle Contrast Analysis (LASCA) technology [15]. In the pelvis, intestines of similar length were chosen to conduct the PSI test. A piece of black paper was placed under the intestines to avoid irrelevant blood flow signals: sample rate of 1 frame per second and detecting distance of 10.5 ± 0.5 cm with the whole monitoring area of 3×3 cm^2. Perfusion data was recorded in real time, and the date of the Region of Interest (ROI) was calculated and analyzed by the PSI system [15].

2.7. Western Blot Analysis. Tissue samples of the upper genital tract were homogenized and lysed in ice-cold RIPA lysis buffer (C1053+; Applygen Technologies, Beijing, China) supplemented with protease inhibitor (P1265; Applygen Technologies). The proteins were in the supernatants after the homogenates were centrifuged at $12000 \times$g for 20 min at 4°C. The proteins were quantified with bicinchoninic acid (BCA) (P1511; Applygen Technologies) and resolved in SDS-PAGE loading buffer at 95°C for 10 min. After loading (20 μg protein), proteins were separated in 10% Tris-Bis gel and then transferred to nitrocellulose membranes by electroblotting. After blotting in 5% of nonfat dry milk in TBST for 30 min at room temperature, the membranes were incubated with anti-VEGF (1 : 1000, ab46154; Abcam, Cambridge, UK) or anti-Ang-2 (1 : 1000, SC-20718; Santa Cruz Biotechnology, Heidelberg, Germany) or anti-OPN (1 : 1000, ab8448; Abcam, Cambridge, UK) antibodies overnight at 4°C, followed by incubation with goat anti-rabbit horseradish peroxidase-labeled secondary antibody (1 : 5000, C1309; Applygen Technologies) for 1 hour at room temperature. The blots were visualized using the Super ECL Plus detection reagent (P1010; Applygen Technologies). The enhanced chemiluminescence signals were detected using Quantity One software (Bio Rad).

2.8. Immunohistochemistry. The upper genital tract tissues were immersed in 4% paraformaldehyde. Formalin-fixed tissues were separately paraffin-embedded and cut into 5 μm sections, stained with anti-VEGF (1 : 100) or anti-Ang-2 (1 : 100) or anti-OPN (1 : 200) as mentioned above. DAB was used as chromogen. Negative controls were run by omitting the primary antibodies. Images were photographed with digital camera (E4500; Nikon, Mississauga, Ontario, Canada) at ×40 magnification on a light microscope (Nikon Eclipse E600). The mean IOD values of VEGF, Ang-2, and OPN were calculated with Image-Pro Plus 6.0.

2.9. Statistical Analyses. Data was presented as the mean $\pm$ SEM. Statistical analysis was performed using SPSS 19.0 and one-way ANOVA was used to compare the data between the 6 groups. Correlation coefficients were calculated to identify the relationship between CPP and hemodynamics of the pelvis. Difference was considered significant at $P < 0.05$.

TABLE 2: MGS score and hemodynamic parameters in each group.

	Control group	Model group	Aspirin group	DZD-H group	DZD-M group	DZD-L group
MGS	1.367 ± 1.245	5.633 ± 1.847^a	$3.167 \pm 1.315^{a,b}$	$2.033 \pm 1.098^{b,c}$	$1.667 \pm 1.093^{b,c}$	$2.900 \pm 1.242^{a,b,d,e}$
Blood flow of internal genital tract						
PSV of ovarian artery	58.288 ± 11.853	45.772 ± 10.880^a	55.219 ± 15.668^b	60.400 ± 16.312^b	58.326 ± 9.813^b	$46.538 \pm 6.393^{a,c,d,e}$
PSV of internal iliac artery	51.176 ± 7.778	44.685 ± 9.038^a	51.516 ± 12.975^b	$59.286 \pm 14.137^{a,b,c}$	$51.431 \pm 10.211^{b,d}$	$44.069 \pm 8.650^{a,c,d,e}$
Microvascular perfusion of pelvic wall	53.783 ± 7.454	31.596 ± 7.682^a	60.992 ± 11.219^b	$70.380 \pm 15.757^{a,b,c}$	$56.901 \pm 9.801^{b,d}$	$37.735 \pm 6.219^{a,c,d,e}$
Mesenteric blood flow perfusion	90.596 ± 13.594	61.029 ± 21.219^a	91.209 ± 22.603^b	$107.375 \pm 22.902^{a,b,c}$	$85.818 \pm 17.079^{b,d}$	$58.926 \pm 15.59^{a,c,d,e}$

$^a P < 0.05$ compared with the control group; $^b P < 0.05$ compared with the model group; $^c P < 0.05$ compared with the aspirin group; $^d P < 0.05$ compared with the DZD-H group; $^e P < 0.05$ compared with the DZD-M group.

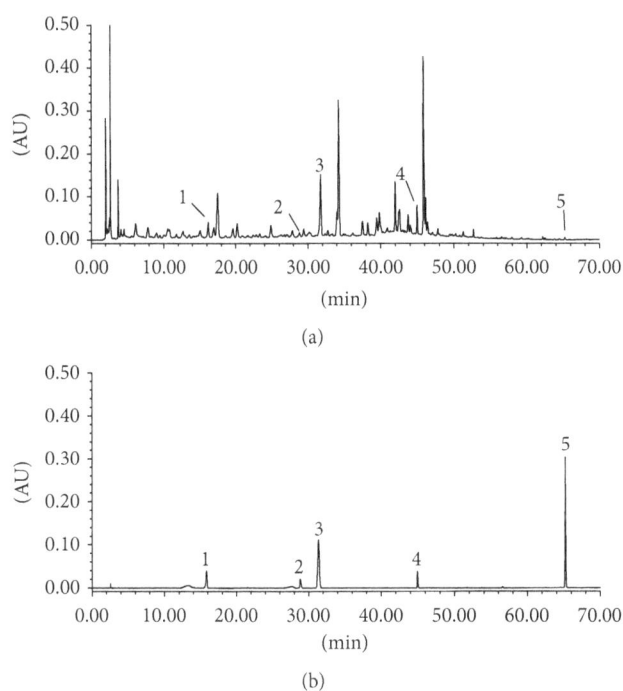

FIGURE 1: The HPLC-based fingerprint of DZD. (a) DZD of 0.9 g/mL; (b) mixed reference compounds. 1: mulberroside A; 2: tetrahydropalmatine; 3: ferulic acid; 4: phillyrin; 5: tanshinone IIA.

3. Result

3.1. Identification of Compounds.
As shown in Figure 1, these compounds of DZD were identified as mulberroside A; tetrahydropalmatine; ferulic acid; phillyrin; tanshinone IIA. The established method could identify the bioactive compounds in DZD at the same time.

3.2. Verification of Infection.
7 days after infection, vaginal swabs were collected from 30 mice randomly. The $\log_{10}$ IFUs/swab was significantly different with the data before infection (4.70 ± 0.64 versus 0). It verified that mice were successfully infected with *C. muridarum* intrauterinely.

3.3. Treatment with DZD Relieved CPP in Mice with SPID.
The result was shown in Table 2. Based on the data, it could be stated that CPP formed in the infected mice, as the MGS score was significantly different between the control group and the model group. High-dose and mid-dose DZD could obviously relieve CPP and were superior to aspirin. Low-dose DZD had similar effect with aspirin, which could not completely relieve CPP in SPID mice.

3.4. Treatment with DZD Accelerated Hemodynamics in Mice with SPID.
The result was shown in Table 2 and Figures 2–5. Blood flows, involving PSV of the ovarian artery and the internal iliac artery, blood flow perfusion of the pelvic wall, and mesentery in the pelvis, were significantly different between the mice in the model group and the control group. It could be concluded that the pelvis was in blood-stasis microenvironment in SPID mice. Treatment with high-dose and mid-dose DZD accelerated blood flow in the pelvis; the blood-stasis environment could be improved significantly by dose-dependent DZD compared with the placebo (CMC). High-dose DZD increased blood flow significantly, even in excess of the level of the control group, which might cause other problems; mid-dose DZD had a similar positive effect with aspirin on blood circulation, while low-dose DZD could not significantly increase blood flow in the pelvis. So in SPID mice, mid-dose DZD could properly improve hemodynamics of the pelvic blood-stasis microenvironment.

3.5. Correlation between MGS and Hemodynamics of the Pelvis in the SPID Murine Model.
The MGS score statistically showed a significant negative correlation with PSV of the ovarian artery and the internal iliac artery, blood perfusion of microvessels of pelvic wall, and mesentery ($r = -0.311$, $P = 0.000$; $r = -0.166$, $P = 0.026$; $r = -0.349$, $P = 0.000$; $r = -0.363$, $P = 0.000$, resp.).

3.6. Treatment with DZD Decreased Ang-2, VEGF, and OPN Levels in the Upper Genital Tract.
The results were evaluated by Western blot and immunochemistry.

3.6.1. Western Blot Analysis Results.
The protein expressions of VEGF, Ang-2, and OPN in the upper genital tract were

(a)

(b)

(c)

(d)

(e)

(f)

(g)

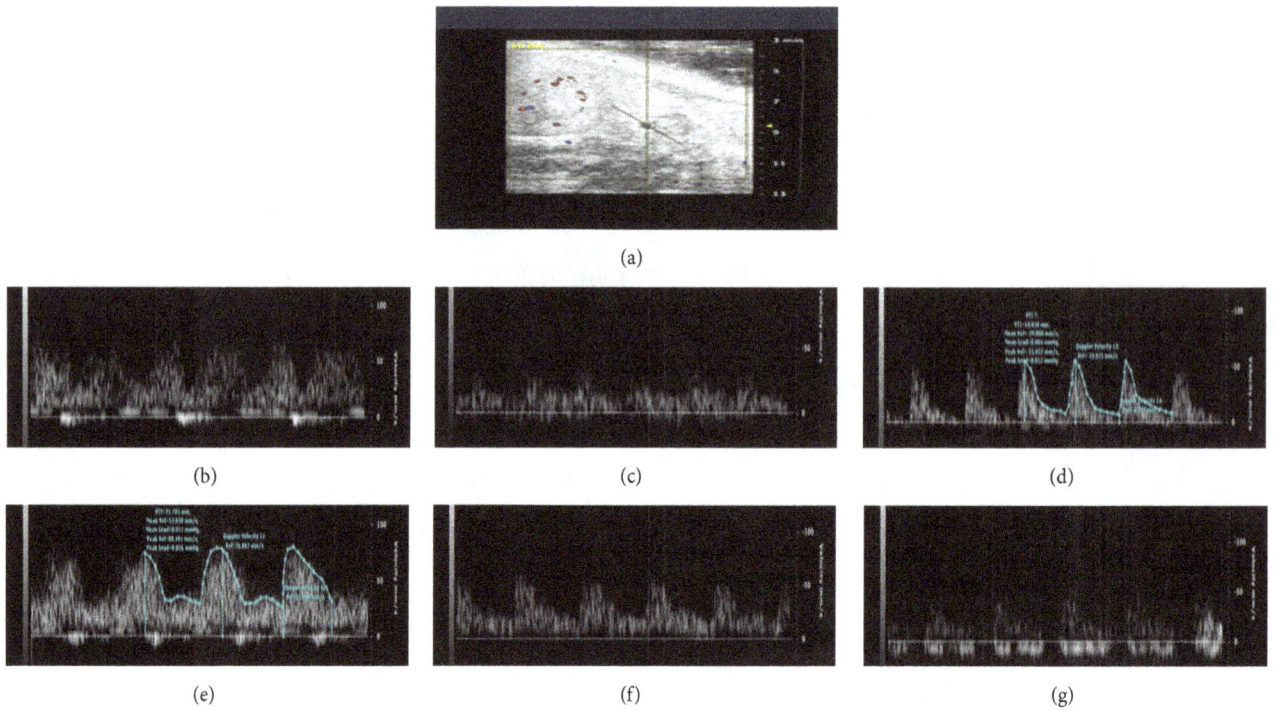

FIGURE 2: Representative Doppler waveforms of the ovarian artery. (a) The image of the ovary; (b) the control group; (c) the model group; (d) the aspirin group; (e) the DZD-H group; (f) the DZD-M group; (g) the DZD-L group.

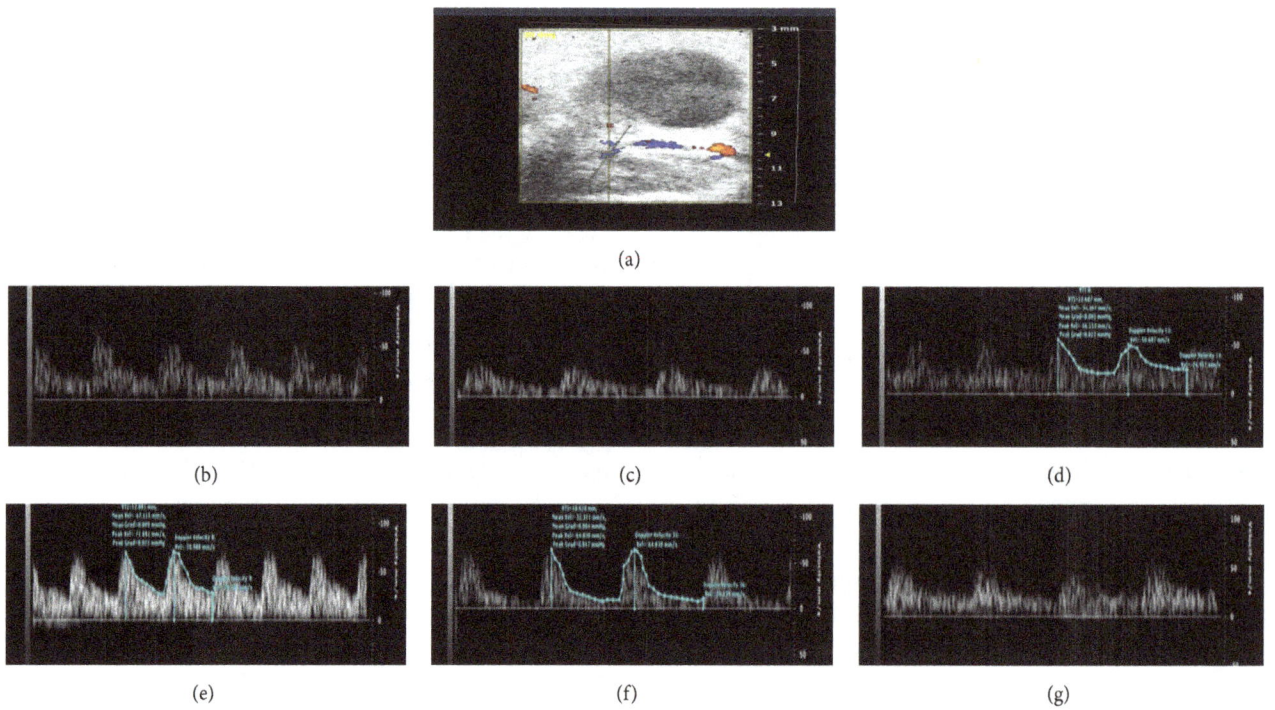

(a)

(b)

(c)

(d)

(e)

(f)

(g)

FIGURE 3: Representative Doppler waveforms of the internal iliac artery. (a) The image of measurement of the internal iliac artery in color mode; (b) the control group; (c) the model group; (d) the aspirin group; (e) the DZD-H group; (f) the DZD-M group; (g) the DZD-L group.

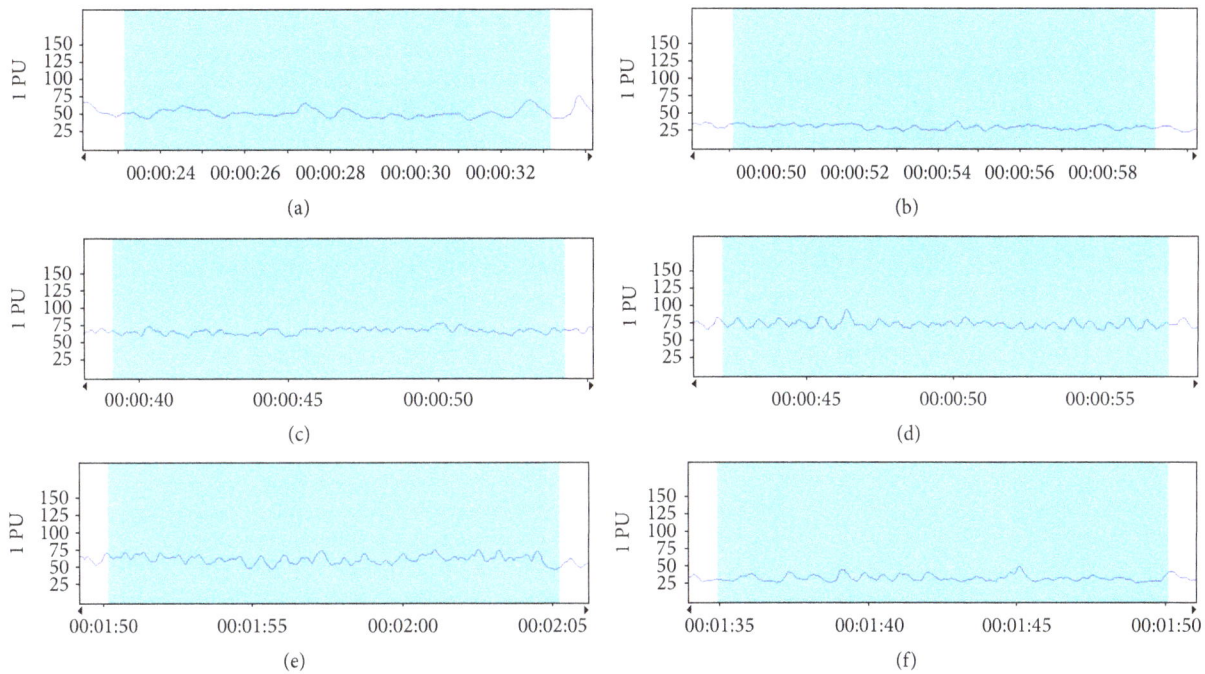

FIGURE 4: Representative blood perfusion curves of the pelvic microvessels. (a) The control group; (b) the model group; (c) the aspirin group; (d) the DZD-H group; (e) the DZD-M group; (f) the DZD-L group.

confirmed by Western blot (Figure 6). The protein levels were normalized by β-actin. Among the 6 groups, VEGF, Ang-2, and OPN levels in the model groups were significantly higher than those in the control groups in the upper genital tract (including the uterine horn, ovary, oviduct, and connective tissue). These protein levels decreased in the aspirin, DZD-H, DZD-M, and DZD-L groups compared with those in the model groups, but significant differences were more common in the DZD-H and DZD-M groups. There were no significant differences between the DZD-H and DZD-M groups.

3.6.2. Immunochemical Analysis Results. To verify the changes of the protein levels, the mean IOD values of VEGF, Ang-2, and OPN expressions were measured using immunochemistry. The results were shown in Table 3. The mean IOD of VEGF, Ang-2, and OPN in the model groups was significantly increased compared with those in the control groups. The mean IOD of these protein expressions was lower in DZD and aspirin groups compared with the model groups, but more significant differences were found in the DZD-H and DZD-M groups. Significant intergroup differences were not seen in the 2 groups.

3.7. Gastrointestinal Adverse Effects. During the study, mice were not observed any gastrointestinal symptoms in all groups (including dyspepsia, gastrointestinal bleeding, etc.). After being sacrificed, the digestive tract of mice was checked and none of gastrointestinal mucosal defects were detected either.

4. Discussions

SPID is increased by delayed antimicrobial treatment of PID [16] and its occurrence cannot be excluded by short-term

clinical and/or microbiologic cure [17]. Its manifestations include infertility, ectopic pregnancy, and chronic pelvic pain as described before and can cause considerable physical and emotional problem, in addition to significant cost on healthcare services [18].

For SPID, early prevention is essential, mainly involving health-care education that emphasizes the importance of safe sex and encourages early presentation for the diagnosis [19] and timely and normative use of broad-spectrum antibiotics in accordance with current management guidelines in acute episode. Once SPID forms, nonsteroid anti-inflammatory drugs (NSAIDs) play a limited role in the treatment because of pelvic adhesion and fibrosis [20]. Also, a long-time, repeating, and excessive use of NSAIDs in SPID has obvious adverse effects in the body, mainly involving gastrointestinal injury, such as dyspepsia, ulcer, and gastrointestinal bleeding. Besides these, renal impairment, interactions with other commonly prescribed medications, weakened immunity, and drug resistance could be observed [21, 22]. Traditional Chinese formula, acupuncture and moxibustion, short wave diathermy, acupoint injection, retention enema, and so forth are effective on the treatment of SPID as reported in lots of researches. Among these therapies, traditional Chinese formula for oral administration is relatively more commonly used in China.

As mentioned above, blood stasis is considered the main pathogenesis of SPID. It is caused by interruption of qi and blood in the pelvis because of invasion and retention of external or internal pathogenic factors in the pelvic collaterals [23]. At the meantime, blood stasis exacerbates stagnant movement of qi and blood. As a pathogenic factor, it causes persistent pelvic pain and other dysfunctions of the genital

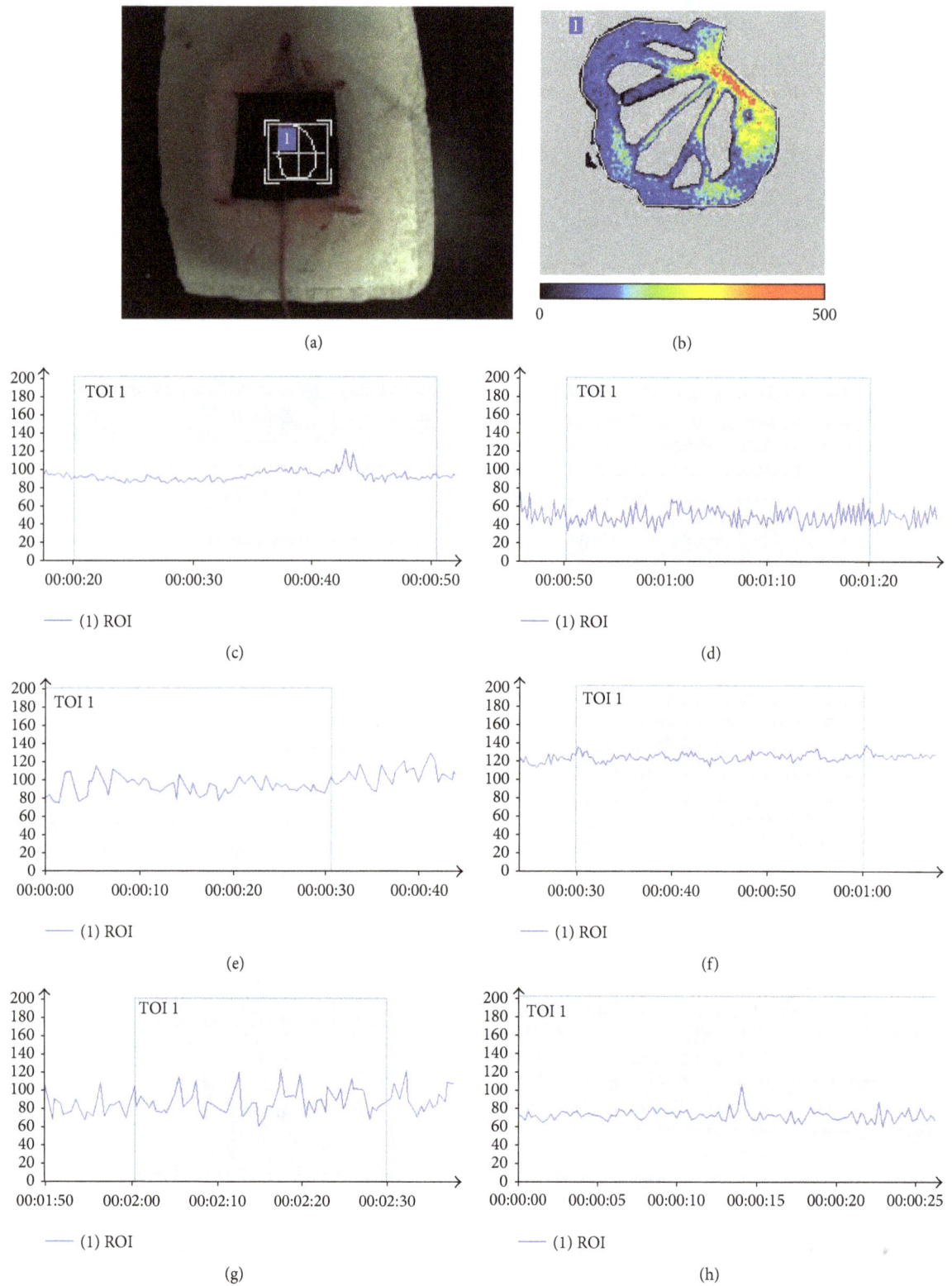

FIGURE 5: Representative blood perfusion curves of the mesentery. (a) The image of measurement of a mouse; (b) the image of Doppler signals of blood flow; (c) the control group; (d) the model group; (e) the aspirin group; (f) the DZD-H group; (g) the DZD-M group; (h) the DZD-L group.

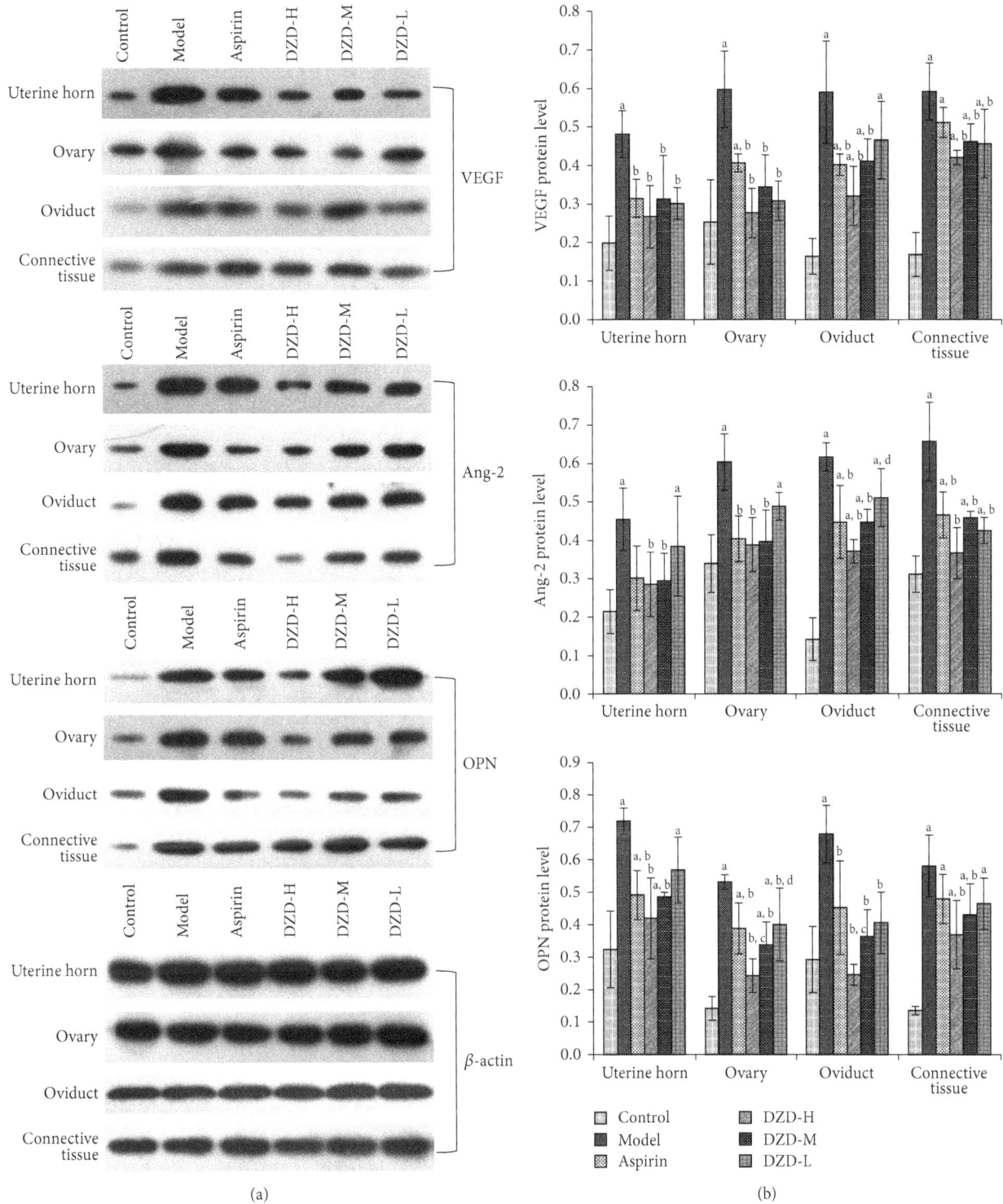

(a)   (b)

FIGURE 6: Protein expressions in the upper genital tract. Western blot was used to measure VEGF, Ang-2, and OPN protein levels in the upper genital tract of different groups ($n = 5$). [a]$P < 0.05$ compared with the control group; [b]$P < 0.05$ compared with the model group; [c]$P < 0.05$ compared with the aspirin group; [d]$P < 0.05$ compared with the DZD-H group.

tract [24]. Therefore, the principle of SPID treatment is to disperse blood stasis and dredge collaterals.

DZD was formulated in accordance with the principle and in combination of herbs with doctors' individual experience. *Salvia miltiorrhiza Bge.* and *Morus alba L.* are main components of DZD. Both of them have antibacterial effect [25, 26] in modern pharmacological studies. The former also plays a role in expansion of arteries and

TABLE 3: The mean IOD in each group.

	Control group	Model group	Aspirin group	DZD-H group	DZD-M group	DZD-L group
VEGF						
Uterine horn	54.505 ± 16.039	135.296 ± 29.325[a]	51.799 ± 12.086[b]	51.742 ± 15.186[b]	54.220 ± 14.616[b]	57.915 ± 16.543[b]
Ovary	59.378 ± 17.142	144.959 ± 37.763[a]	96.791 ± 15.833[a,b]	57.886 ± 15.867[b,c]	59.343 ± 16.402[b,c]	69.018 ± 20.919[b]
Oviduct	94.771 ± 41.003	529.083 ± 236.206[a]	157.738 ± 32.198[b]	145.077 ± 45.462[b]	150.045 ± 45.070[b]	462.198 ± 173.323[a,c,d,e]
Connective tissue	73.784 ± 14.413	602 ± 160.033[a]	563.536 ± 198.160[a]	244.358 ± 123.487[b,c]	207.859 ± 75.754[b,c]	216.703 ± 132.329[b,c]
Ang-2						
Uterine horn	23.019 ± 7.897	45.572 ± 3.830[a]	35.053 ± 12.983	26.587 ± 7.638[b]	27.498 ± 11.256[b]	40.213 ± 10.506[a,d,e]
Ovary	20.383 ± 4.929	97.899 ± 59.154[a]	27.711 ± 11.785[b]	21.635 ± 6.463[b]	31.504 ± 10.090[b]	79.445 ± 30.283[a,c,d,e]
Oviduct	27.482 ± 11.808	1443.231 ± 300.789[a]	364.597 ± 65.823[a,b]	330.218 ± 89.037[a,b]	416.294 ± 170.433[a,b]	1261.075 ± 244.432[a,c,d,e]
Connective tissue	65.812 ± 15.765	210.132 ± 56.290[a]	132.163 ± 52.801[a,b]	84.020 ± 13.940[b]	114.405 ± 36.019[b]	114.298 ± 41.990[b]
OPN						
Uterine horn	27.591 ± 5.723	81.30 ± 32.775[a]	54.024 ± 5.950[a,b]	33.113 ± 5.556[b]	52.330 ± 3.519[b]	81.801 ± 31.474[a,c,d,e]
Ovary	142.331 ± 39.000	416.631 ± 84.065[a]	228.653 ± 67.869[b]	162.881 ± 19.448[b]	225.215 ± 75.143[b]	302.368 ± 122.731[a,b,d]
Oviduct	198.387 ± 127.226	532.347 ± 172.325[a]	195.368 ± 86.126[b]	166.968 ± 58.035[b]	206.683 ± 74.969[b]	205.345 ± 67.066[b]
Connective tissue	110.077 ± 48.041	482.171 ± 135.153[a]	415.074 ± 84.211[a]	241.861 ± 103.486[a,b,c]	218.142 ± 65.258[b,c]	434.350 ± 126.390[a,d,e]

[a] $P < 0.05$ compared with the control group; [b] $P < 0.05$ compared with the model group; [c] $P < 0.05$ compared with the aspirin group; [d] $P < 0.05$ compared with the DZD-H group; [e] $P < 0.05$ compared with the DZD-M group.

improvement of microcirculation. The other herbs assist in anti-inflammatory effect or increasing blood flow in vessels or alleviating pain [27–32]. Combination of herbs is thought to increase therapeutic efficacy and reduce adverse effects through multiple targets and biological pathway [33], which can be confirmed by identification of bioactive compounds in the formula. As a result, waste products, such as prostaglandin [34], are removed from the blood circulation; pain threshold is lifted; nutrition and oxygen supply is increased; metabolism is enhanced to facilitate absorption and elimination of inflammation; tissue fibrosis is softened. Thus series of symptoms can be relieved.

CPP is a common symptom of SPID. It occurred in about 36% PID patients in the PEACH trial [35]. In clinical trials, pain could be graded by Visual Analogue Scale (VAS) [36] or Chronic Pain Grade developed by Von Korff et al. [37], both of which were based on patients' language expression. In animal experiments, the severity of pain cannot be expressed, so normal methods are unsuitable to be applied [38]. In the study, MGS, standardized behavioral coding system involving noxious stimuli of moderate duration accompanied by facial expressions of pain [11], was used to assess CPP in mice. The results of MGS in the control, high-dose, and mid-dose DZD groups had no significant difference between each other and were significantly lower than those of the low-dose DZD and the aspirin groups. It suggested that certain dose of DZD could dramatically relieve CPP in SPID mice.

Hemodynamics is an important parameter in many conditions of gynecology and obstetrics, so as to predict the risk of pregnancy [39], judge the severity of adnexal torsion [40], assess the function of pelvic floor [41], and so forth. In this study, we analyzed (1) peak systolic velocity (PSV) of the ovarian artery and the internal iliac artery and (2) blood perfusion of microvessels of pelvic wall and mesentery, to observe the hemodynamics of SPID and to evaluate the effect of DZD on pelvic blood flow. According to the present results, especially the results of the model group, we concluded that, in SPID, pelvis was in the blood-stasis microenvironment, which is consistent with TCM theory as mentioned above. By eliminating blood stasis and promoting blood circulation, DZD could improve hemodynamics and blood-stasis microenvironment in the pelvis of SPID when it was in a suitable dose (mid-dose).

The results also indicated a negative correlation between CPP and hemodynamics of the pelvis in SPID mice. It was confirmed that CPP was related to obstructed blood circulation. Eliminating blood stasis and promoting blood circulation are a selectable option for the treatment of SPID, especially the symptom, CPP.

VEGF, Ang-2, and OPN are well-known proinflammatory factors, distributed in a variety of tissues, including the reproductive tracts [42–44]. These factors are increased during inflammation, and the expression levels are positively correlated with the severity of inflammatory responses [45]. In this study, VEGF, Ang-2, and OPN expressions were significantly higher in the model groups. After the treatment of drugs, these factors declined to varying degrees, especially in the DZD-H and DZD-M groups, and all of the differences are statistically significant compared with the model groups. It

was indicated that DZD might play a positive role in the anti-inflammatory process.

Aspirin is the positive control drug in this study, as it is a well-known NSAID, also widely used for its analgesic and platelet antiaggregation properties [46] to relieve pain and improve blood circulation. We observed that aspirin had similar effect with mid-dose DZD on the aspect of hemodynamics in the pelvis, but it was less effective than mid-dose DZD in terms of alleviating CPP and downregulating proinflammatory factors.

Our study explained the following results: (1) DZD could relieve CPP in SPID; (2) the pelvis was in blood-stasis microenvironment in SPID mice; (3) DZD could improve the blood-stasis microenvironment by accelerating hemodynamics in the pelvis, including arteries of upper genital tract, microvessels in the pelvic wall, and mesentery; (4) CPP had correlation with obstructed blood flow in some ways and promoting blood circulation could relieve CPP; (5) DZD could reduce the expressions of VEGF, Ang-2, and OPN in the upper genital tract.

In conclusion, dose-dependent DZD relieved CPP and improved the blood-stasis microenvironment of SPID by ameliorating the hemodynamics in the pelvis. Moreover, it might play a positive role in the anti-inflammatory process by downregulating proinflammatory factors. A further clinical evaluation needs to be conducted to confirm these results in human subjects.

Additionally, in clinical setting, PID patients are firstly prescribed with sensitive antibiotics in the acute phase. However, in the chronic stage, antibiotics' effect is limited. Furthermore, aspirin is more effective on blood flow. So the study did not set a control group of antibiotics. This may be limitation to completely mimic the real world. Gastrointestinal adverse effects of both DZD and aspirin have not been found in this animal experiment. In clinical practice, patients should be monitored mindfully to ensure medication safety.

Disclosure

Xiaoling Bu and Yanxia Liu are co-first authors.

Conflict of Interests

The authors declare that they have no conflict of interests.

Authors' Contribution

Xiaoling Bu and Yanxia Liu contributed equally to this work.

Acknowledgments

The authors thank Wu Yan and Yuan Yueying of Beijing University of Chinese Medicine for their help in operating ultrasonic machine. The study was supported by a grant from the National Natural Science Foundation of China [81373677].

References

[1] S. Simmons, "Understanding pelvic inflammatory disease," *Nursing*, vol. 45, no. 2, pp. 65–66, 2015.

[2] D. E. Greydanus and C. Dodich, "Pelvic inflammatory disease in the adolescent: a poignant, perplexing, potentially preventable problem for patients and physicians," *Current Opinion in Pediatrics*, vol. 27, no. 1, pp. 92–99, 2015.

[3] K.-J. Chen, "Blood stasis syndrome and its treatment with activating blood circulation to remove blood stasis therapy," *Chinese Journal of Integrative Medicine*, vol. 18, no. 12, pp. 891–896, 2012.

[4] B.-Q. Liu, X. Gong, and Z. Jin, "Effect of Danzhi decoction on expression of angiogenesis factors in patients with sequelae of pelvic inflammatory disease," *Asian Pacific Journal of Tropical Medicine*, vol. 7, no. 12, pp. 985–990, 2014.

[5] W.-W. Li, H. Guo, and X.-M. Wang, "Relationship between endogenous hydrogen sulfide and blood stasis syndrome based on the Qi-blood theory of chinese medicine," *Chinese Journal of Integrative Medicine*, vol. 19, no. 9, pp. 701–705, 2013.

[6] X. Zhang, C. Zhang, J. Sai et al., "Xueshuan xinmaining tablet treats blood stasis through regulating the expression of F13a1, Car1, and Tbxa2r," *Evidence-Based Complementary and Alternative Medicine*, vol. 2015, Article ID 704390, 8 pages, 2015.

[7] M. Tuffrey, F. Alexander, C. Woods, and D. Taylor-Robinson, "Genetic susceptibility to *Chlamydial* salpingitis and subsequent infertility in mice," *Journal of Reproduction and Fertility*, vol. 95, no. 1, pp. 31–38, 1992.

[8] N. R. Roan, T. M. Gierahn, D. E. Higgins, and M. N. Starnbach, "Monitoring the T cell response to genital tract infection," *Proceedings of the National Academy of Sciences of the United States of America*, vol. 103, no. 32, pp. 12069–12074, 2006.

[9] S. Pal, T. J. Fielder, E. M. Peterson, and L. M. De la Maza, "Analysis of the immune response in mice following intrauterine infection with the *Chlamydia trachomatis* mouse pneumonitis biovar," *Infection and Immunity*, vol. 61, no. 2, pp. 772–776, 1993.

[10] Z. Li, C. Lu, B. Peng et al., "Induction of protective immunity against *Chlamydia muridarum* intravaginal infection with a chlamydial glycogen phosphorylase," *PLoS ONE*, vol. 7, no. 3, Article ID e32997, 2012.

[11] D. J. Langford, A. L. Bailey, M. L. Chanda et al., "Coding of facial expressions of pain in the laboratory mouse," *Nature Methods*, vol. 7, no. 6, pp. 447–449, 2010.

[12] P. Pallares and A. Gonzalez-Bulnes, "The feasibility of ultrasound biomicroscopy for non-invasive and sequential assessment of ovarian features in rodents," *Reproductive Biology*, vol. 8, no. 3, pp. 279–284, 2008.

[13] Z. Rowinska, S. Zander, A. Zernecke et al., "Non-invasive *in vivo* analysis of a murine aortic graft using high resolution ultrasound microimaging," *European Journal of Radiology*, vol. 81, no. 2, pp. 244–249, 2012.

[14] G. Vana and J. G. Meingassner, "Morphologic and immunohistochemical features of experimentally induced allergic contact dermatitis in Göttingen minipigs," *Veterinary Pathology*, vol. 37, no. 6, pp. 565–580, 2000.

[15] Y. Li, X. Li, D. Zhou et al., "Microcirculation perfusion monitor on the back of the health volunteers," *Evidence-Based Complementary and Alternative Medicine*, vol. 2013, Article ID 590698, 6 pages, 2013.

[16] S. D. Hillis, R. Joesoef, P. A. Marchbanks, J. N. Wasserheit, W. Cates Jr., and L. Westrom, "Delayed care of pelvic inflammatory disease as a risk factor for impaired infertility," *American Journal of Obstetrics & Gynecology*, vol. 168, no. 5, pp. 1503–1509, 1993.

[17] G. M. Trautmann, K. E. Kip, H. E. Richter et al., "Do short-term markers of treatment efficacy predict long-term sequelae of pelvic inflammatory disease?" *American Journal of Obstetrics & Gynecology*, vol. 198, no. 1, pp. 30.e1–30.e7, 2008.

[18] D. Dhasmana, E. Hathorn, R. McGrath, A. Tariq, and J. D. Ross, "The effectiveness of nonsteroidal anti-inflammatory agents in the treatment of pelvic inflammatory disease: a systematic review," *Systematic Reviews*, vol. 3, no. 1, pp. 79–84, 2014.

[19] D. Newton, C. Bayly, C. K. Fairley et al., "Women's experiences of pelvic inflammatory disease: implications for health-care professionals," *Journal of Health Psychology*, vol. 19, no. 5, pp. 618–628, 2014.

[20] L. L. Fan, W. H. Yu, X. Q. Liu et al., "Meta-analysis on effectiveness of acupuncture and moxibustion for chronic pelvic disease," *Acupuncture Research*, vol. 39, no. 2, pp. 156–163, 2014.

[21] X.-F. Cai, L.-F. Chen, Z.-L. Wang, and Y.-E. Gu, "Effect of acupoint injection by astragalus injection on local SIgA and pathomorphology changes in rats with chronic pelvic inflammatory disease," *China Journal of Chinese Materia Medica*, vol. 31, no. 16, pp. 1361–1364, 2006.

[22] J. A. Baron, S. Senn, M. Voelker et al., "Gastrointestinal adverse effects of short-term aspirin use: a meta-analysis of published randomized controlled trials," *Drugs in R and D*, vol. 13, no. 1, pp. 9–16, 2013.

[23] D. N. Cao, "Clinical thinking of chronic pelvic inflammatory disease treated with TCM," *ACTA Chinese Medicine and Pharmacology*, vol. 31, no. 2, 2003.

[24] Y. H. Hou, "Chenying's experience in the treatment of chronic pelvic inflammation," *Liaoning Journal of Traditionl Chinese Medicine*, vol. 34, no. 10, 2007.

[25] X.-D. Wen, C.-Z. Wang, C. Yu et al., "Salvia miltiorrhiza (dan shen) significantly ameliorates colon inflammation in dextran sulfate sodium induced colitis," *The American Journal of Chinese Medicine*, vol. 41, no. 5, pp. 1097–1108, 2013.

[26] C. Guo, T. Liang, Q. He, P. Wei, N. Zheng, and L. Xu, "Renoprotective effect of ramulus mori polysaccharides on renal injury in STZ-diabetic mice," *International Journal of Biological Macromolecules*, vol. 62, no. 11, pp. 720–725, 2013.

[27] Q. Zengyong, M. Jiangwei, and L. Huajin, "Effect of Ligusticum wallichii aqueous extract on oxidative injury and immunity activity in myocardial ischemic reperfusion rats," *International Journal of Molecular Sciences*, vol. 12, no. 3, pp. 1991–2006, 2011.

[28] Y. B. Niu, Y. H. Li, X. H. Kong et al., "The beneficial effect of *Radix Dipsaci* total saponins on bone metabolism in vitro and in vivo and the possible mechanisms of action," *Osteoporosis International*, vol. 23, no. 11, pp. 2649–2660, 2012.

[29] H. Y. Zhang, X. S. Piao, Q. Zhang et al., "The effects of *Forsythia suspensa* extract and berberine on growth performance, immunity, antioxidant activities, and intestinal microbiota in broilers under high stocking density," *Poultry Science*, vol. 92, no. 8, pp. 1981–1988, 2013.

[30] T. Ichinose, T. M. Musyoka, K. Watanabe, and N. Kobayashi, "Evaluation of antiviral activity of Oligonol, an extract of Litchi chinensis, against betanodavirus," *Drug Discoveries and Therapeutics*, vol. 7, no. 6, pp. 254–260, 2013.

[31] H. Ma, Q. Zhao, Y. Wang, T. Guo, Y. An, and G. Shi, "Design and evaluation of self-emulsifying drug delivery systems of *Rhizoma corydalis* decumbentis extracts," *Drug Development and Industrial Pharmacy*, vol. 38, no. 10, pp. 1200–1206, 2012.

[32] H. G. Kim, J. Hong, Y. Huh et al., "Cyperi Rhizoma inhibits the 1-methyl-4-phenyl-1,2,3,6-tetrahydropyridine-induced reduction in nigrostriatal dopaminergic neurons in estrogen-deprived mice," *Journal of Ethnopharmacology*, vol. 148, no. 1, pp. 322–328, 2013.

[33] L. Wang, G.-B. Zhou, P. Liu et al., "Dissection of mechanisms of Chinese medicinal formula Realgar-*Indigo naturalis* as an effective treatment for promyelocytic leukemia," *Proceedings of the National Academy of Sciences of the United States of America*, vol. 105, no. 12, pp. 4826–4831, 2008.

[34] S. Lamina, S. Hanif, and Y. S. Gagarawa, "Short wave diathermy in the symptomatic management of chronic pelvic inflammatory disease pain: a randomized controlled trial," *Physiotherapy Research International*, vol. 16, no. 1, pp. 50–56, 2011.

[35] C. Mitchell and M. Prabhu, "Pelvic inflammatory disease," *Infectious Disease Clinics of North America*, vol. 27, no. 4, pp. 793–809, 2013.

[36] K. Özbay and S. Deveci, "Relationships between transvaginal colour Doppler findings, infectious parameters and visual analogue scale scores in patients with mild acute pelvic inflammatory disease," *European Journal of Obstetrics Gynecology & Reproductive Biology*, vol. 156, no. 1, pp. 105–108, 2011.

[37] M. Von Korff, J. Ormel, F. J. Keefe, and S. F. Dworkin, "Grading the severity of chronic pain," *Pain*, vol. 50, no. 2, pp. 133–149, 1992.

[38] H. Peng and D. Huang, "Research progress in the assessment of pain in rodent animals," *Chinese Journal of Pain Medicine*, vol. 20, no. 7, pp. 505–508, 2014.

[39] L. Guedes-Martins, A. Cunha, J. Saraiva, R. Gaio, F. Macedo, and H. Almeida, "Internal iliac and uterine arteries Doppler ultrasound in the assessment of normotensive and chronic hypertensive pregnant women," *Scientific Reports*, vol. 4, article 3785, 2014.

[40] S. Kupesic and B. M. Plavsic, "Adnexal torsion: color Doppler and three-dimensional ultrasound," *Abdominal Imaging*, vol. 35, no. 5, pp. 602–606, 2010.

[41] C. E. Constantinou, "Dynamics of female pelvic floor function using urodynamics, ultrasound and Magnetic Resonance Imaging (MRI)," *European Journal of Obstetrics Gynecology & Reproductive Biology*, vol. 144, no. 1, pp. S159–S165, 2009.

[42] Y. Kuwabara, A. Katayama, R. Tomiyama et al., "Gonadotropin regulation and role of ovarian osteopontin in the periovulatory period," *Journal of Endocrinology*, vol. 224, no. 1, pp. 49–59, 2015.

[43] U. Fiedler, Y. Reiss, M. Scharpfenecker et al., "Angiopoietin-2 sensitizes endothelial cells to TNF-α and has a crucial role in the induction of inflammation," *Nature Medicine*, vol. 12, no. 2, pp. 235–239, 2006.

[44] X. Gong, Q. Tong, Z. Chen, Y. Zhang, C. Xu, and Z. Jin, "Microvascular density and vascular endothelial growth factor and osteopontin expression during the implantation window in a controlled ovarian hyperstimulation rat model," *Experimental and Therapeutic Medicine*, vol. 9, no. 3, pp. 773–779, 2015.

[45] H. Y. Park, C. R. Hahm, K. Jeon et al., "Serum vascular endothelial growth factor and angiopoietin-2 are associated with the severity of systemic inflammation rather than the presence of hemoptysis in patients with inflammatory lung disease," *Yonsei Medical Journal*, vol. 53, no. 2, pp. 369–376, 2012.

[46] S. Y. Tang, M. Sivakumar, A. M.-H. Ng, and P. Shridharan, "Anti-inflammatory and analgesic activity of novel oral aspirin-loaded nanoemulsion and nano multiple emulsion formulations generated using ultrasound cavitation," *International Journal of Pharmaceutics*, vol. 430, no. 1-2, pp. 299–306, 2012.

Oleanolic Acid Attenuates Insulin Resistance via NF-κB to Regulate the IRS1-GLUT4 Pathway in HepG2 Cells

Ming Li, Zongyu Han, Weijian Bei, Xianglu Rong, Jiao Guo, and Xuguang Hu

Key Unit of Modulating Liver to Treat Hyperlipemia SATCM (State Administration of Traditional Chinese Medicine),
Level 3 Lab of Lipid Metabolism SATCM, Guangdong TCM Key Laboratory for Metabolic Diseases,
Guangdong Pharmaceutical University, Guangzhou Higher Education Mega Centre, Guangzhou 510006, China

Correspondence should be addressed to Jiao Guo; gyguoyz@163.com and Xuguang Hu; hxguang21@163.com

Academic Editor: Yuewen Gong

The aim of our study is to elucidate the mechanisms of oleanolic acid (OA) on insulin resistance (IR) in HepG2 cells. HepG2 cells were induced with FFA as the insulin resistance model and were treated with OA. Then the glucose content and the levels of tumor necrosis factor-α (TNF-α) and interleukin-6 (IL-6) were analyzed. Moreover, protein expression of nuclear factor kappa B (NF-κB), insulin receptor substrate 1(IRS1), and glucose transporter 4 (GLUT4) in cells treated with OA were measured by Western blot analysis. Additionally, IRS1 protein expression exposed to OA was detected after using pyrrolidine dithiocarbamate (PDTC).Our results revealed that OA decreased the glucose content in HepG2 cells in vitro. Moreover, OA reduced the levels of TNF-α and IL-6 and upregulated IRS1 and GLUT4 protein expression. Furthermore, OA also reduced NF-κB protein expression in insulin-resistant HepG2 cells. After blocking NF-κB, the expression of IRS1 protein had no obvious changes when treated with OA. OA attenuated insulin resistance and decreased the levels of TNF-α and IL-6. Meanwhile, OA decreased NF-κB protein expression and upregulated IRS1 and GLUT4 protein expression. Therefore, regulating the IRS1-GLUT4 pathway via NF-κB was the underlying mechanism of OA on insulin resistance.

1. Introduction

Most pathology ultimately arises from obesity's characteristic milieu of chronic low-grade inflammation and insulin resistance [1]. The inability of insulin to perform normal biological functions in vivo is called insulin resistance. In general, insulin resistance occurs when a certain concentration of insulin cannot effectively stimulate glucose uptake and utilization in the peripheral target organs. Thus the organism suffers from impaired glucose tolerance that ultimately leads to diabetes or other diseases [2–4]. Many studies have demonstrated that patients with insulin resistance (IR) have displayed an increased risk of developing diabetes, cardiovascular disease, and other diseases [5, 6].

Recent studies have found that metabolic diseases including obesity are a common cause of insulin resistance. Meanwhile, increases in FFA (sodium oleate, Figure 1) levels have been shown to occur in metabolic diseases [7–9]. Higher FFA levels could induce the body to secrete inflammatory cytokines, such as TNF-α or IL-6, which would be a low-grade inflammatory state. Inflammation induced by FFA plays a key role in insulin resistance [10, 11]. As the important target of the inflammatory pathways, NF-κB could disrupt IRS1 and downregulate the expression of IRS1 under conditions of insulin resistance [12, 13].

Oleanolic acid (OA), a naturally occurring triterpenoid (Figure 2), is the main effective active ingredient in many herbs such as glossy privet fruit and exists largely in food products (vegetable oils) [14].

Preliminary study found that OA had blood glucose-reducing effect and inhibited insulin resistance in diabetic rats [15]. OA decreased blood glucose, improved insulin resistance, and enhanced insulin signaling by inhibition of ROS and anti-inflammatory effect in diabetic mice [16]. OA also regulated the NF-κB signaling which exhibits high anti-inflammatory activity and was regarded as a potential NF-κB inhibitor [17]. Recently a study conducted by Li et al. demonstrated that OA ameliorated insulin resistance via

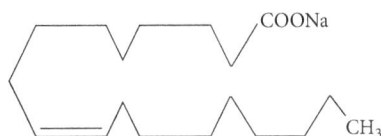

FIGURE 1: Chemical structure of sodium oleate.

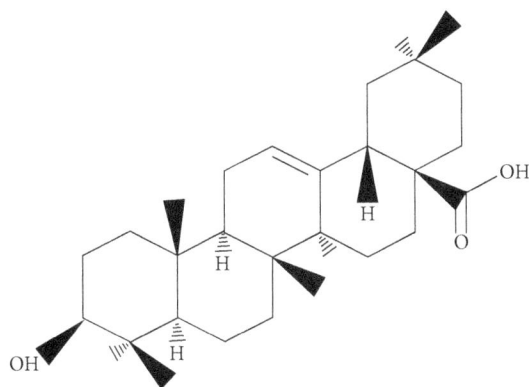

FIGURE 2: Chemical structure of oleanolic acid.

the IRS-1/PI3k/Akt pathway in rats [18]. Although previous evidence showed that OA attenuated insulin resistance in part through inhibiting inflammation and enhancing the IRS-1 signal, the role of NF-κB in attenuating insulin resistance by OA remains essentially unknown.

To further elucidate the molecular mechanisms of OA on insulin resistance and investigate the role of NF-κB in regulating IRS-1 signal by OA, the levels of TNF-α and IL-6 were analyzed and protein expression of nuclear factor kappa B (NF-κB), insulin receptor substrate 1 (IRS1), and glucose transporter 4 (GLUT4) in insulin-resistant HepG2 cells treated with OA was measured. In addition, IRS1 protein expression exposed to OA was detected after NF-κB was blocked using pyrrolidine dithiocarbamate (PDTC).

2. Methods and Materials

HepG2 cells were purchased from Landbiology (Guangzhou, China, lot: HB-8065). Dulbecco's modified Eagle's medium (DMEM) was bought from GIBCO (Gibco, Grand Island, NY, USA, lot: 8114176). Fetal bovine serum (FBS) was purchased from Biological Industries (Israel, lot: 1415878). NF-κB, IRS1, and GLUT4 antibodies were from Abcam Inc. (Cambridge, UK, lot: GR165665-1; GR95405-9; GR56566-1). Rosiglitazone (RSG) was bought from Sigma (St. Louis, MO, USA, lot: R2408-10 mg). Sodium oleate was bought from Tokyo Chemical Industry (Tokyo, Japan, lot: W76EC-0J). All other reagents were analytical grade. A GOD-POD kit was purchased from Biosino Bio-Technology and Science Inc. (Beijing, China, lot: 143271). ELISA kits were bought from Raybiotech Inc. (Norcross, GA, USA, Human TNF-α, lot: 0926140193; human IL-6, lot: 0926140140). Oleanolic acid (OA) was purchased from the National Institutes for Food and Drug Control (Beijing, China, lot: 110709-200505).

2.1. Cell Culture. The human hepatocellular carcinoma cell line HepG2 was purchased from Land Unicomed. Cells were cultured in DMEM supplemented with 10% heat-inactivated FBS at 37°C in a 5% CO_2 atmosphere. In all experiments, the cells were grown to 80–90% confluence.

2.2. Cell Viability Assay. The cytotoxicity of OA against the HepG2 cells was assessed by the MTT assay. The MTT viability assay was described previously [19]. Briefly, HepG2 cells were plated in 96-well plates at 1×10^5 cells per well. After 24 h, HepG2 cells were treated with indicated dose of OA at 37°C for 24 h; MTT stock solution (20 μL; 5 mg/mL in PBS) was added to each well to achieve a total reaction volume of 220 μL. After 4 h of incubation at 37°C and 5% CO_2, the media were then removed and 150 μL dimethyl sulfoxide (DMSO) was added to every well. After shaking for 10 min, the amount of purple formazan was assessed by measuring the absorbance at 490 nm.

2.3. Induction of Insulin Resistance in HepG2 Cells and Glucose Utilization Experiments. The HepG2 cells were cultured and determination of glucose utilization was performed as previously described [20]. Briefly, HepG2 cells were seeded on 24-well plates at 1×10^5 cells/well and incubated for 24 h to reach maximal confluence. The cells were then incubated for 24 h in serum-free DMEM, 0.2% BSA, and 200 μmol/L sodium oleate in the absence or presence of OA (OA was dissolved in DMSO) or RSG. Next, cells were washed twice with PBS and incubated for 3 h in serum-free DMEM containing 25 mmol/L d-glucose and 1×10^{-9} mol/L insulin. The culture medium was collected. The content of glucose was quantified using a GOD-POD kit.

2.4. Enzyme-Linked Immunosorbent Assay of TNF-α and IL-6 Levels. Insulin resistance was induced in HepG2 cells as previously described. The culture medium was centrifuged at 14000 ×g for 10 minutes at 4°C. The supernatant was then collected and stored at −80°C until analysis. The levels of TNF-α and IL-6 in the supernatant were determined using ELISA kits according to the manufacturer's instructions.

2.5. Western Blot Analysis. Insulin resistance was induced in HepG2 cells as previously described. Cells were washed with ice-cold PBS and lysed with a RIPA lysis buffer. For Western blotting, protein samples (20 μg) of sodium oleate induced insulin-resistant HepG2 cells were separated via 10% sodium dodecyl sulfate-polyacrylamide gel electrophoresis (SDS-PAGE). The proteins were transferred to a PVDF membrane and incubated with primary antibody (anti-NF-κB, anti-IRS1, anti-GLUT4, or anti-GAPDH), followed by a secondary antibody (horseradish peroxidase-conjugated anti-rabbit IgG). The intensity of the immunoblot signal was assayed using Western Bright ECL spray and analyzed quantitatively using GeneTools software from Syngene (Syngene, Cambridge, UK).

To choose the most effective concentration of PDTC, the cells were incubated for 26 h in serum-free DMEM at the different dosages of PDTC or 0.2% BSA and 200 μmol/L sodium

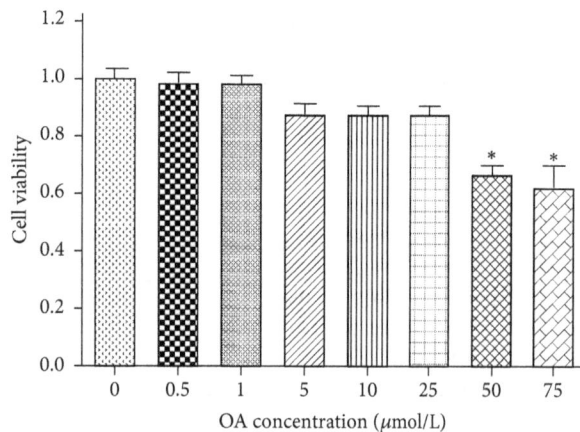

FIGURE 3: Influence of OA on the cell viability in HepG2 cells. 1 × 10^5 cells per well were seeded into a 96-well plate; cells were stimulated with various concentrations of OA (1–75 μmol L^{-1}) for 24 h; cell viability was measured by MTT. $^*P < 0.05$.

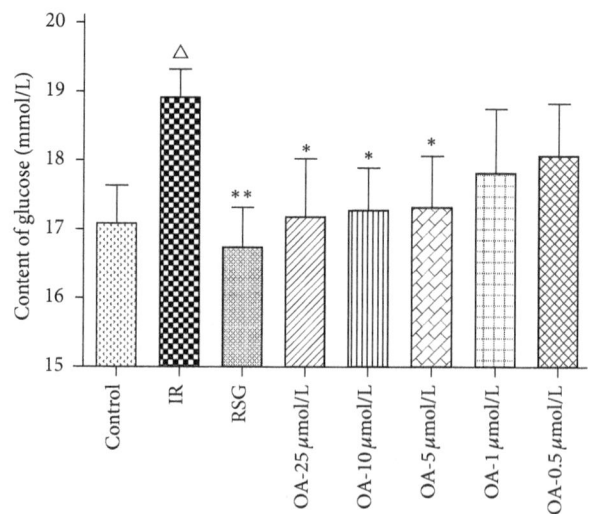

FIGURE 4: Effect of OA on the glucose content of the culture media in HepG2 cells. $^{\triangle}P < 0.01$ compared with the control cells; $^{**}P < 0.01$, $^*P < 0.05$ compared with the IR cells.

oleate. The protein samples were prepared for Western blot experiments and incubated with anti-NF-κB.

Then, the cells were incubated for 2 h in serum-free DMEM and PDTC with the most effective concentration (all PDTC groups). After that, 0.2% BSA and 200 μmol/L sodium oleate and three dosages of OA were added. Next, the cells were incubated for an additional 24 h after preparing the protein samples in Western blot experiments and incubated with anti-IRS1.

2.6. Statistics Analysis. The statistical analyses were conducted using SPSS16.0 software. All results are presented as the mean ± standard deviation (SD). Statistical analyses were performed using analysis of variance (one-way ANOVA) followed by the Student-Newman-Keuls test for significance. The differences were considered to be statistically significant at $P < 0.05$.

3. Result

3.1. Influence of OA on the Cell Viability in HepG2 Cells. The influence of OA on the cell viability in HepG2 cells was examined using the MTT reduction assay. The MTT assay results demonstrated no significant difference in cell viability of cells treated with OA at the concentrations of lower than 50 μmol/L. As the concentration of OA was 75 μmol/L, the cell viability was reduced by approximately 40% when compared to the control treatment (Figure 3).

3.2. Effect of OA on the Glucose Content of the Culture Media in Insulin-Resistant HepG2 Cells. The HepG2 cells were incubated for 24 h in serum-free DMEM containing 200 μmol/L sodium oleate, in either 0.5, 1, 5, 10, and 25 μmol/L OA or RSG (10 μmol/L). Next, the cells were incubated for 3 h in insulin. The glucose content in the insulin-resistant HepG2 cells in culture medium was significantly increased compared with

the control cells ($P < 0.01$). After treatment with OA (5, 10, and 25 μmol/L), the glucose content in the culture medium significantly reduced compared with the IR cells ($P < 0.05$). Rosiglitazone (RSG), which is the insulin sensitizer as a positive control drug, decreased the glucose content in the culture medium compared with the IR cells ($P < 0.01$). These results showed that OA attenuated insulin resistance in a dose-dependent manner (Figure 4).

3.3. Effect of OA on the Levels of TNF-α and IL-6 in Insulin-Resistant HepG2 Cells. To examine the effect of OA on inflammatory cytokines, the levels of TNF-α and IL-6 in the culture media of insulin-resistance HepG2 cells were measured by ELISA. The HepG2 cells were incubated for 24 h in serum-free DMEM containing 200 μmol/L sodium oleate, in the 5, 10, and 25 μmol/L OA, or in RSG (10 μmol/L). The levels of TNF-α and IL-6 in insulin-resistant HepG2 cells were significantly higher compared with the control cells ($P < 0.01$). After treatment with OA (5, 10, and 25 μmol/L), the level of IL-6 in the culture medium was significantly lower compared with the IR cells ($P < 0.01$). Moreover, treatment with OA at the dosages of 10 and 25 μmol/L significantly lowered the levels of TNF-α in the culture medium compared with the IR cells ($P < 0.05$; $P < 0.01$). Moreover, after treatment with OA at a dosage of 5 μmol/L, the level of TNF-α in the culture medium did not obviously decrease compared with the IR cells. RSG was also able to decrease all of the levels of TNF-α and IL-6 in the culture medium compared with the IR cells ($P < 0.01$) (Figure 5).

3.4. Effect of OA on the Protein Expression of NF-κB, IRS1, and GLUT4 in Insulin-Resistant HepG2 Cells. To elucidate the mechanism of OA on insulin resistance in HepG2 cell, a

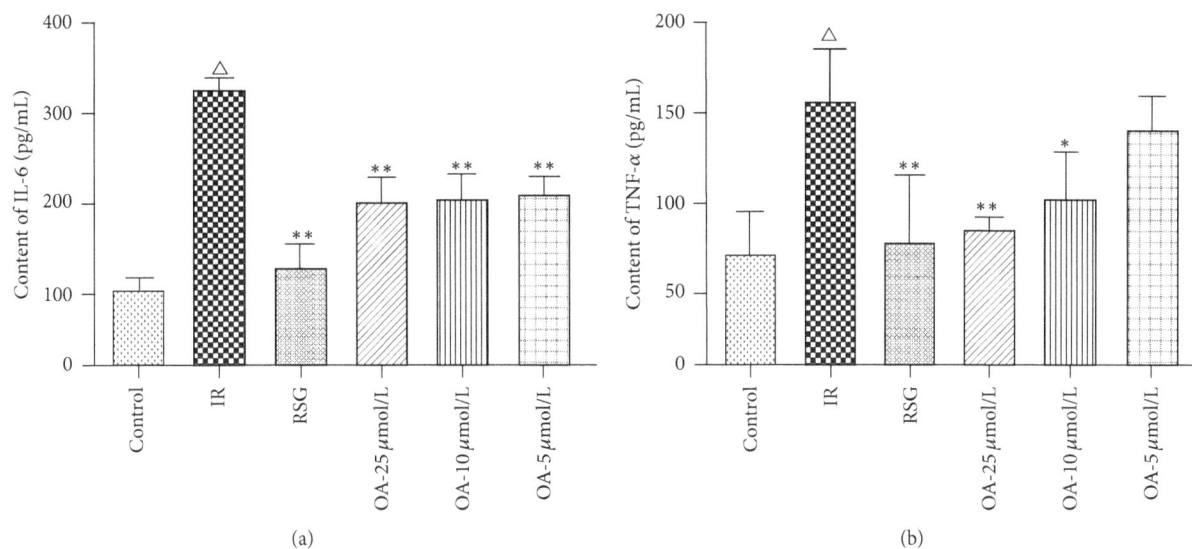

FIGURE 5: Effect of OA on TNF-α and IL-6 levels in HepG2 cells. $^{\triangle}P < 0.01$ compared with the control cells; $^{**}P < 0.01$, $^{*}P < 0.05$ compared with the IR cells.

Western blot analysis was used to measure the protein expression of NF-κB, IRS1, and GLUT4 in HepG2 cells. The cells were divided into six groups, including a Control group, IR group (200 μmol/L sodium oleate), RSG group (200 μmol/L sodium oleate and RSG 10 μmol/L), OA-25 μmol/L group (200 μmol/L sodium oleate, OA 25 μmol/L), OA-10 μmol/L group (200 μmol/L sodium oleate, OA 10 μmol/L), and OA-5 μmol/L group (200 μmol/L sodium oleate, OA 5 μmol/L). As shown in Figure 4, the expression of NF-κB protein in the IR group was significantly greater than the Control group ($P < 0.01$). IRS1 and GLUT4 protein expression in the IR group was significantly reduced compared with the Control group ($P < 0.01$). After treatment with OA at three dosages, the protein expression of NF-κB was significantly reduced compared with the IR group ($P < 0.01$). In addition, the expression of IRS1 and GLUT4 protein with OA at three dosages was significantly higher compared with the IR group ($P < 0.01$). RSG was also able to increase the expression of IRS1 and GLUT4 protein and reduce the expression of NF-κB protein compared with the IR group ($P < 0.01$) (Figure 6).

3.5. Effect of PDTC on NF-κB Protein Expression in HepG2 Cells.
To select the most effective concentration of PDTC that blocked NF-κB expression using Western blot analysis, HepG2 cells were divided into six groups, including a Control group, 100 μmol/L PDTC group, 300 μmol/L PDTC group, 500 μmol/L PDTC group, 1000 μmol/L PDTC group, and IR group (200 μmol/L sodium oleate). The levels of NF-κB expression in all groups that were treated with PDTC were significantly lower than the Control group ($P < 0.01$). The expression of NF-κB in the IR group was significantly greater than the Control group ($P < 0.01$). As shown in Figure 5, the most effective concentration of PDTC that blocked NF-κB expression was 300 μmol/L (Figure 7).

3.6. Effect of OA on the Expression of IRS1 Protein in Insulin-Resistant HepG2 Cells with Blocking of the Expression of NF-κB

Figure 8(a). To study the IRS1 protein expression when PDTC exists or not, HepG2 protein samples were divided into four groups as follows: Control group, IR group (200 μmol/L sodium oleate), P + Control group (300 μmol/L PDTC), and P + IR group (300 μmol/L PDTC and 200 μmol/L sodium oleate). As shown in Figure 6(a), the expression of IRS1 protein in the P + Control group was significantly greater than the Control group ($P < 0.01$). In addition, the expression of IRS1 protein in P + IR group was significantly increased compared with the IR group ($P < 0.01$) and significantly reduced compared with the P + Control group ($P < 0.05$).

Figure 8(b). To evaluate the effect of OA on the IRS1 protein expression when PDTC exists or not, HepG2 protein samples were divided into nine groups as follows: Control group, IR group (200 μmol/L sodium oleate), OA-25 μmol/L group (200 μmol/L sodium oleate, 25 μmol/L OA), OA-10 μmol/L group (200 μmol/L sodium oleate, 10 μmol/L OA), OA-5 μmol/L group (200 μmol/L sodium oleate, 5 μmol/L OA), P + IR group (300 μmol/L PDTC, 200 μmol/L sodium oleate), P + OA-25 μmol/L group (300 μmol/L PDTC, 200 μmol/L sodium oleate and 25 μmol/L OA), P + OA-10 μmol/L group (300 μmol/L PDTC, 200 μmol/L sodium oleate and 10 μmol/L OA), and P + OA-5 μmol/L group (300 μmol/L PDTC, 200 μmol/L sodium oleate and 5 μmol/L OA). As shown in Figure 6(b), the expression of IRS1 protein in the IR group was significantly lower than the Control group ($P < 0.01$); the expression of IRS1 protein in the OA-25 μmol/L group, OA-10 μmol/L group, OA-5 μmol/L group, P + IR group, P + OA-25 μmol/L group, P + OA-10 μmol/L group, and P +

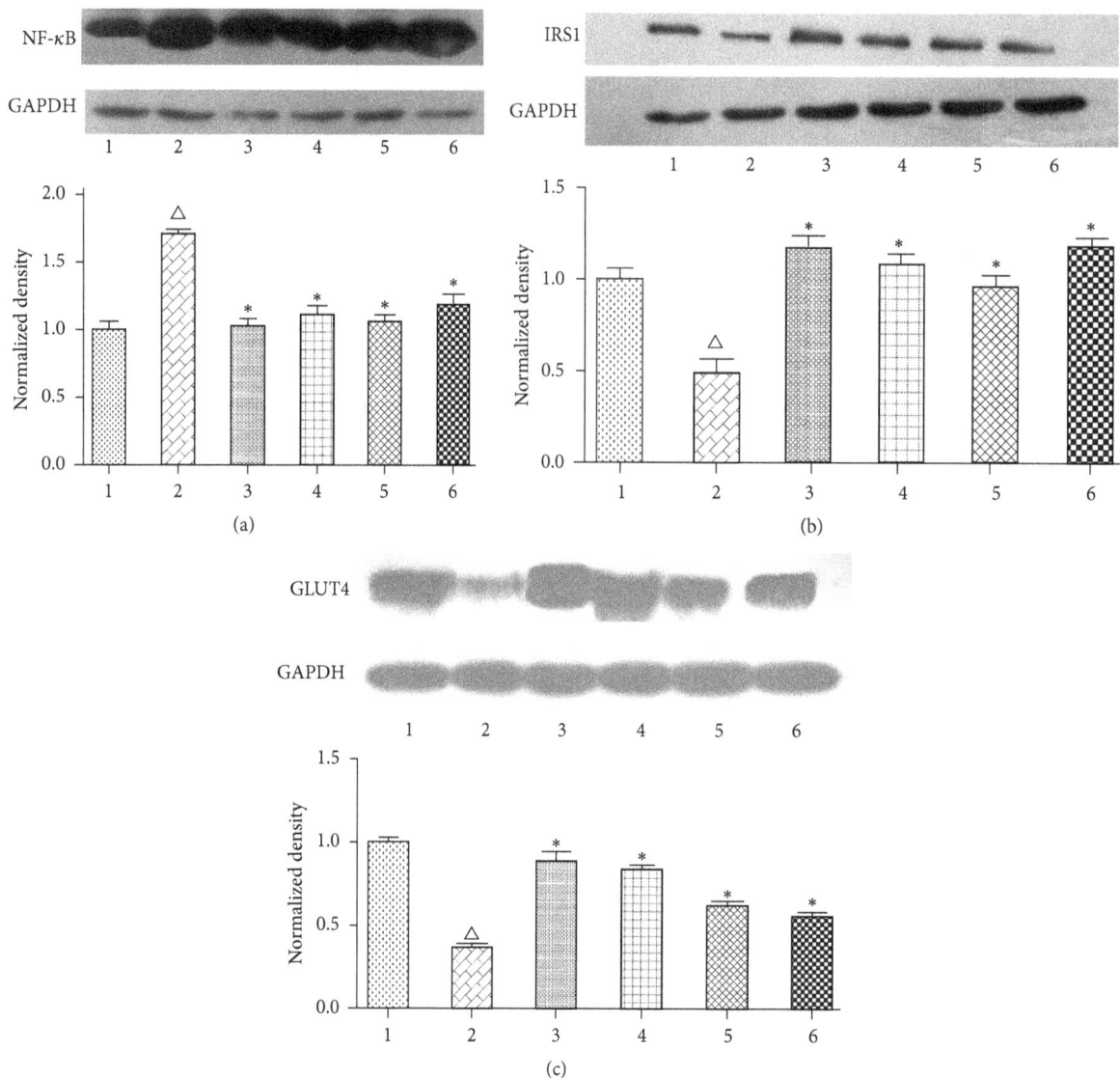

(a)

(b)

(c)

FIGURE 6: Effect of OA on NF-κB, IRS1, and GLUT4 protein expression. (1) Control; (2) IR; (3) RSG; (4) OA-25 μmol/L; (5) OA-10 μmol/L; (6) OA-5 μmol/L. The protein expression of NF-κB, IRS1, and GLUT4 was measured via Western blotting as described in the text. The figures represent one of three experiments with similar results. $^{\triangle}P < 0.01$ compared with the Control group; $^{*}P < 0.01$ compared with the IR group.

OA-5 μmol/L group was significantly greater than the IR group ($P < 0.01$). When compared to the three dosages of OA without PDTC, the expression of IRS1 protein in three dosages of OA with PDTC was reduced ($P < 0.05$) (Figure 8).

4. Discussion

This study demonstrated that OA attenuated insulin resistance in HepG2 cells, whose effect is possibly mediated through decreasing the levels of TNF-α and IL-6 and regulating the expression of IRS1 and GLUT4 protein via the NF-κB protein.

Elevated levels of free fatty acids are thought to be the pathogenic factors causing metabolic disorders such as obesity and diabetes [21]. Oleate, an unsaturated fatty acid,

can induce insulin resistance in HepG2 cells [22]. HepG2 cells were wildly used for studying insulin resistance [23]. When HepG2 cells were induced with insulin resistance, their responses to glucose were affected. The glucose content in insulin-resistant cells in culture medium increased compared with healthy cells [24]. In the present study, we used 200 μmol/L sodium oleate to induce insulin resistance in HepG2 cells. The glucose content in the IR group in culture medium was significantly greater than the Control groups. It showed that it is a suitable model of insulin resistance.

Oleanolic acid (OA) exerts multiple pharmacological actions including glycoregulatory, hepatoprotective, anti-inflammatory, and antioxidant effects and is used to treat chronic diseases, such as diabetes, liver injury, and hepatitis [25]. A study conducted by Wang et al. found that OA decreased the glucose content in the culture medium,

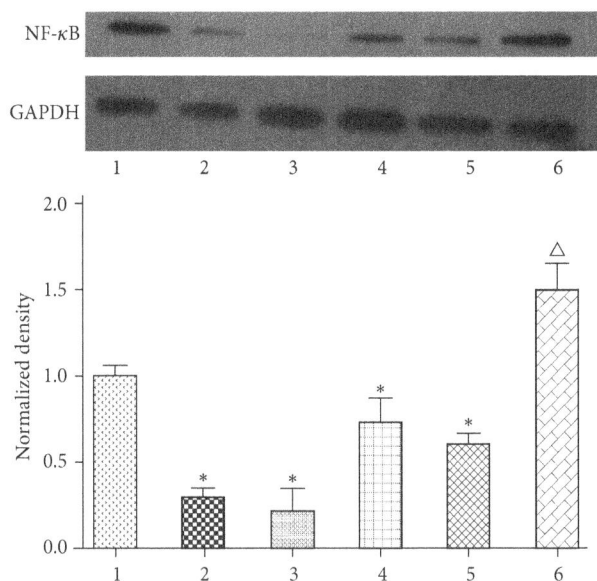

FIGURE 7: Effect of PDTC on NF-κB protein expression. (1) Control; (2) PDTC-100 μmol/L; (3) PDTC-300 μmol/L; (4) PDTC-500 μmol/L; (5) PDTC-1000 μmol/L; (6) IR. The protein expression of NF-κB was measured via Western blotting as described in the text. The figures represent one of three experiments with similar results. $^{\triangle}P < 0.01$ compared with the Control group; $^{*}P < 0.01$ compared with the Control group.

improved insulin resistance, protected beta-cell, and inhibited the mitochondrial apoptosis in beta-TC3 cells [26]. de Melo et al.'s study [27] showed that OA reduced blood glucose and improved glucose tolerance in mice. Our study results showed that OA decreased the glucose content in the culture medium at variable dosage in HepG2 cells. It demonstrated that OA affected the glucose utilization and attenuated insulin resistance in dose-dependent manner (Figure 2). Consistence with our study, Teodoro et al. [28] found that OA enhanced insulin secretion and increased the glucose utilization in pancreatic beta-cells in vitro.

High levels of FFA could induce insulin resistance as well as inflammation [29]. Much research has shown that OA had an anti-inflammatory effect and reduced the content of inflammatory cytokines, such as TNF-α and IL-6. Chai et al. found that OA decreased the level of IL-6 and TNF-α in the serum and liver of db/db mice [30]. Liu et al. showed that OA could inhibit the generation of the inflammatory factors TNF-α and IL-6 [31]. Nkeh-Chungag et al. found that OA exerted potent anti-inflammatory effects by inhibiting NO and PGE2 in RAW 264.7 cells [32]. Our results showed that OA decreased the levels of IL-6 and TNF-α in insulin-resistant HepG2 cells (Figure 3).

Mounting evidence has suggested that inflammatory processes were related to the pathogenesis of insulin resistance [33]. The NF-κB is a pivotal molecular mediator of insulin resistance [34]. Various inflammatory cytokines, including IL-6 and TNF-α, have been shown to activate NF-κB to cause insulin resistance [35]. Insulin resistance causes the impairment of IRS1 and GLUT4, which lead to obstacle

of glucose utilization [36]. As mentioned above, OA has anti-inflammatory effects. It not only reduced the content of inflammatory cytokines but also reduced the expression of NF-κB and upregulated IRS1 protein expression. Kim et al. found that OA could disturb NF-κB activation in 3T3-L1 adipocytes by inhibiting inflammatory responses during adipocyte differentiation through blocking IL-6-TRAF6-NF-κB signaling [37]. Li et al.'s results showed that OA could upregulate IRS1 protein expression in adipose tissue in insulin-resistant rats. Our studies showed that insulin resistance induced by sodium oleate could lead to overexpression of NF-κB protein and that IRS1 and GLUT4 proteins were impaired. After treatment with OA, the expression of NF-κB protein was significantly reduced and the expression of IRS1 and GLUT4 protein was partially restored.

Pyrrolidine dithiocarbamate (PDTC) is a specific NF-κB inhibitor that becomes widely used [38]. In Zheng et al.'s study, PDTC was used to block NF-κB to explain the protective effects of chronic resveratrol treatment on vascular inflammatory injury in streptozotocin-induced type 2 diabetic rats [39]. To illustrate the point that OA could relieve the expression of the IRS1 and GLUT4 by blocking the expression of NF-κB, PDTC was used to block NF-κB in our study. We found that the expression of IRS1 protein in the cells of the IR group that were previously blocked by PDTC was significantly elevated compared with IR group cells without PDTC. After the addition of OA at three dosages, the expression of IRS1 protein in the OA groups was significantly higher than those in the IR group. The expression of IRS1 protein in the OA groups with PDTC was not increased as obviously as the OA groups that were not exposed to PDTC. Therefore, we thought that NF-κB was the potential key target of OA that relieved insulin resistance. According to the results of Figure 4, OA could reduce the expression of NF-κB protein and directly increase the expression of IRS1. As mentioned above, PDTC is a specific NF-κB inhibitor. Meanwhile, the expression of IRS1 would increase when NF-κB was blocked. Based on the above knowledge, we speculated that OA can relieve insulin resistance by directly affecting the expression of IRS1 protein. OA also affected the expression of IRS1 protein indirectly by regulating NF-κB. When NF-κB was blocked by PDTC, OA could not affect IRS1 by NF-κB. Thus, the effect of OA on the expression of IRS1 protein in cells was attenuated compared to those without PDTC.

5. Conclusions

In conclusion, our study indicated that OA could decrease insulin resistance by reducing the content of inflammatory cytokines in culture medium. Regulating the IRS1-GLUT4 pathway via NF-κB was the underlying mechanism of the effects of OA on insulin resistance. Our findings may provide new insights into the mechanisms underlying the effect of oleanolic acid in insulin-resistant cells.

Abbreviations

IR: Insulin resistance
OA: Oleanolic acid

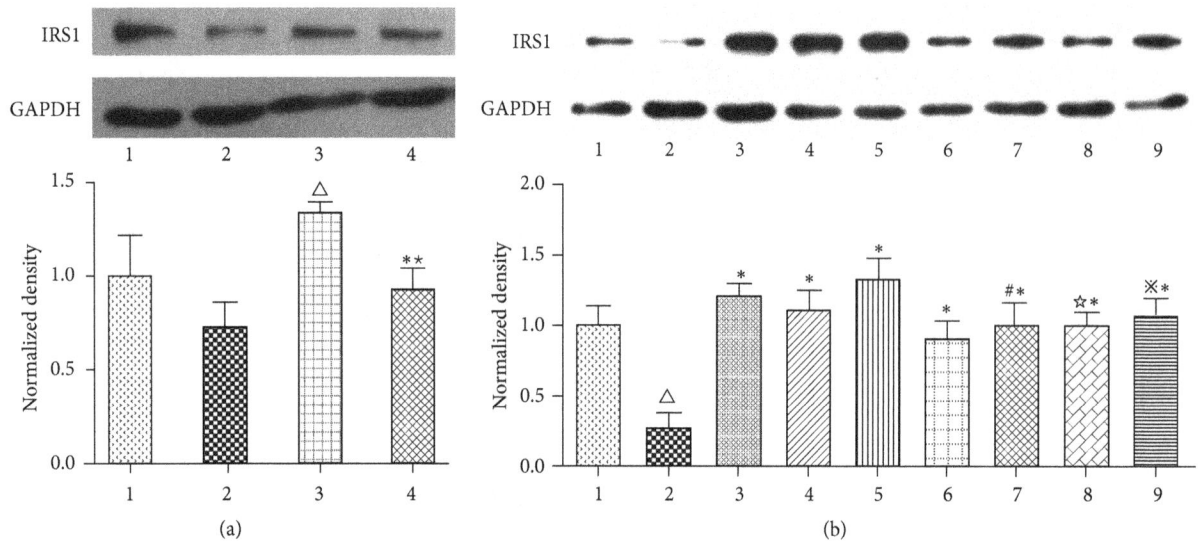

FIGURE 8: Effect of OA on IRS1 protein expression with blocking of the expression of NF-κB. (a) (1) Control; (2) IR; (3) P + Control; (4) P + IR. (b) (1) Control; (2) IR; (3) OA-25 μmol/L; (4) OA-10 μmol/L; (5) OA-5 μmol/L; (6) P + IR; (7) P + OA-25 μmol/L; (8) P + OA-10 μmol/L; (9) P + OA-5 μmol/L. The protein expression of IRS1 was measured via Western blotting as described in the text. The figures represent one of three experiments with similar results. $^{\triangle}P < 0.01$ compared with the Control group; $^{*}P < 0.01$ compared with the IR group; $^{*}P < 0.05$ compared with the P + Control group; $^{\#}P < 0.05$ compared with the OA-25 μmol/L group; $^{\star}P < 0.05$ compared with the OA-10 μmol/L group; $^{\times}P < 0.05$ compared with the OA-5 μmol/L group.

FFA: Free fatty acid
TNF-α: Tumor necrosis factor-α
IL-6:   Interleukin-6
NF-κB: Nuclear factor kappa B
IRS1:   Insulin receptor substrate 1
GLUT4: Glucose transporter 4
PDTC: Pyrrolidine dithiocarbamate
ELISA: Enzyme-linked immunosorbent assay
RSG: Rosiglitazone
DMEM: Dulbecco's modified Eagle's medium
FBS: Fetal bovine serum
DMSO: Dimethyl sulfoxide.

Disclosure

This paper does not contain any studies on human or animal subjects performed by any of the authors.

Conflict of Interests

The authors declare that they have no conflict of interests.

Authors' Contribution

Dr. Jiao Guo and Xuguang Hu designed the study. Ming Li and Zongyu Han carried out experiments. Weijian Bei and Xianglu Rong participated in the design of study. Dr. B. Han, MC Fang, L. Wan, and M. Wang have provided a lot of support and help. All authors have read and approved the final paper.

Acknowledgments

This study was supported by grants from the Natural Sciences Funds, China (no. 81173626, 2011), Guangdong Province-Chinese Education Ministry Industry, Education and Research Cooperation Project (no. 2011B090400379), and Guangdong Province Natural Sciences Funds Research Team Project (no. 10351022401000000).

References

[1] J. I. Odegaard and A. Chawla, "Pleiotropic actions of insulin resistance and inflammation in metabolic homeostasis," *Science*, vol. 339, no. 6116, pp. 172–177, 2013.

[2] G. M. Reaven, "Role of insulin resistance in human disease," *Diabetes*, vol. 37, no. 12, pp. 1595–1607, 1988.

[3] K. Choi and Y.-B. Kim, "Molecular mechanism of insulin resistance in obesity and type 2 diabetes," *Korean Journal of Internal Medicine*, vol. 25, no. 2, pp. 119–129, 2010.

[4] K. Makki, P. Froguel, and I. Wolowczuk, "Adipose tissue in obesity-related inflammation and insulin resistance: cells, cytokines, and chemokines," *ISRN Inflammation*, vol. 2013, Article ID 139239, 12 pages, 2013.

[5] L. Pedersen, M. Nybo, M. Poulsen, J. Henriksen, J. Dahl, and L. Rasmussen, "Plasma calprotectin and its association with cardiovascular disease manifestations, obesity and the metabolic syndrome in type 2 diabetes mellitus patients," *BMC Cardiovascular Disorders*, vol. 14, article 196, 2014.

[6] S. K. Panchal, H. Poudyal, A. Iyer et al., "High-carbohydrate, high-fat diet-induced metabolic syndrome and cardiovascular remodeling in rats," *Journal of Cardiovascular Pharmacology*, vol. 57, no. 5, pp. 611–624, 2011.

[7] J. M. Castellano, A. Guinda, T. Delgado, M. Rada, and J. A. Cayuela, "Biochemical basis of the antidiabetic activity of oleanolic acid and related pentacyclic triterpenes," *Diabetes*, vol. 62, no. 6, pp. 1791–1799, 2013.

[8] E. Fjære, U. L. Aune, K. Røen et al., "Indomethacin treatment prevents high fat diet-induced obesity and insulin resistance but not glucose intolerance in C57BL/6J mice," *The Journal of Biological Chemistry*, vol. 289, no. 23, pp. 16032–16045, 2014.

[9] G. Boden, "Obesity, insulin resistance and free fatty acids," *Current Opinion in Endocrinology, Diabetes and Obesity*, vol. 18, no. 2, pp. 139–143, 2011.

[10] Q. Huang, J. Xue, R. Zou et al., "NR4A1 is associated with chronic low-grade inflammation in patients with type 2 diabetes," *Experimental and Therapeutic Medicine*, vol. 8, no. 5, pp. 1648–1654, 2014.

[11] B.-C. Lee and J. Lee, "Cellular and molecular players in adipose tissue inflammation in the development of obesity-induced insulin resistance," *Biochimica et Biophysica Acta—Molecular Basis of Disease*, vol. 1842, no. 3, pp. 446–462, 2014.

[12] D. Zhang and P. S. Leung, "Potential roles of GPR120 and its agonists in the management of diabetes," *Drug Design, Development and Therapy*, vol. 8, pp. 1013–1027, 2014.

[13] G. Boden, P. She, M. Mozzoli et al., "Free fatty acids produce insulin resistance and activate the proinflammatory nuclear factor-κb pathway in rat liver," *Diabetes*, vol. 54, no. 12, pp. 3458–3465, 2005.

[14] K. Xu, F. Chu, G. Li et al., "Oleanolic acid synthetic oligoglycosides: a review on recent progress in biological activities," *Pharmazie*, vol. 69, no. 7, pp. 483–495, 2014.

[15] X. Wang, Y.-L. Li, H. Wu et al., "Antidiabetic effect of oleanolic acid: a promising use of a traditional pharmacological agent," *Phytotherapy Research*, vol. 25, no. 7, pp. 1031–1040, 2011.

[16] X. Wang, R. Liu, W. Zhang et al., "Oleanolic acid improves hepatic insulin resistance via antioxidant, hypolipidemic and anti-inflammatory effects," *Molecular and Cellular Endocrinology*, vol. 376, no. 1-2, pp. 70–80, 2013.

[17] Y.-J. Hwang, J. Song, H.-R. Kim, and K.-A. Hwang, "Oleanolic acid regulates NF-κB signaling by suppressing MafK expression in RAW 264.7 cells," *BMB reports*, vol. 47, no. 9, pp. 524–529, 2014.

[18] Y. Li, J. Wang, T. Gu, J. Yamahara, and Y. Li, "Oleanolic acid supplement attenuates liquid fructose-induced adipose tissue insulin resistance through the insulin receptor substrate-1/phosphatidylinositol 3-kinase/Akt signaling pathway in rats," *Toxicology and Applied Pharmacology*, vol. 277, no. 2, pp. 155–163, 2014.

[19] Z. Song, H. Wang, L. Zhu et al., "Curcumin improves high glucose-induced INS-1 cell insulin resistance via activation of insulin signaling," *Food & Function*, vol. 6, no. 2, pp. 461–469, 2015.

[20] D. Gao, S. W. Nong, X. Q. Huang et al., "The effects of palmitate on hepatic insulin resistance are mediated by NADPH oxidase 3-derived reactive oxygen species through JNK and p38 MAPK pathways," *The Journal of Biological Chemistry*, vol. 285, no. 39, pp. 29965–29973, 2010.

[21] Y. Luo, P. Rana, and Y. Will, "Palmitate increases the susceptibility of cells to drug-induced toxicity: an in vitro method to identify drugs with potential contraindications in patients with metabolic disease," *Toxicological Sciences*, vol. 129, no. 2, pp. 346–362, 2012.

[22] A. Chabowski, M. Zendzian-Piotrowska, K. Konstantynowicz et al., "Fatty acid transporters involved in the palmitate and oleate induced insulin resistance in primary rat hepatocytes," *Acta Physiologica*, vol. 207, no. 2, pp. 346–357, 2013.

[23] A. Aravinthan, B. Challis, N. Shannon, M. Hoare, J. Heaney, and G. J. M. Alexander, "Selective insulin resistance in hepatocyte senescence," *Experimental Cell Research*, vol. 331, no. 1, pp. 38–45, 2015.

[24] X. G. Hu, M. Wang, W. J. Bei, Z. Y. Han, and J. Guo, "The Chinese herbal medicine FTZ attenuates insulin resistance via IRS1 and PI3K in vitro and in rats with metabolic syndrome," *Journal of Translational Medicine*, vol. 12, no. 1, article 47, 2014.

[25] J. Pollier and A. Goossens, "Oleanolic acid," *Phytochemistry*, vol. 77, pp. 10–15, 2012.

[26] X. Wang, H. L. Chen, J. Z. Liu et al., "Protective effect of oleanolic olic acid against beta cell dysfunction and mitochondrial apoptosis: crucial role of ERK-NRF2 signaling pathway," *Journal of Biological Regulators and Homeostatic Agents*, vol. 27, no. 1, pp. 55–67, 2013.

[27] C. L. de Melo, M. G. R. Queiroz, S. G. C. Fonseca et al., "Oleanolic acid, a natural triterpenoid improves blood glucose tolerance in normal mice and ameliorates visceral obesity in mice fed a high-fat diet," *Chemico-Biological Interactions*, vol. 185, no. 1, pp. 59–65, 2010.

[28] T. Teodoro, L. Zhang, T. Alexander, J. Yue, M. Vranic, and A. Volchuk, "Oleanolic acid enhances insulin secretion in pancreatic β-cells," *FEBS Letters*, vol. 582, no. 9, pp. 1375–1380, 2008.

[29] P. Han, Y.-Y. Zhang, Y. Lu, B. He, W. Zhang, and F. Xia, "Effects of different free fatty acids on insulin resistance in rats," *Hepatobiliary and Pancreatic Diseases International*, vol. 7, no. 1, pp. 91–96, 2008.

[30] J. Chai, X. Du, S. Chen et al., "Oral administration of oleanolic acid, isolated from Swertia mussotii Franch, attenuates liver injury, inflammation, and cholestasis in bile duct-ligated rats," *International Journal of Clinical and Experimental Medicine*, vol. 8, no. 2, pp. 1691–1702, 2015.

[31] J. Liu, X. Wang, R. Liu et al., "Oleanolic acid co-administration alleviates ethanol-induced hepatic injury via Nrf-2 and ethanol-metabolizing modulating in rats," *Chemico-Biological Interactions*, vol. 221, pp. 88–98, 2014.

[32] B. N. Nkeh-Chungag, O. O. Oyedeji, A. O. Oyedeji, and E. J. Ndebia, "Anti-inflammatory and membrane-stabilizing properties of two semisynthetic derivatives of oleanolic acid," *Inflammation*, vol. 38, no. 1, pp. 61–69, 2015.

[33] D. P. Arçari, W. Bartchewsky Jr., and T. W. dos Santos, "Anti-inflammatory effects of yerba maté extract (Ilex paraguariensis) ameliorate insulin resistance in mice with high fat diet-induced obesity," *Molecular and Cellular Endocrinology*, vol. 335, no. 2, pp. 110–115, 2011.

[34] M. K. Moon, M. Kim, S. S. Chung et al., "S-Adenosyl-L-methionine ameliorates TNFα-induced insulin resistance in 3T3-L1 adipocytes," *Experimental and Molecular Medicine*, vol. 42, no. 5, pp. 345–352, 2010.

[35] S. E. Shoelson, J. Lee, and A. B. Goldfine, "Inflammation and insulin resistance," *The Journal of Clinical Investigation*, vol. 116, no. 7, pp. 1793–1801, 2006.

[36] S. Schinner, W. A. Scherbaum, S. R. Bornstein, and A. Barthel, "Molecular mechanisms of insulin resistance," *Diabetic Medicine*, vol. 22, no. 6, pp. 674–682, 2005.

[37] H.-S. Kim, S.-Y. Han, H.-Y. Sung et al., "Blockade of visfatin induction by oleanolic acid via disturbing IL-6-TRAF6-NF-κB signaling of adipocytes," *Experimental Biology and Medicine*, vol. 239, no. 3, pp. 284–292, 2014.

[38] R. Madonna, Y.-J. Geng, R. Bolli et al., "Co-activation of nuclear factor-κB and myocardin/serum response factor conveys the hypertrophy signal of high insulin levels in cardiac myoblasts," *Journal of Biological Chemistry*, vol. 289, no. 28, pp. 19585–19598, 2014.

[39] X. Zheng, S. Zhu, S. Chang et al., "Protective effects of chronic resveratrol treatment on vascular inflammatory injury in streptozotocin-induced type 2 diabetic rats: role of NF-κ B signaling," *European Journal of Pharmacology*, vol. 720, no. 1–3, pp. 147–157, 2013.

19

Chemical Components and Cardiovascular Activities of *Valeriana* spp.

Heng-Wen Chen,[1] Ben-Jun Wei,[2] Xuan-Hui He,[3] Yan Liu,[4] and Jie Wang[1]

[1]*Guang'anmen Hospital, China Academy of Chinese Medical Sciences, Beijing 100053, China*
[2]*Hubei University of Traditional Chinese Medicine, Wuhan, Hubei 430062, China*
[3]*Department of Pharmaceutical Chemistry, Beijing Institute of Radiation Medicine, Beijing 100850, China*
[4]*Key Laboratory of Chinese Materia Medica, Heilongjiang University of Chinese Medicine, Ministry of Education,
 Harbin, Heilongjiang 150036, China*

Correspondence should be addressed to Jie Wang; jiewang1001@126.com

Academic Editor: William C. Cho

Valeriana spp. is a flowering plant that is well known for its essential oils, iridoid compounds such as monoterpenes and sesquiterpenes, flavonoids, alkaloids, amino acids, and lignanoids. *Valeriana* spp. exhibits a wide range of biological activities such as lowering blood pressure and heart rate, antimyocardial ischemia reperfusion injury, antiarrhythmia, and regulation of blood lipid levels. This review focuses on the chemical constituents and cardiovascular activities of *Valeriana* spp.

1. Introduction

Valeriana officinalis Linn, perennial herbaceous plant belonging to the Valerianaceae family, is widely distributed in temperate regions. It comprises approximately 250 species, and 11 out of the 28 (including 1 variant) Chinese varieties are used as herbal medicines [1–4]. Most research studies have focused on six species: *V. officinalis* L., *V. jatamansi* Jones, *V. officinalis* L. var. *latifolia* Miq., *V. amurensis* Smir. ex Kom., *V. fauriei* Briq., and *V. alternifolia* var. *stolonifera* Bar. et Skv.

The roots and rhizomes of *Valeriana* spp. are rich in essential oils, iridoids, flavonoids, alkaloids, amino acids, and lignanoids [5–9], which possess characteristic fragrance or off-flavor and are used as medicines based on their inherent bioactivities that include inducing sedation, promoting sleep, antidepression, and antianxiety [10–18]. *Valeriana* spp. is now listed in the European and USA pharmacopeias. It is also sold as a diet supplement in the USA and is one of the highest selling natural medicines in Europe and the USA [19]. In addition, *Valeriana* spp. is of high medical and economic value in the food, drink, and cosmetic industries due to its distinct flavor, and current research efforts are aimed at further exploiting other features of the plant [20, 21]. This review focuses on the chemical constituents and cardiovascular activities of *Valeriana* spp., aiming at providing a theoretical foundation for further research and evaluation of its medicinal value.

2. Chemical Constituents

2.1. Essential Oils. Approximately 0.5%–2.0% of *Valeriana* spp. consists of essential oils by gas chromatography-mass spectrometry (GC-MS), which varies with species, climate, and growing environment. Valerian plants from high-altitude fertile and sandy soil have significantly higher essential oil content and yield similar to that of biennials compared to annuals. Valerian plants that produce a higher amount of essential oil are cultivated between September and November, although the content of essential oils decreases with longer periods of propagation.

A total of 150 compounds have been identified in the essential oils of Valerian plants, mainly including monoterpenes and sesquiterpenes. Most monoterpenes, namely, borneol, bornyl acetate, and isobornyl acetate, exhibit various bioactivities. Around 30 sesquiterpenes have also been detected in the Valerian essential oils. These have been

TABLE 1: The list of essential oil constituents from *V. officinalis* L. var. *latifolia* Miq.

Signal	Compounds	Molecular format	Molecular weight	Retention time (min)	Content (%)
1	Carene	$C_{10}H_{16}$	136	6.100	0.29
2	α-Thujene	$C_{10}H_{16}$	136	6.473	4.18
3	6-Isopropyl-1-methyl bicycles [3,1,0] hexane	$C_{10}H_{16}$	136	6.983	14.19
4	Sabinene	$C_{10}H_{16}$	136	7.736	2.55
5	p-Cymene	$C_{10}H_{14}$	134	9.143	0.43
6	Limonene	$C_{10}H_{16}$	136	9.281	1.26
7	Camphor	$C_{10}H_{16}O$	152	12.596	0.19
8	Borneol	$C_{10}H_{18}O$	154	13.671	3.54
9	L-Myrtanol	$C_{11}H_{16}O$	164	14.584	0.81
10	α-Methyl 4($1'$, $1'$-methyl ethyl) phenol	$C_{11}H_{16}O$	164	15.432	2.49
11	Bornyl acetate	$C_{12}H_{20}O_2$	196	17.311	23.93
12	Sabinol	$C_{10}H_{16}O$	152	18.270	1.70
13	α-Terpineol	$C_{10}H_{18}O$	154	18.944	1.20
14	β-Caryophyllene	$C_{15}H_{24}$	204	20.989	0.82
15	β-Gurjunene	$C_{15}H_{24}$	204	21.343	1.16
16	Humulene	$C_{15}H_{24}$	204	21.891	0.40
17	Unidentified	$C_{15}H_{22}$	202	22.045	1.32
18	*trans*-caryophyllene	$C_{15}H_{24}$	204	22.450	0.28
19	Nerolidol	$C_{15}H_{24}O$	220	22.838	0.78
20	Elemene	$C_{15}H_{24}$	204	22.977	0.45
21	Bornyl isovalerianate	$C_{15}H_{26}O$	238	23.441	0.36
22	Azulene furan	$C_{15}H_{10}O_2$	222	23.867	0.58
23	Stereoisomer of ramie enol	$C_{10}H_{16}O$	152	24.485	1.46
24	4a,8-Dimethyl-α-isopropyl naphthyl ketone	$C_{15}H_{24}O$	220	25.155	2.77
25	Tetramethyl-4-hydroxyl cyclopropane naphthalene	$C_{15}H_{24}O$	220	25.294	1.26
26	Unidentified	$C_{15}H_{24}O$	220	25.790	1.72
27	Ledol	$C_{15}H_{26}O$	222	27.011	1.22
28	Guaiol	$C_{15}H_{26}O$	222	27.150	4.73
29	Valerone	$C_{15}H_{26}O$	222	27.493	1.14
30	Nootkatone	$C_{15}H_{22}O$	218	29.031	14.79
31	Nootkatone isomer 1	$C_{15}H_{22}O$	218	29.467	1.06
32	Nootkatone isomer 2	$C_{15}H_{22}O$	218	30.333	0.90
33	1,2,3,4,4a,5,6,8,8a-Eight hydrogen-4a,8-dimethyl-α-Propenyl [α] naphthyl alcohol	$C_{15}H_{24}O$	220	35.174	0.83
34	Unidentified			36.500	0.83

classified to be of the guaiane type and valerian type. Despite the low contents of these essential oils, their biological activities have drawn the attention of researchers around the world [22–24].

Long et al. [25], Ming et al. [26], Wang et al. [27], and Yu et al. [28] previously investigated essential oils from *Valeriana* by GC-MS, showing its content was 1%, and 20%–60% of it was bornyl acetate. Wang et al. [27] detected 34 compounds by GC-MS, which comprised 91.75% of the total content of the essential oil of *V. officinalis* L. var. *latifolia* Miq. (Table 1

and Figure 1). Compared to the standard spectrum, bornyl acetate showed the highest content level at 23.93%, followed by nootkatone (14.79%) and 6-isopropyl-1-methyl bicycles [3,1,0] hexane (14.19%).

Yu et al. [28] analyzed essential oils from cultivated *V. officinalis* L. var. *latifolia* Miq. by GC-MS and identified 6 compounds, bornyl acetate (60.19%), (−)-acetic acid *Rhodomyrtus* enol ester (3.87%), α-terpinyl acetate (1.55%), acetyl carene (1.68%), α-selinene (26.07%), and (Z,E)-α-farnesene (1.56%), comprising 94.92% of the total content.

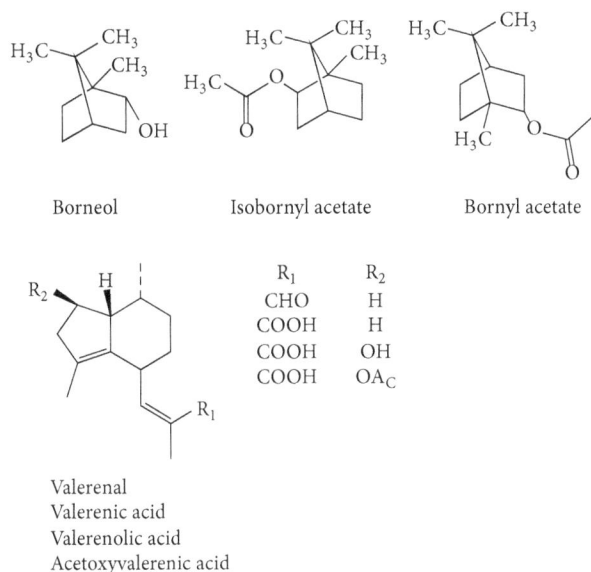

Borneol   Isobornyl acetate   Bornyl acetate

	R_1	R_2
	CHO	H
	COOH	H
	COOH	OH
	COOH	OA_C

Valerenal
Valerenic acid
Valerenolic acid
Acetoxyvalerenic acid

FIGURE 1: Major essential oil constituents from *V. officinalis* L. var. *latifolia* Miq.

TABLE 2

Number	R_1	R_7	R_{11}	Compounds	References
1-1	a	a	b	Valtrate	[6]
1-2	a	f	b	Acevaltrate	[6]
1-3	a	b	a	Isovaltrate	[35]
1-4	a	H	b	7-Epi-deacetylisovaltrate	[36]
1-5	a	H	a	Deacetylisovaltrate	[37]
1-6	d	a	b	Homovaltrate 1	[35]
1-7	a	b	d	Homovaltrate 2	[35]
1-8	f	a	b	1-β-Acevaltratum	[38]
1-9	g	a	b	1-Seneciovaltrate	[39]
1-10	a	b	b	Diavaltrate	[40]
1-11	f	f	b	1-β-Aceacevaltrate	[40]
1-12	c	b	a	Homoisovaltrate	[41]
1-13	c	c	b	1,7-Dihomovaltrate	[41]
1-14	e	a	b	1-α-Acevaltrate	[41]
1-15	e	c	b	Homo-A	[41]
1-16	c	b	b	Homo-B	[41]
1-17	a	c	k	Homo-Z	[41]
1-18	e	b	a	1-α-Aceisovaltrate	[42]
1-19	a	c	b	Homovaltrate	[43]
1-20	c	f	b	1-Homovaltrate	[44]
1-21	c	b	e	1-Homoisoacevaltrate	[44]
1-22	g	a	a	Sorbifolivaltrate A	[45]
1-23	g	c	b	Sorbifolivaltrate B	[45]
1-24	a	a	H	Deacetlyvaltrate	[46]
1-25	a	c	b	7-Homovaltrate	[46]
1-26	c	a	b	1-Homovaltrate	[46]
1-27	a	b	e	11-Acevaltrate	[46]
1-28	a	i	b	Homoacevaltrate	[46]
1-29	a	k	b	Hydroxyvaltrate	[47]
1-30	a	h	b	Isohomovaltrate	[47]

Cultivated *V. officinalis* L. var. *latifolia* Miq. consisted of a higher number of simple components, which was predominated by bornyl acetate relative to that of wild *V. officinalis* L.

2.2. Iridoids.

Valepotriate was first isolated from *V. wallichii* and preliminary studies by Thies and Funke [29] have confirmed the presence of a sedation ingredient. The study drew the attention of researchers from around the world. To date, over 130 iridoids from *Valeriana* spp. have been identified, possibly contributing their sedative, antidepressant, and antitumor activities.

Chen et al. [30] studied the levels of valepotriate, dihydrovalepotriate, and acetyl-valepotriate from *V. jatamansi* Jones, *V. officinalis* L., and *V. officinalis* L. var. *latifolia* Miq. by using the reverse phase high-performance liquid chromatography (RP-HPLC) method. The highest levels were observed in *V. jatamansi* Jones, followed by *V. officinalis* L. and *V. officinalis* L. var. *latifolia* Miq. In addition, the content of iridoid varied significantly among different parts and habitats.

The main iridoids in *Valeriana* comprised didrovaltrate and valepotriates derivatives (0.5%–9.0%), including valepotriate, isovalepotriate, acetoxyvalepotriate, and isovalemxy-hydroxy-dihydrovatrate. These were characterized by a hemiacetal fragment, which leads to the decomposed productions of isopentoic acid and valerienal at a specific pH or 60°C. C-1, C-7, C-10, or C-11 of compounds were mainly substituted by acyl groups such as acetyl, isovaleryl, α-acetoxyisovaleryl, β-acetoxyisovaleryl, and β-hydroxyisovaleryl. Furthermore, iridoids could be further divided into diethenoid-type, monoethenoid-type, and other types based on the parent structure.

2.2.1. Diethenoid-Type Iridoids.

Diethenoid-type iridoids were characterized by the following molecular structures: (1) two C-C double bonds often presented between C-3 and

C-4, C-5, and C-6 and occasionally presented between C-4 and C-5, C-6, and C-7; (2) an oxacyclopropane was often presented between C-8 and C-10, and C-10 was usually in a β-configuration; (3) H-1 (α-configuration) and H-9 (β-configuration) were preferentially located on different sides of the ring, and the C-7 acyl group usually was determined to be in the β-configuration (Figure 2 and Table 2 and Figure 3 and Table 3).

2.2.2. Monoethenoid-Type Iridoids.

Monoethenoid-type iridoids were predominantly aglycones, which are characterized by the following structures: (1) a carbon double bond occurring mostly between C-3 and C-4; (2) H-1 (α-configuration), H-5 or 5-OH (β-configuration), H-7 (β-configuration), and H-9 (β-configuration); (3) a triatomic heterocyclic structure occurring between C-8 and C-10, and C-10 is usually a β-methylene, which is called monoene closed-loop iridoids. When C-8 and C-10 were not in ring formation, the structure is classified as a monoene open-loop iridoid (Figure 4 and Table 4).

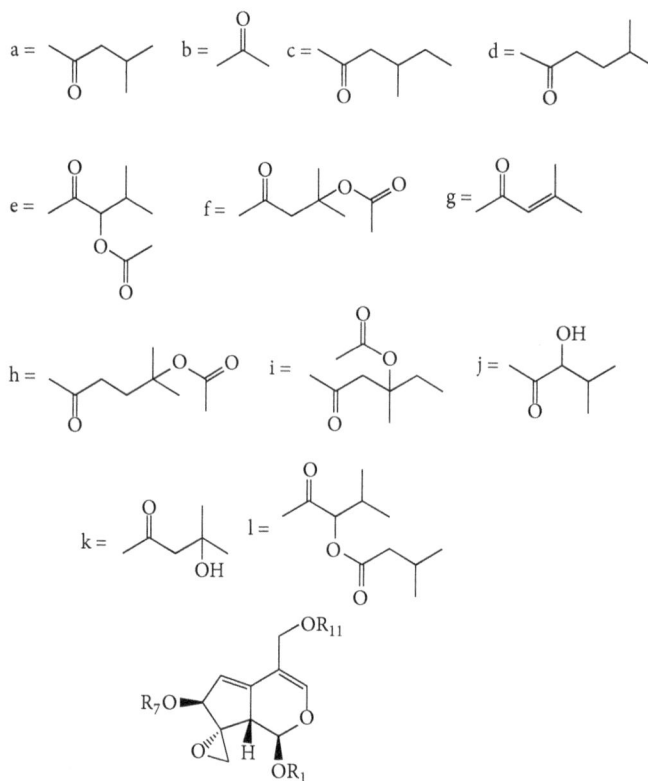

FIGURE 2: Compounds of diethenoid epoxy-type iridoids from *Valeriana* spp. (see Table 2).

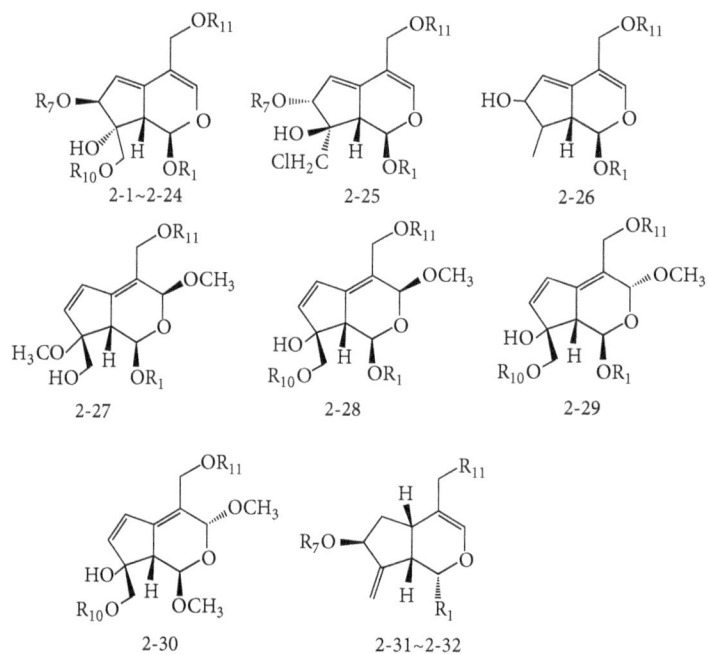

FIGURE 3: Compounds of diethenoid open ring-type iridoids from *Valeriana* spp. (see Table 3).

TABLE 3

Number	R_1	R_7	R_{10}	R_{11}	Compounds	References
2-1	a	a	a	b	Valtrate-isovaleroxyhydrin	[37]
2-2	a	a	a	b	Valtrate hydrin B1	[47]
2-3	a	a	b	b	Valtrate hydrin B2	[47]
2-4	j	a	a	b	Valtrate hydrin B3	[47]
2-5	a	b	a	a	Valtrate hydrin B4	[39]
2-6	a	a	c	b	Valtrate hydrin B5	[39]
2-7	a	b	c	b	Valtrate hydrin B6	[39]
2-8	g	a	a	b	Valtrate hydrin B7	[39]
2-9	e	a	a	b	Valtrate hydrin B8	[39]
2-10	e	b	b	a	Acetoxydesiovaleroxy-1-α-acetoxy-isovaleroxy isovaltratehydrine	[42]
2-11	c	a	b	b	10-Acetoxy-1-homovaltrate hydrin	[44]
2-12	f	a	b	b	10-Acetoxy-1-acevaltrate hydrin	[44]
2-13	k	a	a	a	Sorbifolivaltrate C	[45]
2-14	g	c	a	b	Sorbifolivaltrate D	[45]
2-15	a	e	l	b	Valeriandoid F	[48]
2-16	a	b	X	a	Jatamanvaltrate I	[49]
2-17	a	H	a	b	Jatamanvaltrate J	[49]
2-18	a	a	H	a	Jatamanvaltrate K	[49]
2-19	a	a	b	b	10-Acetoxyvaltrahedrin	[49]
2-20	a	b	Cl	a	Rupesin B	[50]
2-21	b	H	Cl	a	Valeriandoids A	[51]
2-22	a	f	Cl	b	Valeriandoids B	[51]
2-23	a	b	a	a	Isovaltrate isovaleroyloxyhydrin	[51]
2-24	a	a	Me	b	Valeriandoids F	[52]
2-25	a	a	—	b	Volechlorine	[36]
2-26	a	—	—	a	Nardostachin	[53]
2-27	a	—	—	b	Jatamanvaltrate N	[50]
2-28	a	—	l	b	Jatamanvaltrate O	[50]
2-29	a	—	l	b	Valeriandoids D	[52]
2-30	—	—	l	b	Valeriandoids E	[52]
2-31	a	b	—	a	8,11-Desoidodidrovaltrate	[37]
2-32	d	b	—	a	8,11-Desoidohomoddidrovaltrate	[37]

2.2.3. Other Types of Iridoids. Iridoids from *Valeriana* spp. were mostly of the two above-mentioned types (Figure 5). In addition, other types were also identified: (1) most of one type having free hydroxyl groups and ester groups, with a lactone structure between C-1 and C-3 and a double bond between C-4 and C-1, (2) an oxygen bridge between C-3 and C-8, C-3 and C-10, or C-8 and C-11, (3) cleaved Ring-A of other types forming a free hydroxyl or aldehyde group between C-1 and C-3 (e.g., see Lin et al. [31]).

2.3. Lignanoids. Recent researches have indicated that lignanoids are 7,9-monoepoxy lignin and a glycoside or bisepoxy lignin. Britta Schumacher isolated eight lignanoids from *Valeriana officinalis*, namely, pinoresinol-4-O-D-glucoside, lignans 8′-hydro-xypinoresinol, 7,9′-monoepoxylignans

massoniresinol-4′-O-beta-D-glucoside, berchemol-4′-O-D-glucoside, 8′-hydroxy-pinoresinol-4′-O-D-glucoside, and 8-hydroxypinoresinol-4′-O-D-glucoside [32]. Piccinelli et al. isolated two novel lignan glycosides from *Valeriana priono-phylla*, including fraxireslnol-4′-O-D-glucopyranoside and prinse-piol-4-O-D-glucopy-ranoside [33].

2.4. Alkaloids. Alkaloids in *Valeriana* spp. included chatinine, nordelporphine, norphoebine, thaliperphine, nantenine, phenanthrene, phoebine, dehydroaphine, valerine, valeriane, and oxoaporphine, which occupy the low level of 1% [3, 34].

2.5. Flavonoids. Flavonoids in *Valeriana* spp. were mainly acacetin, apigenin, diosmetin, luteolin, quercetin,

TABLE 4

Number	R_1	R_5	R_7	R_{10}	R_{11}	Compounds	References
3-1	a	H	a	—	b	Didrovaltrate	[6, 37, 53]
3-2	a	OH	b	—	l	Isovaleroxyhydroxydihydrovaltrate	[43]
3-3	a	H	b	—	a	Isodidrovaltrate	[54]
3-4	a	OH	b	—	e	AHD-valtrate	[40]
3-5	a	OH	b	—	c	11-Homohydroxyldihydrovaltrate	[44]
3-6	c	H	b	—	a	Homodidrovaltrate	[37]
3-7	a	OH	H	—	l	Jatamanvaltrate L	[49]
3-8	a	OH	b	—	Et	Jatamanvaltrate M	[49]
3-9	a	OH	b	—	a	5-Hydroxydidrovaltrate	[49]
3-10	a	OH	H	b	l	Valeriotriate B	[55]
3-11	a	OH	b	l	l	Valeriotertrate A	[56]
3-12	a	OH	b	f	l	Jatamanvaltrate A	[49]
3-13	a	OH	b	a	l	Jatamanvaltrate B	[49]
3-14	a	OH	b	b	l	Jatamanvaltrate C	[49]
3-15	a	OH	b	X	l	Jatamanvaltrate D	[49]
3-16	a	OH	b	Me	l	Jatamanvaltrate E	[49]
3-17	a	H	b	f	a	Jatamanvaltrate F	[49]
3-18	a	H	H	b	a	Jatamanvaltrate J	[49]
3-19	a	H	b	H	a	Jatamanvaltrate K	[49]
3-20	a	H	b	b	a	Didrovaltrate acetoxyhydrin	[49]
3-21	a	OH	b	Cl	l	Volvatrate B	[57]
3-22	a	OH	H	Cl	l	Jatamandoid A	[58]

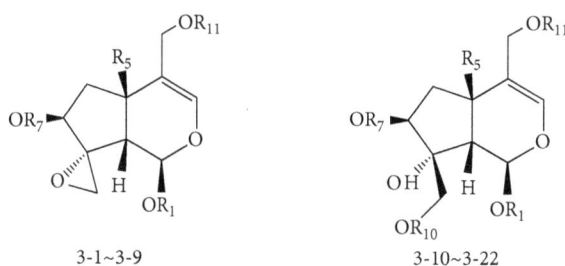

3-1~3-9   3-10~3-22

FIGURE 4: Compounds of monoethenoid-type iridoids from *Valeriana* spp. (see Table 4).

kaempferol, linarin, and luteolin [10, 33, 34], which occurred at low levels.

2.6. Amino Acids. Free amino acids in the water extracts of *Valeriana* spp. included γ-amino butyric acid (GABA), tyrosine, refined ammonia acid, glutamine, caffeic acid, chlorogenic acid, tannins, and sitosterol. GABA, a well-studied inhibitory neurotransmitter, is involved in lots of metabolic activities [59–62].

3. Research Advances on the Cardiovascular Activities of *Valeriana*

3.1. Reduction in Blood Pressure Level and Heart Rate. The increase of peripheral resistance in blood circulation was the common characteristic for primary hypertension, whose pathological mechanism was related to an increase of peripheral vascular tone and structural change of vessel walls.

Additionally, structure and function disorders of vascular smooth muscle cells (VSMC) also contributed largely to this abnormal change. Therefore, improving the contract status of VSMC, expending the peripheral vessels, and inhibiting abnormal growth of VSMC preventing or alleviating vessel reconstruction at the same time were the keys to treating hypertension. Wang et al. [63] cultured aortic medial smooth muscle cells from a 6-month-old aborted fetus and examined the migration of cultured cells by Boyden Chamber. They found essential oil (VOL) could significantly inhibit the migration of human VSMC in a dose-dependent manner. Yang et al. [64] observed the effect of VOL and L-nitro arginine methyl ester (L-NAME) on the contraction of VSMC through the analogous experiment and investigated changes of ^{3}H-thymidine (^{3}H-TdR) and ^{3}H-Leucine caused by angiotensin II (Ang II) and different concentrations of VSMC. VOL markedly inhibited the Ang II-stimulated contraction and growth of VSMC, which was not affected

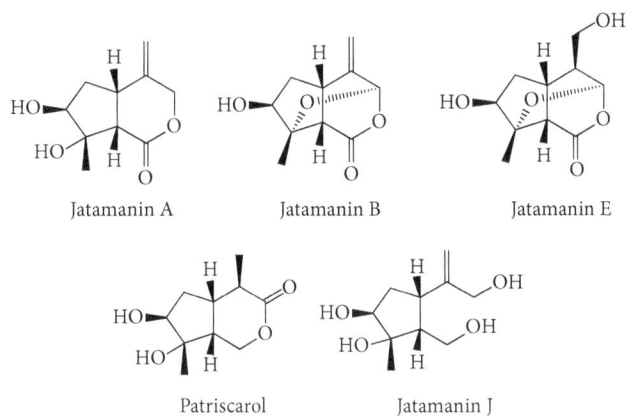

Jatamanin A   Jatamanin B   Jatamanin E

Patriscarol   Jatamanin J

FIGURE 5: Compounds of other types of iridoids from *Valeriana* spp.

by L-NAME. In addition, VOL inhibited the incorporation of ^{3}H-TdR and ^{3}H-leucine. Zhou et al. [65] found that VOL could decrease the heart rate and blood pressure (priority to diastolic pressure) of rabbit and prolonged the duration of ST segment and T wave in a dose-dependent manner. VOL could decrease heart rate and blood pressure stimulated by adrenaline, which might be related to relaxing VSMC, enlarging vessel diameter, and decreasing blood resistance. VOL also observably inhibited contraction of VSMC stimulated by adrenaline, dilated coronary arteries, and decreased myocardial oxygen consumption. The vasorelaxant effects of the EtOH extract ($1 \, mg \cdot mL^{-1}$) and 8-hydroxypinoresinol ($100 \, \mu m$) from the roots of *Valeriana prionophylla* have been already shown [66]. Fields et al. [66] reported that VOL could dilate pulmonary vessels in felines via a nonselective GABA mechanism and inhibited contraction of isolated frog hearts stimulated by cardenolide. It has already been shown that hexanic extracts (HEVe) from *V. edulis* ssp. *procera* enriched in valepotriates present vasorelaxant properties by blocking calcium channels. HEVe induced a significant concentration-dependent and endothelium-independent relaxation on isolated rat aorta precontracted with noradrenaline ($0.1 \, \mu m$). HEVe, the most potent extract (0.15–$50 \, \mu g/mL$), induced relaxation in aortic rings precontracted with KCl ($80 \, mm$), with IC_{50} value of $34.61 \, \mu g/mL$ and E_{max} value of 85.0% [67].

3.2. Antimyocardial Ischemia Reperfusion Injury.

As early as the 1980s, Zhang et al. [68] reported that the ethanol extract of valerian could dilate the coronary artery and reduce myocardial oxygen consumption in anesthetized cats. Yang et al. [69] reported that its essential oil and iridoids enhance microcirculation perfusion of the heart and kidney. The valerian extract can prevent injuries to myocardial ischemia reperfusion model in the rabbit by decreasing the levels of xanthine oxidase (XOD), malondialdehyde (MDA), and tumor necrosis factor-α (TNF-α), thereby increasing the 6-keto-prostaglandin F1α/thromboxane B2 (6-keto-PGF1α/TXB2) ratio. Huang et al. [70] conducted a study to investigate myocardial protection mechanism of monoterpene oxide of valerian (VMO). Compared to the control group, VMO showed a maximum change rate of left ventricular pressure, with a maximal rate of the increase of the left ventricular

pressure ($+d_{ip}/t_{max}$) and maximal rate of the decrease of the left ventricular pressure ($-d_{ip}/t_{max}$) by 25.1% and 25.3%, respectively. Adenosine triphosphate (ATP) and energy charge (E_C) increased by 72.8% and 20.9%, respectively, whereas myocardial creatine kinase-myocardial band (CK-MB) decreased by 20.7%. These results demonstrated the analogical performance between VMO and ischemic preconditioning pretreatment on cardio protection, which indicated a mobilizing myocardial endogenesis protective mechanism and an exoteric ATP-sensitive potassium channel. Yang et al. [71] set up an isolated rat ischemia reperfusion (I/R) heart model using a Langendorff-perfusion system, observing the effects of VOL pretreatment on I/R injury and related biochemical factors and cytosolic free calcium. The results indicated that VOL pretreatment markedly prevented I/R injury, weakened vasospasm perfusion, sustained the heartbeat, and reduced ventricular arrhythmic events in a dose-dependent manner. Simultaneously, VOL significantly lowered lactate dehydrogenase (LDH), creatine phosphokinase (CK), and MDA levels. The activities of superoxide dismutase (SOD), adenosine triphosphatase (ATPase), and glutathione peroxidase (GSH-Px) were enhanced. VOL reduced intracellular calcium in a concentration-dependent manner. The mechanism of action for VOL's aforementioned activities potentially involved preventing the increase in concentration of free Ca^{2+} and decrease in lipid peroxidation.

3.3. Antiarrhythmia.

Arrhythmia is a common disease that involves various pathological mechanisms. Although western medicines have considerable efficiency, the adverse reactions at different levels and the development of arrhythmia caused by the drug itself have been reported. Therefore, it is imperative to discover an antiarrhythmic drug that features efficiency, stability, and the absence of adverse effects; these properties are inherent to traditional Chinese medicine, which are also of scientific and societal significance.

Arrhythmia induced by aconitine might be caused by myocardium excitability, which opens Na^+ channel of the cardiac muscle and promotes sodium currents, resulting in a ventricular and supraventricular ectopic rhythm and ventricular tachycardia. Ventricular fibrillation induced by chloroform could be related to the release of neurotransmitters or adrenaline secretion in the adrenal medulla, as well as stimulation of β receptors [72, 73].

Jia and Zhang [74] found that chloroform extract of ethanol extract (v3d) could effectively prevent atrial fibrillation in mice induced by acetylcholine-calcium chloride and ventricular fibrillation induced by chloroform. It also protected rats from ischemia arrhythmia induced by ligation of the left anterior descending coronary artery. In addition, it effectively prevents dog auricular and renal vessels contraction induced by high K^+ levels. Therefore, v3d prevents arrhythmia in various animal species partly by inhibiting Ca^{2+} channel from opening, which was induced by high K^+ level.

Huang [75] found valerian extract (monoterpene and sesquiterpene oxides from essential oils) could dose-dependently reduce the duration of an action potential and inhibit

Na current (I_{Na}), L-type calcium current (I_{Ca-L}), and transient outward potassium current (I_{to}). It interacts with inactivated I_{Na} and I_{Ca-L}, although various concentrations of v3d had no detectable effect on the delayed rectifier potassium current (I_K) or inward rectifier potassium current (I_{KI}) or direct interference with adenosine triphosphate sensitive potassium current (I_{KATP}). The impacts of the valerian extract on these ion pathways might have contributed to its antiarrhythmia activity.

Wen et al. [76] reported the water, essential oil, and other fractions of valerian could protect a rat model from arrhythmia caused by aconitine or chloroform. Water extract at a dose of 50 and 25 g·kg^{-1} (calculated as raw herb) effectively decreased the occurrence of ventricular fibrillation, delayed the occurrence of arrhythmia, and decreased the mortality rate. The essential oil at a dose of 50 and 25 g·kg^{-1} (calculated as raw herb) effectively inhibited arrhythmia that was induced by chloroform; other fractions also demonstrated antiarrhythmia activities at different levels. Duan [77] found two active compounds from *V. officinalis* L., prinsepiol-4-O-β-D-glucoside and 8-hydroxy pinoresinol-4-O-β-D-glucoside; both showed antiarrhythmia activities. The former imparted an inhibitory effect on the Kv1.5 channel, which is the key mechanism for antiarrhythmia activity.

It was shown that didrovaltrate blocks L-type calcium current in a concentration-dependent manner and probably inhibited these currents in its inactive state. Didrovaltrate at concentrations of 30 μg/L and 100 μg/L significantly decreased peak I_{Ca-L} ($I_{Ca-Lmax}$) from 6.01 to 3.45 pA/pF and 2.16 pA/pF, respectively. Didrovaltrate shifted upwards the current-voltage curves of I_{Ca-L} without changing their active, peak, and reverse potentials. Didrovaltrate affected the steady-state inactivation of I_{Ca-L}. The half activation potential ($V_{1/2}$) was significantly shifted from -26 to -36 mV, with a significant change in the slope factor (k) (from 8.8 to 11.1) [78].

Liu et al. [79] studied antiarrhythmia effective substances in serum of *V. officinalis* L. The study showed that borneol and bornyl acetate from Valerian essential oils and another unidentified compound from ethyl acetate extract could be absorbed into the blood in its original form, which indicated that this unidentified compound might be the main substance that contributes to the antiarrhythmia activity of the ethyl acetate extract.

3.4. Regulation of Blood Lipid Levels. Reports on *V. officinalis* L. var. *latifolia* Miq. (VOL) and its constituents in lipid regulation are limited. Hu et al. [80] examined the effects of VOL on blood lipid metabolism in rabbits with hyperlipidemia. VOL imparts a remarkable antilipid peroxidation effect, reduces the levels of serum total cholesterol (TC), triglyceride (TG), low-density lipoprotein cholesterol (LDL-C), and MDA, and elevates the levels of high-density lipoprotein cholesterol (HDL-C) and SOD. The results prove that it is imperative to further investigate the underlying mechanisms in regulating lipid metabolism. Si et al. [81] also demonstrated VOL could reduce the serum levels of total cholesterol, low-density lipoprotein, urinary albumin, and serum creatinine. Light

microscopy and immunohistochemical stain revealed that, in the same time of lowering serum lipid, mesangial matrix index was significantly reduced, accompanied by decreased expression of TGF-β_1 and type IV collagen.

4. Conclusions

Valeriana spp. possesses a wide range of bioactivities, which have been conferred by its complex and diverse active ingredients. Although the effects of *Valeriana* spp. mainly affected the cardiovascular system in Section 3, its mechanism of action needs to be further investigated.

Abbreviations

$+d_{ip}/t_{max}$:	Maximal rate of the increase of the left ventricular pressure
^{3}H-TdR:	^{3}H-Thymidine
6-keto-PGF1α/TXB2:	6-Keto-prostaglandin F1α/thromboxane B2
Ang II:	Angiotensin II
ATP:	Adenosine triphosphate
CK:	Creatine phosphokinase
CK-MB:	Creatine kinase-myocardial band
$-d_{ip}/t_{max}$:	Maximal rate of the decrease of the left ventricular pressure
E_C:	Energy charge
GABA:	γ-Amino butyric acid
GC-MS:	Chromatography-mass spectrometry
GSH-Px:	Glutathione peroxidase
HDL-C:	High-density lipoprotein cholesterol
HEVe:	Hexanic extracts
I/R:	Ischemia reperfusion
I_{Ca-L}:	L-type calcium current
I_K:	Delayed rectifier potassium current
I_{KATP}:	Adenosine triphosphate sensitive potassium current
I_{KI}:	Inward rectifier potassium current
I_{Na}:	Na current
I_{to}:	Transient outward potassium current
LDH:	Lactate dehydrogenase
LDL-C:	Low-density lipoprotein cholesterol
L-NAME:	L-nitro arginine methyl ester
MDA:	Malondialdehyde
RP-HPLC:	Reverse phase high-performance liquid chromatography
SOD:	Superoxide dismutase
TC:	Total cholesterol
TG:	Triglyceride
TNF-α:	Tumor necrosis factor-α
v3d:	Chloroform extract of ethanol extract
VMO:	Monoterpene oxide of valerian
VOL:	Essential oil
VSMC:	Vascular smooth muscle cells
XOD:	Xanthine oxidase.

Conflict of Interests

The authors declare that there is no conflict of interests regarding the publication of this paper.

Authors' Contribution

Heng-Wen Chen and Ben-Jun Wei contributed equally to this work.

Acknowledgment

This study was supported by a research grant from the National Natural Science Foundation of China (no. 81503421).

References

[1] H.-B. Chen and J.-R. Cheng, "Taxonomic revision of the relative species of *Valeriana officinalis* Linn. from China," *Bulletin of Botanical Research*, vol. 3, pp. 29–40, 1991.

[2] H. B. Chen and J. R. Cheng, "Studies on the medicinal plants of *Valerianaceae* in China," *China Journal of Chinese Materia Medica*, vol. 2, no. 3, pp. 67–70, 1994.

[3] P.-J. Houghton, "The biological activity of *valerian* and related plants," *Journal of Ethnopharmacology*, vol. 22, no. 2, pp. 121–142, 1988.

[4] P. J. Houghton, "The scientific basis for the reputed activity of *Valerian*," *The Journal of Pharmacy and Pharmacology*, vol. 51, no. 5, pp. 505–512, 1999.

[5] D. Muller, T. Pfeil, and V. von den Driesch, "*Valeriana officinalis* (monograph)," *Alternative Medicine Review*, vol. 9, no. 4, pp. 438–441, 2004.

[6] P.-W. Thies, "Zur Konstitution der isovalerian saureester valepotriat, acetoxyvalepotriat und dihydrovalepotriat," *Tetrahedron Letters*, vol. 7, no. 11, pp. 1163–1170, 1966.

[7] H. Hendriks, H.-J. Geertsma, and T.-M. Malingre, "The occurrence of valeranone and crytofauronol in the essential oil of *Valeriana officinalis cinalis* L. collected in the northern part of the Netherlands," *Pharmaceutisch Weekblad Scientific Edition*, vol. 116, pp. 1316–1320, 1981.

[8] P. D. Leathwood, F. Chauffard, E. Heck, and R. Munoz-Box, "Aqueous extract of valerian root (*Valeriana officinalis* L.) improves sleep quality in man," *Pharmacology, Biochemistry and Behavior*, vol. 17, no. 1, pp. 65–71, 1982.

[9] T. Sakamoto, Y. Mitani, and K. Nakajima, "Psychotropic effects of Japanese *Valerian* root extract," *Chemical and Pharmaceutical Bulletin*, vol. 40, no. 3, pp. 758–761, 1992.

[10] M.-S. Santos, F. Ferreira, C. Faro et al., "The amount of GABA present in aqueous extracts of valerian is sufficient to account for [^{3}H] GABA release in synaptosomes," *Planta Medica*, vol. 60, no. 5, pp. 475–476, 1994.

[11] Z.-X. Zhang and X.-S. Yao, "The advance of chemical study on the medicinal plant *Valeriana officinalis* L.," *Chinese Journal of Medicinal Chemistry*, no. 3, pp. 226–229, 2000.

[12] X.-G. Liu, P.-Y. Gao, G.-S. Wang et al., "*In vivo* antidepressant activity of sesquiterpenes from the roots of *Valeriana faurieiBriq*," *Fitoterapia*, vol. 83, no. 3, pp. 599–603, 2012.

[13] Q.-H. Wang, C.-F. Wang, Y.-M. Zuo, Z.-B. Wang, B.-Y. Yang, and H.-X. Kuang, "Compounds from the roots and rhizomes of *Valeriana amurensis* protect against neurotoxicity in PC12 cells," *Molecules*, vol. 17, no. 12, pp. 15013–15021, 2012.

[14] S. M. Nam, J. H. Choi, D. Y. Yoo et al., "*Valeriana officinalis* extract and its main component, valerenic acid, ameliorate d-galactose-induced reductions in memory, cell proliferation, and neuroblast differentiation by reducing corticosterone levels and lipid peroxidation," *Experimental Gerontology*, vol. 48, no. 11, pp. 1369–1377, 2013.

[15] F. Felgentreff, A. Becker, B. Meier, and A. Brattström, "Valerian extract characterized by high valerenic acid and low acetoxy valerenic acid contents demonstrates anxiolytic activity," *Phytomedicine*, vol. 19, no. 13, pp. 1216–1222, 2012.

[16] Q.-H. Wang, C.-F. Wang, Z.-P. Shu et al., "*Valeriana amurensis* improves Amyloid-beta 1-42 induced cognitive deficit by enhancing cerebral cholinergic function and protecting the brain neurons from apoptosis in mice," *Journal of Ethnopharmacology*, vol. 153, no. 2, pp. 318–325, 2014.

[17] S. Sridharan, K. Mohankumar, S. P. Jeepipalli et al., "Neuroprotective effect of Valeriana wallichii rhizome extract against the neurotoxin MPTP in C57BL/6 mice," *Neurotoxicology*, vol. 51, pp. 172–183, 2015.

[18] W. Letchamo, W. Ward, B. Heard, and D. Heard, "Essential oil of *Valeriana officinalis* L. cultivars and their antimicrobial activity as influenced by harvesting time under commercial organic cultivation," *Journal of Agricultural and Food Chemistry*, vol. 52, no. 12, pp. 3915–3919, 2004.

[19] Y.-D. Chen and C.-H. Gu, "Study on the chemical composition of essential oil from *Valeriana Officinalis* L.," *Chemistry and Industry of Forest Products*, vol. 9, pp. 59–64, 1989.

[20] C.-H. Gu, L. Gu, and Y.-K. Zhang, "Comparison study on essential oil from wild and cultivated *Valeriana pseudofficinalis* by GC/MS anaylsis," *Chemistry and Industry of Forest Products*, vol. 19, pp. 64–69, 1999.

[21] B.-K. Huang, L.-P. Qin, Q.-C. Chu, Q.-Y. Zhang, L.-H. Gao, and H.-C. Zheng, "Comparison of headspace spme with hydrodistillation and sfe for analysis of the volatile components of the roots of *Valeriana officinalis* var. *latifolia*," *Chromatographia*, vol. 69, no. 5-6, pp. 489–496, 2009.

[22] J.-L. Shi, Y. Liu, and P.-G. Xiao, "The chemical constituents and bioactivities of *Valeriana officinlais* L.," *World Phytomedicines*, vol. 18, no. 6, pp. 231–239, 2003.

[23] M. Pavlovic, N. Kovacevic, O. Tzakou, and M. Couladis, "The essential oil of *Valeriana officinalis* L. *s.l.* growing wild in Western Serbia," *Journal of Essential Oil Research*, vol. 16, no. 5, pp. 397–399, 2004.

[24] R. Bos, H. Hendriks, N. Pras, A.-S. Stojanova, and E. V. Georgiev, "Essential oil composition of *Valeriana officinalis* ssp. *collina* cultivated in Bulgaria," *Journal of Essential Oil Research*, vol. 12, no. 3, pp. 313–316, 2000.

[25] C.-Z. Long, H.-L. Xiao, and J.-Q. Peng, "Chemical constituents of the volatile oil from *Valeriana officinalis* Linn. var. *Latifolia Miq* grown in guizhou province," *Acta Botanica Yunnanica*, vol. 9, no. 1, pp. 109–112, 1987.

[26] D.-S. Ming, J.-X. Guo, and Q.-S. Shun, "Determination of chemical composition of the essential oil from four kinds of *Valeriana officinalis* L. by GC/MS," *Chinese Traditional Patent Medicine*, vol. 16, no. 1, pp. 41–42, 1994.

[27] L.-Q. Wang, Y.-T. Xiong, F.-H. Tao, and N.-Q. Li, "Chemical constituents of essential oil from *Valeriana officinalis* Linn. var. *Latifolia Miq*," *China Journal of Chinese Materia Medica*, vol. 22, no. 6, pp. 298–299, 1999.

[28] Z.-W. Yu, Z.-N. Yang, and Y. Yi, "Analysis of chemical constituents of essential oil from cultured *Valeriana officinalis* L.," *Chinese Journal of Spectroscopy Laboratory*, vol. 28, no. 4, pp. 1672–1674, 2011.

[29] P.-W. Thies and S. Funke, "Active principles of baldrian. I. Detection and isolation of the sedative active isovalerianic acid esters from roots and rhizomes of various *Valerian* and *Centranthus* species," *Tetrahedron Letters*, vol. 7, no. 11, pp. 1155–1162, 1966.

[30] L. Chen, L.-P. Qin, and H.-C. Zheng, "Chemical constituents, plant resource and pharmacology-activity on the *Valeriana officinalis* L," *Journal of Pharmaceutical Practice*, vol. 18, no. 5, pp. 277–279, 2000.

[31] S. Lin, T. Chen, X.-H. Liu et al., "Iridoids and lignans from *Valeriana jatamansi*," *Journal of Natural Products*, vol. 73, no. 4, pp. 632–638, 2010.

[32] B. Schumacher, S. Scholle, J. Hölzl, N. Khudeir, S. Hess, and C. E. Müller, "Lignans isolated from valerian: identification and characterization of a new olivil derivative with partial agonistic activity at A_1 adenosine receptors," *Journal of Natural Products*, vol. 65, no. 10, pp. 1479–1485, 2002.

[33] A. L. Piccinelli, S. Arana, A. Caceres, R. D. di Villa Bianca, R. Sorrentino, and L. Rastrelli, "New lignans from the roots of *Valeriana prionophylla* with antioxidative and vasorelaxant activities," *Journal of Natural Products*, vol. 67, no. 7, pp. 1135–1140, 2004.

[34] I.-P. Nazarova, A.-I. Glushenkova, and A.-U. Umarov, "Gossypol-like compounds of the cotton plant. Methods of determining gossypol," *Chemistry of Natural Compounds*, vol. 17, no. 2, pp. 87–102, 1981.

[35] P.-W. Thies, E. Finner, and F. Rosskopf, "Über die wirkstoffe des baldrians—X: die konfiguration des valtratum und anderer valepotriate," *Tetrahedron*, vol. 29, no. 20, pp. 3213–3226, 1973.

[36] S. Popov, N. Handjieva, and N. Marekov, "A new valepotriate, 7-epi-deacetylisovaltrate from *Valeriana officinalis*," *Phytochemistry*, vol. 13, no. 12, pp. 2815–2818, 1974.

[37] P.-W. Thies, "Constitution of valepotriates. Report on active agents of valerian," *Tetrahedron*, vol. 24, no. 1, pp. 313–347, 1968.

[38] J. Holzl and U. Koch, "The compounds of *Valeriana alliariifolia*. 1-β-acevaltratum, a new valepotriate," *Planta Medica*, vol. 50, no. 5, p. 458, 1984.

[39] U. Koch and J. Hoelzl, "Constituents of *Valeriana alliariifolia*. 2. Valepotriathydrines," *Planta Medica*, vol. 51, no. 2, pp. 172–173, 1985.

[40] L.-A. Salles, A. L. Silva, S. B. Rech, N. Zanatta, and G. L. Von Poser, "Constituents of *Valeriana glechomifolia* Meyer," *Biochemical Systematics and Ecology*, vol. 28, no. 9, pp. 907–910, 2000.

[41] H. Becker and S. Chavadej, "Tissue cultures of *Valerianaceae*. 7. Valepotriate production of normal and colchicine-treated cell-suspension cultures of *Valeriana Wallichii*," *Journal of Natural Products*, vol. 48, no. 1, pp. 17–21, 1985.

[42] Y. Amanzadeh, N. Ghassemi-Dehkordi, S. E. Sadat-Ebrahimi, and M. Pirali-Hamedani, "Two new valepotriates from the roots of *Valeriana sisymbriifolia*," *DARU Journal of Pharmaceutical Sciences*, vol. 10, no. 2, pp. 63–66, 2002.

[43] N. Fuzzati, J. L. Wolfender, K. Hostettmann, J. D. Msonthi, S. Mavi, and L. P. Molleyres, "Isolation of antifungal valepotriates from *Valeriana capense* and the search for valepotriates in crude *Valerianaceae* extracts," *Phytochemical Analysis*, vol. 7, no. 2, pp. 76–85, 1996.

[44] Y. Tang, X. Liu, and B. Yu, "Iridoids from the rhizomes and roots of *Valeriana jatamansi*," *Journal of Natural Products*, vol. 65, no. 12, pp. 1949–1952, 2002.

[45] Y.-M. Xu, S.-P. McLaughlin, and A. A. L. Gunatilaka, "Sorbifolivaltrates A-D, diene valepotriates from *Valeriana sorbifolia*," *Journal of Natural Products*, vol. 70, no. 12, pp. 2045–2048, 2007.

[46] P.-W. Thies, E. Finner, and S. David, "On the active agents of valerian.14. assignment of type and location of the acyloxy substituents in valepotriates via ^{13}C-NMR spectroscopy," *Planta Medica*, vol. 41, no. 1, pp. 15–20, 1981.

[47] J. Holzl, V.-M. Chari, and O. Seligmann, "Structure of 3 genuine valtrate hydrines from *Valeriana tiliaefolia*," *Tetrahedron Letters*, vol. 17, no. 15, pp. 1171–1174, 1976.

[48] R. Wang, D. Xiao, Y.-H. Bian et al., "Minor iridoids from the roots of *Valeriana wallichii*," *Journal of Natural Products*, vol. 71, no. 7, pp. 1254–1257, 2008.

[49] S. Lin, Y.-H. Shen, H.-A. Li et al., "Acylated iridoids with cytotoxicity from *Valeriana jatamansi*," *Journal of Natural Products*, vol. 72, no. 4, pp. 650–655, 2009.

[50] J. Xu, P. Guo, L.-Z. Fang, Y.-S. Li, and Y.-Q. Guo, "Iridoids from the roots of *Valeriana jatamansi*," *Journal of Asian Natural Products Research*, vol. 14, no. 1, pp. 1–6, 2012.

[51] J. Xu, P. Zhao, Y.-Q. Guo et al., "Iridoids from the roots of *Valeriana jatamansi* and their neuroprotective effects," *Fitoterapia*, vol. 82, no. 7, pp. 1133–1136, 2011.

[52] J. Xu, Y.-Q. Guo, D.-Q. Jin et al., "Three new iridoids from the roots of *Valeriana jatamansi*," *Journal of Natural Medicines*, vol. 66, no. 4, pp. 653–657, 2012.

[53] K.-K. Bach, F. Ghia, and K.-B.-G. Torssell, "Valtrates and lignans in *Valeriana microphylla*," *Planta Medica*, vol. 59, no. 5, pp. 478–479, 1993.

[54] W. Kucaba, P.-W. Thies, and E. Finner, "Isodidrovaltratum, ein neues valepotriat aus *Valeriana vaginata*," *Phytochemistry*, vol. 19, no. 4, pp. 575–577, 1980.

[55] L. Yu, R. Huang, C. Han, Y. Lv, Y. Zhao, and Y. Chen, "New iridoid triesters from *Valeriana jatamansi*," *Helvetica Chimica Acta*, vol. 88, no. 5, pp. 1059–1062, 2005.

[56] L.-L. Yu, C.-R. Han, R. Huang, Y.-P. Lv, S.-H. Gui, and Y.-G. Chen, "A new iridoid tetraester from *Valeriana jatamansi*," *Pharmazie*, vol. 61, no. 5, pp. 486–488, 2006.

[57] P.-C. Wang, J.-M. Hu, X.-H. Ran et al., "Iridoids and sesquiterpenoids from the roots of *Valeriana officinalis*," *Journal of Natural Products*, vol. 72, no. 9, pp. 1682–1685, 2009.

[58] J. Xu, P. Guo, Y. Guo et al., "Iridoids from the roots of *Valeriana jatamansi* and their biological activities," *Natural Product Research*, vol. 26, no. 21, pp. 1996–2001, 2011.

[59] B.-K. Huang, H.-C. Zheng, and L.-P. Qin, "Material basis of the sedative and hypnotic activities of *Valeriana officinalis*," *Pharmaceutical Care and Research*, vol. 6, no. 3, pp. 165–168, 2006.

[60] B. Wu, Y.-M. Fu, A.-H. Huang, and Y.-J. Ma, "Changes of GABA and Glu content in hippocampus of PTZ-induced epileptic rats treated with volatile oil of *Valeriana*," *Chinese Archives of Traditional Chinese Medicine*, vol. 26, no. 11, pp. 2476–2477, 2008.

[61] J.-S. Chen, J.-K. Wu, L. Liu, Y. Zhang, F.-J. Wang, and X.-W. Du, "Studies on improving sleep function and relative mechanism of mice by petroleum extract of *Valeriana amurensis*," *Chinese Journal of Experimental Traditional Medical Formulae*, vol. 19, no. 24, pp. 245–249, 2013.

[62] Z.-X. Zhang and X.-S. Yao, "The development and research advances in bio-activity for the medicinal plant *Valeriana officinalis*," *Journal of Shenyang Pharmaceutical University*, no. 1, pp. 222–225, 2000.

[63] J.-F. Wang, G.-Y. Yang, and J.-N. Wang, "Effects of *Valeriana officinalis* var *Latifolia Miq* on the migration of cultured human vascular smooth muscle cells," *Journal of Yunyang Medical College*, vol. 18, no. 4, pp. 196–197, 1999.

[64] G.-Y. Yang, Q. Xu, and J.-F. Wang, "*Valeriana officinalis* var. *Latifolia Miq* regulates vascular smooth muscle cell contraction and growth," *Journal of Yunyang Medical College*, vol. 21, no. 6, pp. 324–326, 2002.

[65] X.-Z. Zhou, L. Kang, Y. Kang, L. Li, and S.-H. Xiong, "Effect of *Valeriana Officinalis* Var *Latifolia Miq* on heart rat and arterial blood pressure of rabbit," *Journal of Liaoning University of TCM*, vol. 11, no. 12, pp. 188–189, 2009.

[66] A.-M. Fields, T.-A. Richards, J.-A. Felton et al., "Analysis of responses to valerian root extract in the feline pulmonary vascular bed," *Journal of Alternative and Complementary Medicine*, vol. 9, no. 6, pp. 909–918, 2003.

[67] S. Estrada-Soto, J. Rivera-Leyva, J.-J. Ramírez-Espinosa, P. Castillo-España, F. Aguirre-Crespo, and O. Hernández-Abreu, "Vasorelaxant effect of *Valeriana edulis* ssp. procera (Valerianaceae) and its mode of action as calcium channel blocker," *Journal of Pharmacy and Pharmacology*, vol. 62, no. 9, pp. 1167–1174, 2010.

[68] B.-H. Zhang, H.-P. Meng, T. Wang et al., "Effects of *Valeriana officinalis* L. extract on cardiovascular system," *Acta Pharmaceutica Sinica*, vol. 17, no. 5, pp. 382–384, 1982.

[69] J. Yang, C.-K. Xue, X.-Z. Zhu et al., "Evaluate the effect of some TCMs extracts on improving micro circulation reperfusion volume of both cardiac and renal tissues by ^{86}Rb tracer," *Chinese Journal of Microcirculation*, vol. 8, no. 1, pp. 15–17, 1998.

[70] Z.-R. Huang, Q.-Z. Tang, W.-H. Li, L.-J. Zhang, Q. Xie, and G. Wu, "Study of monoterpene oxide pretreatment on donor heart preservation," *Chinese Heart Journal*, vol. 18, no. 2, pp. 182–184, 2006.

[71] S.-H. Yang, F. Chen, H.-M. Ma, and T. Wang, "Protection of *Valeriana officinalis* L. extract preconditioning on ischemia-reperfusion injury in rat hearts in vitro," *Medical Journal of Wuhan University*, vol. 33, no. 5, pp. 639–643, 2012.

[72] H. Wang, S.-D. Luo, H.-S. Cai, F. Wang, and J. Yang, "Antiarrhythmic effect of diacetyl-linesinine," *Chinese Journal of Hospital. Pharmacy*, vol. 21, no. 6, pp. 326–330, 2001.

[73] D.-M. Gong, H.-L. Shan, D.-L. Dong, H.-Y. Zhou, and B.-F. Yang, "Study of ion targets in Ouabain-induced rat arrhythmia," *Journal of Harbin Medical University*, vol. 36, no. 2, pp. 87–90, 2002.

[74] J.-N. Jia and B.-H. Zhang, "Effects of extract of *Valeriana officinalis* L. (V3d) on cardiovascular system," *Journal of Guangxi University of Chinese Medicine*, vol. 16, no. 1, pp. 40–42, 1999.

[75] Z.-R. Huang, *Effect of Valerian Extract on Ionic Channels of Rabbit Ventricular Myocytes*, Wuhan University, Wuhan, China, 2004.

[76] L. Wen, Y. Zhou, W. Zhou, X.-Y. Duan, and Y. Fang, "Effect of extracts of *Valeriana officinalis* L. on cardiac arrhythmias," *Chinese Journal of Hospital Pharmacy*, vol. 29, no. 3, pp. 191–194, 2009.

[77] X.-Y. Duan, *Study on the Drug Effect Substances and the Mechanism of Arrhythmic Effects of Valeriana officinalis L.*, Hubei College of TCM, Wuhan, China, 2009.

[78] Q. Xie, W.-H. Li, Z. R. Huang, and Z. Zhang, "Effect of didrovaltrate on l-calcium current in rabbit ventricular myocytes," *Journal of Traditional Chinese Medicine*, vol. 32, no. 3, pp. 442–445, 2012.

[79] J.-F. Liu, Y. Fang, Z.-F. Gong, Y.-W. Liu, and J.-F. Jiu, "Study on the anti-arrhythmia effective substances and serum pharmacochemistry of *Valeriana officinalis* L.," *Hubei Journal of Traditional Chinese Medicine*, vol. 35, no. 1, pp. 72–73, 2013.

[80] C.-X. Hu, D.-B. Zhang, H. Li et al., "Effects of *Valeriana officinalis* L. var *Latifolia Miq* on blood-lipid metabolism in rabbits with hyperlipidemia," *Journal of Nanjing Military Medical College*, vol. 21, no. 2, pp. 65–68, 1999.

[81] X.-Y. Si, R.-H. Jia, C.-X. Huang, G.-H. Ding, and H.-Y. Liu, "Effects of *Valeriana officinalis* var. *latifolia* on expression of transforming growth factor β_1 in hypercholesterolemic rats," *China Journal of Chinese Materia Medica*, vol. 28, no. 9, pp. 845–848, 2003.

20

Antibacterial and Cytotoxic Activity of Compounds Isolated from *Flourensia oolepis*

Mariana Belén Joray,[1] **Lucas Daniel Trucco,**[2] **María Laura González,**[1]
Georgina Natalia Díaz Napal,[1] **Sara María Palacios,**[1] **José Luis Bocco,**[2]
and María Cecilia Carpinella[1]

[1]*Fine Chemicals and Natural Products Laboratory, School of Chemistry, Catholic University of Córdoba,*
Avda Armada Argentina 3555, X5016DHK Córdoba, Argentina
[2]*CIBICI CONICET and Department of Clinical Biochemistry, Faculty of Chemical Science, National University of Córdoba,*
Haya de la Torre and Medina Allende, Córdoba, Argentina

Correspondence should be addressed to María Cecilia Carpinella; ceciliacarpinella@ucc.edu.ar

Academic Editor: Jairo Kennup Bastos

The antibacterial and cytotoxic effects of metabolites isolated from an antibacterial extract of *Flourensia oolepis* were evaluated. Bioguided fractionation led to five flavonoids, identified as $2',4'$-dihydroxychalcone (**1**), isoliquiritigenin (**2**), pinocembrin (**3**), 7-hydroxyflavanone (**4**), and $7,4'$-dihydroxy-$3'$-methoxyflavanone (**5**). Compound **1** showed the highest antibacterial effect, with minimum inhibitory concentration (MIC) values ranging from 31 to 62 and 62 to 250 μg/mL, against Gram-positive and Gram-negative bacteria, respectively. On further assays, the cytotoxic effect of compounds **1**–**5** was determined by MTT assay on acute lymphoblastic leukemia (ALL) and chronic myeloid leukemia (CML) cell lines including their multidrug resistant (MDR) phenotypes. Compound **1** induced a remarkable cytotoxic activity toward ALL cells (IC$_{50}$ = 6.6–9.9 μM) and a lower effect against CML cells (IC$_{50}$ = 27.5–30.0 μM). Flow cytometry was used to analyze cell cycle distribution and cell death by PI-labeled cells and by Annexin V/PI staining, respectively. Upon treatment, **1** induced cell cycle arrest in the G$_2$/M phase accompanied by a strong induction of apoptosis. These results describe for the first time the antibacterial metabolites of *F. oolepis* extract, with **1** being the most effective. This chalcone also emerges as a selective cytotoxic agent against sensitive and resistant leukemic cells, highlighting its potential as a lead compound.

1. Introduction

Since the discovery of chemotherapy, scientists have developed a vast arsenal of bioactive agents enabling the successful treatment of a huge variety of diseases, including bacterial infections and cancer. However, over time, the treatment of these ailments is frequently associated with side effects and the development of resistance, rendering the drugs useless [1, 2]. This has increased the importance of the search for new entities with antibacterial and anticancer properties.

The role of natural products in drug discovery remains critical. Sixty-five percent of the 118 new chemical entities (NCE) approved between 1981 and 2010 for indication as antibacterial drugs and 34% of the 128 approved as anticancer drugs corresponded to natural products and semisynthetic derivatives obtained from these natural precursors [3]. The fact that natural products have 40% more chemical scaffolds than synthetic chemistry means that they have a considerable advantage in continuing to provide new commercial drug leads [4]. The key is to efficiently and effectively access this diversity [4]. Among sources of natural active compounds, plants are a promising starting point [5]. Approximately one-third of the top-selling drugs have been derived from plant metabolites [6] and there are 190 examples of clinical trials involving pure or combined plant compounds for treating different ailments currently reported (https://www.clinicaltrials.gov/, US Institute of Health, query "plant drugs"; only herbal extracts or plant-derived pure compounds administered as therapeutic agents were considered). The plant world is still far from being totally explored, however, particularly the native flora from Argentina [7]. *Flourensia oolepis* S. F. Blake (Asteraceae), commonly known as "chilca," is a woody bush widely distributed in the high areas of the provinces of Córdoba and San Luis, in central Argentina [8]. The antibacterial activity of the ethanol extract obtained from this plant was previously reported by our group [7]. The current study aims to gain insight into the metabolites responsible for this effect.

The cytotoxic activity of the compounds isolated against leukemic cell lines and their multidrug resistant (MDR) counterparts was also investigated, and this was extended to determine the mechanism involved in leukemic cell toxicity.

To our knowledge, this is the first detailed study about the constituents of *F. oolepis* that show these pharmacological properties.

2. Materials and Methods

2.1. Plant Material and Extract Preparation. Aerial parts of the native plant *F. oolepis* S. F. Blake were collected from the hills of Córdoba Province, Argentina, in December 2005. A voucher specimen was deposited in the "Marcelino Sayago" Herbarium of the School of Agricultural Science, Catholic University of Córdoba (UCCOR 23). The authorization for the use of the plant is available from the authors. Crushed air-dried material (200 g) was extracted by 48 h maceration with 700 mL of ethanol, and the yield of the extract, obtained after solvent removal and expressed as percentage weight of air-dried crushed plant material, was 23 g%.

2.2. Chemicals, Equipment, and Reagents. 3-(4,5-dimethylthiazol-2-yl)-2,5-diphenyltetrazolium bromide (MTT) was purchased from Sigma-Aldrich CO (St Louis, MO, USA). Doxorubicin hydrochloride 99.8% (DOX, Synbias Pharma Ltd.) was purchased from Nanox Release Technology (Buenos Aires, Argentina).

Gentamicin sulfate (potency: 550–590 μg/mg) and erythromycin (potency: 863 μg/mg) were provided by Laboratorio Fabra S.A, Buenos Aires, Argentina, and Unifarma, Buenos Aires, Argentina, respectively.

^{1}H- and ^{13}C-NMR and two-dimensional spectra were recorded with a Bruker AVANCE II 400 spectrometer (Bruker Corporation, Ettlingen, Germany) with tetramethylsilane (TMS) as the internal reference. HPLC was performed on a Shimadzu LC-10 AS (Shimadzu Corp., Tokyo, Japan), equipped with a Phenomenex Prodigy 5 μ ODS (4.6 mm i.d. × 250 mm) reversed-phase column. The mobile phase was water/methanol/trifluoroacetic acid 65 : 35 : 1 with detection at 365 nm.

Flow cytometry analysis was performed in a Becton-Dickinson (BD) FACS Canto II flow cytometer (BD Biosciences, USA).

2.3. Bioguided Isolation of the Active Principles from Flourensia oolepis. The antibacterial ethanol extract of *F. oolepis* (12 g) was initially subjected to vacuum liquid chromatography on

silica gel (622 g, 63–200 μm, 11.0 × 24.0 cm; Macherey & Nagel) eluted with a step gradient of hexane/diethyl ether (Et$_2$O)/methanol (MeOH) to yield 26 fractions, which were combined in 6 groups according to their thin layer chromatography (TLC) profile (F1 to F6). Of these, fraction F3 eluted with hexane/Et$_2$O 50 : 50 and F5, eluted with 100% Et$_2$O, demonstrated bactericidal activity at 2 mg/mL and were therefore submitted to additional separation methods for further purification. F3 was processed by radial preparative chromatography using an isocratic mobile phase of hexane/Et$_2$O 70 : 30. The fractions obtained were combined in 5 groups in accordance with the TLC analysis (F$_3$1 to F$_3$5). From fraction F$_3$4, compound **3** was obtained by spontaneous crystallization (97.8% purity, by HPLC). The pure compound, the remaining F$_3$4 containing traces of **3** and another substance, as well as the rest of the fractions, were tested for antibacterial activity. Only **3** and the remaining F$_3$4 exerted bactericidal effects at 2 mg/mL. The latter was further fractionated by preparative TLC (Analtech DE, USA; mobile phase: toluene/ethyl acetate/glacial acetic acid 8 : 2.5 : 0.4) to finally obtain compound **1** (99.9% purity, by HPLC).

Fraction F5 was subjected to column chromatography (130 g, 35–70 μm, 3.0 × 60 cm; Fluka) using 100% Et$_2$O as the mobile phase. The resulting fractions were placed in 14 groups according to TLC monitoring (F$_5$1 to F$_5$14). Of these, F$_5$2 showed bactericidal activity and was further fractionated by column chromatography on silica gel (60 g, 35–70 μm, 3.0 × 60 cm; Fluka) performed with hexane/Et$_2$O/glacial acetic acid 8 : 2 : 0.4. The fractions obtained were combined in 7 groups according to their TLC profile (F$_{5.2}$1–F$_{5.2}$7). Their antibacterial activity was evaluated at 2 mg/mL, and F$_{5.2}$2 and F$_{5.2}$5 were seen to be active. Both groups were separately submitted to solid phase extraction (Sep-Pak plus C18, Waters, Ireland) using water/MEOH/trifluoroacetic acid 65 : 35 : 1 as the mobile phase, to afford compound **2** (99.1% purity, by HPLC) from F$_{5.2}$2 and compounds **4** (96.4% purity, by HPLC) and **5** (97.2% purity, by HPLC) from F$_{5.2}$5.

Compounds **1–5** were identified by ^{1}H NMR and ^{13}C NMR, comparing their spectra (copies of the original spectra are obtainable from the corresponding author) with reference data from literature, as 2$'$,4$'$-dihydroxychalcone C$_{15}$H$_{12}$O$_3$ (**1**; *m/z* 240.2) [9, 10], isoliquiritigenin C$_{15}$H$_{12}$O$_4$ (**2**; *m/z* 256.2) [11], pinocembrin C$_{15}$H$_{12}$O$_4$ (**3**; *m/z* 256.2) [8], 7-hydroxyflavanone C$_{15}$H$_{12}$O$_3$ (**4**; *m/z* 240.2) [12], and 7,4$'$-dihydroxy-3$'$-methoxyflavanone C$_{16}$H$_{14}$O$_5$ (**5**; *m/z* 286.3) [13]. The compounds were quantified by HPLC and their yields in g per 100 g of dried and crushed plant material were 1.24, 0.06, 1.14, 0.3, and 0.06 for **1–5**, respectively.

2.4. Microorganisms and Preparation of Inocula. The antibacterial activity assays were carried out on strains of *Enterococcus faecalis* (Andrews and Horder) Scheifer and Klipper-Balz (ATCC 29212), *Escherichia coli* (Migula) Castellani and Chalmers (ATCC 25922), *Pseudomonas aeruginosa* (Schroeter) Migula (ATCC 27853), and *Staphylococcus aureus* subsp. *aureus* Rosenbach (ATCC 6538) and on a clinical isolate of tetracycline, erythromycin, and polymyxin-resistant *Proteus mirabilis* (Pr2921) [14]. This isolate was identified by conventional biochemical assays and by the commercial system API20E (bioMérieux SA, Mercy L'Etoile, France). Antimicrobial resistances were determined by disk diffusion susceptibility testing (Kirby-Bauer Method) according to CLSI [15]. Bacterial suspensions were prepared on sterile saline from each organism grown overnight. Turbidity was spectrophotometrically adjusted to the McFarland 0.5 standard. Dilutions were carried out with sterile saline to give an adjusted concentration of 1.5×10^7 colony-forming units/mL.

2.5. Antibacterial Activity Test and Determination of MICs and MBCs. MICs were determined by the agar dilution test according to CLSI [15] with some modifications [7]. Briefly, the plate count agar medium (PCA, Oxoid Ltd, UK) was added in duplicate to the suitable amount of fraction or pure compound previously dissolved in ethanol. The final concentration of solvent was 2% (no adverse effects were observed at this concentration). After solidification of the agar in 6-well plates (Greiner Bio-One, Germany), $2 \mu L$ of each bacterial suspension was placed on the agar surface. Three independent experiments were carried out. Plates were incubated in ambient air at $37°C$ for 24 h. For reading, visual observations were carried out. Nitro blue tetrazolium (NBT, Sigma-Aldrich CO, USA) solution in saline phosphate buffer (PBS) was applied on one spot for confirmation. Plates containing only the culture medium, with or without the addition of the dissolution solvent, were used as controls. Positive controls with commercial gentamicin sulfate or erythromycin dissolved in sterile water or ethanol, respectively, were simultaneously carried out. The minimum inhibitory concentration (MIC) was defined as the lowest concentration that completely inhibits growth of the microorganism.

The bactericidal effect was further studied from each concentration of product showing growth inhibition. For this study, 0.5 mm portions of agar, coincident with the place at which inocula had been placed and showing negative growth at 24 hr (without NBT), were cut and transferred to brain-heart infusion broth (BHI, Oxoid Ltd, UK). Tubes were incubated in ambient air at $37°C$ for five days. At the end of this period, the minimum bactericidal concentration (MBC) values, defined as the lowest concentration with absence of turbidity, were recorded.

2.6. Cell Lines and Culture Conditions. CCRF-CEM acute lymphoblastic leukemia (ALL) [16] and K562 chronic myeloid leukemia (CML) [17] cells and their MDR P-glycoprotein overexpressing variants [18, 19], CEM/ADR5000 and Lucena 1, respectively, were a generous gift from Dr. T. Efferth (Institute of Pharmacy and Biochemistry, Johannes Gutenberg University, Mainz, Germany) and Dr. V. Rumjanek (Instituto de Bioquímica Médica Leopoldo de Meis, Universidade Federal do Rio de Janeiro, Rio de Janeiro, Brazil), respectively. The HEK293T non-tumor derived cell line [20] and human isolated mononuclear cells (PBMC) were also tested. Leukemic and PBMC cells were grown in Roswell Park Memorial Institute (RPMI) 1640 medium (Invitrogen Life Technologies, CA, USA) while the HEK293T cell line was grown in Dulbecco's Modified Eagle's medium (DMEM,

Invitrogen Life Technologies, CA, USA), both of these media supplemented with 10% heat-inactivated fetal bovine serum (FBS, PAA Laboratories, Pasching, Austria), 2 mM glutamine (Invitrogen Life Technologies, CA, USA), and penicillin (100 units/mL) streptomycin (100 μg/mL) (Invitrogen Life Technologies, CA, USA). Cells were cultured at $37°C$ in a 5% CO_2 humidified environment.

CEM/ADR5000 cells were exposed once a week to gradually increasing doses of DOX from 1.7 to 8.6 μM. The latter concentration was then used for maintenance of the cells. Lucena 1 were continuously cultured in the presence of 60 nM DOX. Both cell lines were grown in drug-free medium 3-4 days before the experiments. Overexpression of P-glycoprotein (P-gp) in both MDR variants was verified by flow cytometry using FITC-labeled mouse anti-human P-gp (BD Pharmingen, USA). Cells were subcultured twice a week from frozen stocks and used before the 20th passage. All experiments were performed with cells in the logarithmic growth phase with cell viabilities over 90%, determined by trypan blue staining.

2.7. Isolation of Human Mononuclear Cells from Peripheral Blood. Peripheral blood mononuclear cells (PBMC) were collected from fresh heparinized blood and separated by density gradient centrifugation (Ficoll) as described by Rennó et al. [21]. As the current study required samples from healthy human volunteer donors, ethical approval was provided by the Catholic University of Córdoba Research Ethics Board. Written signed consents were obtained from donors.

2.8. Cell Proliferation Assay. To investigate the cytotoxic potential of the isolated compounds, the MTT colorimetric assay was performed [22]. Briefly, 5×10^4 cells suspended in 100 μL of growth medium were seeded in 96-well plates (Greiner Bio-One, Germany) containing 100 μL of medium in the presence of serial twofold dilutions of each tested compound previously dissolved in ethanol (1% v/v, no adverse effects on cell growth were observed at this concentration). The compounds were evaluated at a final maximum concentration of 100 μM. After 72 hours, 20 μL of 5 mg/mL solution of MTT in sterile PBS was added to each well and further incubated for 4 h. Then, the supernatants were removed and replaced with 100 μL DMSO to solubilize the resulting purple formazan crystals produced from metabolically viable cells. Absorbance was measured with an iMark micro-plate reader (Bio-Rad, USA) at 595 nm. Two wells were used for each concentration of the products assayed and three independent experiments were performed. Untreated and ethanol (1%) treated cells were used as controls while DOX (maximum tested concentration 69 μM) was used as reference. The percentage of cytotoxic activity of the assayed compounds was determined by the following formula: cytotoxicity (%) = [1 − (optical density of treated cells − optical density DMSO)/(optical density of ethanol control cells − optical density DMSO)] × 100.

Medium inhibitory concentrations (IC_{50}) represent the concentrations of the tested samples required to inhibit 50% cell proliferation and were calculated from the mean values of data from wells.

To confirm the effect of compound **1** on the proliferation of CCRF-CEM and K562, cell suspensions (5×10^4 cells/well) were treated in culture medium with different concentrations of **1** (final volume of 200 μL) and incubated in triplicate for 24, 48, and 72 h. Two independent experiments were performed. The number of viable cells at the different time points was counted by the trypan blue dye exclusion method using a hemocytometer (Neubaur, USA).

2.9. Cell Cycle Distribution by Flow Cytometry. CCRF-CEM and K562 cells placed in supplemented RPMI 1640 medium in 12-well plates (Greiner Bio-One, Germany) at a density of 5×10^5/mL were treated with **1** at a concentration equivalent to two times its IC$_{50}$ for 72 h. Control cells were devoid of **1** and negative controls contained 1% ethanol. After treatment, cells were harvested and washed twice with ice cold PBS. Then, cells were fixed with 70% cold ethanol and kept at 4°C for 24 h. Before analysis, the cells were washed twice with PBS and stained with a solution containing propidium iodide (PI, 50 μg/mL, Sigma-Aldrich CO, USA) and RNase A (100 μg/mL, Sigma-Aldrich CO, USA) in PBS (pH 7.4) for 30 min in the dark. DNA content was evaluated by flow cytometry. The relative distribution of at least 20,000 cells was analyzed using FlowJo software version 7.6.2 (Tree Star, Inc. OR, USA).

2.10. Assessment of Apoptosis by Annexin V/PI Double Staining Assay. CCRF-CEM and K562 cells (5×10^5 cells/mL) placed in supplemented RPMI 1640 medium in 12-well plates (Greiner Bio-One, Germany) were treated for 72 h with compound **1** at two times its IC$_{50}$ value. After incubation, cells were harvested, washed, and suspended in cold PBS. The proportion of cells undergoing apoptosis was examined by double staining using allophycocyanin (APC) conjugated Annexin-V (BD Pharmingen, USA) and propidium iodide (Sigma-Aldrich CO, USA). Over the following hour, the fluorescence of ten thousand cells, including that of control groups, was assayed and populations were analyzed with FlowJo software version 7.6.2 (Tree Star, Inc., OR, USA). Percentages of Annexin-V positive cells (PI− or PI+) indicate early or late apoptosis, respectively.

2.11. Statistical Analysis. Data were analyzed by one-way analysis of variance (ANOVA) and means were compared using Bonferroni's comparison test, with $p \leq 0.05$ considered as statistically significant. The inhibitory concentration (IC$_{50}$) was calculated by log-Probit analysis responding to at least five concentrations at the 95% confidence level with upper and lower confidence limits.

3. Results and Discussion

In the current study, five compounds $2'$,$4'$-dihydroxychalcone (**1**), isoliquiritigenin (**2**), pinocembrin (**3**), 7-hydroxyflavanone (**4**), and 7,$4'$-dihydroxy-$3'$-methoxyflavanone (**5**) (Figure 1) were obtained by bioguided fractionation from the ethanol extract of the aerial parts of *Flourensia oolepis*. This extract was selected among 51 extracts assayed by our group,

after demonstrating an effective growth inhibition of a panel of pathogenic bacteria [7]. As far as we know, there was no information up to now about the metabolites responsible for the antibacterial activity of this extract. These results support the popular use of *F. oolepis* as an herb used for the treatment of respiratory tract infections such as bronchitis [23].

The presence of compounds **1**, **3**, and **4** in *F. oolepis* has been previously reported [8, 24], but the presence of compounds **2** and **5** is reported here for the first time. It should be noted that while compounds **1–4** have been frequently described in nature, this is not the case for compound **5**. In fact, although there is considerable information available about the presence of its corresponding flavone (geraldone) [25, 26], there is very little describing the presence of **5** in plants and there is a total absence of information concerning species native to Argentina.

As shown in Table 1, compound **1** was the most effective, followed by **3**. Both metabolites showed inhibitory effects against Gram-positive referents, with remarkable MIC values ranging from 15 to 62 μg/mL. In relation to their bactericidal activity, it should be noted that the MBCs of **1** and **3** against *S. aureus* were similar to those obtained with the commercial antibiotics (31, 62, 10, and 60 μg/mL, for **1**, **3**, gentamicin, and erythromycin, resp.).

As previously established in the literature, metabolites with MICs ≤ 100 μg/mL are considered noteworthy [27, 28]. Based on this criterion, compound **1** was clearly active against *E. faecalis, S. aureus,* and *P. mirabilis,* while **3** was effective against both positive strains (Table 1). Since *S. aureus* is associated with respiratory diseases like bronchitis [29], the activity of compounds **1** and **3** against this pathogen supports the popular use of *F. oolepis* for the treatment of these affections [30].

On the other hand, the bacteriostatic activity of **1** against the resistant strain of *P. mirabilis,* which was comparable to or even better than that of the commercial antibiotics used as referents, is highly encouraging. It should be pointed out that *P. mirabilis* is an important pathogen that has acquired resistance to clinically used antibiotics being the second most common cause of urinary tract infections [14].

The antibacterial activity of compounds **1–4** has been previously described [31–34]; however, as far as we know, there are no reports of this inhibitory property for **5**.

Certain structural features can be linked to the major antibacterial efficacy displayed by the chalcone **1**. It has been reported that the carbonyl region is part of the active site of flavonoids [31], with the hydroxylations at positions $2'$ and $4'$ being important structural features for the antibacterial effect of chalcones [31, 35]. Interestingly, the other chalcone isolated, $2'$,$4'$,4-trihydroxychalcone, commonly known as isoliquiritigenin (**2**), showed lower activity than its dihydroxylated counterpart (Table 1), demonstrating that the presence of a hydroxyl group at position 4 reduces effectiveness, a phenomenon that was also described by M. A. Alvarez et al. [35]. In addition, **1** was more active for inhibiting bacterial growth than its respective flavanone **4**.

With respect to flavanones, when comparing the activity of **3** and **4** against the Gram-positive strains, it was observed that the presence of a hydroxyl group at position 5 in

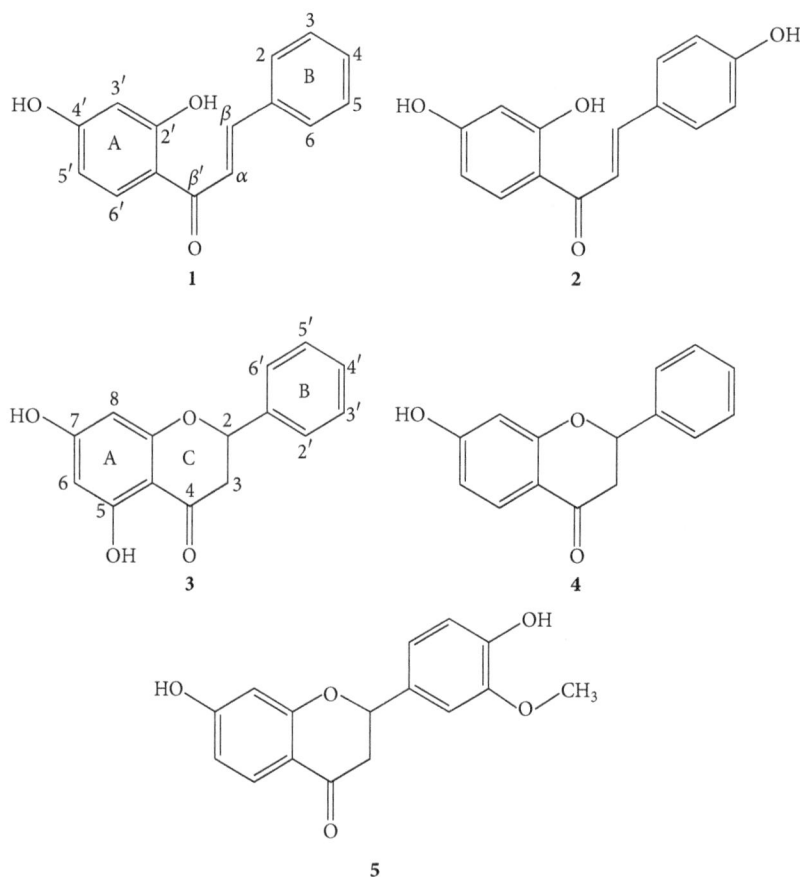

FIGURE 1: Chemical structures of 2′,4′-dihydroxychalcone (**1**), isoliquiritigenin (**2**), pinocembrin (**3**), 7-hydroxyflavanone (**4**), and 7,4′-dihydroxy-3′-methoxyflavanone (**5**).

TABLE 1: Antibacterial activity of compounds **1–5** isolated from *Flourensia oolepis* extract.

Compound	MIC (MBC) (μg/mL)				
	E. coli	*P. aeruginosa*	*P. mirabilis*	*E. faecalis*	*S. aureus*
2′,4′-Dihydroxychalcone (**1**)	250 (500)	250 (>500)	62 (125)	62 (125)	31 (31)
Isoliquiritigenin (**2**)	>500 (>500)	>500 (>500)	>500 (>500)	500 (>500)	250 (500)
Pinocembrin (**3**)	500 (500)	>500 (>500)	>500 (>500)	62 (125)	15 (62)
7-Hydroxyflavanone (**4**)	500 (500)	500 (>500)	>500 (>500)	250 (500)	250 (250)
7,4′-Dihydroxy-3′-methoxyflavanone (**5**)	>500 (>500)	>500 (>500)	>500 (>500)	500 (>500)	250 (>500)
Gentamicin	4 (8)	4 (4)	10 (10)	8 (10)	8 (10)
Erythromycin	125 (>500)	62 (500)	500 (>500)	1 (30)	1 (60)

compound **3** may be responsible for its improved activity, since this substitution pattern constitutes the only structural difference with respect to **4**. This agrees with a study of a number of structurally different flavonoids, which showed that hydroxylation at position 7 of flavanones is important for their antibacterial activity and the presence of an additional hydroxyl group at position 5 enhances the activity [31]. On the other hand, it was also reported that the presence of methoxy groups drastically reduces the antibacterial activity of flavonoids [31, 36]. This may be the reason why compound **5** showed the weakest bacteriostatic activity among the flavanones.

TABLE 2: Anticancer effects of compounds 1–5 isolated from *Flourensia oolepis* extract toward sensitive and resistant leukemic cells.

Compounds	IC$_{50}$ (μM) values and 95% confidence limits (lower, upper)			
	CCRF-CEM	CEM/ADR5000	K562	Lucena 1
2′,4′-Dihydroxychalcone (1)	6.6 (3.3–14.1)	9.9 (5.8–18.3)	27.5 (14.6–52.0)	30.0 (14.6–64.9)
Isoliquiritigenin (2)	58.1 (22.6–148.7)	51.9 (26.9–99.1)	>100	>100
Pinocembrin (3)	58.9 (16.4–210.3)	53.5 (19.5–145.9)	>100	>100
7-Hydroxyflavanone (4)	72.8 (30.0–175.2)	66.2 (27.5–160.7)	>100	>100
7,4′-Dihydroxy-3′-methoxyflavanone (5)	24.8 (10.8–57.3)	30.4 (15.4–60.1)	>100	>100
Doxorubicin	0.133 (0.0–0.3)	>69	4.1 (1.6–11.4)	>69

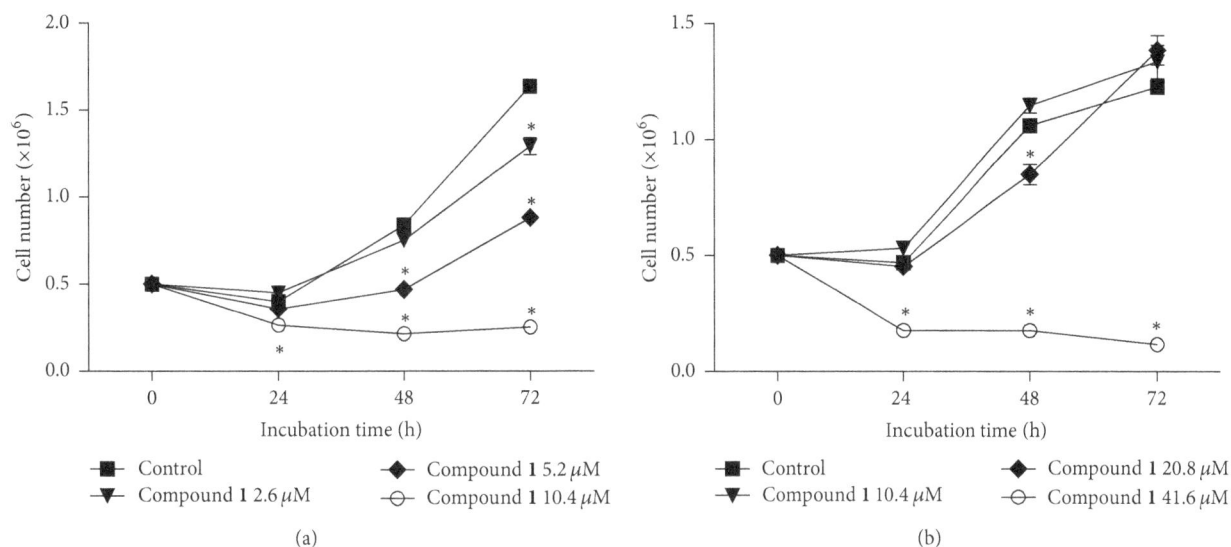

(a)

(b)

FIGURE 2: Time- and dose-dependent effects of compound 1 on CCRF-CEM (a) and K562 (b) cells. Cell viability was quantified by using the trypan blue dye exclusion method. The results are expressed as mean ± SEM. Significant differences were labeled with asterisks ($p < 0.05$) compared to 1% ethanol control group at each time (ANOVA followed by Bonferroni's test).

The anticancer activity of compounds 1–5 against a panel of two leukemia cell lines and their respective drug-resistant phenotypes was further evaluated by conducting MTT cell viability assays. As observed in Table 2, compound 1 showed a strong cytotoxic effect against CCRF-CEM cells and their MDR counterpart CEM/ADR5000, as is evident from the IC$_{50}$ values obtained, which were below 10 μM, the value established by the US National Cancer Institute plant screening program for considering a pure compound as cytotoxic [37]. It is interesting to note that 1 also showed a moderate inhibitory effect against K562 and Lucena 1 (Table 2) with IC$_{50}$ values lower than 30 μM. As observed, a lack of cross-resistance on P-gp-overexpressing cell lines was evidenced by the toxic effect exerted by 1 over these (resistant index (RI) = IC$_{50}$ resistant cells/IC$_{50}$ sensitive cells = 1.5 and 1.1 against CEM/ADR5000 and Lucena 1 cells, resp.), in contrast to that found when cells were exposed to DOX (RI ≥ 518.8 and 16.8 against CEM/ADR5000 and Lucena 1, resp.). These results highlight the potential of 1 as a therapeutic agent for the treatment of resistant phenotypes. Although its toxic effects toward different human and murine tumor cell types, such as MCF-7 (breast) [38], MGC-803 (gastric) [39], 26-L5 (colon), B16-BL6 (melanoma), A549 and LLC (lung), HeLa (cervix), HT-1080 (fibrosarcoma), HL 60 (promyelocytic leukemia),

and PANC-1 (pancreatic) [40–42], have been described, this is the first report about the cytotoxicity of 1 against ALL and CML cells and particularly against their MDR/P-gp sublines as a way to circumvent the reduced response of these resistant phenotypes to chemotherapy.

The toxic effect of 1 was also determined against the noncancerous rapidly dividing cell line HEK293T [43] and against PBMC. From the IC$_{50}$ values obtained, we saw that 1 was highly selective against ALL cells, as evidenced by the selectivity indexes calculated (SI, ratio between IC$_{50}$ value in nontarget cells to the IC$_{50}$ value in tumor cells), with values greater than 6, taking into consideration previous classifications [44, 45]. When the medium growth inhibitory concentration of 1 toward HEK293T (IC$_{50}$ = 67.0 μM) and PBMC (IC$_{50}$ = 82.8 μM) was compared to that of CCRF-CEM (IC$_{50}$ = 6.6 μM), SIs of 10.1 and 12.5 were, respectively, observed, while in the case of CEM/ADR5000 (IC$_{50}$ 9.9 μM), the IC$_{50}$ ratios were 6.8 and 8.4, respectively. On the other hand, compounds with SIs between 3 and 6 were rated as moderately selective [44, 45]. According to the ratios between the IC$_{50}$ obtained for PBMC and those obtained for K562 cells (IC$_{50}$ = 27.5 μM) and for Lucena 1 (IC$_{50}$ = 30.0 μM) cells, compound 1 meets this criterion (SI = 3.0 and 2.8, resp.). It is worth noting that 1 also showed a low toxic effect when

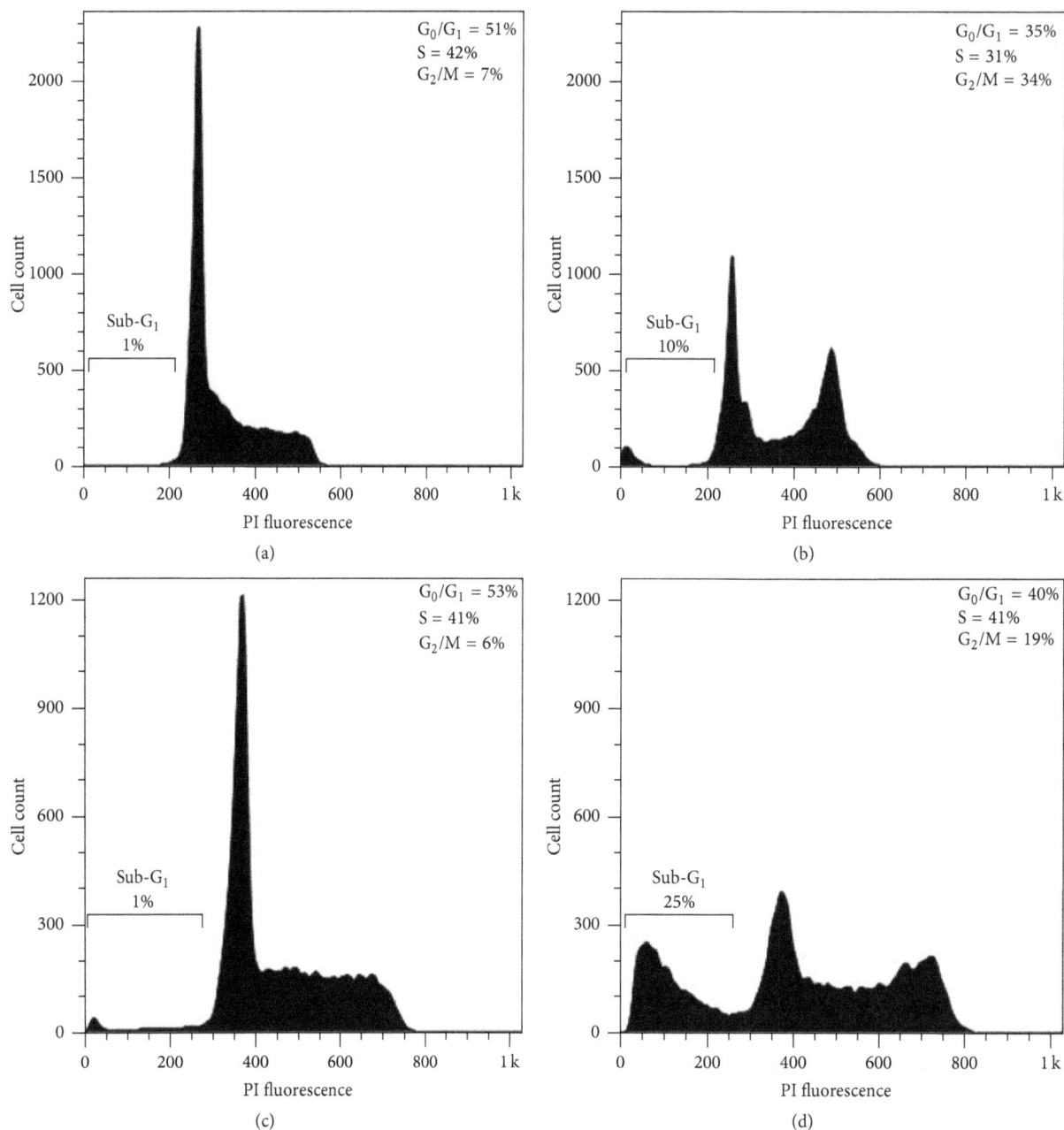

FIGURE 3: CCRF-CEM and K562 cells treated with 1% ethanol (controls (a) and (c), resp.) or with **1** at $2 \times IC_{50}$ ((b) and (d), resp.) for 72 h were stained with PI for cell cycle phase distribution analysis by flow cytometry. The percentages of cells in each phase, including sub-G1 (hypodiploid), are indicated.

assayed against normal hepatocytes (IC_{50} 34 μg/mL, by the trypan blue exclusion method) [46].

The selective activity of **5** is also interesting, showing moderate toxicity against CCRF-CEM and CEM/ADR5000 in contrast to its complete lack of effectiveness (IC_{50} > 100 μM) on the rest of the assayed cells.

Comparing the cytotoxic activity of chalcones **1** and **2**, the presence of an additional hydroxyl group at position 4 of compound **2** would not prove favorable for its toxicity, as reflected by its higher IC_{50} values (51.9–>100 μM) with respect to **1** (6.6–30.0 μM). This is in complete agreement with

Li et al. [40], who tested these compounds against a panel of different tumor cell lines and reported that the toxicity exerted by **1** broadly exceeded that of compound **2**. From our results, we can infer that the presence of 4-OH negatively influences both cytotoxic and antibacterial activity.

The strong cytotoxic activity exhibited by **1** in comparison to the low potency exerted by **4** matches that reported by Pouget et al. [38], who found that **1** was more effective at inhibiting MCF-7 cell proliferation than its corresponding flavanone **4**. The presence of a hydroxyl group at position C-5 made no difference to the activity of compounds **3** and **4**,

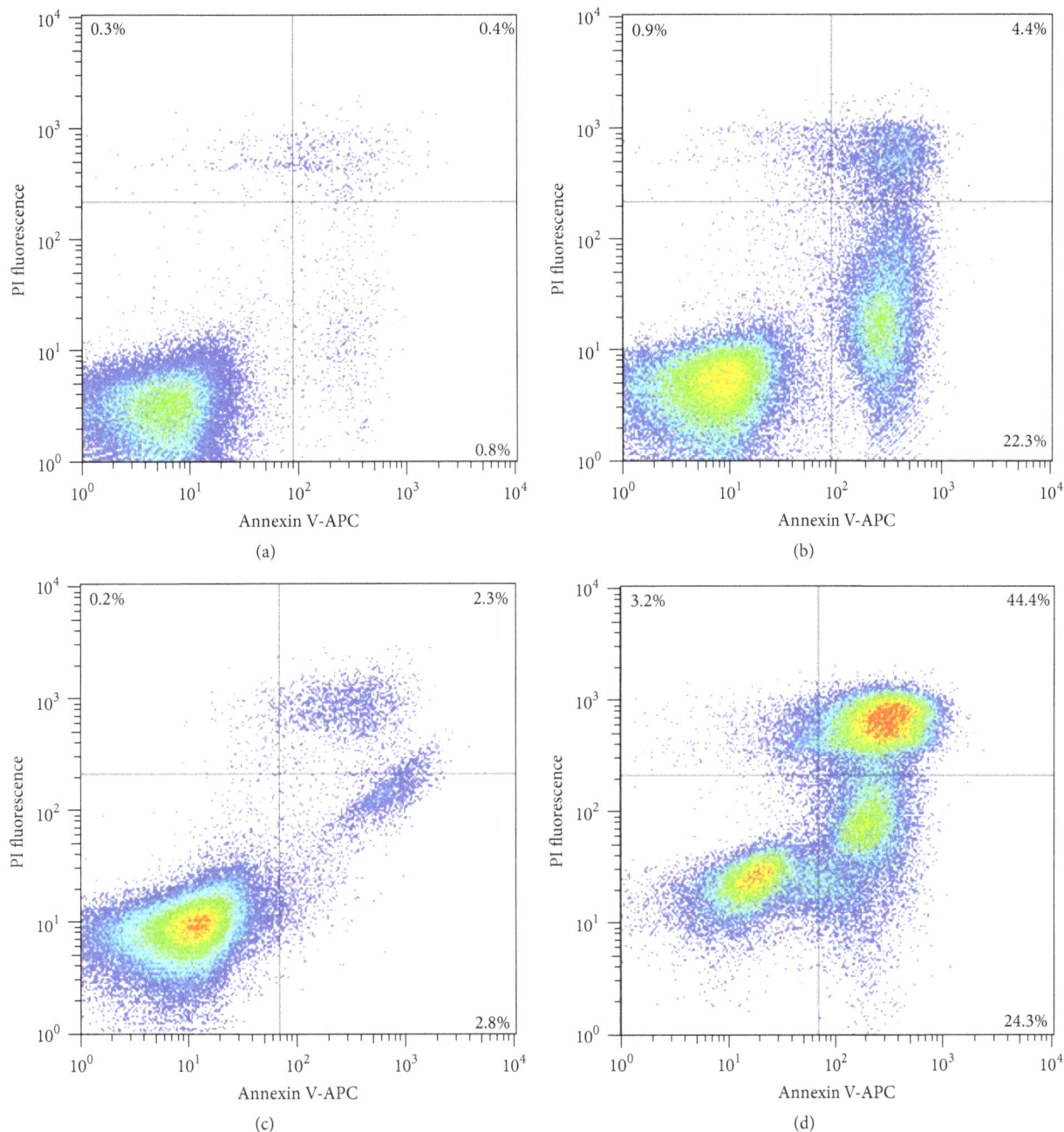

FIGURE 4: Effects of compound 1 on cell death process. CCRF-CEM and K562 cells were incubated for 72 h with 1% ethanol (controls (a) and (c), resp.) or with $2 \times IC_{50}$ of 1 ((b) and (d), resp.). Apoptotic effect of 1 was evaluated by flow cytometry analysis after double staining with Annexin V-APC and PI. Annexin V-APC intensity is represented on the x-axis and PI fluorescence intensity is represented on the y-axis.

in contrast to that observed with respect to the antibacterial effect exerted by these compounds. The substitution pattern of the B-ring in flavanone 5 with respect to 4 increased the compound's toxicity against CCRF-CEM and its MDR counterpart (see Table 2).

When the number of viable cells was determined at different time points by a trypan blue exclusion test, it was observed that 1 exerted a negative effect on normal cell proliferation of both CCRF-CEM (Figure 2(a)) and K562 (Figure 2(b)) cell lines in a time- and dose-dependent manner. As shown

in Figure 2(a), compound 1 at 2.6 μM showed a significant difference ($p < 0.05$) in the number of CCRF-CEM viable cells with respect to the ethanol control at 72 h from the beginning, while this effect was already observed at 48 h when 5.2 μM of 1 was added. When K562 cells were treated with 1 at 20.8 μM for 48 h, a significant decrease ($p < 0.05$) was observed in the number of viable cells compared to the ethanol control and, when the concentration of 1 was increased to 41.6 μM, this difference ($p < 0.05$) was already observed at 24 h (Figure 2(b)).

When exposed to cytotoxic agents, cells may suffer death or a stop in their cell cycle, which in turn can trigger death by apoptosis if cells cannot overcome the damage [47]. Apoptosis is a common mechanism involved in the toxicity of many anticancer drugs, including those from natural origin [48]. Hence, due to the strong compound **1**-induced cytotoxicity and since the mechanism underlying this effect in the leukemic cells, CCRF-CEM, and K562 cells was uncertain, we performed flow cytometric experiments to dissect the possible mode of action beyond the toxic effect of **1**. As depicted in Figure 3(b), analysis of the DNA contents of CCRF-CEM cells indicated that treatment with **1** at $2 \times$ IC_{50} for 72 h produced a cell cycle arrest of 34% of the cells in the G_2/M phase compared to 7% of cells in this phase in the ethanol control (Figure 3(a)). K562 cells also showed an increase in the proportion of cells in the G_2/M phase (19%) (Figure 3(d)) compared to the ethanol control (6%) (Figure 3(c)). Given the key role that the G_2/M checkpoint plays in the maintenance of chromosomal integrity, allowing cells to repair DNA damage before entering mitosis [49], blockage of the cell cycle at this stage by compound **1** emerges as a potential pharmacological strategy for the treatment of leukemia. The arrest observed was also accompanied by an increase in the hypodiploid sub-G1 population from 1% in the ethanol controls (Figures 3(a) and 3(c)) to 10% and 25% for CCRF-CEM and K562 cells, respectively (Figures 3(b) and 3(d)), indicating the presence of cell death.

To further determine the induction of apoptosis, the flipping of phosphatidylserine to the outer membrane as a hallmark of apoptosis was analyzed using Annexin V staining. As shown in Figures 4(b) and 4(d), compound **1** at $2 \times IC_{50}$ induced apoptosis in CCRF-CEM and in K562 at 72 h of treatment, reaching 26.7% and 68.7%, respectively, of early and late apoptotic cells.

In agreement with our results, Lou et al. [50, 51] reported that the exposure of the human gastric cancer cell line MGC-803 to **1** resulted in a dose-dependent G_2/M phase cell cycle arrest, accompanied by apoptosis, but these effects have not been described yet for ALL and CML cells.

4. Conclusions

This work extends the currently available information about the chemical composition and activity of *F. oolepis* and offers a set of bioactive molecules that can be used as a model for the design of improved antibacterial and cytotoxic compounds. The antibacterial activity observed for compound **1**, in addition to its strong and selective cytotoxicity, highlights its potential as a lead compound to fight against pathogenic bacteria and ALL and CML cells, including their MDR phenotypes.

Conflict of Interests

The authors declare that there is no conflict of interests regarding the publication of this paper.

Acknowledgments

This work was supported by the Catholic University of Córdoba, FONCYT (BID 1728 33593, PICTO CRUP 6-31396 and PICT 0141), MINCyT Córdoba (GRF 2008), and CONICET (PIP 11220100100236). The authors thank Joss Heywood for revising the English language. They also thank Dr. V. Rumjanek and Dr. T. Efferth for providing K562 and its derivate Lucena 1 and CCRF-CEM and CEM/ADR5000 cells, respectively.

References

[1] V. Kuete, S. Alibert-Franco, K. O. Eyong et al., "Antibacterial activity of some natural products against bacteria expressing a multidrug-resistant phenotype," *International Journal of Antimicrobial Agents*, vol. 37, no. 2, pp. 156–161, 2011.

[2] L. Hu, Z.-R. Li, J.-N. Li, J. Qu, J.-D. Jiang, and D. W. Boykin, "3-(2′-Bromopropionylamino)-benzamides as novel S-phase arrest agents," *Bioorganic & Medicinal Chemistry Letters*, vol. 17, no. 24, pp. 6847–6852, 2007.

[3] D. J. Newman and G. M. Cragg, "Natural products as sources of new drugs over the 30 years from 1981 to 2010," *Journal of Natural Products*, vol. 75, no. 3, pp. 311–335, 2012.

[4] A. Harvey, "Strategies for discovering drugs from previously unexplored natural products," *Drug Discovery Today*, vol. 5, no. 7, pp. 294–300, 2000.

[5] M. C. Carpinella and M. Rai, *Novel Therapeutic Agents from Plants*, Science Publishers, Enfield, NH, USA, 2009.

[6] X. H. Ma, C. J. Zheng, L. Y. Han et al., "Synergistic therapeutic actions of herbal ingredients and their mechanisms from molecular interaction and network perspectives," *Drug Discovery Today*, vol. 14, no. 11-12, pp. 579–588, 2009.

[7] M. B. Joray, M. R. del Rollán, G. M. Ruiz, S. M. Palacios, and M. C. Carpinella, "Antibacterial activity of extracts from plants of central Argentina—isolation of an active principle from *Achyrocline satureioides*," *Planta Medica*, vol. 77, no. 1, pp. 95–100, 2011.

[8] G. N. D. Napal, M. C. Carpinella, and S. M. Palacios, "Antifeedant activity of ethanolic extract from *Flourensia oolepis* and isolation of pinocembrin as its active principle compound," *Bioresource Technology*, vol. 100, no. 14, pp. 3669–3673, 2009.

[9] A. F. Barrero, M. M. Herrador, P. Arteaga, I. Rodriguez-Garcia, and M. Garcia-Moreno, "Resorcinol derivatives and flavonoids of *Ononis natrix* subspecies ramosissima," *Journal of Natural Products*, vol. 60, no. 2, pp. 65–68, 1997.

[10] E. Wollenweber and D. S. Seigler, "Flavonoids from the exudate of *Acacia neovernicosa*," *Phytochemistry*, vol. 21, no. 5, pp. 1063–1066, 1982.

[11] Z.-P. Zheng, K.-W. Cheng, J. Chao, J. Wu, and M. Wang, "Tyrosinase inhibitors from paper mulberry (*Broussonetia papyrifera*)," *Food Chemistry*, vol. 106, no. 2, pp. 529–535, 2008.

[12] E. Kostrzewa-Susłow and T. Janeczko, "Microbial transformations of 7-hydroxyflavanone," *The Scientific World Journal*, vol. 2012, Article ID 254929, 8 pages, 2012.

[13] C. A. Calanasan and J. K. MacLeod, "A diterpenoid sulphate and flavonoids from *Wedelia asperrima*," *Phytochemistry*, vol. 47, no. 6, pp. 1093–1099, 1998.

[14] M. C. Carpinella, L. De Bellis, M. B. Joray, V. Sosa, P. M. Zunino, and S. M. Palacios, "Inhibition of development, swarming differentiation and virulence factors in *Proteus mirabilis* by an

extract of *Lithrea molleoides* and its active principle (Z,Z)-5-(trideca-4′,7′-dienyl)-resorcinol," *Phytomedicine*, vol. 18, no. 11, pp. 994–997, 2011.

[15] CLSI, *Methods for Dilution Antimicrobial Susceptibility Tests for Bacteria That Grow Aerobically; Approved Standard*, Clinical and Laboratory Standards Institute, Wayne, Pa, USA, 2012.

[16] T. Efferth, M. Davey, A. Olbrich, G. Rücker, E. Gebhart, and R. Davey, "Activity of drugs from traditional chinese medicine toward sensitive and MDR1- or MRP1-overexpressing multidrug-resistant human CCRF-CEM leukemia cells," *Blood Cells, Molecules, and Diseases*, vol. 28, no. 2, pp. 160–168, 2002.

[17] V. M. Rumjanek, R. S. Vidal, and R. C. Maia, "Multidrug resistance in chronic myeloid leukaemia: how much can we learn from MDR-CML cell lines?" *Bioscience Reports*, vol. 33, no. 6, Article ID e00081, 2013.

[18] A. Kimmig, V. Gekeler, M. Neumann et al., "Susceptibility of multidrug-resistant human leukemia cell lines to human interleukin 2-activated killer-cells," *Cancer Research*, vol. 50, no. 21, pp. 6793–6799, 1990.

[19] M. A. M. Moreira, C. Bagni, M. B. de Pinho et al., "Changes in gene expression profile in two multidrug resistant cell lines derived from a same drug sensitive cell line," *Leukemia Research*, vol. 38, no. 8, pp. 983–987, 2014.

[20] L. D. Trucco, V. Andreoli, N. G. Núñez, M. Maccioni, and J. L. Bocco, "Krüppel-like factor 6 interferes with cellular transformation induced by the H-ras oncogene," *The FASEB Journal*, vol. 28, no. 12, pp. 5262–7276, 2014.

[21] M. N. Rennó, G. M. Barbosa, P. Zancan et al., "Crude ethanol extract from babassu (*Orbignya speciosa*): cytotoxicity on tumoral and non-tumoral cell lines," *Anais da Academia Brasileira de Ciencias*, vol. 80, no. 3, pp. 467–476, 2008.

[22] M. B. Joray, M. L. González, S. M. Palacios, and M. C. Carpinella, "Antibacterial activity of the plant-derived compounds 23-methyl-6-O-desmethylauricepyrone and (Z,Z)-5-(trideca-4,7-dienyl)resorcinol and their synergy with antibiotics against methicillin-susceptible and -resistant *Staphylococcus aureus*," *Journal of Agricultural and Food Chemistry*, vol. 59, no. 21, pp. 11534–11542, 2011.

[23] A. Sersic, A. Cocucci, S. Vieiras et al., *Flores del Centro de Argentina. Una Guía Ilustrada Para Conocer 141 Especies Típicas*, Academia Nacional de Ciencias, Córdoba, Argentina, 2006.

[24] E. Guerreiro, J. Kavka, O. S. Giordano, and E. G. Gros, "Sesquiterpenoids and flavonoids from *Flourensia oolepis*," *Phytochemistry*, vol. 18, no. 7, pp. 1235–1237, 1979.

[25] E. Wong and G. Latch, "Effect of fungal diseases on phenolic contents of white clover," *New Zealand Journal of Agricultural Research*, vol. 14, no. 3, pp. 633–638, 1971.

[26] E. Wong and C. M. Francis, "Flavonoids in genotypes of *Trifolium subterraneum*—I. The normal flavonoid pattern of the Geraldton variety," *Phytochemistry*, vol. 7, no. 12, pp. 2123–2129, 1968.

[27] J. L. Ríos and M. C. Recio, "Medicinal plants and antimicrobial activity," *Journal of Ethnopharmacology*, vol. 100, no. 1-2, pp. 80–84, 2005.

[28] T. P. T. Cushnie and A. J. Lamb, "Recent advances in understanding the antibacterial properties of flavonoids," *International Journal of Antimicrobial Agents*, vol. 38, no. 2, pp. 99–107, 2011.

[29] J.-F. T. K. Akoachere, R. N. Ndip, E. B. Chenwi, L. M. Ndip, T. E. Njock, and D. N. Anong, "Antibacterial effect of *Zingiber officinale* and *Garcinia kola* on respiratory tract pathogens," *East African Medical Journal*, vol. 79, no. 11, pp. 588–592, 2002.

[30] A. Sérsic, A. Cocucci, S. Benítez-Vieyra et al., *Flores del Centro de Argentina. Una Guía Ilustrada Para Conocer 141 Especies Típicas*, Academia Nacional de Ciencias, Córdoba, Argentina, 2006.

[31] L. E. Alcaráz, S. E. Blanco, O. N. Puig, F. Tomás, and F. H. Ferretti, "Antibacterial activity of flavonoids against methicillin-resistant *Staphylococcus aureus* strains," *Journal of Theoretical Biology*, vol. 205, no. 2, pp. 231–240, 2000.

[32] I. C. Zampini, M. A. Vattuone, and M. I. Isla, "Antibacterial activity of *Zuccagnia punctata* Cav. ethanolic extracts," *Journal of Ethnopharmacology*, vol. 102, no. 3, pp. 450–456, 2005.

[33] H. Koo, P. L. Rosalen, J. A. Cury, Y. K. Park, and W. H. Bowen, "Effects of compounds found in propolis on *Streptococcus mutans* growth and on glucosyltransferase activity," *Antimicrobial Agents and Chemotherapy*, vol. 46, no. 5, pp. 1302–1309, 2002.

[34] H. P. Ávila, E. D. F. A. Smânia, F. D. Monache, and A. Smânia Jr., "Structure-activity relationship of antibacterial chalcones," *Bioorganic and Medicinal Chemistry*, vol. 16, no. 22, pp. 9790–9794, 2008.

[35] M. A. Alvarez, V. E. P. Zarelli, N. B. Pappano, and N. B. Debattista, "Bacteriostatic action of synthetic polyhydroxylated chalcones against *Escherichia coli*," *Biocell*, vol. 28, no. 1, pp. 31–34, 2004.

[36] T. P. T. Cushnie and A. J. Lamb, "Antimicrobial activity of flavonoids," *International Journal of Antimicrobial Agents*, vol. 26, no. 5, pp. 343–356, 2005.

[37] V. Kuete, P. Y. Ango, S. O. Yeboah et al., "Cytotoxicity of four *Aframomum* species (*A. arundinaceum*, *A. alboviolaceum*, *A. kayserianum* and *A. polyanthum*) towards multi-factorial drug resistant cancer cell lines," *BMC Complementary and Alternative Medicine*, vol. 14, no. 1, article 340, 2014.

[38] C. Pouget, F. Lauthier, A. Simon et al., "Flavonoids: structural requirements for antiproliferative activity on breast cancer cells," *Bioorganic and Medicinal Chemistry Letters*, vol. 11, no. 24, pp. 3095–3097, 2001.

[39] C. Lou, M. Wang, G. Yang et al., "Preliminary studies on anti-tumor activity of 2′,4′-dihydroxychalcone isolated from Herba Oxytropis in human gastric cancer MGC-803 cells," *Toxicology in Vitro*, vol. 23, no. 5, pp. 906–910, 2009.

[40] F. Li, S. Awale, Y. Tezuka, and S. Kadota, "Cytotoxic constituents from Brazilian red propolis and their structure-activity relationship," *Bioorganic and Medicinal Chemistry*, vol. 16, no. 10, pp. 5434–5440, 2008.

[41] S. Awale, T. Miyamoto, T. Z. Linn et al., "Cytotoxic constituents of *Soymida febrifuga* from Myanmar," *Journal of Natural Products*, vol. 72, no. 9, pp. 1631–1636, 2009.

[42] A. S. Sufian, K. Ramasamy, N. Ahmat, Z. A. Zakaria, and M. I. M. Yusof, "Isolation and identification of antibacterial and cytotoxic compounds from the leaves of *Muntingia calabura* L.," *Journal of Ethnopharmacology*, vol. 146, no. 1, pp. 198–204, 2013.

[43] J. McNulty, J. J. Nair, C. Codina et al., "Selective apoptosis-inducing activity of crinum-type Amaryllidaceae alkaloids," *Phytochemistry*, vol. 68, no. 7, pp. 1068–1074, 2007.

[44] C. M. Viau, D. J. Moura, V. A. Facundo, and J. Saffi, "The natural triterpene 3β,6β,16β-trihydroxy-lup-20(29)-ene obtained from the flowers of *Combretum leprosum* induces apoptosis in MCF-7 breast cancer cells," *BMC Complementary and Alternative Medicine*, vol. 14, no. 1, article 280, 2014.

[45] E. M. Acton, V. L. Narayanan, P. A. Risbood, R. H. Shoemaker, D. T. Vistica, and M. R. Boyd, "Anticancer specificity of some

ellipticinium salts against human brain tumors in vitro," *Journal of Medicinal Chemistry*, vol. 37, no. 14, pp. 2185–2189, 1994.

[46] O. Sabzevari, G. Galati, M. Y. Moridani, A. Siraki, and P. J. O'Brien, "Molecular cytotoxic mechanisms of anticancer hydroxychalcones," *Chemico-Biological Interactions*, vol. 148, no. 1-2, pp. 57–67, 2004.

[47] L. G. León, O. J. Donadel, C. E. Tonn, and J. M. Padrón, "Tessaric acid derivatives induce G2/M cell cycle arrest in human solid tumor cell lines," *Bioorganic and Medicinal Chemistry*, vol. 17, no. 17, pp. 6251–6256, 2009.

[48] C. Pieme, S. Kumar, M. Dongmo et al., "Antiproliferative activity and induction of apoptosis by *Annona muricata* (Annonaceae) extract on human cancer cells," *BMC Complementary and Alternative Medicine*, vol. 14, no. 1, article 516, 2014.

[49] J.-G. Lee, J.-H. Kim, J.-H. Ahn, K.-T. Lee, N.-I. Baek, and J.-H. Choi, "Jaceosidin, Isolated from dietary mugwort (*Artemisia princeps*), Induces G2/M cell cycle arrest by inactivating cdc25C-cdc2 via ATM-Chk1/2 activation," *Food and Chemical Toxicology*, vol. 55, pp. 214–221, 2013.

[50] C. Lou, M. Wang, G. Yang et al., "Preliminary studies on anti-tumor activity of 2′,4′-dihydroxychalcone isolated from Herba Oxytropis in human gastric cancer MGC-803 cells," *Toxicology in Vitro*, vol. 23, no. 5, pp. 906–910, 2009.

[51] C. Lou, G. Yang, H. Cai et al., "2′,4′-Dihydroxychalcone-induced apoptosis of human gastric cancer MGC-803 cells via down-regulation of survivin mRNA," *Toxicology in Vitro*, vol. 24, no. 5, pp. 1333–1337, 2010.

21

Identification of a Potential Target of Capsaicin by Computational Target Fishing

Xuan-yi Ye,[1] Qing-zhi Ling,[2] and Shao-jun Chen[2]

[1]*College of Ecology, Lishui University, Lishui, Zhejiang 323000, China*
[2]*Department of Traditional Chinese Medicine, Zhejiang Pharmaceutical College, Ningbo 315100, China*

Correspondence should be addressed to Shao-jun Chen; chenshaojun@hotmail.com

Academic Editor: Ki-Wan Oh

Capsaicin, the component responsible for the pungency of chili peppers, shows beneficial effects in many diseases, although the underlying mechanisms remain unclear. In the present study, the potential targets of capsaicin were predicted using PharmMapper and confirmed via chemical-protein interactome (CPI) and molecular docking. Carbonic anhydrase 2 was identified as the main disease-related target, with the pharmacophore model matching well with the molecular features of capsaicin. The relation was confirmed by CPI and molecular docking and supported by previous research showing that capsaicin is a potent inhibitor of carbonic anhydrase isoenzymes. The present study provides a basis for understanding the mechanisms of action of capsaicin or those of other natural compounds.

1. Introduction

Capsaicin (Figure 1), the component responsible for the pungency of chili peppers, is an alkaloid from the *Capsicum* species, which is used worldwide in foods, spices, and medicines [1–4]. Capsaicin has been used as traditional medicine to treat muscular pain and headaches, to improve circulation, for its gastrointestinal protective effects, and to fight against many types of cancer [4, 5]. It is commonly added to herbal formulations because it acts as a catalyst for other herbs and aids in their absorption [4]. As a result, capsaicin has become an exciting pharmacological agent and its utility in different clinical conditions is being explored [1]. However, the mechanisms underlying the therapeutic effects of capsaicin remain unclear [1].

Target fishing, or target identification, is an important step in modern drug development that explores the mechanism of action of bioactive small molecules by identifying their interacting proteins [6, 7]. In recent years, a large number of computational target fishing methods have been developed [8]. For example, reverse or inverse docking represents a useful tool that involves docking a small-molecule drug/ligand into the potential binding cavities of a set of clinically relevant macromolecular targets [9]. Identification

of the top-ranking targets based on their binding affinity with the drug/ligand may be relevant for drug repositioning and/or rescue [9]. In recent work from our group, computational tools were used to identify targets of Danshensu and Tanshinone IIA [10, 11]. Computational target fishing technologies have increased our ability to efficiently and effectively screen for targets in a high-throughput format, which is expected to have a large impact on drug development [6, 8].

In the present study, potential targets of capsaicin were predicted by reverse docking and confirmed via chemical-protein interactome (CPI) and molecular docking. The present study describes a computational drug repositioning method and explores its potential for elucidating the mechanism of action of natural compounds.

2. Methods

2.1. Targets Predicted by PharmMapper. PharmMapper is a web server for potential drug target identification based on the use of a pharmacophore mapping approach [12]. It automatically finds the best mapping poses of the query molecule against all the pharmacophore models in PharmTargetDB and lists the top N best-fitted hits with appropriate target

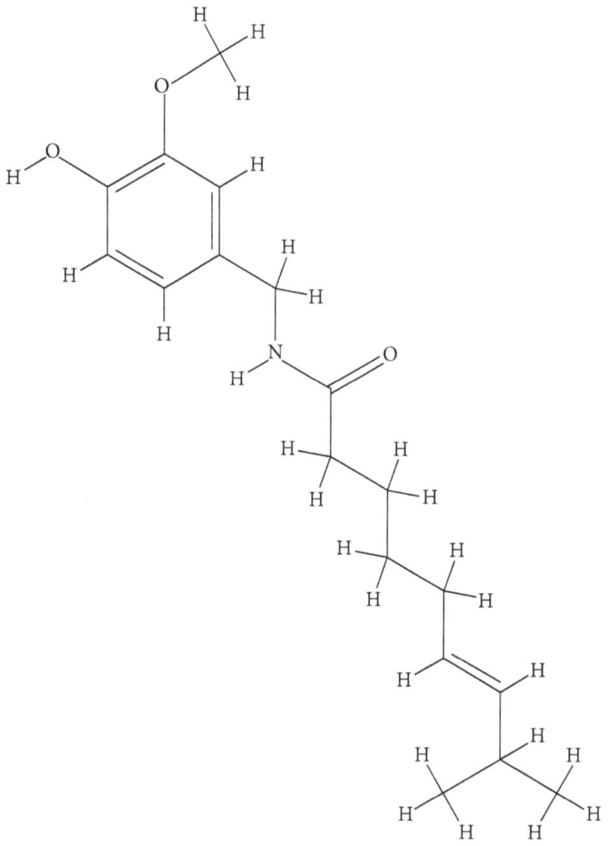

FIGURE 1: The chemical structure of capsaicin (PubChem CID: 1548943).

annotations, as well as the aligned poses of the respective molecules [12].

The molecular file of capsaicin was downloaded from the PubChem database (CID: 1548943) and uploaded to the PharmMapper server. The search started using the maximum generated conformations at 300 by selecting "all targets (7302)" option and default value of 300 for the number of reserved matched targets as described previously [10, 11, 13]. The default settings were used for other parameters.

2.2. Targets Checked by the CPI. The CPI refers to the interaction information of a panel of chemicals across a panel of target proteins in terms of binding strength and binding conformation for each chemical-protein pocket pair [14]. Both DRAR-CPI and DDI-CPI are the servers for computational drug repositioning via the CPI [15, 16].

The molecular file of capsaicin was downloaded and pretreated following the web instructions as described previously [11, 15]. Then, it was submitted to the DRAR-CPI and DDI-CPI servers. Parameters were set to default values.

2.3. Molecular Docking. Molecular docking is a computational procedure that attempts to predict noncovalent binding of macromolecules or a macromolecule (receptor) and a small molecule (ligand) efficiently [17]. Autodock Vina in PyRx 0.8 is a new program for molecular docking and virtual screening that has been widely used [17–19].

The target protein was prepared using the protein preparing tool in TCM Database@Taiwan (http://dock.cmu.edu.tw/ligand.php), which can extract ligands from binding sites, protonate protein structures, and show ligand coordinates and radius information as described previously [10, 11]. Then, the ligand capsaicin was pretreated through OpenBabel in PyRx 0.8. During the docking procedure, the grid box was centered to cover the binding site residues and to allow the ligand to move freely [10, 11]. The box was set to $10 \times 10 \times 10$ nm, and the center coordinates are shown in Table 2. Other parameters were set to default values.

2.4. Visualization. The 3D visualizations of the complex structure were performed using soft PyMol, and the diagrams of chemical-protein interactions were prepared using Ligplot software.

3. Results

3.1. Target Prediction by PharmMapper. Ranking by fit score in descending order and the top ten disease-related targets are shown in Table 1. Carbonic anhydrase 2 (CA2) (PDB ID: 1BNV, 1I9Q, and 1I9O) ranked number one, three, and nine respectively. The pharmacophore model (1BNV) shows three hydrophobic sites, one donor, and three acceptors (Figure 2). Moreover, the pharmacophore model showed that CA2 is well matched with capsaicin (Figure 2). These results indicate that

TABLE 1: Top ten potential disease-related targets of capsaicin predicted by PharmMapper.

Rank	PDB ID	Name	Fit score	Disease
1	1BNV	Carbonic anhydrase 2	4.856	Autosomal recessive osteopetrosis type 3
2	1IZ2	Alpha-1-antitrypsin	4.727	Chronic obstructive pulmonary disease
3	1I9Q	Carbonic anhydrase 2	4.581	Autosomal recessive osteopetrosis type 3
4	5P21	GTPase HRas	4.447	Costello syndrome, cancer
5	1B0F	Leukocyte elastase	4.301	Cyclic hematopoiesis
6	2DUX	Aldose reductase	4.228	Diabetes, galactosemia
7	3BYS	Protooncogene tyrosine-protein kinase LCK	4.225	Leukemias
8	1RLB	Transthyretin	4.028	Amyloidosis
9	1I9O	Carbonic anhydrase 2	4.002	Autosomal recessive osteopetrosis type 3
10	1R1H	Neprilysin	3.982	Acute lymphocytic leukemia

TABLE 2: Results of capsaicin-CA interactome by DRAR-CPI and DDI-CPI.

DRAR-CPI				DDI-CPI		
PDB ID	Name	Docking score	Z'-score	PDB ID	Name	Docking score
1JD0	CA 12	−45.9539	1.48099	3CZV	CA 13	−6.4
				2FOY	CA 1	−6.1
1Z93	CA 3	−41.1238	1.79532	2FOU	CA 2	−5.9
				3FW3	CA 4	−5.7

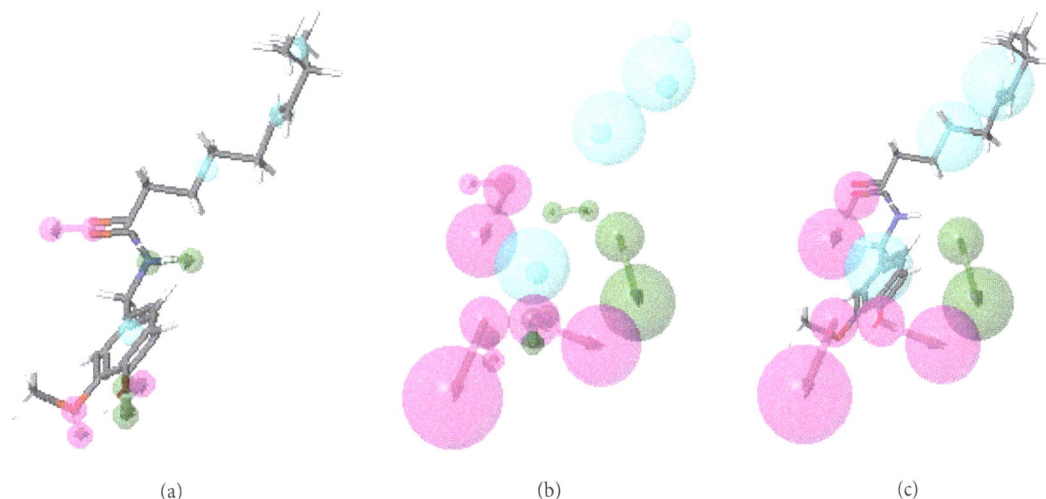

FIGURE 2: Alignment of capsaicin and pharmacophore model of CA2. (a) Capsaicin features. (b) Pharmacophore model of CA2. (c) Molecular and pharmacophore model. Note: pharmacophore features are indicated by color as follows: hydrophobic, cyan; positive, blue; negative, red; donor, green; and acceptor, magenta.

CA2 may be a potential target of capsaicin. Therefore, CA2 was selected for further investigation.

3.2. Targets Verified by Chemical-Protein Interactome.

When a drug is uploaded to the DRAR-CPI server, it is "hybridized" with all targets using the DOCK program [15]. Table 2 shows the results of DRAR-CPI for capsaicin-CA (12 and 3), including the docking score and Z'-score.

When a molecule is submitted to DDI-CPI, the server will dock it across 611 human proteins, generating a CPI profile that can be used as a feature vector of the preconstructed prediction model [16]. As shown in Table 2, four CA isoforms, including CA1, 2, 4, and 13, docked with capsaicin. The docking score of capsaicin-CA2 was −5.9 kcal/mol. Furthermore, the binding pattern of capsaicin-CA2 complex can be visualized in Figure 3.

3.3. Molecular Docking.

Upon docking using Autodock Vina in PyRx 0.8, the lowest binding energy of the capsaicin-CA2 complex was −6.2 kcal/mol (Table 3). As shown in Figure 4, the ligand capsaicin formed four hydrogen bonds with the active site residues (Gln92, Thr199, and Thr200). A number

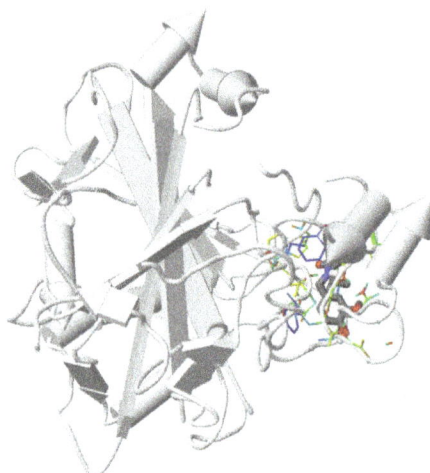

FIGURE 3: Visualization of a capsaicin-CA2 complex captured from the DDI-CPI server. Note: protein chain: rocket; drug: stick; key residues: colorful line.

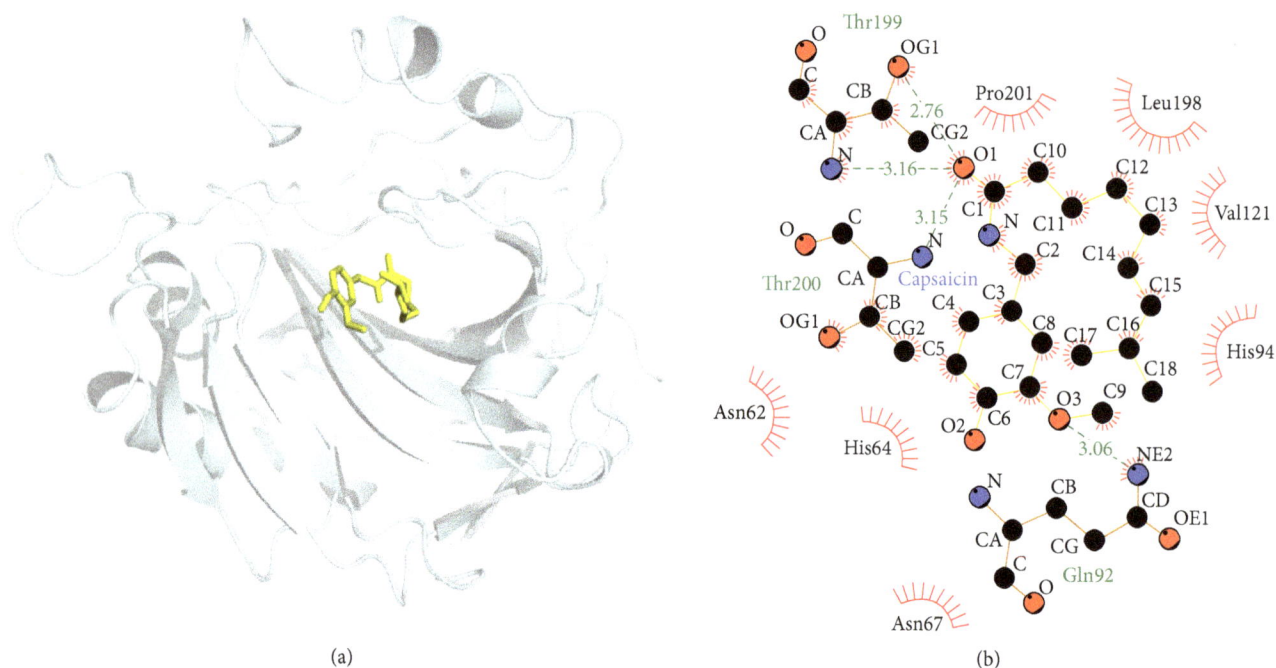

(a)

(b)

FIGURE 4: Molecular interactions between capsaicin and CA2. (a) 3D structure of the CA2 (1BVN)-capsaicin complex by PyMol. Capsaicin: yellow; hydrogen bond: red dash line. (b) 2D interaction scheme by Ligplot. Capsaicin: yellow; C, N, and O atoms are represented in black, blue, and red; hydrophobic contacts are presented in brick red.

TABLE 3: The center coordinates of the binding site and the lowest binding energy by molecular docking.

PDB ID	Name	Center ($x \times y \times z$)	Binding affinity
1BNV	Carbonic anhydrase 2	$-4.03 \times 4.83 \times 14.43$	-6.2 kcal/mol

of hydrophobic interactions are depicted in Figure 4(b). Many residues, including Asn62, His64, Asn67, His94, Val121, Leu198, and Pro201, formed hydrophobic contacts with capsaicin.

4. Discussion

The identification of drug targets in the human genome is important for the development of new pharmaceutical products and the allocation of resources in academic and industrial biomedical research [20]. Various innovative computational tools have been developed to integrate biological data such as regulatory networks, molecular pathways, and cell phenotypes, which facilitates the interpretation and prediction of the biological activities of drugs and their targets [8, 21]. Reverse or inverse docking is a powerful tool for drug repositioning and drug rescue [9]. Recently, PharmMapper, a reverse docking server, was used to identify potential targets of small molecules derived from *Indigofera* species [22] and for the computational prediction of breast cancer targets for 6-methyl-1,3,8-trichlorodibenzofuran [13]. In our previous reports, we used the PharmMapper server to identify potential targets of active compounds from Danshen, a traditional Chinese medicine [10, 11]. We therefore used PharmMapper, a powerful computational tool, to identify CA2 as the main disease-related target of capsaicin in the present study (Table 1). The CA2 pharmacophore confirmed the alignment of molecular features with capsaicin (Figure 2).

The use of CPI together with systems biology-based integrative computational strategies is an essential complement, if not an alternative, to current drug evaluation methods [14]. In a DRAR-CPI job, potential drug targets with Z'-score <-1 are considered as the favorable targets and those with Z'-score >1 are considered as the unfavorable targets [15]. In a DDI-CPI job, the docking scores for each drug in the training set are generated against the 611 library targets [16]. In the present study, Z'-score in DRAR-CPI and docking score in DDI-CPI indicated that CA2 is a target of capsaicin and should be further investigated. These results were consistent with the reverse docking results (Table 1).

Understanding the interactions between proteins and biologically relevant ligands is an important step towards identifying the functions of proteins [23]. The hydrophobic surface of the active site cavity of CA2 contains the residues Ala121 and 135; Val207; Phe91; Leu131, 138, 146, and 109; and Pro201 and 202; and the hydrophilic surface consists of His64, 67, and 200; Asn69; Gln92; Thr199; Tyr7; and Val62 [24]. Thr199 plays a significant role by forming two hydrogen bonds with the carboxyl group of Glu106 and zinc hydroxide [24]. Residues Asn67 and Leu198 protrude towards the Zn^{2+} ion and reduce the volume of the active site cavity considerably [24]. His64, Asn67, and Gln92 residues are involved in histidine recognition [24]. In short, these residues play key roles in ligand-protein interactions. The original ligand sulfonamide forms hydrogen bonds with residues Gln92, His119, Thr199, and Thr200 and forms hydrophobic interactions with Phe131 [25]. Figure 4(b) shows that capsaicin can form hydrogen bonds with Gln92, Thr199, and Thr200 and has hydrophobic interactions with Asn62, His64, Asn67, His94, Val121, Leu198, and Pro201. The structural details indicate that capsaicin may interact with CA2 via these key residues [24]. A previous study reported that capsaicin has K_i of 696.15 μM against hCA I and of 208.37 μM against hCA II, showing unique inhibition profiles against both CA isoforms I and II and suggesting that capsaicin is a selective inhibitor of both cytosolic CA isoenzymes [26].

CAs, a group of ubiquitously expressed metalloenzymes, are involved in numerous physiological and pathological processes, including gluconeogenesis, lipogenesis, ureagenesis, tumorigenicity, and the growth and virulence of various pathogens [27]. In addition to the established role of CA inhibitors (CAIs) as diuretics and antiglaucoma drugs, the potential of CAIs as novel antiobesity, anticancer, anti-infective, and anti-Alzheimer's drugs was recently shown [27]. Taken together with previous results, our findings suggest that capsaicin may play a role in these diseases through its effect on CA2.

In the present study, potential targets of capsaicin were identified using PharmMapper and confirmed via CPI and Autodock Vina. Our results identified CA2 as a potential target of capsaicin, although further studies are necessary to determine their precise interaction. The present study demonstrated that computational drug repositioning is a useful strategy to screen for targets of capsaicin or other natural compounds and suggested a mechanism of action of capsaicin.

Conflict of Interests

The authors declare that there is no conflict of interests regarding the publication of this paper.

Acknowledgments

This work was supported by Zhejiang Provincial Natural Science Foundation of China (LY15H280009), Ningbo Municipal Natural Science Foundation (2015A610280), and the Administration of Traditional Chinese Medicine of Zhejiang Province (2014ZB110).

References

[1] S. K. Sharma, A. S. Vij, and M. Sharma, "Mechanisms and clinical uses of capsaicin," *European Journal of Pharmacology*, vol. 720, no. 1–3, pp. 55–62, 2013.

[2] M. De Lourdes Reyes-Escogido, E. G. Gonzalez-Mondragon, and E. Vazquez-Tzompantzi, "Chemical and pharmacological aspects of capsaicin," *Molecules*, vol. 16, no. 2, pp. 1253–1270, 2011.

[3] J. Szolcsányi, "Forty years in capsaicin research for sensory pharmacology and physiology," *Neuropeptides*, vol. 38, no. 6, pp. 377–384, 2004.

[4] X.-F. Huang, J.-Y. Xue, A.-Q. Jiang, and H.-L. Zhu, "Capsaicin and its analogues: structure-activity relationship study," *Current Medicinal Chemistry*, vol. 20, no. 21, pp. 2661–2672, 2013.

[5] I. Díaz-Laviada and N. Rodríguez-Henche, "The potential antitumor effects of capsaicin," *Progress in Drug Research*, vol. 68, pp. 181–208, 2014.

[6] L. Wang and X.-Q. Xie, "Computational target fishing: what should chemogenomics researchers expect for the future of in silico drug design and discovery?" *Future Medicinal Chemistry*, vol. 6, no. 3, pp. 247–249, 2014.

[7] B. Lomenick, R. W. Olsen, and J. Huang, "Identification of direct protein targets of small molecules," *ACS Chemical Biology*, vol. 6, no. 1, pp. 34–46, 2011.

[8] A. Cereto-Massagué, M. J. Ojeda, C. Valls, M. Mulero, G. Pujadas, and S. Garcia-Vallve, "Tools for in silico target fishing," *Methods*, vol. 71, pp. 98–103, 2015.

[9] P. S. Kharkar, S. Warrier, and R. S. Gaud, "Reverse docking: a powerful tool for drug repositioning and drug rescue," *Future Medicinal Chemistry*, vol. 6, no. 3, pp. 333–342, 2014.

[10] S.-J. Chen and J.-L. Ren, "Identification of a potential anticancer target of Danshensu by inverse docking," *Asian Pacific Journal of Cancer Prevention*, vol. 15, no. 1, pp. 111–116, 2014.

[11] S.-J. Chen, "A potential target of Tanshinone IIA for acute promyelocytic leukemia revealed by inverse docking and drug repurposing," *Asian Pacific Journal of Cancer Prevention*, vol. 15, no. 10, pp. 4301–4305, 2014.

[12] X. Liu, S. Ouyang, B. Yu et al., "PharmMapper server: a web server for potential drug target identification using pharmacophore mapping approach," *Nucleic Acids Research*, vol. 38, no. 2, pp. W609–W614, 2010.

[13] K. N. Chitrala and S. Yeguvapalli, "Computational prediction and analysis of breast cancer targets for 6-methyl-1, 3, 8-trichlorodibenzofuran," *PLoS ONE*, vol. 9, no. 11, Article ID e109185, 2014.

[14] L. Yang, K. J. Wang, L. S. Wang et al., "Chemical-protein interactome and its application in off-target identification," *Interdisciplinary Sciences: Computational Life Sciences*, vol. 3, no. 1, pp. 22–30, 2011.

[15] H. Luo, J. Chen, L. Shi et al., "DRAR-CPI: a server for identifying drug repositioning potential and adverse drug reactions via the chemical-protein interactome," *Nucleic Acids Research*, vol. 39, supplement 2, pp. W492–W498, 2011.

[16] H. Luo, P. Zhang, H. Huang et al., "DDI-CPI, a server that predicts drug-drug interactions through implementing the chemical-protein interactome," *Nucleic Acids Research*, vol. 42, no. 1, pp. W46–W52, 2014.

[17] O. Trott and A. J. Olson, "AutoDock Vina: improving the speed and accuracy of docking with a new scoring function, efficient optimization, and multithreading," *Journal of Computational Chemistry*, vol. 31, no. 2, pp. 455–461, 2010.

[18] A. Sridhar, S. Saremy, and B. Bhattacharjee, "Elucidation of molecular targets of bioactive principles of black cumin relevant to its anti-tumour functionality—an Insilico target fishing approach," *Bioinformation*, vol. 10, no. 11, pp. 684–688, 2014.

[19] S. Kumar, L. Jena, K. Mohod, S. Daf, and A. K. Varma, "Virtual screening for potential inhibitors of high-risk human papillomavirus 16 E6 protein," *Interdisciplinary Sciences: Computational Life Sciences*, vol. 7, no. 2, pp. 136–142, 2015.

[20] M. Rask-Andersen, M. S. Almén, and H. B. Schiöth, "Trends in the exploitation of novel drug targets," *Nature Reviews Drug Discovery*, vol. 10, no. 8, pp. 579–590, 2011.

[21] J. N. Y. Chan, C. Nislow, and A. Emili, "Recent advances and method development for drug target identification," *Trends in Pharmacological Sciences*, vol. 31, no. 2, pp. 82–88, 2010.

[22] S. K. Paramashivam, K. Elayaperumal, B. B. Natarajan, M. Ramamoorthy, S. Balasubramanian, and K. Dhiraviam, "In silico pharmacokinetic and molecular docking studies of small molecules derived from *Indigofera aspalathoides* Vahl targeting receptor tyrosine kinases," *Bioinformation*, vol. 11, no. 2, pp. 73–84, 2015.

[23] J. Yang, A. Roy, and Y. Zhang, "BioLiP: a semi-manually curated database for biologically relevant ligand-protein interactions," *Nucleic Acids Research*, vol. 41, no. 1, pp. D1096–D1103, 2013.

[24] M. Imtaiyaz Hassan, B. Shajee, A. Waheed, F. Ahmad, and W. S. Sly, "Structure, function and applications of carbonic anhydrase isozymes," *Bioorganic and Medicinal Chemistry*, vol. 21, no. 6, pp. 1570–1582, 2013.

[25] P. A. Boriack-Sjodin, S. Zeitlin, H.-H. Chen et al., "Structural analysis of inhibitor binding to human carbonic anhydrase II," *Protein Science*, vol. 7, no. 12, pp. 2483–2489, 1998.

[26] B. Arabaci, I. Gulcin, and S. Alwasel, "Capsaicin: a potent inhibitor of carbonic anhydrase isoenzymes," *Molecules*, vol. 19, no. 7, pp. 10103–10114, 2014.

[27] C. T. Supuran, "Carbonic anhydrases: novel therapeutic applications for inhibitors and activators," *Nature Reviews Drug Discovery*, vol. 7, no. 2, pp. 168–181, 2008.

22

Tiao He Yi Wei Granule, a Traditional Chinese Medicine, against Ethanol-Induced Gastric Ulcer in Mice

Jinfu Yao

Changchun University of Chinese Medicine, Changchun 130117, China

Correspondence should be addressed to Jinfu Yao; yaojinfuch@126.com

Academic Editor: Yoshiji Ohta

Tiao He Yi Wei granule (DHYW), a traditional Chinese medicine, has been used for the treatment of gastric ulcer in clinical setting. The purpose of the present study was to investigate the possible effect of DHYW and explore the underlying mechanism against ethanol-induced gastric ulcer in mice. The model of ethanol-induced gastric ulcer in mice was induced by ethanol (0.2 mL/kg). Administration of DHYW at the doses of 250, 500 mg/kg body weight prior to the ethanol ingestion could effectively protect the stomach from ulceration. The gastric lesions were significantly ameliorated in the DHYW group compared with that in the model group. Treatment with DHYW markedly decreased the levels of interleukin-6 (IL-6), IL-1β, and tumor necrosis factor-α (TNF-α). In addition, DHYW treatment elevated myeloperoxidase (MPO) level in stomach, increased superoxide dismutase (SOD) activity, and decreased malonaldehyde (MDA) content in serum and stomach compared with those in the model group. DHYW significantly inhibited NF-κB pathway expressions in the gastric mucosa ulcer group. Taken together, DHYW exerted a gastroprotective effect against gastric ulceration and the underlying mechanism might be associated with NF-κB pathway.

1. Introduction

Peptic ulcer is one of the most pervasive gastrointestinal diseases which affect 4-5% people in the society [1]. The gastric ulcer is characterized by the reduction in blood flow, induction of oxidative stress, infiltration of neutrophils, and secretion of proinflammatory cytokines [2, 3]. A variety of factors such as *Helicobacter pylori* infection, alcohol consumption, smoking, excessive use of nonsteroidal anti-inflammatory drugs (NSAIDs), and psychological and physiological stress contribute to gastric ulcer [4]. Alcohol consumption increased the risk for major upper gastrointestinal bleeding [5]. As alcohol is one of the major abused agents, thus the alcohol-induced peptic ulcer is the common disorder of the gastrointestinal tract [6].

The nuclear factor kappa B (NF-κB) signaling pathway is one of the most widely recognized intracellular signaling pathways in inflammatory responses [7]. Expressed in almost all cells, NF-κB is involved in the mediation of various genes governing immune response and acute phase inflammatory reaction [8]. Various proinflammatory stimulus can lead to the activation of NF-κB via the phosphorylation of inhibitors of κB (IκBs) by the IκB kinase (IKK) complex [9]. Then the free NF-κB translocates into the nucleus and ultimately leads to the transcriptional activation of several proinflammatory mediators including TNF-α, IL-1β, and IL-6 [10].

Traditional Chinese medicine has been used for several centuries around the world and was considered as a main source of medicine [11, 12]. Tiao He Yi Wei granule (DHYW), a traditional Chinese medicine, contains eleven herbs, which are as follows: *Citrus medica* L., the fruit of *Polygonum orientale* L., the fruit of *Raphanus sativus* L., *Fructus Amomi*, inner membrane of chicken gizzard, *Rhizoma Smilacis Glabrae*, *Atractylodes macrocephala*, *Lindera aggregata* (Sims) Kosterm, *Bletilla striata* (Thunb.) Reichb. f., *Citrus aurantium* L., and *Glycyrrhiza uralensis*. DHYW has been used for the treatment of gastric ulcer in clinical setting. However, few reports focused on the ethanol-induced gastric ulcer and the effects of DHYW. The aim of the study was to investigate the antigastric ulcer effects of DHYW on ethanol-induced mice and explore its possible mechanisms.

2. Materials and Methods

2.1. Reagents. *Citrus medica* L., the fruit of *Polygonum orientale* L., the fruit of *Raphanus sativus* L., *Fructus Amomi*, inner membrane of chicken gizzard, *Rhizoma Smilacis Glabrae*, *Atractylodes macrocephala*, *Lindera aggregata (Sims) Kosterm*, *Bletilla striata* (Thunb.) *Reichb. f.*, *Citrus aurantium* L., and *Glycyrrhiza uralensis* were purchased from Jilin Drug Store (Changchun, China). As the positive control, omeprazole (OME) was supplied by Shanghai Xinyi Jiahua Pharmaceutical Company Limited (Shaanxi, China). All biochemical indicator kits were provided by the Institute of Jiancheng Bioengineering (Nanjing, China). The enzyme-linked immunosorbent assay (ELISA) kits for determination of IL-6, IL-1β, and TNF-α were produced by BioLegend (San Diego, CA, USA). All antibodies were supplied by Cell Signaling Technology.

2.2. Animals. A total of 50 female specific pathogen-free female BALB/c mice, aged 6–8 weeks, were obtained from the Center of Experimental Animals of Changchun University of Chinese Medicine (Changchun, China). Mice were kept in an animal facility under standard laboratory conditions for 1 week prior to the experiments and provided with water and standard chow *ad libitum*. All experimental procedures were performed in accordance with the NIH Guidelines for the Care and Use of Laboratory Animals and the National Animal Welfare Law of China.

2.3. HPLC Analysis of DHYW. An agilent 1100 liquid chromatography system (Agilent, Santa Clara, California, USA), equipped with a quaternary solvent delivery system, an autosampler and DAD detector, was used. A Zorbax Extend-C18 (250 mm × 4.6 mm, 5 μm) column connected with a Zorbax Extend guard column (20 mm × 4.6 mm, 5 μm) was used. The column temperature was set at 25°C. The mobile phase consisted of (A) acetonitrile and (B) 0.1% formic acid-water (V/V) using a linear gradient elution of 5%–55% A at 0–5 min, 55%–80% A at 6–10 min, 80%–95% A at 11–15 min, and 95%–5% A at 16–17 min. The flow rate was 1.0 mL·min^{-1} and 10 μL of samples was injected. Ultraviolet detection was performed on a UV-2450 spectrometer (Shimadzu, Kyoto, Japan). The chromatograms were monitored at 280 nm and the absorption spectra of compounds were recorded from 200 to 400 nm.

2.4. Induction of Gastric Ulcer and Treatment. Five groups of mice were assigned: groups 1 and 2 were orally given PBS (vehicle). Group 3 was administered omeprazole (OME) 20 mg/kg; Group 4 and 5 were given DHYW (250 mg/kg and 500 mg/kg, resp.). After an additional hour, the mice in groups 2–5 intragastrically received ethanol (0.2 mL/kg) while group 1 received PBS at the same volume. Mice were sacrificed after 4 h. The serum and stomach tissues were harvested for the further studies.

2.5. Determinations of MPO in Stomach Tissue and SOD and MDA in Serum and Stomach. At the end of the experiment, the blood was centrifuged at 3000 rpm for 8 min and then the serum samples were stored at −80°C for pending tests.

Stomach tissues were homogenized with cold normal saline and centrifuged at 12,000 rpm for 10 min at 4°C; the supernatant of the homogenate was collected and stored at −80°C. The protein content of stomach sample was determined using a BCA protein assay kit. The levels of SOD and MDA in serum and stomach as well as MPO activity in stomach tissue were determined using test kits purchased from Nanjing Jiancheng Bioengineering Institute (China, Nanjing) according to the manufacturer's protocols.

2.6. Determinations of the Levels of IL-1β, IL-6, and TNF-α in Serum. IL-1β, IL-6, and TNF-α levels in serum were determined with ELISA kits purchased from BioLegend (San Diego, CA, USA). All procedures were carried out according to the manual. Then the absorbance of each well was read at 450 nm by a microplate spectrophotometer.

2.7. Histological Analysis. Stomach sample removed from each mouse was fixed in 10% buffered formalin for more than 48 h. After dehydrating in graded alcohol and embedding in paraffin wax, the sections were cut to a thickness of 4 μm. Then the samples were stained with hematoxylin and eosin (H&E) for histological evaluation. The pathological changes in the gastric tissues were observed under a light microscope.

2.8. Western Blot of NF-κB Pathway. The stomach tissues were homogenized, washed with PBS, and lysed in a RIPA buffer (Beyotime, Nanjing, China). After the determination of the protein concentration using an enhanced BCA kit (Beyotime, China), the samples were loaded to 10% SDS-PAGE gels and then electrotransferred to a polyvinylidene difluoride membrane (Millipore, MA, USA). The blots were incubated with the appropriate concentrations of specific antibodies at 4°C overnight. After washing, the blots were incubated with horseradish peroxidase-conjugated second antibodies. The membrane was stripped and reblotted to verify the equal loading of protein in each lane. Quantification of protein expression was normalized to GAPDH or Histone H3 using a densitometer (Imaging System).

2.9. Statistical Analysis. All values were expressed as the means ± SDs and analyzed with one-way analysis of variance (ANOVA) with Tukey's multiple comparison test. $P < 0.05$ was considered significant and $P < 0.01$ was considered to be statistically very significant.

3. Results

3.1. HPLC Analysis of DHYW. As shown in Figure 1, two compounds which have gastroprotective action were determinate: one is hesperidin; another is glycyrrhizic acid, and the contents are 0.43 mg/g and 0.69 mg/g, respectively.

3.2. Effect of DHYW on Gastric Lesions. Acute gastric lesions were induced by intragastric administration of ethanol. As revealed in Figure 2, the ethanol-stimulated mice presented extensive elongated thick, dark red and black bands of hemorrhagic lesions on the glandular part of the stomach compared with that of control animals. By contrast, treatment with

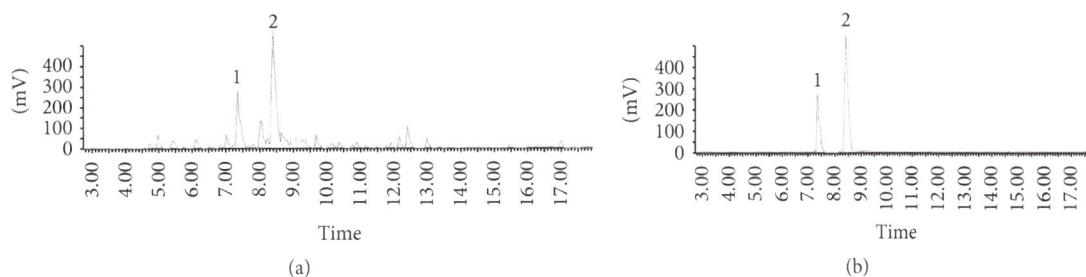

FIGURE 1: HPLC analysis of DHYW. (a) Sample of DHYW. (b) Sample of hesperidin and glycyrrhizic acid. 1: hesperidin, 2: glycyrrhizic acid.

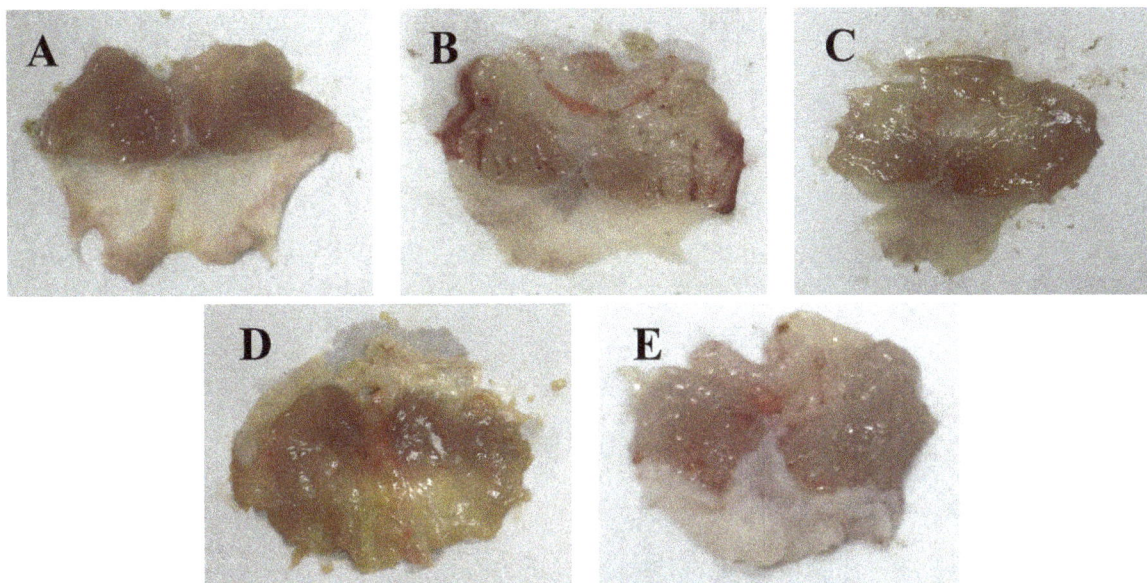

FIGURE 2: Macroscopic evaluation of the effect of DHYW on ethanol-induced gastric ulcer. Mice were intragastrically administered with DHYW (250 mg/kg, 500 mg/kg) or OME (20 mg/kg). 1 h later, the mice were intragastrically given ethanol (0.2 mL/kg) and were sacrificed at 4 h after ethanol challenge. These are representative photos from (A) control group, (B) ethanol group, (C) ethanol + OME (20 mg/kg) group, (D) ethanol + DHYW (250 mg/kg) group, and (E) ethanol + DHYW (500 mg/kg) group.

DHYW (250 and 500 mg/kg) or OME effectively attenuated the severe gastric mucosal damage caused by ethanol.

3.3. Effect of DHYW on SOD and MDA Levels in the Ethanol-Treated Mice. To evaluate the effect of DHYW on lipid peroxidation in gastric ulcer, the levels of SOD and MDA were measured using commercial kits. As revealed in Figure 3, ethanol stimulation significantly declined the SOD activity in serum and stomach tissues, while DHYW (250 and 500 mg/kg) treatment effectively restored the level of SOD. In addition, exposure to ethanol displayed strikingly high MDA contents in both serum and stomach tissue, whereas the oral administration with DHYW (250 and 500 mg/kg) significantly ameliorated these situations. The experimental data clearly demonstrated that DHYW was capable of mediating the oxidative stress in ethanol-stimulated gastric ulcer.

3.4. Effects of DHYW on Inflammatory Cytokines. Next, we detected the levels of TNF-α, IL-6, and IL-1β in serum by ELISA kits to confirm the anti-inflammatory properties. As expected, inflammatory cytokines were remarkably increased in serum of the ethanol-induced mice compared with those in control mice. However, treatment with DHYW (500 mg/kg) and OME (20 mg/kg) significantly reduced the levels of the TNF-α, IL-6, and IL-1β, which were slightly more potent than those in DHYW (250 mg/kg) group. The results displayed that DHYW inhibited the generations of inflammatory cytokines in gastric ulcer animals (Figure 4).

3.5. Histological Evaluations. The histopathology of stomach tissues also confirmed the protective effect of DHYW. As illustrated in Figure 5, animals with ethanol-induced ulcer showed more extensive damage to the gastric mucosa, edema, and leucocyte infiltration compared with those of control mice. On the contrary, treatments with DHYW (250 and 500 mg/kg) and OME proved comparatively better protection of the gastric mucosa as evidenced by less submucosal edema, reduction in ulcer area, and suppression of leucocyte infiltration. The analytical data displayed that DHYW obviously attenuated the histopathology situation in ethanol-induced gastric ulcer.

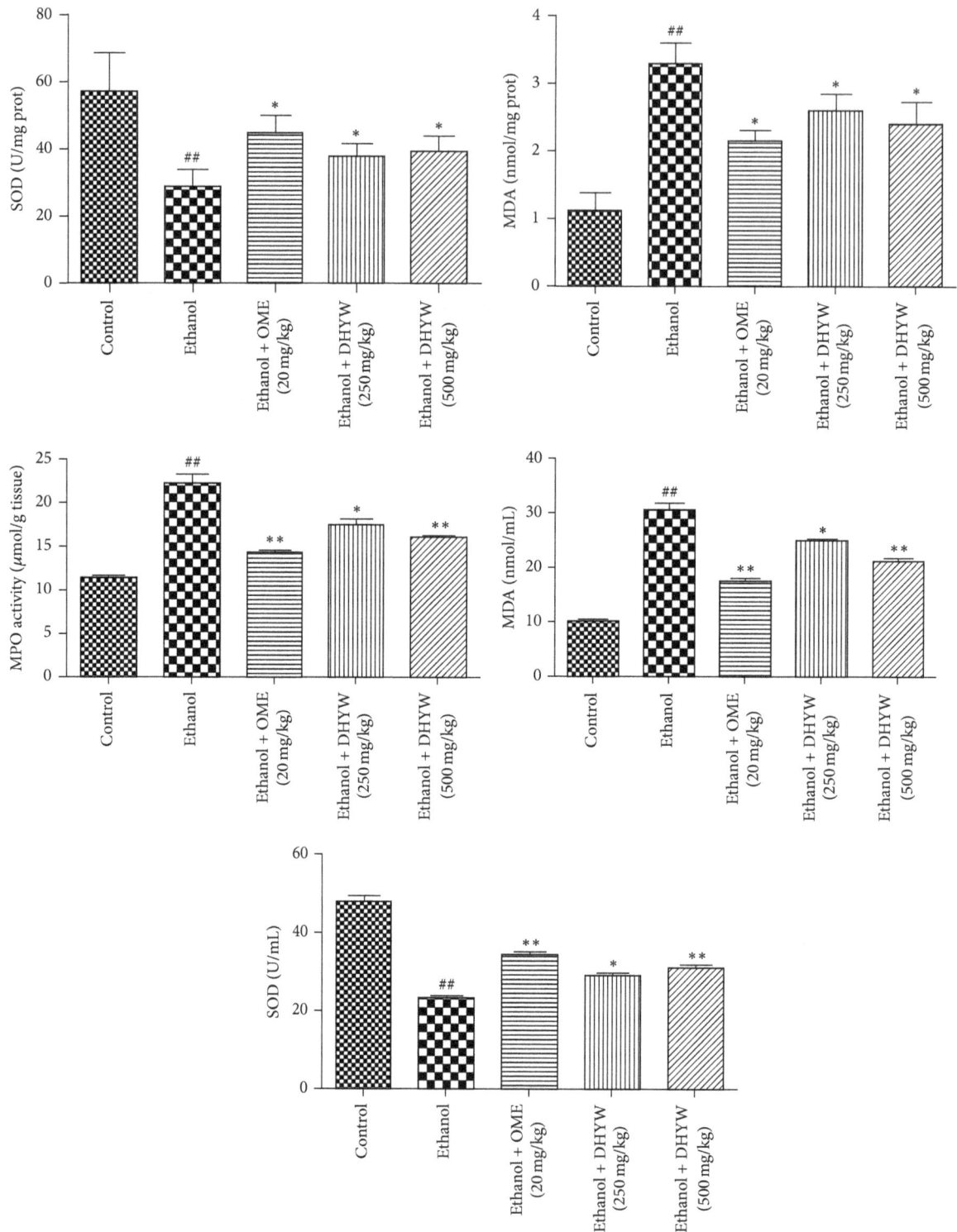

FIGURE 3: Effects of EVD on SOD and MDA levels in the serum and MPO activity in stomach tissue of the ethanol-treated mice. Mice were intragastrically administered with DHYW (250 mg/kg, 500 mg/kg) or OME (20 mg/kg). 1 h later, the mice were intragastrically given ethanol (0.2 mL/kg) and were sacrificed at 4 h after ethanol challenge. Values are expressed as means ± SEM. Compared with control: $^{#}P < 0.05$, $^{##}P < 0.01$; compared with model: $^{*}P < 0.05$, $^{**}P < 0.01$.

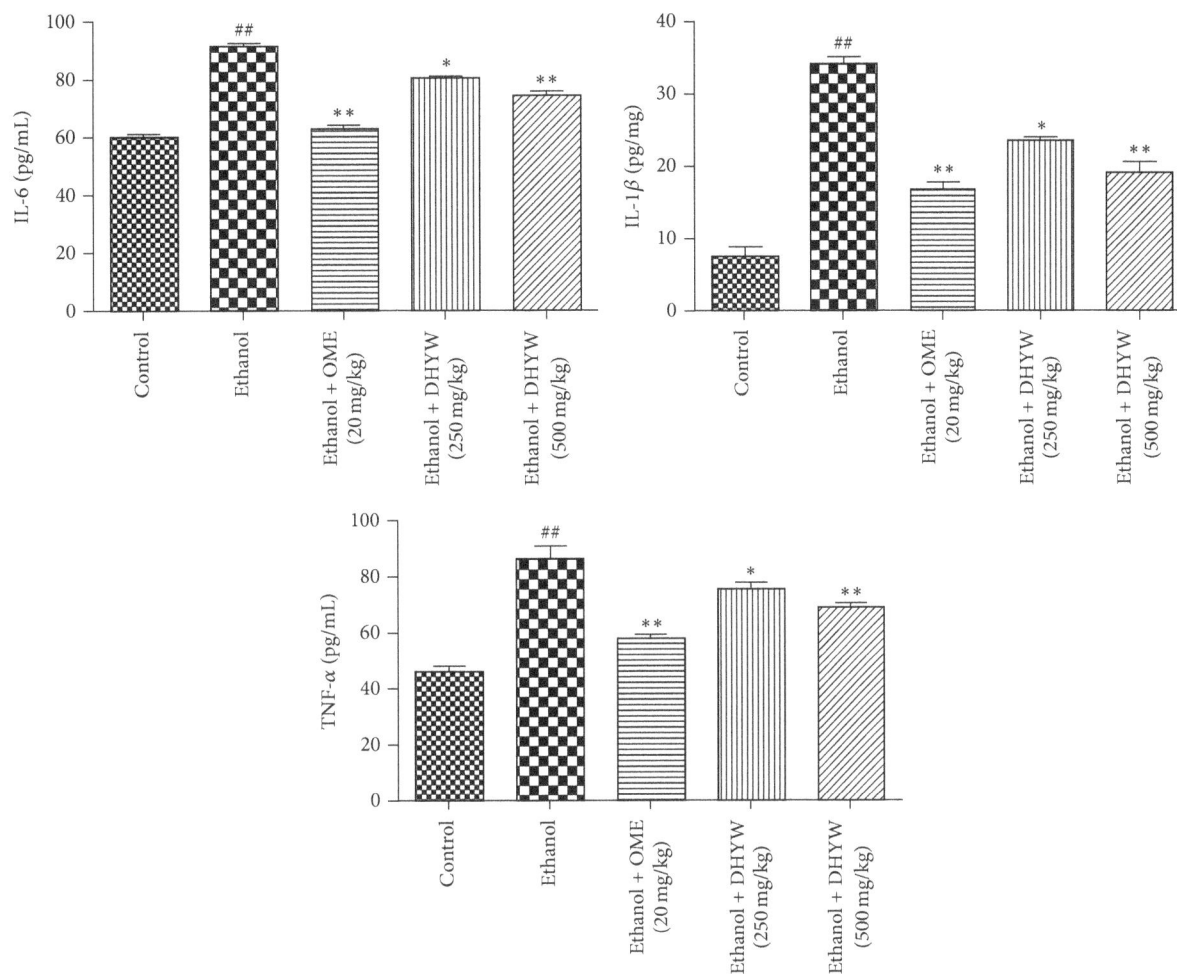

FIGURE 4: Effects of DHYW on inflammatory cytokine. Mice were intragastrically administered with DHYW (250 mg/kg, 500 mg/kg) or OME (20 mg/kg). 1 h later, the mice were intragastrically given ethanol (0.2 mL/kg) and were sacrificed at 4 h after ethanol challenge. Values are expressed as means ± SEM. Compared with control: $^{#}P < 0.05$, $^{##}P < 0.01$; compared with model: $^{*}P < 0.05$, $^{**}P < 0.01$.

3.6. Effects of DHYW on NF-κB. To further detect the underlying mechanism of DHYW, we evaluated the protein expression of NF-κB signaling. As depicted in Figure 6, ethanol significantly upregulated the expressions of p-IκB and p-NF-κB. However, the administrations of DHYW (500 mg/kg) and OME effectively inhibited the phosphorylations of IκB and NF-κB, which were slightly more potent than that of DHYW (250 mg/kg) group. Our results suggested that DHYW might exert its gastroprotective effects via the activation of NF-κB signaling.

4. Discussion

With the risk of human health in daily life, gastrointestinal problems have been a global issue which was always ignored at early stage. In general, gastric ulcer is a common disease triggered by various etiologies including free oxygen radicals. Ethanol is widely acknowledged as an abused agent to gastric ulceration [13]. Thus, the gastric ulcer model induced by ethanol in mice was applied to examine the effect of the compounds against gastric ulcer in our study. As the incentive

of gastric ulcer, ethanol ingestion in the model mice led to an obvious pathological process compared with that of control mice, which was elucidated by acute gastric mucosal lesions through the neutrophil infiltration, release of proinflammatory cytokines, and the expression of nuclear factor-κB (NF-κB). Despite taking into consideration the relation between efficacy and dose, omeprazole (OME) was proved to possess a more marked inhibition against gastric ulcer in comparison with DHYW. However, the potential role of DHYW was also indicated in the improvement of gastrointestinal problems. On the basis of successful model method, the purpose of the present study was to evaluate the antiulcer activity of DHYW using an ethanol-challenged experimental gastric ulcer model and investigate its potential mechanisms. The above results indicated that DHYW could reverse the lesion of gastric mucosa from ethanol induced ulceration to a degree via anti-inflammatory and antioxidative effects which are probably mediated by inhibiting NF-κB pathway activation.

There is growing evidence that ethanol-induced gastric mucosal injury is highly related to the increased ROS level. ROS mainly comes from neutrophils which were driven by

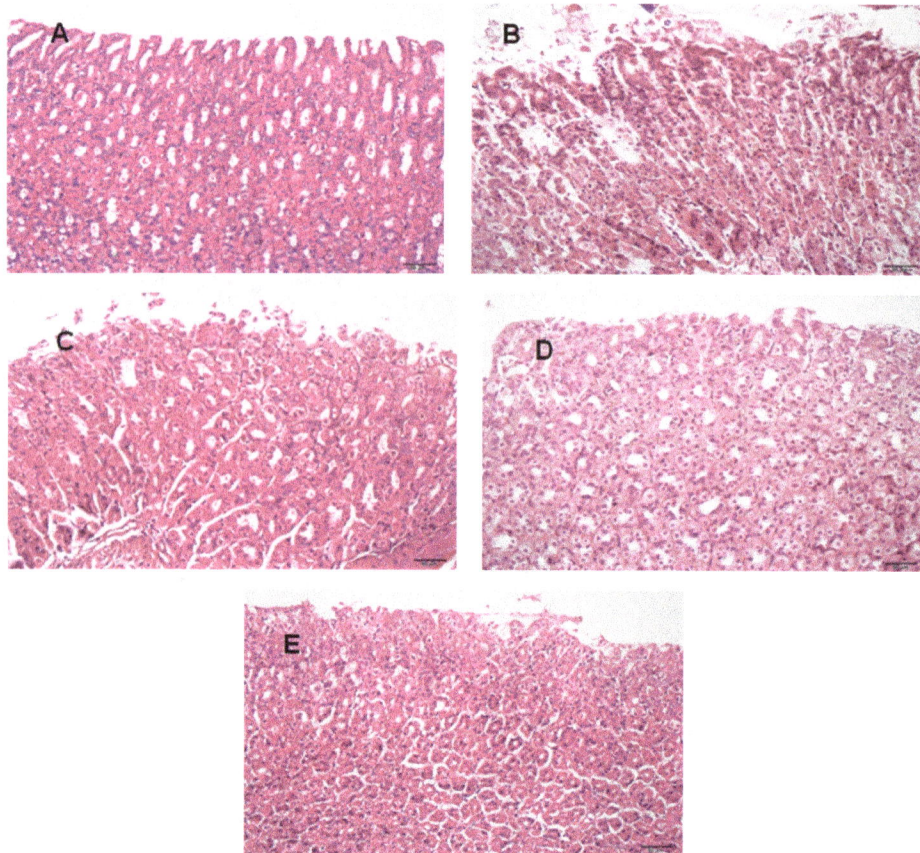

FIGURE 5: Effects of DHYW on ethanol-stimulated histopathologic changes in stomach tissues. (A) The stomach section from the control mice; (B) the stomach section from the mice administered with ethanol; (C) the stomach section from the mice administered with OME (20 mg/kg) and ethanol; (D) the stomach section from the mice administered with DHYW (250 mg/kg) and ethanol; and (E) the stomach section from the mice administered with DHYW (500 mg/kg) and ethanol.

MPO under inflammatory circumstance [14, 15]. Neutrophil infiltration takes the responsibility for prompting reactions in the process of injury by releasing and aggregating tissue-disrupting events in tissues [16, 17]. Therefore, MPO could be treated as a marker to estimate the accumulation of neutrophil infiltration into the gastric mucosal tissues. On the other hand, organisms' enzymatic and nonenzymatic defenses including SOD protect the host against the ROS-induced lipid peroxidation [18]. Generally, SOD exerts multifaceted physiological activities including anti-inflammatory and antioxidant effects [19]. Meanwhile, MDA is the end-product of polyunsaturated fatty acid, which is often used as an indicator for evaluating the lipid peroxidation in gastric mucosal [20, 21]. Our data supported a critical role of oxidative stress in the pathogenesis of the ethanol-induced gastric ulcer. Nevertheless, pretreatment with DHYW resulted in significant increases in the activity of SOD, as well as the decreases in MDA and MPO levels. Hence, our study revealed that DHYW potentially exerted gastroprotective properties alleviating neutrophil infiltration and lipid peroxidation induced by growing ROS level through an antioxidative mechanism, as likewise evidenced by ameliorative consequences in the histological evaluations.

Despite the widely accepted notion that alcohol abuse leads to detrimental consequences in the gastrointestinal tract, the underlying mechanisms still remain obscure. Evidence has emerged indicating that ethanol ingestion may activate the innate immune system to change the levels of proinflammatory cytokines including TNF-α, IL-6, and IL-1β [22]. The generation of inflammatory mediators also plays an important role for the mechanisms of lesions in providing an inflammatory circumstance to facilitate the development of acute gastric mucosal lesions [23]. Previous findings implicated that the productions of proinflammatory cytokines remarkably increased in the serum and gastric tissue of the ethanol-induced ulcer [24]. As a representative inflammatory cytokine with pleiotropic functions, TNF-α is closely associated with the progression of inflammatory disorder and the activation of relevant proinflammatory cytokines such as IL-6 and IL-1β [25]. Previous research showed an aberrant high level of IL-6 in the serum of mice with inflammatory diseases including severe mucosal inflammation [26]. Therefore, the possible alterations of TNF-α, IL-6, and IL-1β contents were investigated. Our experimental results indicated that the serum IL-6 and TNF-α levels were significantly increased due to the necrotizing

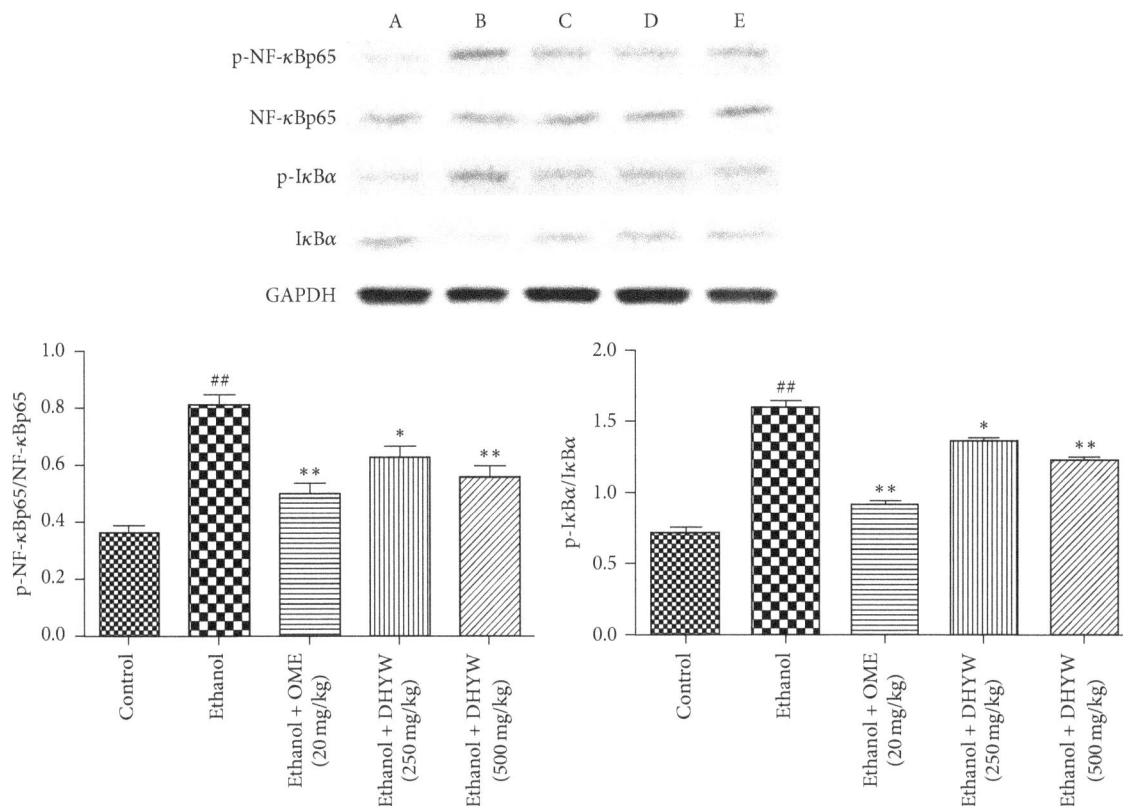

FIGURE 6: Effects of DHYW on NF-κB pathway. Mice were intragastrically administered with DHYW (200 mg/kg, 500 mg/kg) or OME (20 mg/kg). 1 h later, the mice were intragastrically given ethanol (0.2 mL/kg) and were sacrificed at 4 h after ethanol challenge. (A) control group, (B) ethanol group, (C) ethanol + OME (20 mg/kg) group, (D) ethanol + DHYW (250 mg/kg) group, and (E) ethanol + DHYW (500 mg/kg) group. Values are expressed as means ± SEM. Compared with control: $^{#}P < 0.05$, $^{##}P < 0.01$; compared with model: $^{*}P < 0.05$, $^{**}P < 0.01$.

effects of ethanol. However, the inflammatory status had been favorably reduced in the animals pretreated with DHYW, which suggested that the effect of DHYW treatment the effectively inhibited in the generation of proinflammatory cytokines.

NF-κB, well known to mediate the expression of proinflammatory molecules, is a vital transcription factor that regulates many immune and inflammatory processes [27]. NF-κB has been extensively investigated for cytokine regulation and oxidative stress mediation [28]. It was noteworthy that NF-κB pathway was involved in the pathogenesis of ethanol-induced gastric lesion [29]. Therefore, the inhibition of phosphorylated IκB and NF-κB in the gastric tissue might be an important element in the protective effect of DHYW on ethanol-induced gastric lesions. This assumption was confirmed by the suppression of NF-κB signaling observed in animals treated with DHYW in response to ethanol.

In conclusion, our data suggested that DHYW might effectively ameliorate ethanol-induced gastric ulcer by attenuating the inflammatory and oxidative conditions via the NF-κB signaling pathway. Thus, these results supported the notion that DHYW was beneficial for the treatment of ethanol-induced gastric ulcer. Its exact mechanism and clinical application need further investigation in the future.

Conflict of Interests

All author has no conflict of interests.

References

[1] T. Aihara, E. Nakamura, K. Amagase et al., "Pharmacological control of gastric acid secretion for the treatment of acid-related peptic disease: past, present, and future," *Pharmacology & Therapeutics*, vol. 98, no. 1, pp. 109–127, 2003.

[2] A. F. S. C. Viana, H. B. Fernandes, F. V. Silva et al., "Gastroprotective activity of *Cenostigma macrophyllum* Tul. var. *acuminata* Teles Freire leaves on experimental ulcer models," *Journal of Ethnopharmacology*, vol. 150, no. 1, pp. 316–323, 2013.

[3] E. S. D. S. Almeida, V. C. Filho, R. Niero, B. K. Clasen, S. O. Balogun, and D. T. D. O. Martins, "Pharmacological mechanisms underlying the anti-ulcer activity of methanol extract and canthin-6-one of *Simaba ferruginea* A. St-Hil. in animal models," *Journal of Ethnopharmacology*, vol. 134, no. 3, pp. 630–636, 2011.

[4] S. W. Behrman, "Management of complicated peptic ulcer disease," *Archives of Surgery*, vol. 140, no. 2, pp. 201–208, 2005.

[5] G. Riezzo, M. Chiloiro, and S. Montanaro, "Protective effect of amtolmetin guacyl versus placebo diclofenac and misoprostol in healthy volunteers evaluated as gastric electrical activity

in alcohol-induced stomach damage," *Digestive Diseases and Sciences*, vol. 46, no. 8, pp. 1797–1804, 2001.

[6] E. Stermer, "Alcohol consumption and the gastrointestinal tract," *Israel Medical Association Journal*, vol. 4, no. 3, pp. 200–202, 2002.

[7] J. Wang, Y.-T. Liu, L. Xiao, L. Zhu, Q. Wang, and T. Yan, "Anti-inflammatory effects of apigenin in lipopolysaccharide-induced inflammatory in acute lung injury by suppressing COX-2 and NF-kB pathway," *Inflammation*, vol. 37, no. 6, pp. 2085–2090, 2014.

[8] T. Lou, W. Jiang, D. Xu, T. Chen, and Y. Fu, "Inhibitory effects of polydatin on lipopolysaccharide-stimulated RAW 264.7 cells," *Inflammation*, vol. 38, no. 3, pp. 1213–1220, 2015.

[9] W. Jing, M. Chunhua, and W. Shumin, "Effects of acteoside on lipopolysaccharide-induced inflammation in acute lung injury via regulation of NF-κB pathway in vivo and in vitro," *Toxicology and Applied Pharmacology*, vol. 285, no. 2, pp. 128–135, 2015.

[10] T. Chen, Y. Mou, J. Tan et al., "The protective effect of CDDO-Me on lipopolysaccharide-induced acute lung injury in mice," *International Immunopharmacology*, vol. 25, no. 1, pp. 55–64, 2015.

[11] T. Chen, J. Gao, P. Xiang et al., "Protective effect of platycodin D on liver injury in alloxan-induced diabetic mice via regulation of Treg/Th17 balance," *International Immunopharmacology*, vol. 26, no. 2, pp. 338–348, 2015.

[12] T. Chen, L. Xiao, L. Zhu, S. Ma, T. Yan, and H. Ji, "Anti-asthmatic effects of ginsenoside Rb1 in a mouse model of allergic asthma through relegating Th1/Th2," *Inflammation*, vol. 38, no. 5, pp. 1814–1822, 2015.

[13] Z. Zhao, S. Gong, S. Wang, and C. Ma, "Effect and mechanism of evodiamine against ethanol-induced gastric ulcer in mice by suppressing Rho/NF-κB pathway," *International Immunopharmacology*, vol. 28, no. 1, pp. 588–595, 2015.

[14] M. Czygier, Z. Kamocki, S. Ławicki, and M. Szmitkowski, "The plasma level of myeloperoxidase (MPO) and total antioxidant status (TAS) in gastric cancer patients after surgery," *Przegląd Lekarski*, vol. 67, no. 7, pp. 443–445, 2010.

[15] P. Xiang, T. Chen, Y. Mou et al., "NZ suppresses TLR4/NF-κB signalings and NLRP3 inflammasome activation in LPS-induced RAW 264.7 macrophages," *Inflammation Research*, vol. 64, no. 10, pp. 799–808, 2015.

[16] S. A. El-Maraghy, S. M. Rizk, and N. N. Shahin, "Gastroprotective effect of crocin in ethanol-induced gastric injury in rats," *Chemico-Biological Interactions*, vol. 229, pp. 26–35, 2015.

[17] T. Chen, R. Wang, W. Jiang et al., "Protective effect of astragaloside IV against paraquat-induced lung injury in mice by suppressing Rho signaling," *Inflammation*, pp. 1–10, 2015.

[18] Y.-H. Liu, Z.-B. Zhang, Y.-F. Zheng et al., "Gastroprotective effect of andrographolide sodium bisulfite against indomethacin-induced gastric ulceration in rats," *International Immunopharmacology*, vol. 26, no. 2, pp. 384–391, 2015.

[19] L. Zhu, T. Wei, X. Chang et al., "Effects of salidroside on myocardial injury in vivo in vitro via regulation of Nox/NF-κB/AP1 pathway," *Inflammation*, vol. 38, no. 4, pp. 1589–1598, 2015.

[20] W. Jiang, F. Luo, Q. Lu et al., "The protective effect of Trillin LPS-induced acute lung injury by the regulations of inflammation and oxidative state," *Chemico-Biological Interactions*, 2015.

[21] L. Ma and J. Liu, "The protective activity of *Conyza blinii* saponin against acute gastric ulcer induced by ethanol," *Journal of Ethnopharmacology*, vol. 158, part A, pp. 358–363, 2014.

[22] M. S. Salga, H. M. Ali, M. A. Abdulla, and S. I. Abdelwahab, "Gastroprotective activity and mechanism of novel dichlorido-zinc(II)-4-(2-(5-methoxybenzylideneamino)ethyl)piperazin-1-iumphenolate complex on ethanol-induced gastric ulceration," *Chemico-Biological Interactions*, vol. 195, no. 2, pp. 144–153, 2012.

[23] X. Chang, F. Luo, W. Jiang et al., "Protective activity of salidroside against ethanol-induced gastric ulcer via the MAPK/NF-kappaB pathway in vivo and in vitro," *International Immunopharmacology*, vol. 28, no. 1, pp. 604–615, 2015.

[24] X. Mei, D. Xu, S. Xu, Y. Zheng, and S. Xu, "Novel role of Zn(II)-curcumin in enhancing cell proliferation and adjusting proinflammatory cytokine-mediated oxidative damage of ethanol-induced acute gastric ulcers," *Chemico-Biological Interactions*, vol. 197, no. 1, pp. 31–39, 2012.

[25] Q. Jiang, M. Yi, Q. Guo et al., "Protective effects of polydatin on lipopolysaccharide-induced acute lung injury through TLR4-MyD88-NF-κB pathway," *International Immunopharmacology*, vol. 29, no. 2, pp. 370–376, 2015.

[26] Z. N. Ö. Kumral, G. Memi, F. Ercan, and B. Ç. Yeğen, "Estrogen alleviates acetic acid-induced gastric or colonic damage via both ERα- and ERβ-mediated and direct antioxidant mechanisms in rats," *Inflammation*, vol. 37, no. 3, pp. 694–705, 2014.

[27] T. Chen, Q. Guo, H. Wang et al., "Effects of esculetin on lipopolysaccharide (LPS)-induced acute lung injury via regulation of RhoA/Rho Kinase/NF-κB pathways in vivo and in vitro," *Free Radical Research*, vol. 49, no. 12, pp. 1459–1468, 2015.

[28] X. Chang, H. He, L. Zhu et al., "Protective effect of apigenin on Freund's complete adjuvant-induced arthritis in rats via inhibiting P2X7/NF-κB pathway," *Chemico-Biological Interactions*, vol. 236, pp. 41–46, 2015.

[29] J. Wang, T. Zhang, L. Zhu, C. Ma, and S. Wang, "Anti-ulcerogenic effect of Zuojin Pill against ethanol-induced acute gastric lesion in animal models," *Journal of Ethnopharmacology*, vol. 173, pp. 459–467, 2015.

23

Saw Palmetto Extract Inhibits Metastasis and Antiangiogenesis through STAT3 Signal Pathway in Glioma Cell

Hong Ding,[1] **Jinglian Shen,**[2] **Yang Yang,**[3] **and Yuqin Che**[3]

[1]*Department of Nephrology, The Fourth Affiliated Hospital of China Medical University, Shenyang, China*
[2]*Department of Emergency Medicine, The Fourth Affiliated Hospital of China Medical University, Shenyang, China*
[3]*Department of Neurology, The Fourth Affiliated Hospital of China Medical University, Shenyang, China*

Correspondence should be addressed to Yuqin Che; cheyq_cmu4h@126.com

Academic Editor: Giuseppe Morgia

Signal transducer and activator of transcription factor 3 (STAT3) plays an important role in the proliferation and angiogenesis in human glioma. Previous research indicated that saw palmetto extract markedly inhibited the proliferation of human glioma cells through STAT3 signal pathway. But its effect on tumor metastasis and antiangiogenesis is not clear. This study is to further clear the impact of saw palmetto extract on glioma cell metastasis, antiangiogenesis, and its mechanism. TUNEL assay indicated that the apoptotic cells in the saw palmetto treated group are higher than that in the control group ($p < 0.05$). The apoptosis related protein is detected and the results revealed that saw palmetto extract inhibits the proliferation of human glioma. Meanwhile pSTAT3 is lower in the experimental group and CD34 is also inhibited in the saw palmetto treated group. This means that saw palmetto extract could inhibit the angiogenesis in glioma. We found that saw palmetto extract was an important phytotherapeutic drug against the human glioma through STAT3 signal pathway. Saw palmetto extract may be useful as an adjunctive therapeutic agent for treatment of individuals with glioma and other types of cancer in which STAT3 signaling is activated.

1. Introduction

Human gliomas which originate from neural stromal cells are the most common and malignant brain tumor in human [1]. Human gliomas account for 35.26–60.96% of central nervous system tumors (average, 44.69%). The incidence rate in adults is about 6/100,000 and the five-year survival rate is between 20 and 30% [2]. Due to the tumor's infiltrating growth and no evident boundary with the normal brain tissue, it is difficult to be removed completely via surgery. In addition, gliomas are not susceptible to radiotherapy or chemotherapy, which makes it the worst prognoses in systemic tumors [3]. Therefore, it is urgently needed to identify the critical carcinogenic pathways and discover novel treatment strategies for glioma.

The growth and proliferation of glioma cells are highly dependent on angiogenesis [4]. The glioma has a strong ability in promoting the formation of angiogenesis and microvascular network to provide the tumor with nutrients for the sake of further invasion and metastasis. So the treatment of antiangiogenesis therapy has become an important method in glioma.

Signal transducer and activator of transcription factor 3 (STAT3) with tyrosine phosphorylation in signal pathway exists in the cell holder, regulating the expression of a variety of functional protein, cell proliferation, and apoptosis. The present study has proven that there is a close relationship between STAT3 and cell adhesion molecules, extracellular matrix degrading enzymes, tumor angiogenesis, metastasis through MMP, VEGF, and other related gene interactions [5–7].

Saw palmetto (SR) is a kind of palm plant in Southeast American. In in vitro experiments people found that saw palmetto extract can effectively inhibit the proliferation with dose dependent relationship in human breast cancer cells [8]. In previous research, the effect of saw palmetto extract on human glioma U87 and U251 cells was investigated in vivo. The results revealed that saw palmetto extract markedly inhibited the proliferation of human glioma cells. The underlying mechanism may be associated with the inhibition of signal transducer and activator of transcription 3 phosphorylation [9].

As mentioned, saw palmetto extract regulates the proliferation of tumor cells by inhibiting the STAT3 signaling pathway, but its effect on tumor metastasis and antiangiogenesis is not clear. The purpose of this study is through researching the effect of saw palmetto extract on glioma cell migration related protein and marker of angiogenesis to further clear the impact of saw palmetto extract on glioma cell metastasis, antiangiogenesis, and its mechanism.

2. Materials and Methods

2.1. Animals and Cell Lines. 30 healthy SD male rats were purchased from China Medical University Department of Experimental Animal, which weighed 250–300 g. The rats were randomly divided into three groups: control group, low dose SR group, and high dose SR group. Human glioma cell lines U87 and U251 were purchased from Beijing Dingguochangsheng Biotech Co., Ltd. (Beijing, China).

2.2. Reagents and Drug. Saw palmetto extract was purchased from Yongyuan Bio-technology, Co., Ltd. (Xi'an, China). TUNEL kit, rabbit anti-B-cell lymphoma-2 (Bcl-2), anti-CD34, anti-MMP-2, anti-PARP, and anti-pSTAT3 antibodies were purchased from the Beyotime Institute of Biotechnology (Shanghai, China).

2.3. Cell Culture. Human glioma cell lines, U87 and U251, were grown in a $25 \, cm^2$ cell culture bottle containing Dulbecco's modified Eagle's medium (DMEM), supplemented with 10% fetal bovine serum, 100 IU/mL penicillin, and 100 μg/mL streptomycin. The cell was cultured at 37°C and 5% carbon dioxide. The medium was replaced every two days.

2.4. Cell Count. Blood cell counting plate and cover glass were cleaned with 95% alcohol. Take 1 μL of cell suspension on the blood cell counting chamber to count the cell concentration. The cell number was counted with four angles in the grid on the plate. The procedure was performed in triplicate. The cell number was calculated as follows: Cell number (/mL) = (total cell number of the four angles/4) $* 10^4 *$ dilution.

2.5. Establishment of the Rat Glioma Model. The vigorous growing cell was collected; the cell concentration was adjusted to $1 * 10^7$/mL. The cell suspension was subcutaneously injected into rat dorsal to establish glioma model. The control group was injected with equal amount of saline at the same site. SR low dose group and high dose SR group rats received administration of 50 mg/kg and 300 mg/kg saw palmetto extract every day through gastrointestinal tract for 4 weeks; meanwhile the control group rats were given the same amount of drinking water every day. After the last administration, the rats were sacrificed 24 hours later and the glioma specimens were collected.

2.6. TUNEL Assay. TUNEL assay was utilized to detect the apoptosis in glioma tissues. The tissues were fixed with 10% formalin, were dehydrated, were transparent, and were embedded in paraffin; then the specimens were cut into 5–8 μm thick slices. Then the glioma sections were deparaffinized, rehydrated, and pretreated with 20 μg/mL proteinase K. The endogenous peroxidase was blocked by 3% hydrogen peroxide. The specimens were subsequently incubated with terminal deoxynucleotidyl transferase (TdT) and reacted at 37°C for 1 hour, followed by antidigoxigenin antibody at 37°C for 30 min. After washing, slides were incubated with streptavidin-biotin-peroxidase for 20 min, stained with 3,3′-diaminobenzidine tetrahydrochloride, and counterstained with hematoxylin. Finally, the sections were dehydrated, coverslipped, and observed. Five sights of each section were randomly selected under microscope. The number of TUNEL-positive glioma nuclei and the total glioma nuclei in each sight were counted. The ratio of apoptotic cell was calculated by dividing the number of TUNEL-positive glioma nuclei by the number of total glioma nuclei.

2.7. The Expression of STAT3, MMP-2, CD34, and Bcl-2 Was Detected by Immunohistochemistry. All specimens were promptly fixed in 10% buffered formalin and embedded in paraffin. 4 μm section was cut and conventionally dewaxed to water. The section was incubated in 3% of H_2O_2 PBS at room temperature for 10 min and then washed for five minutes with distilled water three times. The sections were immersed in 0.01 mol/L citric acid buffer (pH 6) boiled for 15 minutes with microwave. After cooling the specimen was washed 2 times with PBS. 5% of BSA sealing liquid was dropped on the specimen and left for reaction for 20 min at room temperature. After that the excess liquid was rejected with no washing. Diluted first antibody (rabbit anti-rat pSTAT3 (1 : 300), rabbit anti-rat Bcl-2 (1 : 300), rabbit anti-rat CD34 (1 : 300), rabbit anti-rat MMP-2 (1 : 300), and rabbit anti-rat PARP (1 : 300)) were added and reacted at 4°C in the moisturizing box overnight. The specimen was washed with PBS three times for 2 min the next day. Following primary antibody incubations, sections were incubated with biotin-conjugated secondary antibodies: goat anti-rabbit IgG (Beyotime Institute of Biotechnology, Shanghai, China) at a temperature of 37°C for 30 min in the moisturizing box. Following that the section was washed 3 times for 2 min with PBS. SABC reagents were added on the section and reacted for 20 min at 37°C in the moisturizing box. Then the section was washed 4 times for 5 min with PBS. Visualization of the immune complex involved the DAB kit according to the protocol. At last, the section was washed with distilled water and counterstained with hematoxylin staining.

2.8. Image Analysis. pSTAT3, Bcl-2, CD34, MMP-2, and PARP positive nuclei were brown or dark brown. The immunoreactive positive cells were determined by the average optical density value of ImageJ image analysis software.

2.9. Statistical Analysis. All the experimental data were processed by SPSS 19 statistical analysis software; the values are expressed in mean ± standard deviation. Comparison

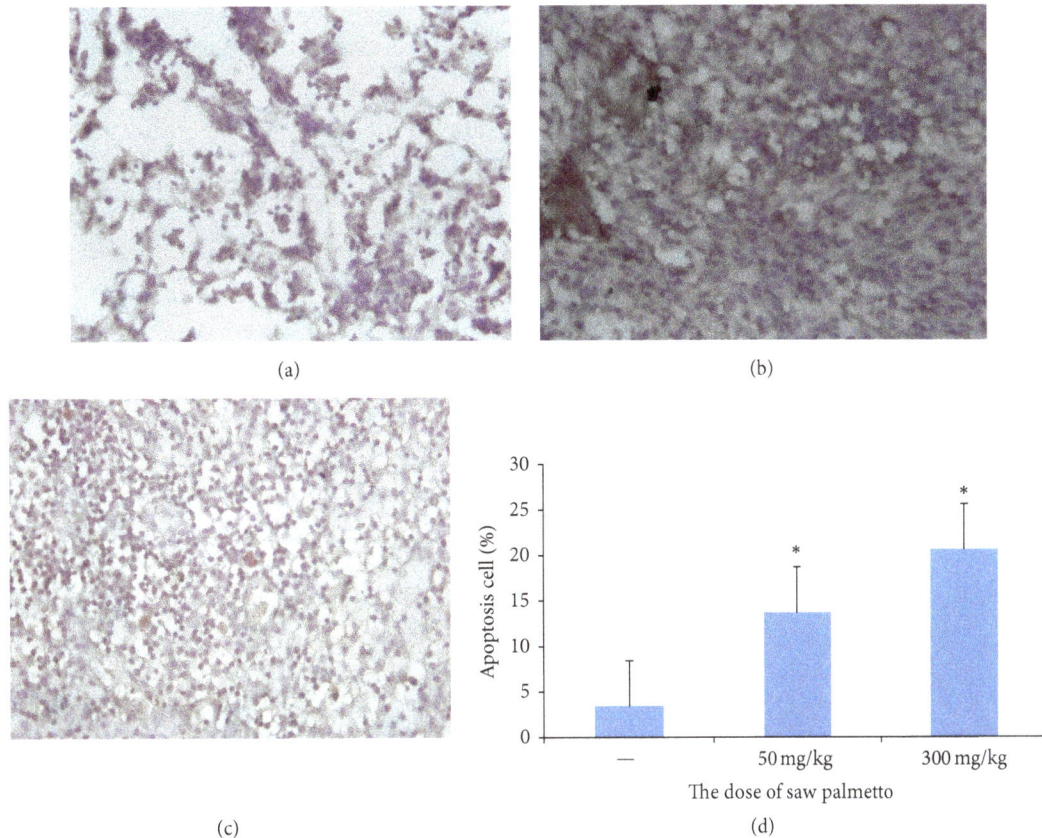

(a)

(b)

(c)

(d)

FIGURE 1: The apoptosis of glioma cell induced by saw palmetto through TUNEL assay. (a) is the control group, (b) is the low dose group in which the rats received administration of 50 mg/kg saw palmetto extract every day for 4 weeks, and (c) is the high dose group in which the rats received administration of 300 mg/kg saw palmetto extract every day for 4 weeks. (d) is the histogram to evaluate the apoptosis cell induced by saw palmetto of above three groups. * means $p < 0.05$.

between groups was analyzed by one-way ANOVA, with statistically significant difference in p less than 0.05.

3. Results

3.1. The Apoptosis of Glioma Tissue Induced by Saw Palmetto Extract. The apoptosis of glioma cell induced by saw palmetto was detected by TUNEL assay. As shown in Figure 1, the apoptosis ratio in the control group is $3.45 \pm 0.48\%$, in the low dose group is $13.67 \pm 0.34\%$, and in the high dose group is $20.58 \pm 1.53\%$. The apoptotic cells in the saw palmetto treated group are higher than that in the control group ($p < 0.05$). In addition, we can conclude that the apoptosis ratio is higher in the high dose group than that in the low dose group ($p < 0.05$).

3.2. The Expression of pSTAT3 in the Glioma Tissue Was Measured by Immunohistochemistry Assay. Previous study suggested that saw palmetto induced growth arrest and apoptosis of prostate cancer cells by the inhibition of STAT3 signal pathway. We adopted immunohistochemistry assay to measure the expression of pSTAT3 in glioma tissue. The results revealed that the optical density value is 0.295 ± 0.007 in the control group, 0.237 ± 0.005 in the low dose group,

and 0.122 ± 0.008 in the high dose group (see Figure 2). The expression of pSTAT3 is lower in the experimental group than that in the control group ($p < 0.05$). At the same time we can see that the expression of pSTAT3 is negative with the concentration of saw palmetto.

3.3. The Expression of MMP-2 in the Glioma Tissue Was Measured by Immunohistochemistry Assay. The previous study certified that MMP-2 is associated with the metastasis of tumor. We detected the expression of MMP-2 to evaluate the effect of saw palmetto on the metastasis of glioma. We adopted immunohistochemistry assay to measure the expression of MMP-2 in glioma tissue. The results revealed that the optical density value is 0.299 ± 0.009 in the control group, 0.222 ± 0.014 in the low dose group, and 0.122 ± 0.009 in the high dose group (see Figure 3). The expression of MMP-2 is lower in the experimental group than that in the control group ($p < 0.05$).

3.4. The Expression of CD34 in the Glioma Tissue Was Measured by Immunohistochemistry Assay. Angiogenesis is very important in the tumor cell proliferation and metastasis. As known, CD34 is a good marker to reflect the density of blood vessels in the tumor. In order to study the effect

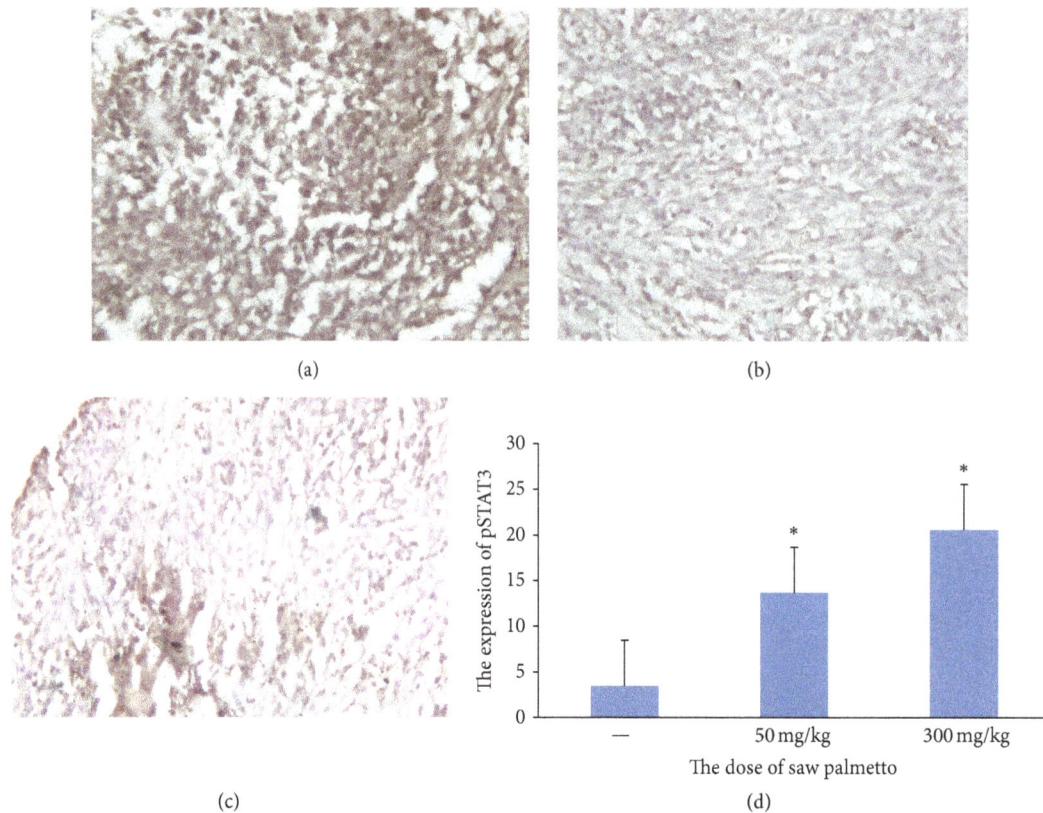

FIGURE 2: The expression of pSTAT3 in the glioma tissue. (a) is the control group, (b) is the low dose group in which the rats received administration of 50 mg/kg saw palmetto extract every day for 4 weeks, and (c) is the high dose group in which the rats received administration of 300 mg/kg saw palmetto extract every day for 4 weeks. (d) is the histogram to evaluate the expression of pSTAT3 in the three groups. ∗ means $p < 0.05$.

of saw palmetto on angiogenesis, we measure the CD34 by immunohistochemistry method. The results revealed that the optical density value is 0.288 ± 0.014 in the control group, 0.224 ± 0.011 in the low dose group, and 0.120 ± 0.115 in the high dose group ($p < 0.05$) (see Figure 4). The results means that the vascular density is lower in the experimental group which indicated that saw palmetto could inhibit the angiogenesis.

3.5. Effect of Saw Palmetto on Expression of Apoptotic Related Protein in Glioma Cells. Furthermore, the proapoptotic effect of saw palmetto was explored by immunohistochemistry assay. The Bcl-2 and PARP (poly ADP-ribose polymerase) were detected in this study. In the study of cell apoptosis, PARP as the DNA repair enzyme which can repair the DNA is a core member of apoptosis. It plays an important role in DNA damage repair and apoptosis. PARP can be used as the hallmark of apoptosis. The average optical density is 0.313 ± 0.137 in control group, 0.238 ± 0.127 in low dose group, and 0.119 ± 0.078 in the high dose group ($p < 0.05$) (see Figure 5). Bcl-2 is an antiapoptosis protein. In this study we also detect the expression of Bcl-2 to further certify the effect of saw palmetto on the glioma cell. The average optical density is 0.116 ± 0.010 in control group, 0.285 ± 0.014 in low dose

group, and 0.335 ± 0.016 in the high dose group ($p < 0.05$) (see Figure 6).

4. Discussion

Human gliomas are tumors of glial origin of central nervous system (CNS) and they are the most common primary tumors, accounting for ~46% of intracranial tumors and ~2% of adult tumors. The glioma is characterized by its invasive growth and is difficult to be treated via surgery. In addition, the human glioma cell is not sensitive to chemotherapy and radiotherapy.

In previous years, studies have focused on chemical compounds which derived from plants that possess pharmacological activity in antitumor therapy [10, 11]. A previous study demonstrated that a number of chemical compounds in herbaceous plant sources can inhibit the proliferation of tumor cells and induce apoptosis through altering the tumor metabolism [12].

The effective ingredients of saw palmetto extract, as matured dry fruit of saw palm, are fatty acids. A foreign study reported that saw palmetto extract could inhibit the proliferation and induction of apoptosis in prostate cancer cells [13]. At the same time, other studies have found that saw

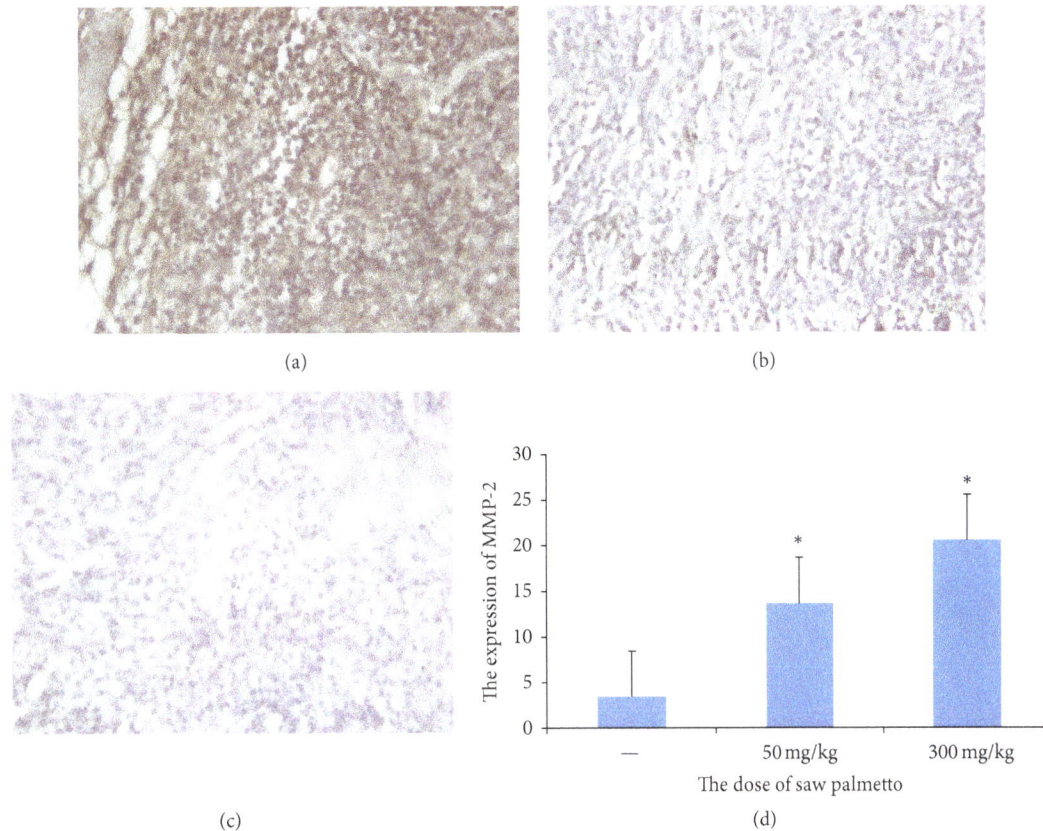

FIGURE 3: The expression of MMP-2 in the glioma tissue. (a) is the control group, (b) is the low dose group in which the rats received administration of 50 mg/kg saw palmetto extract every day for 4 weeks, and (c) is the high dose group in which the rats received administration of 300 mg/kg saw palmetto extract every day for 4 weeks. (d) is the histogram to evaluate the expression of MMP-2 in the three groups. ∗ means $p < 0.05$.

palmetto extract can effectively inhibit multiple myeloma, breast cancer, and another tumor cell proliferation. In this study we detected cell apoptosis by TUNEL method. The number of positive cells in the experimental group was significantly higher than that in the control group. In addition, the apoptosis ratio is higher in the high dose group than the low dose group. The results suggest that saw palmetto extract can increase the apoptosis of glioma cells. At the same time, the presence of some apoptotic related proteins was detected in U87 and U251 glioma cells. *Serenoa repens* significantly increased the level of both cleaved PARP. These results suggest that saw palmetto extract is a kind of antiglioma effect of drugs.

Glioma is one of the most common malignant tumors with the highest degree of vessels in intracranial tumor. It is typical angiogenesis dependent tumor which makes its invasion and recurrence rate significantly higher than those of other intracranial tumors [14–16]. The study found that the brain glioma is involved in vascular endothelial cell activation, proliferation, migration, basement membrane and extracellular matrix degradation, endothelial cell remodeling, and cell interactions with surroundings. In human glioma angiogenesis, proliferation of endothelial cells must break through the barrier of the extracellular basement membrane.

The degradation of matrix in tumor angiogenesis is primarily completed by the metal matrix protease (MMPs) secreted by tumor cells. Many studies have shown that MMPs are directly associated with tumor angiogenesis, tumor invasion, and metastasis of malignant tumor [17, 18]. MMPs can lead to the formation of new blood vessels and enhance the invasion and metastasis ability of tumor. Hamasuna et al. [19] confirmed that MMP-2 can be used as a new index of tumor malignant degree and prognosis. Recent studies have also confirmed that the synthesis and activation of MMP-2 can be induced by glioma. The activation of MMP-2 not only promotes the formation of new blood vessels in the host tissue but also maintains the integrity of the vascular structure. The volume of glioma model cultured by C6 cell line in rats can be significantly reduced, treated by MMP-2 specific inhibitor factor (TIMP-2), and accompanied with the degeneration and necrosis of blood vessel.

Study on the mechanism of glioma angiogenesis and antiangiogenesis has become a new method for the treatment of glioma in recent years. In this study we adopted immuno-histochemistry assay to detect CD34, MMP-2, and other indicators in glioma tissue. The results suggested that CD34 optical density value of the experimental group was higher than that of control group. As is known, CD34 is a good

(a)

(b)

(c)

(d)

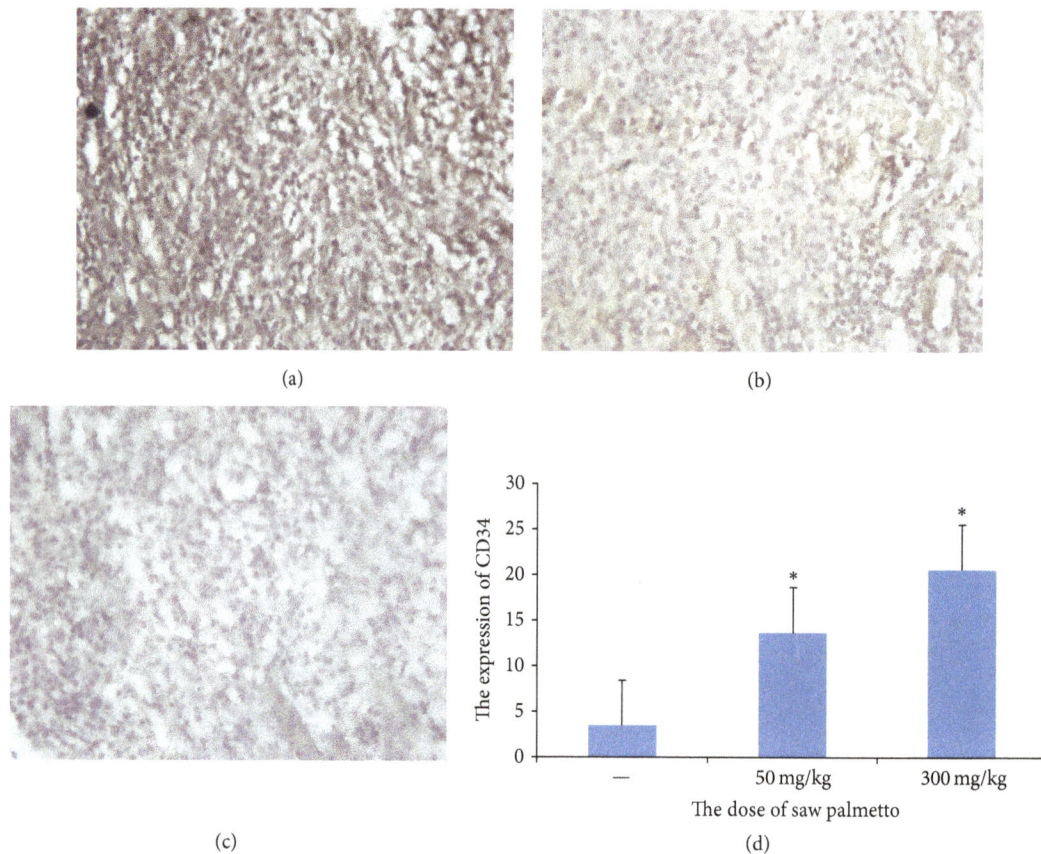

FIGURE 4: The expression of CD34 in the glioma tissue. (a) is the control group, (b) is the low dose group in which the rats received administration of 50 mg/kg saw palmetto extract every day for 4 weeks, and (c) is the high dose group in which the rats received administration of 300 mg/kg saw palmetto extract every day for 4 weeks. (d) is the histogram to evaluate the expression of CD34 in the three groups. $*$ means $p < 0.05$.

marker to reflect the density of blood vessels in the tumor. CD34 is closely related to tumor occurrence, development, and prognosis [20]. This study suggests that saw palmetto extract can effectively reduce the expression of CD34 in tumor cells, so that it can effectively inhibit the tumor angiogenesis. At the same time, we detected the expression of MMP-2 and the results revealed that MMP-2 in the control group was also significantly higher than that in the experimental group. According to the above results it is suggested that saw palmetto extract reduces tumor angiogenesis rough reducing the degradation of extracellular matrix by inhibiting expression of MMP-2 protein.

Signal transducer and activator of transcription factor 3 (STAT3) is a bifunctional protein coupled with tyrosine phosphorylation signal pathway, which exists in the cell holder and regulates the expression of a variety of related functional protein, cell proliferation, and apoptosis [21–23]. STAT3 rarely expresses in normal tissues of the human body and cells, which maintains the normal physiological function of cells and tissues. But the activation of STAT3 is persistent in the tumor tissues and cells. The study finds that STAT3 activation plays an important role in the tumor cell survival, proliferation, angiogenesis, invasion, metastasis, and immune escape [24]. There is high expression of STAT3

in many kinds of tumor cells, so the research of STAT3 in tumors has become a hot topic. The present study has proven that there is a close relationship between STAT3 and cell adhesion molecules, extracellular matrix degrading enzymes, angiogenesis, metastasis, and promotion tumor angiogenesis through MMP [25]. The activation of oncogene STAT3 expression can be induced by antiapoptotic proteins such as Bcl-2, MD-1, and Bcl-XL. All of these are known to promote tumor growth.

The tyrosine of STAT3 is activated under the combination cytokines, growth factors, and hormones with its receptor. STAT3 combined with Janus kinase (JAK) in the cytoplasm caused its tyrosine and JAK tyrosine phosphorylation. The STAT3 is activated after the tyrosine phosphorylation. After STAT3 activated, STAT3 forms homo- or heterodimer in cytoplasm and quickly enters the nucleus to combine with the specific gene promoter on the transcription of target genes, such as the antiapoptotic genes Bcl-2 and Mcl21, cell cycle control genes c-myc and cyclinDl, and angiogenesis related genes VEGF. Studies show that STAT3 phosphorylation at tyrosine 705 is abnormal aggregation in malignant glioma cells, particularly in glioblastoma. The expression of pY705-STAT3 is positively correlated with tumor grade and is one of the poor prognosis factors in survival analysis [26].

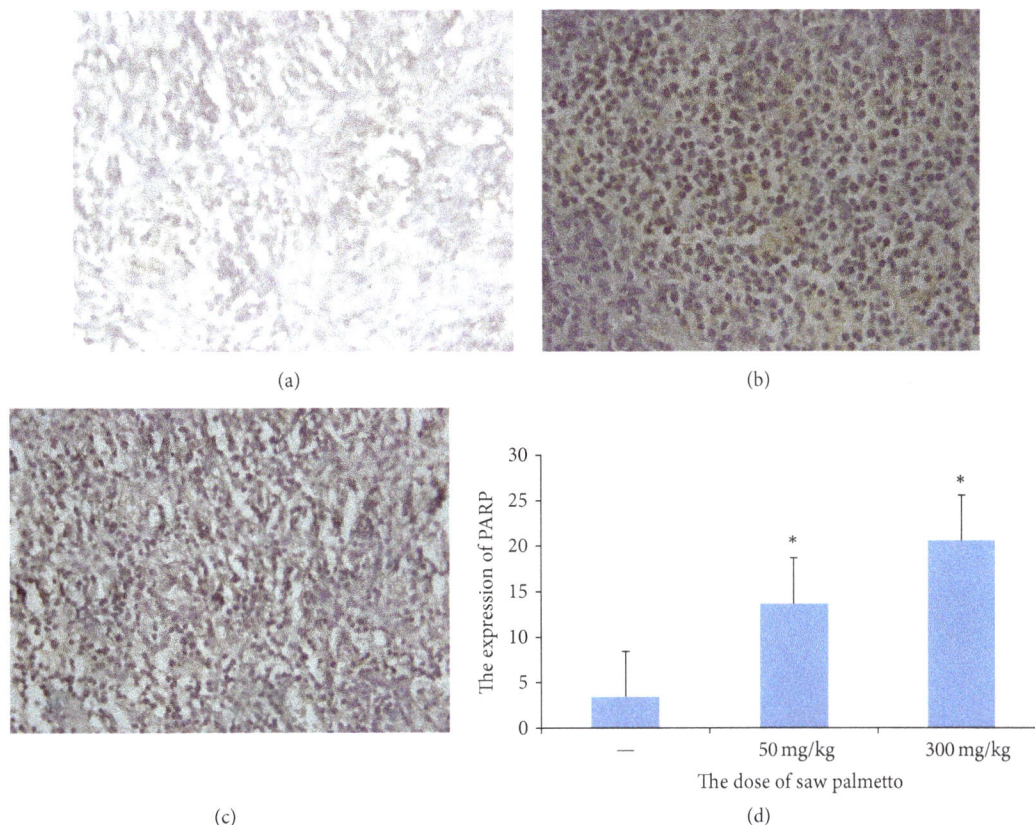

FIGURE 5: The expression of PARP in the glioma tissue. (a) is the control group, (b) is the low dose group in which the rats received administration of 50 mg/kg saw palmetto extract every day for 4 weeks, and (c) is the high dose group in which the rats received administration of 300 mg/kg saw palmetto extract every day for 4 weeks. (d) is the histogram to evaluate the expression of PARP in the three groups. ∗ means $p < 0.05$.

The results show that the abnormal activation of STAT3 plays an important role in the occurrence and development of malignant glioma. Rahaman et al. [27] reported that inhibiting the activity of STAT3 could reduce the proliferation of glioma cells and even promote the apoptosis of glioma cells. Meanwhile inhibition of the activation of STAT3 can decrease the expression of Bcl-2 and Bcl-XL. Abnormal p-STAT3 aggregation can also be observed in the proliferation of vascular endothelial cells which means that p-STAT3 is involved in tumor angiogenesis. In malignant glioma, the expression of activated STAT3 can increase the expression of vascular endothelial growth factor (VEGF). The target genes that have been identified in the STAT3 coding are antiapoptotic proteins Bcl-2 and Bcl-XL, proliferation related proteins Cyclin Dl and Myc, and angiogenesis factor VEGF.

As mentioned, matrix metalloproteinases (MMPs) are a key enzyme in the degradation of extracellular matrix. The study found that STAT3 can bind to MMP-2 promoter to enhance the expression of MMP-2 [28]. Tumor development depends on angiogenesis in order to get the nutrients required for growth and metastasis. It is known that many growth factors and cytokines are involved in the regulation of tumor angiogenesis. Vascular endothelial growth factor plays an important role in the tumor angiogenesis [29]. STAT3 is involved in the regulation of transcription of VEGF. Study has confirmed that the VEGF promoter has the binding site with STAT3. STAT3 can directly bind to the promoter of VEGF further to upregulate the expression of VEGF in tumor cells.

In summary, we found that saw palmetto extract was an important phytotherapeutic drug against the human glioma through STAT3 signal pathway. Saw palmetto extract has been widely used to treat benign prostatic hyperplasia and androgenic alopecia in clinic; the related adverse reactions included ejaculatory disorders, postural hypotension, dizziness, headache, gastrointestinal disorders, rhinitis, fatigue, and asthenia, but the side-effects were limited [30, 31] except for children [32]. So, saw palmetto extract may be useful as an adjunctive therapeutic agent for treatment of individuals with glioma and other types of cancer in which STAT3 signaling is activated.

Conflict of Interests

The authors declare that there are no competing interests regarding the publication of this paper.

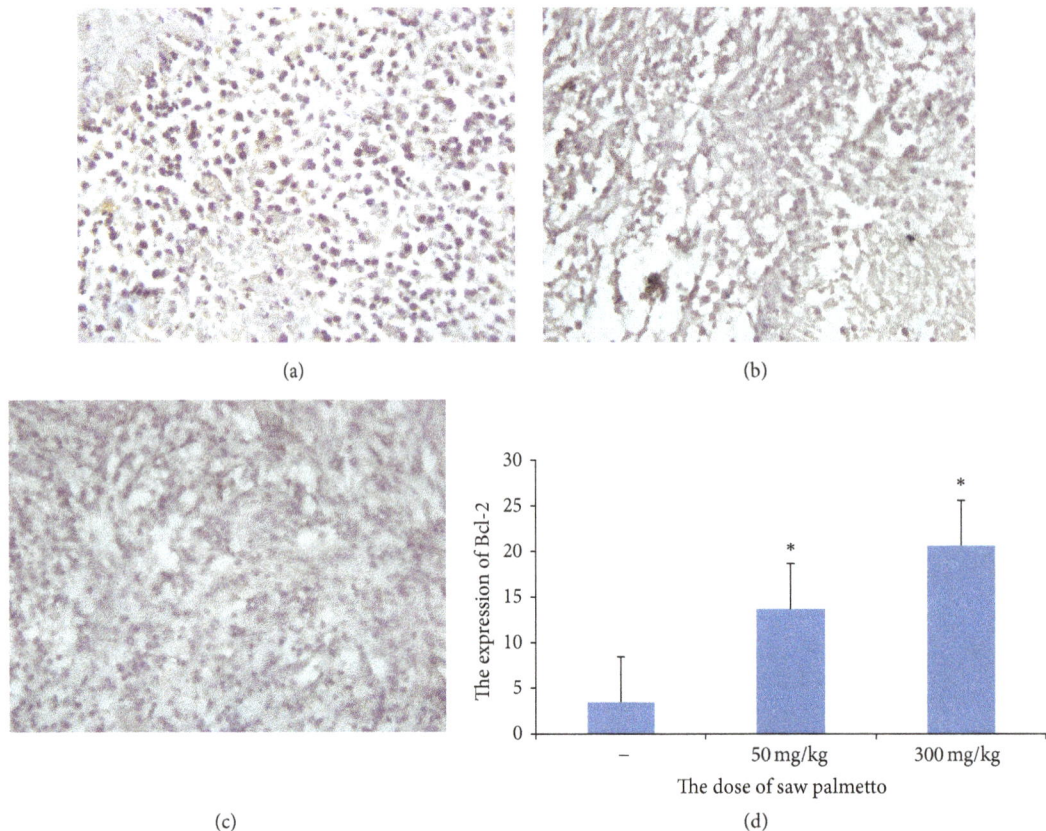

FIGURE 6: The expression of Bcl-2 in the glioma tissue. (a) is the control group, (b) is the low dose group in which the rats received administration of 50 mg/kg saw palmetto extract every day for 4 weeks, and (c) is the high dose group in which the rats received administration of 300 mg/kg saw palmetto extract every day for 4 weeks. (d) is the histogram to evaluate the expression of Bcl-2 in the three groups. $*$ means $p < 0.05$.

Authors' Contribution

Yuqin Che conceived and designed the study. Hong Ding and Jinglian Shen performed immunohistochemistry. Yang Yang dealt with data analysis. Hong Ding and Yuqin Che wrote and revised the paper. All authors read and approved the final paper.

Acknowledgment

This study is supported by a grant from the Liaoning Provincial Natural Science Foundation of China (no. 2013010078-401).

References

[1] T. S. Surawicz, B. J. McCarthy, V. Kupelian, P. J. Jukich, J. M. Bruner, and F. G. Davis, "Descriptive epidemiology of primary brain and CNS tumors: results from the central brain tumor registry of thee United States, 1990–1994," *Neuro-Oncology*, vol. 1, no. 1, pp. 14–25, 1999.

[2] H. Ohgaki and P. Kleihues, "Epidemiology and etiology of gliomas," *Acta Neuropathologica*, vol. 109, no. 1, pp. 93–108, 2005.

[3] P. Y. Wen and S. Kesari, "Malignant gliomas in adults," *The New England Journal of Medicine*, vol. 359, no. 5, pp. 492–507, 2008.

[4] R. C. Curry, S. Dahiya, V. Alva Venur, J. J. Raizer, and M. S. Ahluwalia, "Bevacizumab in high-grade gliomas: past, present, and future," *Expert Review of Anticancer Therapy*, vol. 15, no. 4, pp. 387–397, 2015.

[5] Z. G. Ouédraogo, M. Müller-Barthélémy, J. Kemeny et al., "STAT3 serine 727 phosphorylation: a relevant target to radiosensitize human glioblastoma," *Brain Pathology*, 2015.

[6] X. Feng, J. Wu, X. Xu et al., "A preliminary study about the interaction between basic fibroblast growth factor and signal transducer and activator of transcription 3 in glioma apoptosis," *Zhonghua Wai Ke Za Zhi*, vol. 52, no. 12, pp. 939–944, 2014.

[7] L.-Y. Kong, J. Wei, A. S. Haider et al., "Therapeutic targets in subependymoma," *Journal of Neuroimmunology*, vol. 277, no. 1-2, pp. 168–175, 2014.

[8] A. Fugh-Berman, "Bust enhancing herbal products," *Obstetrics and Gynecology*, vol. 101, no. 6, pp. 1345–1349, 2003.

[9] T. Zhou, Y. Yang, H. Zhang et al., "Serenoa repens induces growth arrest, apoptosis and inactivation of STAT3 signaling in human glioma cells," *Technology in Cancer Research & Treatment*, 2014.

[10] Z. S. Smirnova, K. V. Ermakova, I. Y. Kubasova et al., "Experimental study of combined therapy for malignant glioma,"

Bulletin of Experimental Biology and Medicine, vol. 156, no. 4, pp. 480–482, 2014.

[11] M. Nagane, "Anti-angiogenic therapy for malignant glioma," *Gan To Kagaku Ryoho*, vol. 41, no. 1, pp. 141–147, 2014.

[12] A. K. Taraphdar, M. Roy, and R. K. Bhattacharya, "Natural products as inducers of apoptosis: implication for cancer therapy and prevention," *Current Science*, vol. 80, no. 11, pp. 1387–1396, 2001.

[13] E. Petrangeli, L. Lenti, B. Buchetti et al., "Lipido-sterolic extract of *Serenoa repens* (LSESr, Permixon) treatment affects human prostate cancer cell membrane organization," *Journal of Cellular Physiology*, vol. 219, no. 1, pp. 69–76, 2009.

[14] N. Jhaveri, T. C. Chen, and F. M. Hofman, "Tumor vasculature and glioma stem cells: contributions to glioma progression," *Cancer Letters*, vol. 14, no. 3, pp. 783–786, 2014.

[15] A. L. Cohen and H. Colman, "Glioma biology and molecular markers," *Cancer Treatment and Research*, vol. 163, no. 1, pp. 15–30, 2015.

[16] L. Chen, Z.-X. Lin, G.-S. Lin et al., "Classification of microvascular patterns via cluster analysis reveals their prognostic significance in glioblastoma," *Human Pathology*, vol. 46, no. 1, pp. 120–128, 2015.

[17] Y. Wang, S. Guan, G. Zhao, P. Shi, and J. Wang, "Expressions of aquaporin-4, matrix metallo-proteinase-2 and matrix metallo-proteinase-14 in peritumor edematous zone of glioma and clinical implications," *Zhonghua Yi Xue Za Zhi*, vol. 94, no. 29, pp. 2290–2292, 2014.

[18] J. Zou, L. Xu, Y. Ju, P. Zhang, Y. Wang, and B. Zhang, "Cholesterol depletion induces ANTXR2-dependent activation of MMP-2 via ERK1/2 phosphorylation in neuroglioma U251 cell," *Biochemical and Biophysical Research Communications*, vol. 452, no. 1, pp. 186–190, 2014.

[19] R. Hamasuna, H. Kataoka, T. Moriyama, H. Itoh, M. Seiki, and M. Koono, "Regulation of matrix metalloproteinase-2 (MMP-2) by hepatocyte growth factor/scatter factor (HGF/SF) in human glioma cells: HGF/SF enhances MMP-2 expression and activation accompanying up-regulation of membrane type-1 MMP," *International Journal of Cancer*, vol. 82, no. 2, pp. 274–281, 1999.

[20] K. Majchrzak, W. Kaspera, J. Szymaś, B. Bobek-Billewicz, A. Hebda, and H. Majchrzak, "Markers of angiogenesis (CD31, CD34, rCBV) and their prognostic value in low-grade gliomas," *Neurologia i Neurochirurgia Polska*, vol. 47, no. 4, pp. 325–331, 2013.

[21] H. S. Kim, A. Li, S. Ahn, H. Song, and W. Zhang, "Inositol polyphosphate-5-phosphatase F (INPP5F) inhibits STAT3 activity and suppresses gliomas tumorigenicity," *Scientific Reports*, vol. 4, article 7330, 2014.

[22] X.-F. Wang, G.-S. Lin, Z.-X. Lin et al., "Association of pSTAT3-VEGF signaling pathway with peritumoral edema in newly diagnosed glioblastoma: an immunohistochemical study," *International Journal of Clinical and Experimental Pathology*, vol. 7, no. 9, pp. 6133–6140, 2014.

[23] G. K. Gray, B. C. McFarland, S. E. Nozell, and E. N. Benveniste, "NF-κB and STAT3 in glioblastoma: therapeutic targets coming of age," *Expert Review of Neurotherapeutics*, vol. 14, no. 11, pp. 1293–1306, 2014.

[24] Q. Zheng, L. Han, Y. Dong et al., "JAK2/STAT3 targeted therapy suppresses tumor invasion via disruption of the EGFRvIII/JAK2/STAT3 axis and associated focal adhesion in EGFRvIII-expressing glioblastoma," *Neuro-Oncology*, vol. 16, no. 9, pp. 1229–1243, 2014.

[25] X. Xuan, S. Li, X. Lou et al., "Stat3 promotes invasion of esophageal squamous cell carcinoma through up-regulation of MMP2," *Molecular Biology Reports*, vol. 42, no. 5, pp. 907–915, 2015.

[26] G. Artaş and H. I. Özercan, "The expression of STAT3, BCL-XL and MMP-2 proteins in colon adenocarcinomas and their relationship with prognostic factors," *Turk Patoloji Dergisi*, vol. 30, no. 3, pp. 178–183, 2014.

[27] S. O. Rahaman, M. A. Vogelbaum, and S. J. Haque, "Aberrant Stat3 signaling by interleukin-4 in malignant glioma cells: involvement of IL-13Rα2," *Cancer Research*, vol. 65, no. 7, pp. 2956–2963, 2005.

[28] S. L. Fossey, A. T. Liao, J. K. McCleese et al., "Characterization of STAT3 activation and expression in canine and human osteosarcoma," *BMC Cancer*, vol. 9, article 81, 2009.

[29] T. Qin, C. Wang, X. Chen et al., "Dopamine induces growth inhibition and vascular normalization through reprogramming M2-polarized macrophages in rat C6 glioma," *Toxicology and Applied Pharmacology*, vol. 286, no. 2, pp. 112–123, 2015.

[30] Y. W. Ryu, S. W. Lim, J. H. Kim, S. H. Ahn, and J. D. Choi, "Comparison of tamsulosin plus serenoa repens with tamsulosin in the treatment of benign prostatic hyperplasia in Korean men: 1-year randomized open label study," *Urologia Internationalis*, vol. 94, no. 2, pp. 187–93, 2015.

[31] V. Wessagowit, C. Tangjaturonrusamee, T. Kootiratrakarn et al., "Treatment of male androgenetic alopecia with topical products containing *Serenoa repens* extract," *Australasian Journal of Dermatology*, 2015.

[32] P. Morabito, M. Miroddi, S. Giovinazzo, E. Spina, and G. Calapai, "*Serenoa repens* as an endocrine disruptor in a 10-year-old young girl: a new case report," *Pharmacology*, vol. 96, no. 1-2, pp. 41–43, 2015.

24

Additional Effects of Back-Shu Electroacupuncture and Moxibustion in Cardioprotection of Rat Ischemia-Reperfusion Injury

Seung Min Kathy Lee,[1] **Kang Hyun Yoon,**[1] **Jimin Park,**[1] **Hyun Soo Kim,**[2] **Jong Shin Woo,**[2] **So Ra Lee,**[2] **Kyung Hye Lee,**[2] **Hyun-Hee Jang,**[2] **Jin-Bae Kim,**[2] **Woo Shik Kim,**[2] **Sanghoon Lee,**[1] **and Weon Kim**[2]

[1]*Department of Acupuncture and Moxibustion, College of Korean Medicine, Kyung Hee University, Seoul 02453, Republic of Korea*
[2]*Division of Cardiology, Department of Internal Medicine, Kyung Hee University Hospital, Kyung Hee University, Seoul 02447, Republic of Korea*

Correspondence should be addressed to Sanghoon Lee; shlee777@gmail.com and Weon Kim; mylovekw@hanmail.net

Academic Editor: Hongcai Shang

Many preclinical studies show that electroacupuncture (EA) on PC6 and ST36 can reduce infarct size after ischemia-reperfusion (IR) injury. Yet studies to enhance the treatment effect size are limited. The purpose of this study was to explore whether EA has additional myocardial protective effects on an ischemia-reperfusion (IR) injury rat model when back-shu EA and moxibustion are added. SD rats were divided into several groups and treated with either EA only, EA + back-shu EA (B), or EA + B + moxibustion (M) for 5 consecutive days. Transthoracic echocardiography and molecular and immunohistochemical evaluations were performed. It was found that although myocardial infarct areas were significantly lower and cardiac function was also significantly preserved in the three treatment groups compared to the placebo group, there were no additional differences between the three treatment groups. In addition, HSP20 and HSP27 were expressed significantly more in the treatment groups. The results suggest that adding several treatments does not necessarily increase protection. Our study corroborates previous findings that more treatment, such as prolonging EA duration or increasing EA intensity, does not always lead to better results. Other methods of increasing treatment effect size should be explored.

1. Introduction

Cardiovascular disease, especially acute myocardial infarction (MI), is the leading cause of death around the world [1, 2]. Early revascularization is a critical component of decreasing its damaging effects, but reperfusion itself results in ischemia-reperfusion (IR) injury, which attenuates the overall benefits of reperfusion therapy [3].

Many studies have shown that preexposure to brief cycles of ischemia (i.e., ischemic preconditioning) and/or specific pharmacological stimuli ("pharmacologic preconditioning") can substantially reduce infarct size after IR injury [4, 5]. Postexposure to brief cycles of ischemia (i.e., ischemic

postconditioning) [6] and ischemia at peripheral sites (i.e., remote ischemic preconditioning) can also induce similar attenuation [7]. However, most of the research has focused on uncovering the mechanisms and developing pharmaceuticals while the possibility of developing other treatment methods has remained less explored.

Electroacupuncture (EA) and moxibustion are two treatment modalities that have also been shown to significantly protect rat hearts against IR injury [8, 9]. EA is usually applied for 30 min on PC6, which is located near the median nerve. Stimulation of this point can either precondition or postcondition the heart, depending on the treatment period [8, 10]. Moxibustion, on the other hand, is usually given in the form of local somatic thermal stimulation (LSTS) on PC6, and it is believed to work by increasing the production of protective proteins such as heat shock protein 70 (HSP70) and by activating heat-sensitive neural release of nitric oxide [9]. Other than EA and moxibustion on PC6, acupuncture texts also mention back-shu points, which are a set of special points located about 3 cm apart from the midline of the spine. Each set of points are designated to specific organs, and among them BL14 and BL15 have been frequently cited for use in the treatment of cardiovascular diseases [11]. However, the protective effects of these points on IR injury have not been well investigated.

Although EA, moxibustion, and BL14, and BL15 are all postulated to protect against IR injury, the physiological mechanisms in action are thought to be different. While PC6 and ST36 exert their effects through the central nervous system [12], back-shu points act directly on the dorsal ganglia and spinal nerves that provide sympathetic outflow to the heart [13]. To the best of our knowledge, no previous studies have looked into the effects of all the three combined. Some trials have attempted to enhance the myocardial protective effects of EA or moxibustion, but most of these only added or manipulated stimulation methods. Some used different acupuncture points [14], others prolonged the time of stimulation [15], and one explored moxibustion treatment using different temperatures [16], but none explored added effects.

Therefore, in this trial, we hypothesized that, in order to increase effects, treatment modalities must be appropriately and synergistically combined. As a preliminary study, we aimed to explore the possibility of increasing myocardial protective effects by successively combining standard EA, back-shu EA, and moxibustion in a rat model of IR injury.

2. Materials and Methods

2.1. Study Protocol. Thirty-five Sprague-Dawley rats (8- to 9-week-old males, body weight: 250–300 g, Samtaco Inc., Osan, Korea) were used after a 1-week acclimation period under standard laboratory conditions. They were housed in chip-bedded cages at room temperature $24 \pm 1°C$ and room humidity ($63 \pm 5\%$) in a 12-hour light/dark cycle. Rats were permitted free access to water and standard rat chow. On the day of the experiment, the animals were divided into five groups: (1) the control group ($n = 7$), which received no treatment except 30 min of anesthesia for five consecutive days; (2) the IR + placebo group ($n = 7$), which received 30 min of acupuncture treatment after anesthesia on nonacupuncture points to a shallow depth (5 ± 1 mm) without any electrical stimulation; (3) the IR + EA group (EA) ($n = 7$), which received EA on the left PC5, PC6, ST36, and ST37 with a frequency of 2 Hz for 30 min once daily for 5 days; (4) the IR + EA + back-shu EA group (EA + B) ($n = 7$), which received EA on the left PC5, PC6, ST36, and ST37 and on bilateral BL14 and BL15 with a frequency of 2 Hz for 30 min once daily for 5 days, and (5) the IR + EA + B + moxibustion group (EA + B + M) ($n = 7$), which received EA on the left PC5, PC6, ST36, and ST37 and on bilateral BL14 and BL15 with a frequency of 2 Hz for 30 min, along with moxibustion on left PC6 for 20 ± 5 min (Figure 1).

2.2. Rat IR Injury. All experimental procedures were approved by the Kyung Hee University Hospital Animal Experimentation Committee. The rats were anesthetized via intraperitoneal injection with ketamine (75 mg/kg) and xylazine (2 mg/kg). The neck and chest were shaved. Procedures were performed under endotracheal intubation with mechanical ventilation (Harvard Apparatus, MA, USA). The chest was opened through left intercostal thoracotomy, and the heart was exposed by removing the pericardium. Myocardial ischemia was produced by exteriorizing the heart with a left thoracic incision, followed by placement of a slipknot (5–0 silk) around the left anterior descending coronary artery (LAD). After 40 min of ischemia, the ligature was released and blood flow was restored.

2.3. Electroacupuncture. Acupuncture points for EA were selected through literature research. Many studies utilized bilateral PC6 for stimulation, but ST36 was also frequently used in conjunction with PC6 to increase myocardial protective effects [17]. Among the back-shu points, BL14 and BL15 were the most frequently mentioned acupuncture points for treatment of cardiovascular diseases [11].

All acupuncture needles (0.20 × 30 mm, Dongbang Acupuncture Inc., Gyeonggi-Do, Korea) were inserted to a depth of 5 mm at PC5 and PC6 and to a depth of 1 cm at ST36, ST37, BL14, and BL15. EA was performed with an electric stimulator (ES-160, ITO, Tokyo, Japan). The motor threshold responses of the rat paws and legs were verified by visible muscle twitches of the stimulated area [18, 19]. To make sure the needles were positioned at the same points every day, each area was shaved and marked with a black tip marker. The details of acupuncture points and treatment methods are reported following the Standards for Reporting in Animal Studies of Acupuncture (STRASA) guidelines [20] (Table 1 and Figure 2).

On the day of the surgery, electric clips were connected to the acupuncture points 20 min after ischemia was induced and the snare was loosened 10 min before electrical stimulation was due to end. Additional anesthesia was administered intramuscularly if needed, but to a minimal degree. For the next four days, EA stimulation was given with a frequency of 2 Hz for 30 min under anesthesia.

2.4. Moxibustion. For moxibustion treatment, an indirect moxibustion cone (Ucare Int., Gyeonggi-Do, Korea) was positioned approximately ~5 cm under the left PC6 and its temperature was maintained between 38 and 45°C with a digital thermometer (Giltron GT309, Seoul, Korea).

2.5. Transthoracic Echocardiography. To evaluate LV function, rats were intraperitoneally anesthetized with ketamine (75 mg/kg) and xylazine (10 mg/kg) on day 5. The chest was shaved for two-dimensional transthoracic echocardiography (Vivid Q; GE Medical Systems, Milwaukee, WI, USA) with a 12 MHz probe. M-mode echocardiography of the LV was performed at the papillary muscle level, guided by two-dimensional short-axis images. LV cavity size was measured during at least three beats in each projection and averaged.

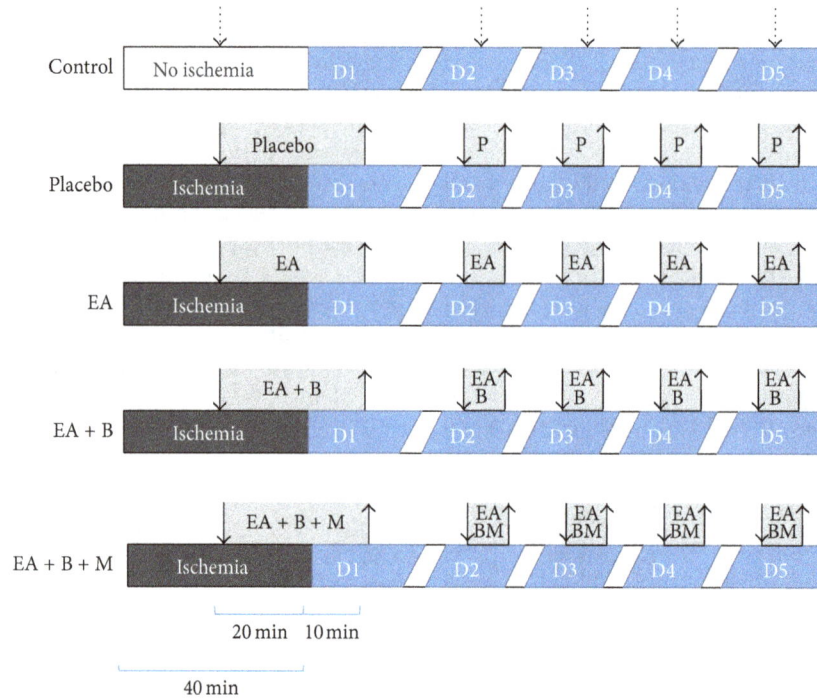

FIGURE 1: Study protocol. The control group received 30 min of anesthesia every day and no other treatment. The placebo group received acupuncture on nonacupuncture points for 20 min at the point of IR injury. The EA group received electroacupuncture on PC5, PC6, ST36, and ST37 for 20 min at the point of IR injury. The EA + B group received electroacupuncture like the EA group but was also treated with electroacupuncture on BL14 and BL15 for 20 min at the point of IR injury. The EA + B + M group received electroacupuncture like the EA + B group but was also treated with moxibustion on PC6 for 15 min for 20 min at the point of IR injury. All treatments were performed every day, and treatment was purposefully designed to overlap with time of reperfusion on the first day (D1). D, day; ischemia, ischemia induced by ligation.

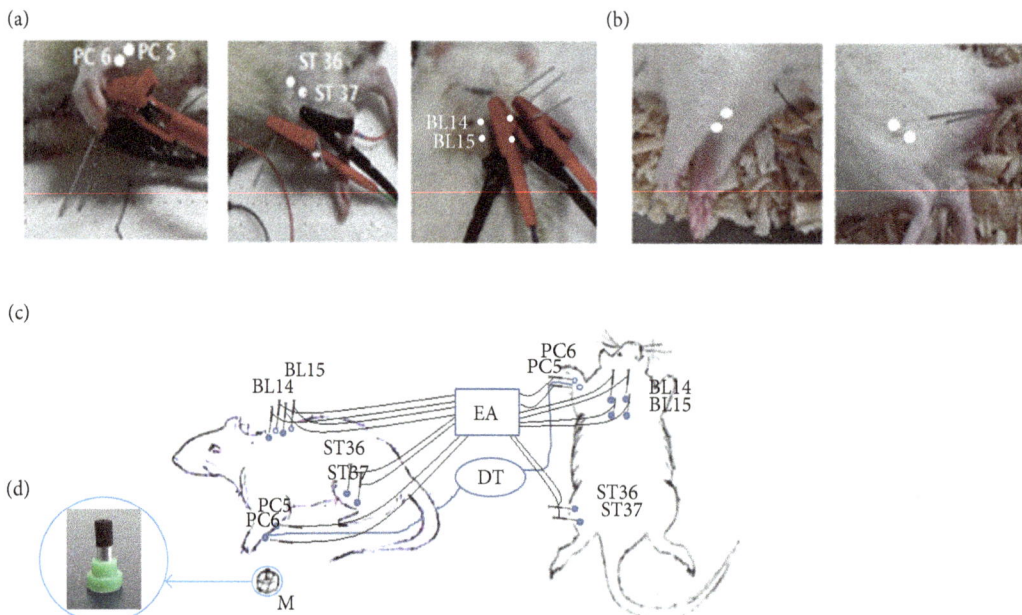

FIGURE 2: Schematic diagram of treatment and acupuncture points. (a) PC5, PC6, ST35, ST36, BL14, and BL15. To needle BL14 and BL15, the back was shaved and the location of the T4/T5 thoracic spine was estimated by palpation of significant anatomical structures. (b) Placebo acupuncture points were located away from any acupuncture points or meridians. (c) Schematic diagram showing electroacupuncture (EA) and moxibustion (M) treatment of the Sprague-Dawley (SD) rats. The temperature was continuously monitored using a digital thermometer (Giltron GT309, Seoul, Korea). (d) For moxibustion treatment, indirect moxibustion (M) was applied on the left PC6.

TABLE 1: Acupuncture treatment according to STRASA*.

Intervention	Item	Description
Experimental animals	(a) Animal model	Nonpain model
	(b) Details for animals	Sprague-Dawley rats of 8 to 9 weeks of age, weighing 250–300 g each
	(c) Experimental environment	Room temperature $24 \pm 1°C$, room humidity $63 \pm 5\%$
Type of acupuncture	(a) Statement about the type of acupuncture used	Electroacupuncture (ES-160, ITO, Tokyo, Japan)
	(b) Rationale for treatment	Literature review and previous studies
List of points	(a) Name of points	PC5, PC6, ST36, ST37, BL14, BL15
	(b) Literature sources to justify rationale	Previous literature and animal studies (listed among references)
		(i) PC5: approximately 2-3 cm proximal to PC6, just above the median nerve
		(ii) PC6: inside the arm, approximately 4 cm proximal to the base of the palmar wrist crease, just above the median nerve
	(c) Location of point	(iii) ST36: on the anterior aspect of the knee, approximately 9 cm below the depression point lateral to the patellar ligament and 5 mm lateral to the anterior tubercle of the tibia
		(iv) ST37: approximately 9 cm below (distal) ST36
		(v) BL14: on the outside dorsal spine corresponding to the 4th thoracic vertebrae
		(vi) BL15: on the outside dorsal spine corresponding to the 5th thoracic vertebrae
Needle stimulation	(a) Depth of insertion	PC5, PC6: 5 mm ST36, ST37, BL14, BL15: 1 cm
	(b) Needle stimulation technique	Electroacupuncture (2 Hz)
	(c) Needle retention time	30 min
	(d) Specification of needle	0.20×30 mm, Dongbang Acupuncture Inc., Gyeonggi-Do, Korea
	(e) Responses elicited	Motor threshold response (movement of the paw and visible muscle twitches of the stimulated leg)
Treatment regimen	(a) Number of treatment sessions	Five sessions
	(b) Frequency of treatment	Once per day
Cointervention	Other interventions	None
Practitioner background	(a) Duration of relevant training	Six years
	(b) Length of clinical experience	Four years
	(c) Expertise in specific condition	None
Control interventions	(a) Active comparison point	Away from acupuncture points and away from near meridians, at a shallower depth of insertion
	(b) Control stimulation	Manual acupuncture
	(c) Details of control intervention	Control points for PC5, PC6: two points located between the Triple Energizer meridian and the Small Intestine meridian
		Control points for ST36, ST37: two points located between the Gall Bladder meridian and the Bladder meridian
	(d) Sources that justify choice of control	Previous studies (the selection of acupuncture points was based on the results of previous studies)

*Standards for Reporting in Animal Studies of Acupuncture (STRASA) guidelines; PC, pericardium; ST, stomach; BL, bladder.

The M-mode images yielded systolic and diastolic wall thicknesses (anterior and posterior) and LV end-systolic and end-diastolic diameters. LV fractional shortening was calculated as (LVEDD minus LVESD)/LVEDD * 100. The ejection fraction was calculated using the Teichholz formula. The following parameters were obtained: left ventricular ejection fraction (LVEF), left ventricular fractional shortening (LVFS), left ventricular internal diameter in diastole (LVIDd), left ventricular internal diameter in systole (LVIDs), LV end-diastolic volume (LVEDV), regional wall thickness, and LV mass.

2.6. Infarct Size and Histological Examination. At day 5, KCl (0.6 mL) was administered intravenously to euthanize the rat. Immediately after euthanasia, the heart was removed and the area at risk was determined by negative staining. Evans blue (0.25%) was administered via the jugular vein to stain the nonoccluded area of the left ventricle (LV). The heart was excised, and the right ventricle and connective tissue were removed, leaving the LV intact. The heart was then frozen at 20°C. The frozen ventricles were sliced transversely from apex to base in 3 mm slices. Slices were incubated in 1% 2,3,4-triphenyltetrazolium chloride (TTC) buffer at pH 7.4 for 20 min at 37°C, washed in flowing water for 30 min, and immersed in 10% formalin. The TTC stained the noninfarcted regions brick red, while the infarcted myocardium remained pale. The infarct area (TTC negative) and area at risk (TTC stained) were measured with the 2000 Visual Image Analysis System, and infarct severity was calculated as a percentage of the infarct size/area at risk (IS/AAR%). The primary end point of the study was myocardial infarct size expressed as IS/AAR. In addition, fibrosis was quantified at the end of the experiment by randomly selecting three heart samples from each group and staining longitudinal 6 μm heart sections with Masson trichrome histochemistry. For each heart section, 5 nonoverlapping areas of the LV immediately proximal to, but not including, the coronary ligation site were imaged using an Olympus BX51 optical microscope (Center Valley, PA, USA). Using ImageJ software, areas of fibrosis within all images were measured. The analysis consisted of determining the MT stained areas (blue) and nonstained myocyte areas from each section via color-based thresholding. A final fibrosis score per heart was achieved by averaging the percentage of total fibrotic areas, calculated as the (total area of collagen/total area of image) × 100%.

2.7. Investigation of Molecular Mechanisms of Action by Western Blot Analysis. The frozen ischemic myocardium was ground to a fine powder using mortar and pestle and the liquid nitrogen was allowed to evaporate. Then, the frozen tissues were homogenized in 500 μL of ice cold lysis buffer (0.5 M Tris-HCl, 150 mM NaCl, 0.1% SDS, 1 mM EDTA, 1% NP-40, 1 mM NaF, 1 mM Na_3VO_4, 1 mM PMSF, and 1 mM aprotinin, containing protease inhibitors) in a glass-Teflon tissue grinder. After homogenization, the samples were centrifuged at 12,000 rpm for 10 min at 4°C and the supernatants were collected. The amount of protein was measured using the BCA assay. For Western blot analysis, the samples (containing 30 μg of total protein) were added

with the same amount of the sample loading buffer (reducing buffer) and then denatured at 100°C with boiling water for 5 min. Protein was then separated by electrophoresis on a 10% sodium dodecyl sulfate-polyacrylamide gel and transferred to a polyvinylidene fluoride membrane (Amersham Biosciences, Buckinghamshire, United Kingdom). The membrane was blocked in 5% skim milk in Tris-buffered saline containing 0.1% Tween-20 (TBS-T) and incubated with primary antibodies overnight at 4°C. The primary antibodies were HSP20 (sc-51955, Santa Cruz Biotechnology Inc.), HSP27 (sc-1049, Santa Cruz Biotechnology Inc.), and HSP70 (sc-1060, Santa Cruz Biotechnology Inc.). The membranes were washed and subsequently incubated with dilutions of secondary antibodies, and the membranes were detected using an enhanced chemiluminescence system (GE Healthcare). The relative intensity of each protein band was normalized to the intensity of GADPH.

2.8. Statistical Analysis. All values are presented as the mean ± standard error of the mean. A one-way analysis of variance followed by the Student-Newman-Keuls multiple comparison test was used to analyze group differences in single point data regarding infarct size. p values less than 0.05 were considered statistically significant. Statistical analyses were performed using SPSS for Windows, version 12.0 (SPSS Inc., Chicago, IL).

3. Results

3.1. Infarct Size/Area at Risk and Myocardial Fibrosis. The infarct size within the percentage of the risk zone was 2.20 ± 2.40% and 23.15 ± 3.71% in the control group and placebo control group, respectively, indicating that the animal model was well established. Myocardial injury was diminished in the EA, EA + B and EA + B + M groups, as seen from the lower infarct area relative to the total area (EA, 8.90±7.13%; EA + B, 7.93±2.95%; EA + B + M, 10.89±2.40%; $p < 0.05$). However, the decrease in infarct size of the EA + B group and the EA + B + M group was not statistically significant compared to the EA group (EA versus EA + B: 8.90±7.1 3% versus 7.93±2.95% and EA versus EA + B + M: 8.90±7.1 3% versus 10.89±2.40%; $p > 0.05$) (Figure 3).

No myocardial fibrosis was observed in the control group, and extensive fibrosis was observed in the placebo group (33.33 ± 3.38%). Mild fibrosis was observed in the EA group (3.03 ± 0.33%), and the EA + B group had less severe fibrosis than the EA group (2.03 ± 0.42%). However, the EA + B + M group had a larger fibrotic area than the other treatment groups (11.73 ± 17.23%). The degree of attenuation of infarct size was not statistically significant between the three treatment groups (EA versus EA + B: 3.03±0.33% versus 2.03 ± 0.42%, $p > 0.05$).

3.2. Cardiac Function. Echocardiography revealed dilated left ventricle and reduced cardiac performance in animals with IR injury. Both EF and FS were improved by the three different treatment modalities compared with placebo treatment (Table 2, Figure 4). However, there were no significant differences between the three treatment groups.

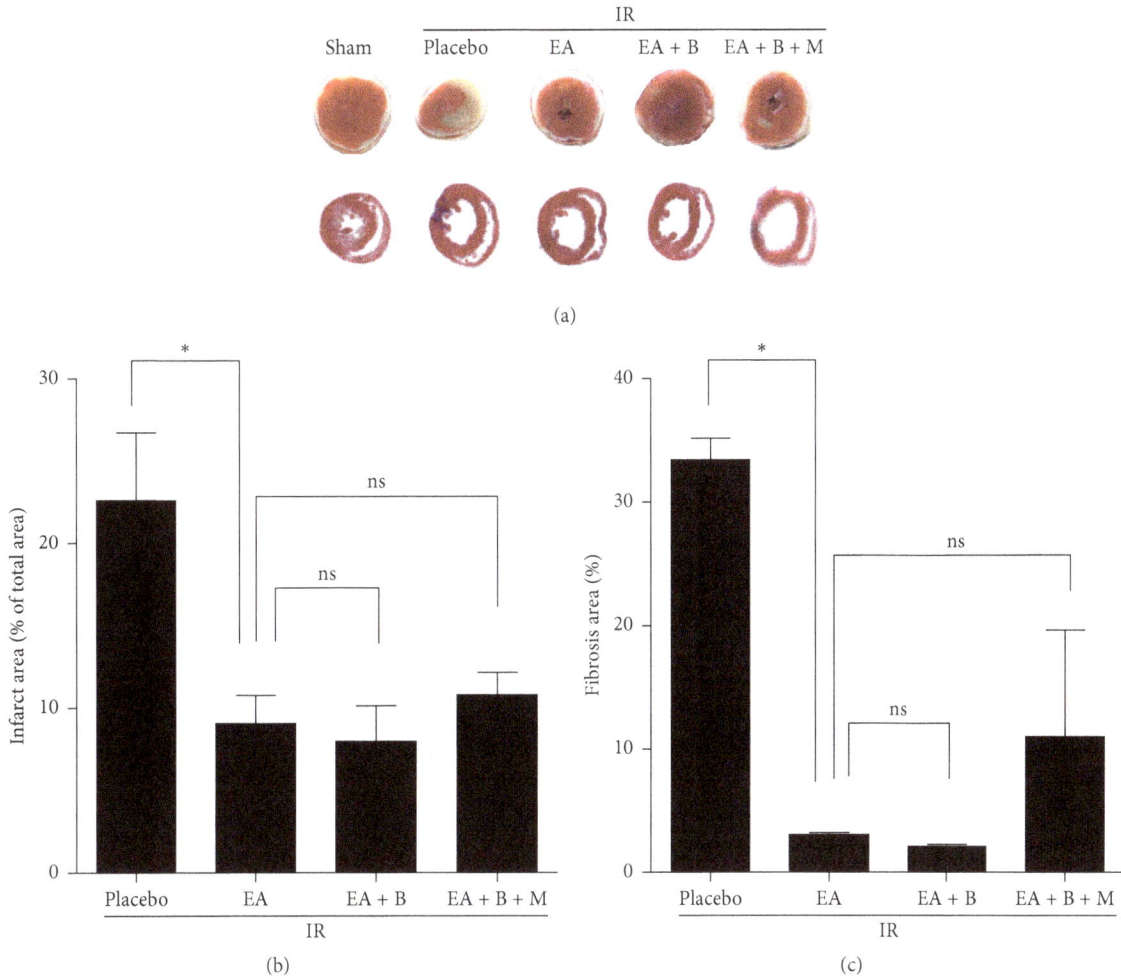

FIGURE 3: Infarct size and fibrosis area. (a) Representative TTC staining and MTC staining heart slices of LV area. (b) Infarct size expressed as a percentage of the area at risk in rats. $^*p < 0.05$ versus the placebo group. (c) Fibrotic area of selected points expressed as a percentage of the total area. $^*p < 0.05$ versus the placebo group. EA, electroacupuncture group; EA + B, electroacupuncture + back-shu electroacupuncture group; and EA + B + M, electroacupuncture + back-shu electroacupuncture + moxibustion group.

3.3. Production of Heat Shock Proteins in the Heart from Rats Subjected to Ischemia and Reperfusion. Western blotting was used to determine the myocardial content of HSP20, HSP27, and HSP70. Figure 5 shows the major peptide band at 65 kDa, representing the specific isoform of each heat shock protein in different groups. We observed significant overexpression of HSP20 in the three treatment groups compared to the placebo group ($p < 0.05$), significant overexpression of HSP27 in the EA group compared to the placebo group ($p < 0.05$), and significant overexpression of HSP70 in the EA + B + M group compared to the placebo group ($p < 0.05$). However, there were no significant differences between the three treatment groups for HSP20, HSP27, and HSP70.

4. Discussion

We investigated possible synergistic effects of three treatment methods (EA, back-shu EA, and moxibustion) that work through different pathways and analyzed the results.

Previous studies in our lab suggested that adding an identical treatment from one to both sides of the body, increasing the number of distal acupuncture points, and increasing the number of treatment sessions in a trial do not strengthen preconditioning effects [not yet published]. This study investigated whether increasing treatment does not lead to increased effects even if the additional treatments worked through different mechanisms. Our results showed that the cardioprotective effects of all three treatment groups were significant compared to the placebo group; however, additional treatment on back-shu points and moxibustion did not significantly decrease infarct size.

We chose these three treatment methods based on literature review and clinical experience. PC6 and ST36 are two of the most frequently investigated acupuncture points for treating cardiovascular problems in the laboratory and in the clinic [21]. PC5 and ST37 were additionally needled in order to conduct EA stimulation on PC6 and ST37, and many cardiovascular studies have used these pairs to

TABLE 2: Results of transthoracic echocardiography.

Group	n	LVEF (%)	LVFS (%)	LVIDd (mm)	LVIDs (mm)	EDV (mL)	ESV (mL)
Control	7	74.91 ± 8.30	39.56 ± 7.80	6.77 ± 0.65	4.13 ± 0.85	0.72 ± 0.18	0.19 ± 0.09
Placebo	7	56.73 ± 3.89#	25.98 ± 2.41#	7.32 ± 0.84	5.42 ± 0.66	0.73 ± 0.34	0.39 ± 0.13
EA	7	69.03 ± 3.68*	34.23 ± 2.83*	7.05 ± 0.76	4.64 ± 0.55	0.81 ± 0.24	0.25 ± 0.08
EA + B	7	67.87 ± 4.19*	33.49 ± 3.03*	7.57 ± 0.79	5.03 ± 0.56	0.98 ± 0.28	0.31 ± 0.09
EA + B + M	7	67.72 ± 11.21*	33.93 ± 7.26*	7.65 ± 0.43	5.05 ± 0.62	1.00 ± 0.16	0.32 ± 0.12

Values are mean ± SE. EA, electroacupuncture group; EA + B, electroacupuncture + back-shu electroacupuncture group; EA + B + M, electroacupuncture + back-shu electroacupuncture + moxibustion group. n, number of rats in each group; LVEF, left ventricular ejection fraction; LVFS, left ventricular fractional shortening; LVIDd, left ventricular internal diameters in diastole; LVIDs, left ventricular internal diameters in systole; EDV, end diastolic volume; ESV, end systolic volume. #p < 0.05 versus the control group. *p < 0.05 versus the placebo group.

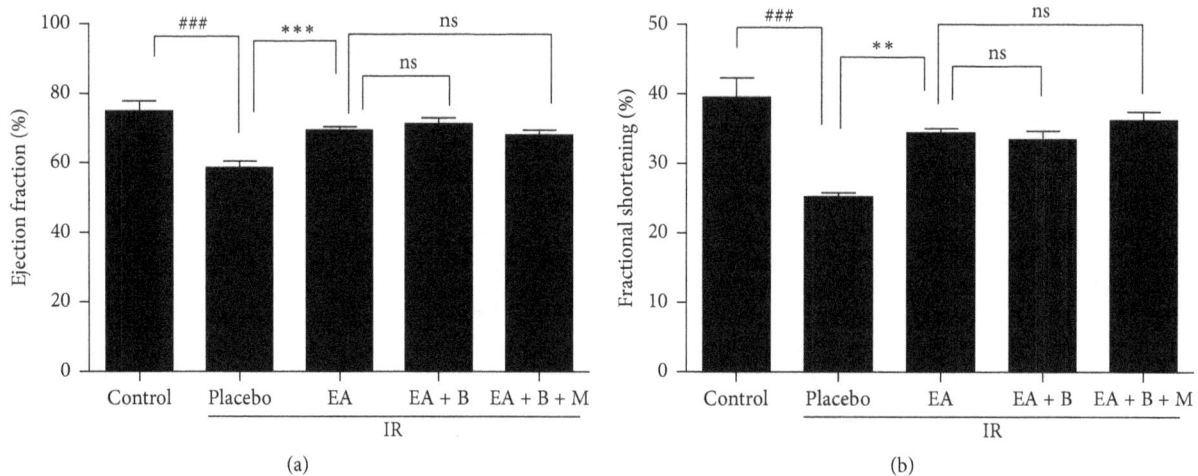

FIGURE 4: Results of 2D echocardiography. (a) Ejection fraction and (b) fractional shortening of the five groups. Both ejection fraction and fractional shortening were significantly different between the placebo group and the three treatment groups. EA, electroacupuncture group; EA + B, electroacupuncture + back-shu electroacupuncture group; and EA + B + M, electroacupuncture + back-shu electroacupuncture + moxibustion group. ###p < 0.05 versus the control group and ***p < 0.05 versus the placebo group. **p < 0.01 versus the placebo group.

produce cardiovascular protective actions [22]. These points send strong signals to the central nervous system via types III and IV sensory nerve fibers on the median and deep peroneal nerves [12]. Suggested mechanisms include the release of endogenous opioids in the brain stem (which leads to a decrease in sympathetic outflow and norepinephrine release in the ischemic area [21]) and the involvement of beta-adrenoceptors [23]. A recent study also showed that acupuncture at PC6 and ST36 improved ECG findings in rats with acute cardiac ischemia by increasing c-fos expression in the nucleus of the solitary tract, which is a center that integrates cardiac functional activity [17].

Back-shu points and moxibustion are hypothesized to exert effects quite differently from PC6 or ST36. Stimulation of back-shu points regulates the autonomic nervous system [24], since they are located above the T4 and T5 sympathetic nerves, close to the dorsal ganglia and the sympathetic innervations to the heart. Studies that looked into the effects of back-shu points for other diseases such as asthma also showed that back-shu points can directly stimulate the dorsal root ganglia to produce substance P [13]. As for moxibustion or LSTS, a recent proteomic analysis study concluded that EA and LSTS specifically act through different myocardial

protective mechanisms [25, 26]. However, we decided to add back-shu points first because using a single treatment modality would make it easier to clarify the mechanisms later on. We added moxibustion as a preliminary investigation of whether the addition of another treatment would increase the effects even further.

The treatment protocol of this trial was intended to be clinically relevant, which is why we chose postconditioning methods over preconditioning. Preconditioning treatments are limited to situations where the onset of ischemia can be predicted, such as planned cardiovascular surgeries. Since most incidences of myocardial infarctions are unpredictable, we focused on conditioning the rats just before reperfusion, which is usually the case in emergency coronary artery bypass surgeries or percutaneous coronary interventions. Measurement of the infarct size 5 days after ischemia provided data on early- and late-phase effects and acute and collective acupuncture effects. In the real world, patients are likely to receive acupuncture treatment more than once and it is necessary to look into the long-term and cumulative effects of these treatments.

There are a few limitations to our study. One limitation that applies to most animal studies related to this subject is

Additional Effects of Back-Shu Electroacupuncture and Moxibustion in Cardioprotection...

241

(a)

(b)

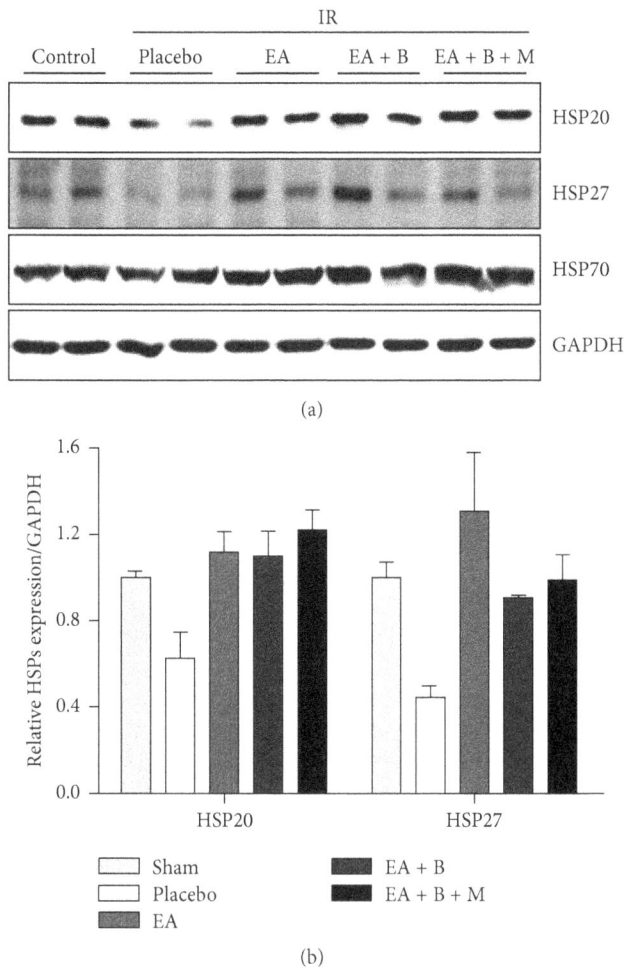

FIGURE 5: HSP20, HSP27, and HSP70 expression. (a) The production of HSP20, HSP27, and HSP70 as detected by Western blotting. (b) Overexpression of HSP20 and HSP27 in the three treatment groups compared to placebo group. EA, electroacupuncture group; EA + B, electroacupuncture group + back-shu electroacupuncture group; EA + B + M, electroacupuncture group + back-shu + moxibustion group.

the fact that these trials are conducted on healthy and young animals. Past studies have shown that preconditioning or postconditioning effects are different between young and old rats [27]. Since the long-term focus of our trial was to design a treatment package suitable for future clinical trials, it would have been more practical to look into additional protective effects in older rats. This is important because previous trials that have investigated age and sex have also shown that the preconditioning effects were more evident in middle-aged rats compared to younger ones [28, 29].

As for the increase in infarct size after additional moxibustion treatment, we believe that either the moxibustion stick that we used had different qualities from the heat generator placed 0.5 cm above PC6, which is more frequently used in LSTS, or more treatment does not always produce better results. This is in agreement with a few other studies that have attempted to increase treatment effects by increasing the stimulation period. In rat ischemic brain injury, 45 min of EA

treatment did not lead to as much improvement as 30 min of EA stimulation [15]. In addition, in human experimental cold thermal pain models, 30 min of EA stimulation resulted in better results than 40 min of stimulation [30]. Myocardial protection with postconditioning was not enhanced by ischemic preconditioning [31].

We postulated that EA on PC6, ST36, BL14, and BL15 and moxibustion on PC6 act through different pathways, but all of these treatments are, in a large sense, external stimulations of the body that aim to activate self-protective mechanisms. Physiologically, the mechanism through which acupuncture is known to work still falls within the category of mechanical stimulation on afferent nerve fibers to elicit local, segmental, or systemic effects. Even if different acupuncture points were utilized, all neural pathways could have reached maximal treatment effects. However, since this was a preliminary investigation, it is necessary to continue to explore conditioning methods that may increase overall effects on the myocardium. This may include investigating acupuncture treatment with other pharmaceuticals, since oral administration of geranylgeranylacetone (GGA) and LSTS doubled the induction of heat shock protein 70 (HSP 70) in rat livers [32]. It is also imperative to carry on related studies onto the bedside, which has already begun [33, 34]. Our trial was an initial attempt to explore potential therapeutic improvements in order to provide better treatment strategies for clinical trials.

Conflict of Interests

The authors have no potential conflict of interests with respect to the research, authorship, and/or publication of this paper to declare.

Acknowledgment

This study was supported by grant from the Korean Government (Ministry of Health; no. HI13C0580).

References

[1] World Health Organization, *Global Status Report on Noncommunicable Diseases*, WHO, Geneva, Switzerland, 2011.

[2] World Health Organization, *Global Atlas on Cardiovascular Disease Prevention and Control*, World Health Organization, Geneva, Switzerland, 2011.

[3] H. K. Eltzschig and T. Eckle, "Ischemia and reperfusion-from mechanism to translation," *Nature Medicine*, vol. 17, no. 11, pp. 1391–1401, 2011.

[4] M. Bayerle-Eder, M. Wolzt, E. Polska et al., "Hypercapnia-induced cerebral and ocular vasodilation is not altered by glibenclamide in humans," *American Journal of Physiology—Regulatory Integrative and Comparative Physiology*, vol. 278, no. 6, pp. R1667–R1673, 2000.

[5] C. E. Murry, R. B. Jennings, and K. A. Reimer, "Preconditioning with ischemia: a delay of lethal cell injury in ischemic myocardium," *Circulation*, vol. 74, no. 5, pp. 1124–1136, 1986.

[6] Z. Q. Zhao, J. S. Corvera, M. E. Halkos et al., "Inhibition of myocardial injury by ischemic postconditioning during reperfusion: comparison with ischemic preconditioning," *American Journal of Physiology—Heart and Circulatory Physiology*, vol. 285, no. 2, pp. H579–H588, 2003.

[7] K. Przyklenk, B. Bauer, M. Ovize, R. A. Kloner, and P. Whittaker, "Regional ischemic 'preconditioning' protects remote virgin myocardium from subsequent sustained coronary occlusion," *Circulation*, vol. 87, no. 3, pp. 893–899, 1993.

[8] M.-T. Tsou, C.-H. Huang, and J.-H. Chiu, "Electroacupuncture on PC6 (Neiguan) attenuates ischemia/reperfusion injury in rat hearts," *American Journal of Chinese Medicine*, vol. 32, no. 6, pp. 951–965, 2004.

[9] J.-H. Chiu, M.-T. Tsou, H.-H. Tung et al., "Preconditioned somatothermal stimulation on median nerve territory increases myocardial heat shock protein 70 and protects rat hearts against ischemia-reperfusion injury," *Journal of Thoracic and Cardiovascular Surgery*, vol. 125, no. 3, pp. 678–685, 2003.

[10] J. Gao, W. Fu, Z. Jin, and X. Yu, "Acupuncture pretreatment protects heart from injury in rats with myocardial ischemia and reperfusion via inhibition of the β1-adrenoceptor signaling pathway," *Life Sciences*, vol. 80, no. 16, pp. 1484–1489, 2007.

[11] S. H. Park and M. R. Cho, "Documentary comparative study on the chief virtues of the Back-Shu points and the Front-Mo points," *Korean Journal of Acupuncture*, vol. 18, no. 1, pp. 117–142, 2001.

[12] J. C. Longhurst, "Central and peripheral neural mechanisms of acupuncture in myocardial ischemia," *International Congress Series*, vol. 1238, pp. 79–87, 2002.

[13] T. F. Jun, P. H. Cheng, and Z. L. Xiao, "Dorsal root ganglion: the target of acupuncture in the treatment of asthma," *Advances in Therapy*, vol. 24, no. 3, pp. 598–602, 2007.

[14] L. Hu, R.-L. Cai, Z.-J. Wu et al., "Effects of electroacupuncture of different acupoints on cardiac function in acute myocardial ischemia rabbits," *Zhen Ci Yan Jiu*, vol. 33, no. 2, pp. 88–92, 2008.

[15] F. Zhou, J. Guo, J. Cheng, G. Wu, and Y. Xia, "Effect of electroacupuncture on rat ischemic brain injury: importance of stimulation duration," *Evidence-Based Complementary and Alternative Medicine*, vol. 2013, Article ID 878521, 12 pages, 2013.

[16] Y.-S. Wang, J.-B. Zhang, J.-F. Jiang, and L.-L. Wang, "Research on effects of the thermal stimulation by moxibustion at different temperatures on cardiac function in rats and on mast cells in the local site of moxibustion," *Evidence-Based Complementary and Alternative Medicine*, vol. 2013, Article ID 545707, 7 pages, 2013.

[17] J.-S. Li, J. Yan, J.-F. He, and N. Peng, "Effects of electroacupuncture on c-fos expression in nucleus of the solitary tract and electrocardiogram ST(II) in myocardial ischemia rats," *Zhen Ci Yan Jiu*, vol. 34, no. 3, pp. 171–174, 2009.

[18] P. Li, K. F. Pitsillides, S. V. Rendig, H.-L. Pan, and J. C. Longhurst, "Reversal of reflex-induced myocardial ischemia by median nerve stimulation: a feline model of electroacupuncture," *Circulation*, vol. 97, no. 12, pp. 1186–1194, 1998.

[19] J. Dow, J. Painovich, S. L. Hale, S. Tjen-A-Looi, J. C. Longhurst, and R. A. Kloner, "Absence of actions of commonly used Chinese herbal medicines and electroacupuncture on myocardial infarct size," *Journal of Cardiovascular Pharmacology and Therapeutics*, vol. 17, no. 4, pp. 403–411, 2012.

[20] Y. H. Hong, *A study on standards for reporting n animal studies of acupuncture [M.S. thesis]*, Kyung Hee University, Seoul, Republic of Korea, 2003.

[21] W. Zhou, Y. Ko, S. Patel, and A. Mahajan, "Electroacupuncture improves left ventricular dysfunction and arrhythmia in a rabbit model of prolonged ischemia/reperfusion," *The FASEB Journal*, vol. 24, meeting abstract supplement, abstract 809.16, 2010.

[22] J. C. Longhurst, "Acupuncture's cardiovascular actions: a mechanistic perspective," *Medical Acupuncture*, vol. 25, no. 2, pp. 101–113, 2013.

[23] J. Gao, W. Fu, Z. Jin, and X. Yu, "A preliminary study on the cardioprotection of acupuncture pretreatment in rats with ischemia and reperfusion: involvement of cardiac β-adrenoceptors," *Journal of Physiological Sciences*, vol. 56, no. 4, pp. 275–279, 2006.

[24] C.-C. Hsu, C.-S. Weng, T.-S. Liu, Y.-S. Tsai, and Y.-H. Chang, "Effects of electrical acupuncture on acupoint BL15 evaluated in terms of heart rate variability, pulse rate variability and skin conductance response," *American Journal of Chinese Medicine*, vol. 34, no. 1, pp. 23–36, 2006.

[25] J.-H. Chiu, "How does moxibustion possibly work?" *Evidence-Based Complementary and Alternative Medicine*, vol. 2013, Article ID 198584, 8 pages, 2013.

[26] M.-T. Tsou, J.-Y. Ho, C.-H. Lin, and J.-H. Chiu, "Proteomic analysis finds different myocardial protective mechanisms for median nerve stimulation by electroacupuncture and by local somatothermal stimulation," *International Journal of Molecular Medicine*, vol. 14, no. 4, pp. 553–563, 2004.

[27] D. Schulman, D. S. Latchman, and D. M. Yellon, "Effect of aging on the ability of preconditioning to protect rat hearts from ischemia-reperfusion injury," *The American Journal of Physiology—Heart and Circulatory Physiology*, vol. 281, no. 4, pp. H1630–H1636, 2001.

[28] K. Boengler, R. Schulz, and G. Heusch, "Loss of cardioprotection with ageing," *Cardiovascular Research*, vol. 83, no. 2, pp. 247–261, 2009.

[29] P. Abete, F. Cacciatore, G. Testa et al., "Clinical application of ischemic preconditioning in the elderly," *Dose-Response*, vol. 8, no. 1, pp. 34–40, 2010.

[30] S.-M. Wang, E. C. Lin, I. Maranets, and Z. N. Kain, "The impact of asynchronous electroacupuncture stimulation duration on cold thermal pain threshold," *Anesthesia & Analgesia*, vol. 109, no. 3, pp. 932–935, 2009.

[31] M. E. Halkos, F. Kerendi, J. S. Corvera et al., "Myocardial protection with postconditioning is not enhanced by ischemic preconditioning," *Annals of Thoracic Surgery*, vol. 78, no. 3, pp. 961–969, 2004.

[32] N. Fan, G.-S. Yang, J.-H. Lu, N. Yang, and H.-B. Zhang, "Oral administration of geranylgeranylacetone plus local somatothermal stimulation: a simple, effective, safe and operable preconditioning combination for conferring tolerance against ischemia-reperfusion injury in rat livers," *World Journal of Gastroenterology*, vol. 11, no. 36, pp. 5725–5731, 2005.

[33] L. F. Yang, J. Yang, Q. Wang et al., "Cardioprotective effects of electroacupuncture pretreatment on patients undergoing heart valve replacement surgery: a randomized controlled trial," *Annals of Thoracic Surgery*, vol. 89, no. 3, pp. 781–786, 2010.

[34] M. Thielmann, E. Kottenberg, P. Kleinbongard et al., "Cardioprotective and prognostic effects of remote ischaemic preconditioning in patients undergoing coronary artery bypass surgery: a single-centre randomised, double-blind, controlled trial," *The Lancet*, vol. 382, no. 9892, pp. 597–604, 2013.

Permissions

List of Contributors

Siti Sarah Mohamad Zaid
Department of Anatomy, Faculty of Medicine, University of Malaya, 50603 Kuala Lumpur, Malaysia
Department of Environmental Sciences, Faculty of Environmental Studies, Universiti Putra Malaysia,

Normadiah M. Kassim
Department of Anatomy, Faculty of Medicine, University of Malaya, 50603 Kuala Lumpur, Malaysia

Shatrah Othman
Department of Molecular Medicine, Faculty of Medicine, University of Malaya, 50603 Kuala Lumpur, Malaysia

Fernanda Coleraus Silva, Juliete Gomes de Lara de Souza, Rodrigo Suzuki, Alana Meira Reichert and Carla Brugin Marek
Laboratory of Cellular Toxicology, State University of Western Paraná, Rua Universitária 1619, 85819110 Cascavel, PR, Brazil

Renata Prestes Antonangelo
Department of Veterinary Medicine, Dynamic Union of the Faculty Falls, 85852010 Foz do Iguaçu, PR, Brazil

Ana Maria Itinose
Assistance Center in Toxicology (CEATOX), Hospital University of Western Paraná, Avenida Tancredo Neves 3224, 85806470 Cascavel, PR, Brazil

Gunasekaran Baskaran, Shamala Salvamani, Siti Aqlima Ahmad,
and Mohd Yunus Shukor
Department of Biochemistry, Faculty of Biotechnology and Biomolecular Sciences, Universiti Putra Malaysia (UPM), 43400 Serdang, Selangor, Malaysia

Azrina Azlan
Department of Nutrition and Dietetics, Faculty of Medicine and Health Sciences, Universiti Putra Malaysia (UPM), 43400 Serdang, Selangor,Malaysia

Swee Keong Yeap
Institute of Bioscience, Universiti Putra Malaysia (UPM), 43400 Serdang, Selangor, Malaysia

Patrícia D. O. de Almeida, Ana Paula de A. Boleti and Emerson S. Lima
Laboratório de Atividade Biológica, Faculdade de Ciências Farmacêuticas, Universidade Federal do Amazonas (UFAM), Avenida Gen. Rodrigo Otavio, No. 6200, 69077 000Manaus, AM, Brazil

André Luis Rüdiger and Valdir Florêncio da Veiga Junior
Instituto de Ciîncias Exatas, Departamento de Qúimica, Universidade Federal do Amazonas, Avenida Gen. Rodrigo Otavio, No. 6200, 69077-000 Manaus, AM, Brazil

Geane A. Lourenço
Laboratório de Farmacologia, Departamento de Ciências Fisiológicas, Instituto de Ciências Biológicas, Universidade Federal do Amazonas, Avenida Gen. Rodrigo Otavio, No. 6200, 69077-000 Manaus, AM, Brazil

Mallappa Kumara Swamy and Uma Rani Sinniah
Department of Crop Science, Faculty of Agriculture, Universiti Putra Malaysia (UPM), 43400 Serdang, Selangor, Malaysia

Mohd. Sayeed Akhtar
Institute of Tropical Agriculture, Universiti Putra Malaysia (UPM), 43400 Serdang, Selangor, Malaysia

You-you Gu and Su Wang
Department of Endocrinology, The Fifth Central Hospital of Tianjin, Tianjin 300450, China

Huan Wang
Community Health Service Center of Hu Jiayuan Street, Binhai New District, Tianjin 300454, China
Graduate School of Tianjin Medical University, Tianjin 300070, China

Hua Gao and Ming-cai Qiu
Department of Endocrinology, General Hospital of Tianjin Medical University, Tianjin 300052, China

Keshav Raj Paudel and Nisha Panth
Department of Pharmacy, School of Health and Allied Science, Pokhara University, P.O. Box 427, Dhungepatan, Kaski, Nepal

Ning-qun Wang
Cerebrovascular Diseases Research Institute, Xuanwu Hospital, Capital Medical University, Ministry of Education, 45 Changchun Street, Beijing 100053, China
Department of Traditional Chinese Medicine, Xuanwu Hospital, Capital Medical University, Ministry of Education, 45 Changchun Street, Beijing 100053, China

Li-ye Wang
Dongfang Hospital, Beijing University of Chinese Medicine, Beijing 100078, China

Hai-ping Zhao, Rong-liang Wang and Yu-min Luo
Cerebrovascular Diseases Research Institute, Xuanwu Hospital, Capital Medical University, Ministry of Education, 45 Changchun Street, Beijing 100053, China

Key Laboratory of Neurodegenerative Diseases (Capital Medical University), Ministry of Education, 45 Changchun Street, Beijing 100053, China

Ping Liu
Cerebrovascular Diseases Research Institute, Xuanwu Hospital, Capital Medical University, Ministry of Education, 45 Changchun Street, Beijing 100053, China
Department of Neurology, Xuanwu Hospital, Capital Medical University, Ministry of Education, 45 Changchun Street, Beijing 100053, China

Jue-xian Song and Li Gao
Department of Neurology, Xuanwu Hospital, Capital Medical University, Ministry of Education, 45 Changchun Street, Beijing 100053, China

Xun-ming Ji
Key Laboratory of Neurodegenerative Diseases (Capital Medical University), Ministry of Education, 45 Changchun Street, Beijing 100053, China

Shinnosuke Murakami, Tomoyoshi Soga, Masaru Tomita and Shinji Fukuda
Systems Biology Program, Graduate School of Media and Governance, Keio University, 5322 Endo, Fujisawa, Kanagawa 252-0882, Japan
Institute for Advanced Biosciences, Keio University, 246-2 Mizukami, Kakuganji, Tsuruoka, Yamagata 997-0052, Japan

Yasuaki Goto and Shigeo Kurihara
Onsen Medical Science Research Center, Japan Health and Research Institute, 1-29-4 Kakigaracho, Nihonbashi, Chuo-ku, Tokyo 103-0014, Japan

Kyo Ito
Ito Medical Office, 7985-5, Nagayu, Naoirimachi, Taketa, Oita 878-0402, Japan

Shinya Hayasaka
Faculty of Human Life Sciences, Tokyo City University, 8-9-18 Todoroki, Setagaya-ku, Tokyo 158-8586, Japan
Onsen Medical Science Research Center, Japan Health and Research Institute, 1-29-4 Kakigaracho, Nihonbashi, Chuo-ku, Tokyo 103-0014, Japan

Yudi Zhang
Department of Combination of Chinese and Western Medicine, The First Affiliated Hospital of Chongqing Medical University, Chongqing 400016, China
College of Laboratory Medicine, Chongqing Medical University, Yuzhong District, Chongqing 400016, China

Rongheng Li, Yu Zhong, Lingyun Zhou and Shike Shang
Department of Combination of Chinese and Western Medicine, The First Affiliated Hospital of Chongqing Medical University, Chongqing 400016, China

Sihan Zhang
Department of Combination of Chinese and Western Medicine,The First Affiliated Hospital of Chongqing Medical University, Chongqing 400016, China
Longgang District People's Hospital of Shenzhen, Longgang District, Shenzhen, Guangdong 518172, China

Xiao-mei Shao, Zui Shen, Jing Sun, Fang Fang, Jun-fan Fang, Yuan-yuan Wu and Jian-qiao Fang
Department of Neurobiology & Acupuncture Research, The Third Clinical College, Zhejiang Chinese Medical University, Hangzhou 310053, China

Hongzhi Tang, Xuebing Yi, Guogang Dai, Junrong Chen, Liugang Tang, Haibo Rong and Junhua Wu
Sichuan Orthopaedic Hospital, Chengdu, Sichuan 610041, China

Huaying Fan, Jiao Chen, Mingxiao Yang and Fanrong Liang
Chengdu University of Traditional Chinese Medicine, Chengdu, Sichuan 610075, China

Li Lu, Huang Zhijian, Li Lei, Chen Wenchuan and Zhu Zhimin
Department of Prosthodontics,West China Hospital of Stomatology, State Key Laboratory of Oral Diseases, Sichuan University, Chengdu 610041, China

Xuan Li Liu, Dan Dan Wang, Zi Hao Wang and Da Li Meng
School of Traditional Chinese Materia Medica, Key Laboratory of Structure-Based Drug Design and Discovery (Shenyang Pharmaceutical University), Ministry of Education, Wenhua Road 103, Shenyang 110016, China

Loretta Olamigoke, Elvedina Mansoor, Vivek Mann, Ivory Ellis and Elvis Okoro
Texas Southern University, Houston, TX 77004, USA

Koji Wakame
Hokkaido School of Pharmacy, Sapporo 004-0839, Japan
Amino Up, Sapporo 004-0839, Japan

Hajime Fuji
Amino Up, Sapporo 004-0839, Japan

Anil Kulkarni, Marie Francoise Doursout and Alamelu Sundaresan
University of Texas Medical School, Houston, TX 77004, USA

Nylane Maria Nunes de Alencar, Rachel Sindeaux Paiva Pinheiro, Patrícia Bastos Luz, Lyara Barbosa Nogueira Freitas, Tamiris de Fátima Goebel de Souza, Luana David do Carmo and Larisse Mota Marques
Departamento de Fisiologia e Farmacologia, UFC, Coronel Nunes de Melo 1127, Rodolfo Teófilo, 60430-270 Fortaleza, CE, Brazil

Ingrid Samantha Tavares de Figueiredo
Departamento de Fisiologia e Farmacologia, UFC, Coronel Nunes de Melo 1127, Rodolfo Téofilo, 60430-270 Fortaleza, CE, Brazil

Marcio Viana Ramos
Departamento de Bioqúimica e Biologia Molecular, UFC, Campus do Pici, Caixa Postal 6033, 60451-970 Fortaleza, CE, Brazil

Xiaoling Bu
Beijing University of Traditional Chinese Medicine, North 3rd Ring Road No. 11 School Range, Chaoyang District, Beijing 100029, China

Yanxia Liu, Qiudan Lu and Zhe Jin
Department of Gynecology, Dongfang Hospital of Beijing University of Traditional Chinese Medicine, No. 6 Fangxingyuan 1 Qu, Fengtai District, Beijing 100078, China

Ming Li, Zongyu Han,Weijian Bei, Xianglu Rong, Jiao Guo and Xuguang Hu
Key Unit of Modulating Liver to Treat Hyperlipemia SATCM (State Administration of Traditional Chinese Medicine), Level 3 Lab of Lipid Metabolism SATCM, Guangdong TCM Key Laboratory for Metabolic Diseases, Guangdong Pharmaceutical University, Guangzhou Higher Education Mega Centre, Guangzhou 510006, China

Heng-Wen Chen and Jie Wang
Guang'anmen Hospital, China Academy of Chinese Medical Sciences, Beijing 100053, China

Ben-Jun Wei
Hubei University of Traditional Chinese Medicine,Wuhan,Hubei 430062, China

Xuan-Hui He
Department of Pharmaceutical Chemistry, Beijing Institute of Radiation Medicine, Beijing 100850, China

Yan Liu
Key Laboratory of Chinese Materia Medica, Heilongjiang University of Chinese Medicine, Ministry of Education, Harbin, Heilongjiang 150036, China

Mariana Belén Joray, María Laura González, Georgina Natalia Díaz Napal, Sara María Palacios and María Cecilia Carpinella
Fine Chemicals and Natural Products Laboratory, School of Chemistry, Catholic University of Córdoba, Avda Armada Argentina 3555, X5016DHK Córdoba, Argentina

Lucas Daniel Trucco and José Luis Bocco
CIBICI CONICET and Department of Clinical Biochemistry, Faculty of Chemical Science, National University of Córdoba, Haya de la Torre and Medina Allende, Córdoba, Argentina

Xuan-yi Ye
College of Ecology, Lishui University, Lishui, Zhejiang 323000, China

Qing-zhi Ling and Shao-jun Chen
Department of Traditional Chinese Medicine, Zhejiang Pharmaceutical College, Ningbo 315100, China

Jinfu Yao
Changchun University of Chinese Medicine, Changchun 130117, China

Hong Ding
Department of Nephrology, The Fourth Affiliated Hospital of China Medical University, Shenyang, China

Jinglian Shen
Department of Emergency Medicine, The Fourth Affiliated Hospital of China Medical University, Shenyang, China

Yang Yang and Yuqin Che
Department of Neurology, The Fourth Affiliated Hospital of China Medical University, Shenyang, China
Seung Min Kathy Lee, Kang Hyun Yoon, Jimin Park and Sanghoon Lee
Department of Acupuncture and Moxibustion, College of Korean Medicine, Kyung Hee University, Seoul 02453, Republic of Korea

Hyun Soo Kim, Jong Shin Woo, So Ra Lee, Kyung Hye Lee, Hyun-Hee Jang, Jin-Bae Kim, Woo Shik Kim and Weon Kim
Division of Cardiology, Department of Internal Medicine, Kyung Hee University Hospital, Kyung Hee University, Seoul 02447, Republic of Korea

www.ingramcontent.com/pod-product-compliance
Lightning Source LLC
Chambersburg PA
CBHW080507200326
41458CB00012B/4122